DATE DUE

DE 15 '97			
MY 20 98			
DE 6 99			
AP 24 00			
AP 7 '03			
OC 09 07			
DE 12 08			
AP 28 09			

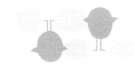

Rheumatoid Arthritis

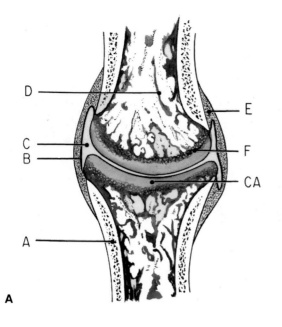

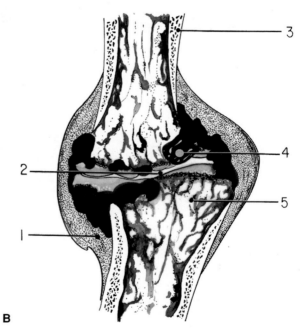

A

B

A coronal view through a normal (**A**) and rheumatoid (**B**) diarthrodial joint. In corticoid bones (*A*), (*B*), is pointing to the normal synovium that is continuous with the sub-synovium and joint capsule (*E*). *C* is the apparent joint space. In the normal joint, this is a "virtual" space containing only a small amount of synovial fluid. *F* is the subchondral bony plate, impervious to fluid and without penetrating blood vessels in adults. CA is articular cartilage.

In the rheumatoid joint, the joint capsule (*1*) becomes enormously thickened, similar to the synovium (*4*) which can increase over 100-fold in weight. The synovium invades under subchondral bone (left) as well as cartilage. The joint space (*2*) contains an excess amount of fluid. Cortical bone can be degraded (*3*) resulting in subluxation.

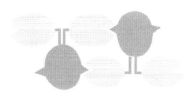

Rheumatoid Arthritis

EDWARD D. HARRIS, JR., M.D.

George DeForest Barnett Professor
Department of Medicine
Stanford University School of Medicine
Palo Alto, California

W.B. SAUNDERS COMPANY
A Division of Harcourt Brace & Company
Philadelphia ■ London ■ Toronto ■ Montreal ■ Sydney ■ Tokyo

Library of Congress Cataloging-in-Publication Data

Harris, Edward D.
    Rheumatoid arthritis / Edward D. Harris, Jr.
      p.   cm.
    ISBN 0–7216–5249–2
    1. Rheumatoid arthritis.   I. Title.
    [DNLM: 1. Arthritis, Rheumatoid.   WE 346 H313rb   1997]
    RC933.H36   1997
    616.7′227--dc21
    DNLM/DLC

                                                     96-40173

RHEUMATOID ARTHRITIS   ISBN 0–7216–5249–2

To Joan, who brings love, joy, and purpose
to my life . . .

To Ned and Edie, Tom and Kate, Tyler, Chandler, and Kyle,
who have optimism, youth, and energy on their side . . .

and to Waldo,
who grew from puppy to dog under the laptop as this book was
written

. . . a very grateful Ted Harris

PREFACE

In 1975 I edited a book titled *Rheumatoid Arthritis*. It was published by MEDCOM Press. Joining me as contributors were Gerald Weissmann, Carwile Leroy, Shawn Ruddy, Allen Myers, Clem Sledge, and Eric Radin. It was an inexpensive book, a paperback, and our copyeditor had an aversion to prepositions. Our galleys had endless examples of nouns modifying nouns! It didn't sell very well. One cold day in March there was a fire in the warehouse where all of the remaindered books were being stored. The activated sprinkler system turned them all into a sodden mass that was carried to the dump. Those who still possess a copy definitely have a collector's item!

As many others have noted, one begins biomedical research in a narrow field, and it is only later that one's interests expand to include understanding of related issues. So it has been with me. When I began to work on collagenase from rheumatoid synovium in Steve Krane's laboratory at the Massachusetts General Hospital in 1968, the pathogenesis of rheumatoid arthritis was a black box about which I knew very little. As I began to appreciate the reality that collagenolysis was an end stage of the rheumatoid process and not a primary factor, my interests grew in the immunogenetics, causation, immunology, clinical manifestations, and treatment of this disease. These interests were enhanced and expanded as I had to tackle these components of rheumatoid arthritis for the first, second, third, and fourth editions of the *Textbook of Rheumatology*.

In August of 1993, we hosted an International Conference on Rheumatoid Arthritis at Stanford. Attending and speaking were many of the best scientists and clinical investigators who are focused on this disease. It was abundantly clear that data were converging sufficiently to generate a believable story about rheumatoid arthritis explaining the rationale for new therapies springing from recombinant and monoclonal antibody technology.

Much of the foundation for this book has been the chapter that I have written and re-written for five editions of the *Textbook of Rheumatology* on "Clinical Manifestations of Rheumatoid Arthritis." I have accepted that fact that there was little that I could do to make this a better chapter, and therefore, with permission of the perspicacious and bright Editor at W.B. Saunders Company, Richard Zorab, I have lifted most of it for the description of clinical disease in this book.

For the experts in cellular immunity, my chapter on T cells in rheumatoid arthritis will seem elementary, and perhaps oversimplified. This will be true for all experts in focused areas as they find descriptions of their work and others in different chapters. But my hope is that the experts in one of the many sub-fields of clinical and basic science discussed in these pages will find the majority of the book a synthesis of information about which they knew less, or little, and can integrate that which they read into their overall views about rheumatoid arthritis.

This book should benefit most the practicing rheumatologist, internist, and general practitioner who would like a scientific rationale for evaluation and treatment of his or her patients with rheumatoid arthritis. For that matter, patients with no science background who have read page proofs of the chapters have said "I want this book—I can understand much of it!" Nothing could be more gratifying to an author.

Writing a single-author text demands time, and I am deeply grateful to David Korn (who was Dean of the Stanford University School of Medicine), Condelezza Rice (Provost at Stanford), and my colleagues in the Department of Medicine at Stanford who provided the permission to take the sabbatical that was essential to begin and finish this book.

There are others, who deserve thanks. Among them are Josh Burnett, the quintessential clinical rheumatologist and teacher at Darmouth. Ted Potter, Bob Porter, Clem Sledge, Pete Hall, and Stu Russell are patient and skilled surgeons who provided my laboratory with rheumatoid synovium from many arthroplasties. Mike Farrell, Sheryl Locke, Peter McCroskery, Carol Vater, Yasunori Okada, Zena Werb, Carlo Mainardi, Connie Brinckerhoff, and Hideake Nagase were my associates who did careful and controlled experiments in our laboratories to test our hypotheses. My coeditors of the very successful *Textbook of Rheumatology*—Bill Kelley, Shaun Ruddy, and Clem Sledge—have given me frank and (usually) helpful critiques of my writing through the years. Richard Zorab and Lew Reines, the duo at W. B. Saunders Company who believed that I would actually write this book, deserve my thanks. Jean Doran-Matua took my crude work from floppy discs and "tweaked" it into good form. Sue Ferguson crafted some figures, and Butch Collier built all of the complex figures in this book. It is essential for me to thank the many investigators and clinicians who have done painstaking and detailed studies on the multiple facets of rheumatoid arthritis; their papers appear in the references to my chapters.

A single author can take much license. I know I have! I have, for example, referenced the papers that have appealed to me. This book is not a traditional, all-reference-encompassing review. In addition, I have used the reference section of each chapter to include material that was best included as annotations rather than textual material. The boldface sentences are for emphasis. The boxes in the text are used to separate out material that is somewhat peripheral to the main text. I have not referenced material from abstracts at the 1995 meeting of the American College of Rheumatology in the usual way; for these, readers will find a name and abstract number in parentheses (e.g., Smith, Abstract 123) and a separate listing of the reference to an abstract in *Arthritis and Rheumatism* placed at the end of the book.

Rheumatoid arthritis is an exciting disease to study. Our patients deserve the best research into the mechanisms and treatment.

CONTENTS

INTRODUCTION

Consider the differences between gout and rheumatoid arthritis, both processes that can destroy joints. Gout has one cause: hyperuricemia. Once specific inhibitors of sodium urate biosynthesis had been developed, hyperuricemia could be controlled, and, when properly managed, there is no reason that gout should be a cause of joint destruction. At the same time, the discovery of the ''cure'' for gout has taken the excitement out of investigative work in gout.

In 1995, the story of rheumatoid arthritis is much different. We are confronted with a disease that we know well in the clinics. Few new manifestations of rheumatoid arthritis have been described in recent years. What has changed are our concepts about how the disease should be treated. Data accumulated in recent years have shown that rheumatoid arthritis is a direct cause of death and severe morbidity more often than has been appreciated, and that destruction of joints in rheumatoid arthritis begins early, in many patients within the first year of disease.

The problem is that our therapeutic approaches are limited because our knowledge of pathogenesis is incomplete. Each year, new pathways of inflammation, tissue proliferation, mechanisms of cell death, or matrix destruction are presented to students of rheumatoid arthritis as being potentially involved in pathogenesis. Similarly, candidates for the direct and primary cause of rheumatoid arthritis have not diminished in number. Aspects of the disease that were apparently clarified, such as the immunogenetics of rheumatoid arthritis, now appear less clear and more complex. Even the best designed of ''designer'' biologics or drugs make only a temporary improvement in the progress of the disease, improvement often rivaled by placebo.

Those are the discouraging facts. However, the optimistic view is that we have accumulated so many good data about the immunogenetics, immunology, and biochemistry of rheumatoid arthritis that we are on the verge of major understandings of how it can be down-regulated enough by therapy to prevent joint destruction, physical impairment, and death.

It is the purpose of this book to provide an up-to-date reveiw of accumulated data about rheumatoid arthritis, and then to attempt a fair synthesis of the facts that can absorb all of the relevant ones and lead to testable hypotheses about how to turn this disease off before joints are programmed for destruction.

IS THERE SOMETHING UNIQUE ABOUT RHEUMATOID ARTHRITIS?

Just as severe hyperuricemia is characteristic of gout, and antibodies against the centromere of dividing cells are characteristic of the CREST syndrome, it would help us in approaching rheumatoid arthritis if there were something characteristic about it not shared by other joint diseases. That ''something'' certainly is not an autoimmune response, nor is it an activated cytokine network or cell adhesion system in vasculature. Not only are these pathways integral parts of other forms of connective tissue disease, but they are activated in diseases of many organ systems other than those of connective tissue.

However, one component—the **synovial lining cell** that becomes a ''pannocyte'' with the capability of invading cartilage, tendon, or bone—is indeed characteristic of rheumatoid arthritis and rarely found in other diseases of joints. This activated synovial lining cell, found two to four layers deep amid an incomplete set of components of basement membrane, is derived

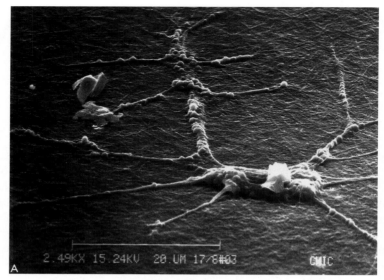

FIGURE 1. A scanning electron photomicrograph of a stellate cell dissociated in vitro from a sample of active rheumatoid synovium and cultured on a bed of collagen. The cell processes stain positively for collagenase. ($\times$2,490). (From Harris, E. D. Jr.: Etiology and pathogenesis of rheumatoid arthritis. *In* Kelley, W. N., Harris, E. D. Jr., Ruddy, S., and Sledge, C. B. [eds.]: Textbook of Rheumatology, 4th ed., Vol. 1. Philadelphia, W. B. Saunders, 1993, pp. 833–873. Used by permission.)

from type A (macrophage-like) or type B (fibroblastic) cells. It expresses cell surface markers characteristic of both. Activated by interleukin-1, tumor necrosis factor α, platelet-derived growth factor, and perhaps other cytokines, the pannocyte changes its appearance to resemble a large stellate cell with long cell processes covered with knobbly excrescences and spade-like terminal extensions that adhere to the connective tissue matrix of cartilage or soft tissue (Fig. 1). These cells form the invasive front that burrows into cartilage. A lacuna forms around

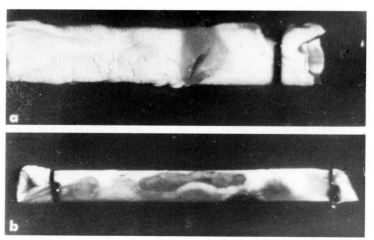

FIGURE 2. In experiments performed in Dr. Judah Folkman's laboratory at Harvard in 1968, sterile samples of invasive adenocarcinoma were placed on inverted sterile rat gut segments and incubated in enriched culture medium (A). Similarly, sterile samples of rheumatoid synovium removed at synovectomy were placed on the same gut preparations (B). The rheumatoid tissue degraded the collagenous bowel wall (black areas) as well as the most invasive of tumors, substantiating the theory that, in the joint, rheumatoid synovium acts as a locally invasive tumor. (From Harris, E. D. Jr., Evanson, J. M., DiBonna, D. R., et al: Collagenase and rheumatoid arthritis. Arthritis Rheum. 13: 83, 1970. Used by permission.)

them as the surrounding collagen and proteoglycans are destroyed. Although individual cells appear isolated in fixed thin histologic sections, it is probable that they are linked by their cell processes to similar cells of the proliferative lining.

This pannocyte is not a primary cell in the pathogenesis of rheumatoid arthritis; rather, it is derived by chronic active stimulation of synovial lining cells by a variety of messages delivered in the form of cytokines from activated fibroblasts, macrophages, and lymphocytes. Once formed, the pannocytes may become autonomous in their ability to degrade cartilage, tendons, and bone. In 1968, experiments were done with rheumatoid synovium that support this. Specimens taken from rheumatoid joints at the time of synovectomy were placed on viable inverted gut segments kept "alive" in enriched and oxygenated medium. It was shown that the rheumatoid tissue was capable of degrading the connective tissue at a rate exceeding that of even the most malignant and invasive of tumors (Fig. 2).[1]

It is these synovial lining cells that synthesize and release collagenase, stromelysin, gelatinase, tumor necrosis factor α, interleukin-1, hyaluronan, and type VI collagen. In addition, they express cell surface glycoproteins that cells under the intima do not. If there were one "target" cell that therapy could down-regulate, it should be these activated synovial lining cells.

RELEVANCE OF PATHOPHYSIOLOGY TO THERAPY

With our current knowledge of rheumatoid arthritis, it is easy to be overwhelmed by the multitude of pathways of inflammation and proliferation that are active concurrently in this disease. One logical conclusion is that our therapies must be aimed at more than one pathway. Because we have no idea about a specific causative agent in rheumatoid arthritis, we must down-regulate as many processes as possible. This is the logic behind "combination therapy." A good case can be made for giving every patient a base therapy of standard anti-inflammatory medication, and then adding second-line drugs in succession, and in doses sufficient to provide their maximal effect. It must be the goal of rheumatologists to determine which second-line drugs can be additive or synergistic in efficacy, but not synergistic in side effects. The same applies to biologic therapy. These products of recombinant DNA technology and monoclonal lymphocyte populations can be highly focused in their beneficial effect, but unfortunately broad in their side effects. For example, anti-CD4 antibodies have a specific and narrow focus, yet the effects of long-lasting depletion of CD4$^+$ cells may be devastating or even fatal to a patient who, for example, acquires an opportunistic infection.

There is no doubt that biologic compounds, cellular therapy,[3] and better use of available drugs have a great potential for treatment, but to discover which would be better and safer will require careful study of many patients with rheumatoid arthritis. If combination therapy is to be studied well, there are multiple permutations of therapy and multiple different protocols that could be designed. It is extraordinarily important for our patients that the protocols chosen represent those drugs, singly or in combination, that have the best potential for success. The danger is that protocols selected will be picked because of the financial resources of the companies producing them, or by choice of combined clinics who control the larger numbers of potential study patients.

NEED FOR A NEW PARADIGM FOR CLINICAL TRIALS

Rheumatologists have become somewhat disillusioned with the term "significant difference" applied to evaluations of one drug or another in clinical trials of rheumatoid arthritis. As pointed out by Fortin et al.[2] what we really want is a demonstration of clinically relevant change brought about by a form of therapy. A change in joint count from 31 to 27 may be statistically significant with a p value of .01, but it also may have no clinical relevance to patients.

At the other end of the scale, it is very likely that many reasonable and potentially useful therapies have been undervalued by trials that insufficiently tested the maximal dose. Trials have concluded without efficacy *or* toxicity. How useful it would be to get unequivocal data from a clinical trial, rather than the conclusion, ''Additional trials are needed''!

A recurrent theme throughout this text is that our patients can no longer be treated in a ''wait and see'' manner. The long-term costs and risks of severe morbidity or death from continually active rheumatoid arthritis are too great to pursue the standard strategy of trying to catch up to the disease process with use of therapeutic pyramid rather than getting on top and in front of it with truly effective treatment.

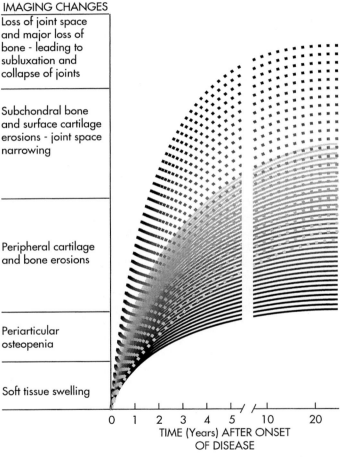

IMAGING CHANGES

Loss of joint space and major loss of bone - leading to subluxation and collapse of joints

Subchondral bone and surface cartilage erosions - joint space narrowing

Peripheral cartilage and bone erosions

Periarticular osteopenia

Soft tissue swelling

TIME (Years) AFTER ONSET OF DISEASE

FIGURE 3. The progression over time of imaging changes of rheumatoid joints. This figure emphasizes two major points about rheumatoid arthritis. One is that there is great variation in the degree of joint destruction among patients. Some (solid black lines) never develop more than periarticular osteopenia. Others, with sustained and aggressive disease, go on to destruction of cartilage, bone, and tendon (dotted lines). Others (dotted/solid mix) have erosions without complete joint destruction. The other point made by this figure is that the rate of destruction is greater in the first 2 years of disease than in later years. For this reason, it is essential that effective therapy be instituted early in hopes of altering the slope of the curves. Measurable determinants of the rate of progression include the mean erythrocyte sedimentation rate, joint count, Health Assessment Questionnnaire results, pain, and a positive rheumatoid factor test. (From Wolfe, F., and Sharp, J. T.: Long term radiographic outcome of patients seen in the course of rheumatoid arthritis [Abstract No. 1056]. Arthritis Rheum. 38 [suppl. 9], 1995. Used by permission.)

A proposal for a new paradigm for clinical trials is to design trials of each therapy with the end-point for each patient being substantial and relevant improvement in arthritis or toxicity severe enough to stop treatment. This premise does not assume that drugs must be initiated in high dose and thus be potentially doomed by toxicity. Escalation of dose and add-on of additional drugs in combination is the best way to achieve definitive end-points. Our patients deserve this approach, and we must educate the Food and Drug Administration and our Human Studies Committees to let us design and implement these studies.

INVOLVING THE PATIENT IN SELECTION OF TREATMENT FOR RHEUMATOID ARTHRITIS

Underscoring the importance of improving our interventions in rheumatoid arthritis is the economic impact of this disease. Patients with rheumatoid arthritis now face three times the cost of medical care, twice the number of hospitalizations, and four times the number of physician visits under the current standards of care. The lifetime cost of rheumatoid arthritis for an individual patient can be as much as $250,000. Patients with more severe disease and disability have much greater costs than those with more mild disease.

Another element must be added to the therapy of rheumatoid arthritis in years ahead. It is *personalization.* No longer should we lump all patients at a certain stage of disease together and conclude that drug *x* or *y* should be used for all of them. The particular expectations of each patient must be factored into therapeutic plans. For example, Mrs. Jones may be more satisfied with limited mobility from her arthritis and be unwilling to risk side effects of therapy, whereas Mr. Smith will want remission of symptoms despite the potential cost of toxic side effects. Even though both patients may be at the same stage and duration of disease, each must be treated differently.

Applicable to all patients is an understanding of how the disease progresses. This is summarized in Figure 3, which demonstrates that, although there is great variation in the activity and severity of rheumatoid arthritis from one patient to another, most joint damage that will occur in every patient happens within the first 2 years of disease. Thus, although each patient must be managed within an individual context, the imperative for treatment is to institute effective therapy soon after the diagnosis has become definite.

REFERENCES

1. Harris, E. D. Jr., Evanson, J. M., DiBona, D. R., et al.: Collagenase and rheumatoid arthritis. Arthritis Rheum. 13:83, 1970.
2. Fortin, P. R., Stucki, G., and Katz, J. N.: Measuring relevant change: an emerging challenge in rheumatologic clinical trials. Arthritis Rheum. 38:1027, 1995.
3. Smith, J. B. and Fort, J. G.: Treatment of rheumatoid arthritis by immunization with monocular white blood cells: results of a preliminary trial. J. Rheumatol. 23:220, 1996.

SECTION I
STRUCTURE AND COMPOSITION OF JOINTS

The diarthrodial (synovial) joints are highly differentiated connective tissues that have evolved to provide support and motion. They are formed of many variations on three basic molecules: collagen, proteoglycans, and other glycoproteins. The manner in which these components are mixed in a tissue determines both its function and its qualities. Collagen that is mineralized is bone. Collagen entwined amid specific proteoglycans becomes articular cartilage. Collagen with minimal associated proteoglycans becomes tendons and ligaments. The cells that make these molecules have the machinery to produce enzymes that degrade them. This well-structured and differentiated system is disturbed by invasion of inflammatory cells and immunocytes in rheumatoid arthritis.

1

Joints and Connective Tissue: The Targets of Rheumatoid Arthritis

A medical student asked me at the close of a lecture, "Why does rheumatoid disease affect the joints?" I had no answer. Indeed, the complete answer would reveal much about the pathogenesis of rheumatoid arthritis. However, we do have some clues. One is that joints "move." Movement is a major part of joint function, and motion of tissues increases inflammation. If a paralyzed patient develops rheumatoid arthritis, joints on the immobile side are less affected.[1] The protective effect is present, albeit less, if a neurologic deficit develops in a patient who already has rheumatoid arthritis.[2]

Another clue may lie in the poorly documented but widely supported observation by orthopedic surgeons that, when all cartilage is removed from a joint during replacement arthroplasty, subsequent flares of rheumatoid arthritis in that patient largely spare the reconstructed joint, even though abundant synovium remains within it. The clue here is that the nature of articular cartilage has something important to do with attraction of inflammatory cells to the joint. Because immunoglobulins and complement components are routinely found in the superficial layers of hyaline cartilage in rheumatoid joints,[3] they may act as cytoattractants for the proliferating synovium.[4]

A third factor may be type II collagen, the major protein in articular cartilage. Normally sequestered from the immune system in its avascular environment, type II collagen could serve as an immunogen after "protective" proteoglycans and other glycoproteins have been stripped away by the initial joint inflammation.[5,6] Although type II collagen can induce arthritis in rats and mice,[7-9] most data in humans are consistent with the hypothesis that rheumatoid arthritis is not caused by an immune response to collagen, but that a cellular and hormonal immune response to collagen helps amplify the ongoing synovitis. A fourth factor in "arthrotropism" could be that chondrocyte cell membrane glycoproteins (e.g., gp 39) are autoantigens, or cross-react with immune reactions against superantigens. Each of these possibilities is explored in later sections of the book. It is appropriate now to examine the nature of joints and how they are formed.

DEVELOPMENTAL BIOLOGY OF SYNOVIAL JOINTS

Condensation within limb buds of a growing mass of embryonic cells to form a **blastema** is the first step in joint development (Fig. 1–1).[1] Areas destined to become cartilage then divide the blastema. **Interzones** develop between these to begin formation of the future joint cavity. Dense layers of type I collagen begin to surround the interzones, eventually forming the joint capsule. The synovium is formed from the **vascular mesenchyme** contained between the capsule and the joint cavity. Modeling and remodeling produces the finely crafted joints that have specialized structure and function appropriate for their role in movement and skeletal support.[10] Of major importance in the development of articular structures is that no epithelial tissue is found in joints; they are composed entirely of mesenchymal tissue and endothelium of blood vessels.

COMPONENTS OF THE MATURE JOINT

The various components of the mature joint are described in the following sections and are illustrated in Figure 1–2.

Articular Cartilage

Articular cartilage is a precisely organized combination of collagens and glycosaminoglycans sur-

3

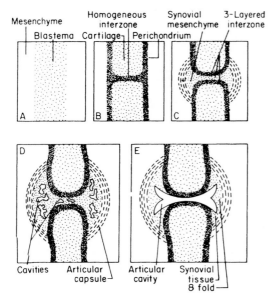

Mesenchyme | Homogeneous interzone | Synovial mesenchyme | 3-Layered interzone

Blastema | Cartilage | Perichondrium

Cavities | Articular capsule | Articular cavity | Synovial tissue 8 fold

FIGURE 1–1. Diagram of the development of a synovial joint. Joints develop from the blastema, not the surrounding mesenchyme (see text for description). (From O'Rahilly, R., and Gardner, E.: The embryology of movable joints. *In* Sokoloff, L. [ed.]: The Joints and Synovial Fluid, Vol. 1. New York, Academic Press, 1978, pp. 49–96. Used by permission.)

rounding isolated chondrocytes. It is terminally differentiated tissue. It is not replaced after injury or destruction in any form resembling the original (Fig. 1–3). The "arcade" organization of type II collagen in articular cartilage facilitates compression during loading and enables a prompt recoil on release of loads. This compression and release allows cellular metabolites to diffuse out of the matrix, and nutrients and oxygen to diffuse into the cartilage after traversing the synovial vessels, synovial lining cell layers, and joint fluid. In adults, no blood vessels penetrate through to cartilage from the subchondral bone; indeed, it is a biologic miracle that chondrocytes can thrive in this avascular environment. Chondrocytes are scattered within individual lacunae in the upper layers and are grouped more densely in lower layers. Collagen fibers are interspersed within the proteoglycan matrix much as steel rods in reinforced concrete (Fig. 1–4).

Another major component of cartilage easy to overlook, is water. Interestingly, when cartilage is damaged enzymatically during inflammation or by osteoarthritis, the water content of the tissue initially *increases*. From this we can infer that the normally tight collagenous structure controls the volume of articular cartilage, limiting the amount of water in the tissue.

Vertebrates have evolved numerous mechanisms to keep the unit load in joints (i.e., force applied

divided by the area over which the load is spread) at around 25 kg/cm.[10] Enabling this are the following factors: (1) transfer of force of impact load into surrounding soft tissue, ligaments, and muscle; (2) a normal surface incongruity of opposing cartilage surfaces that allows increasing surface contact with increasing load; and (3) a cushioning effect of the flared bone regions in the subchondral areas. If the load is increased for sustained periods because of failure of any one or more of the force attenuators mentioned, cartilage begins to deteriorate and osteoarthritis is the result. For example, surgical removal of a meniscal cartilage, or a neuromuscular disease that prevents muscle work in attenuating impact loads, can lead to cartilage degeneration.

Component Parts of Cartilage Matrix

Collagens. Type II collagen fibers, ranging from 30 nm in diameter in the superficial layers of articular cartilage to twice that in deeper zones, make up 40 to 50 per cent of cartilage dry weight. Type IX collagen, although representing less than 10 per cent of dry weight, has an extremely important function of linking the type II collagen fibers and the proteoglycans (e.g., biglycan, aggregan, decorin) in the matrix. Types V, X, and XI also are present. Their functions may be to anchor chondrocytes within the matrix.

The collagens of humans and other vertebrates can be divided into three groups according to size and also into fibrillar, basement membrane, and fiber-associated collagens as outlined here.

FIBRILLAR COLLAGENS. These are formed from monomers of protein tightly packed in a quarter-stagger array to form long, rigid fibers (Fig. 1–5). Single molecules have a triple-helical structure, and amino acid compositions are marked by glycine at every third residue. Large amounts (10 to 15 per cent of total residue) of hydroxyproline are present; this amino acid is formed post-translationally from proline and rarely is found in other proteins. Interestingly, ascorbic acid is an essential cofactor in the hydroxylation process, and its deficiency in scurvy probably explains the failure of wounds to heal. Mutations in collagen genes that impair production are responsible for diseases such as osteogenesis imperfecta, whose victims are plagued by frequent bone fractures.

Type I: This is the most abundant collagen, making up 80 per cent of the dry weight of tendons and ligaments as well as skin and bone; it forms bundles of fibers of high tensile strength.

Type II: Produced by chondrocytes, type II collagen represents approximately 50 per cent of the

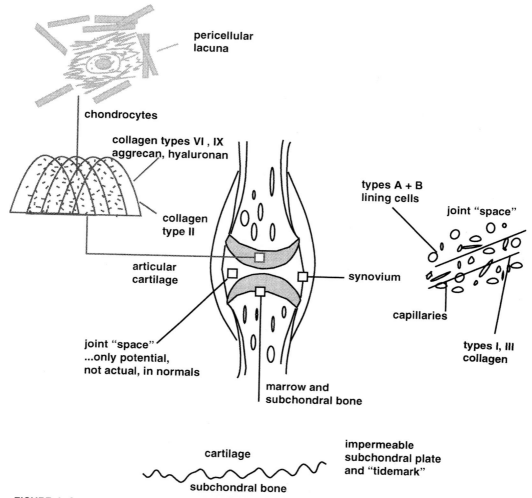

pericellular lacuna

chondrocytes

collagen types VI , IX aggrecan, hyaluronan

collagen type II

articular cartilage

joint "space" ...only potential, not actual, in normals

marrow and subchondral bone

types A + B lining cells

joint "space"

synovium

capillaries

types I, III collagen

cartilage

subchondral bone

impermeable subchondral plate and "tidemark"

FIGURE 1–2. The crucial components of a diarthrodial joint are emphasized in this figure. On the right, is the synovium, with its lining cells that lack a well-defined basement membrane and have a vigorous capillary supply. The subchondral bone (bottom) is impermeable in adults, effectively preventing any flow of nutrients from marrow to articular cartilage. The cartilage (left) is characterized by arcades of type II collagen surrounded by aggrecan and specialized type VI and IX collagens. The chondrocytes in normal cartilage are "hermits," living singly within individual lacunae.

cartilage. It is very similar in structure to type I collagen and is immunogenic in genetically susceptible rats and mice, causing arthritis.

Type III: These thin fibrils are the principal collagen in blood vessels and, with type I collagen, in newly formed connective tissue.

Type V: This collagen is found in small amounts in synovium and a few other tissues.

Type VI: These are found in moderate amounts in rheumatoid synovium among the synovial lining cells and probably help anchor these specialized mesenchymal cells in place at the interface between tissue and joint fluid (Fig. 1–6).

Type XI: These fibers, representing less than 10 per cent of the collagen in cartilage, are distributed uniformly with type II collagen.

BASEMENT MEMBRANE COLLAGENS.

Type IV. These molecules have globular extensions enabling them to link together, forming lattice-like networks resembling chicken wire (Fig. 1–7). They are a major constituent of all basement membranes, serving as a regulator of solute diffusion and as a surface for attachment of cells. Rather than being a single entity, it is useful to think of basement membranes as a complex of biomaterials serving as a diffuse coating over epithelial cells and

Zones

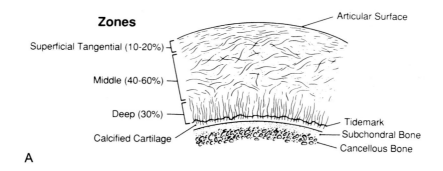

Superficial Tangential (10-20%)
Middle (40-60%)
Deep (30%)
Calcified Cartilage

Articular Surface
Tidemark
Subchondral Bone
Cancellous Bone

A

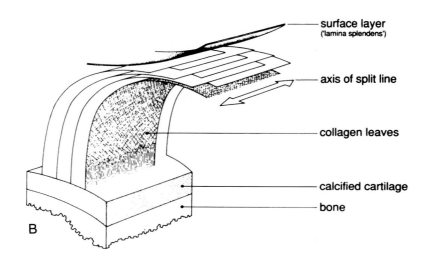

surface layer
('lamina splendens')

axis of split line

collagen leaves

calcified cartilage

bone

B

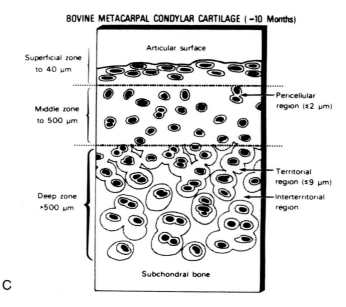

BOVINE METACARPAL CONDYLAR CARTILAGE (~10 Months)

Articular surface

Superficial zone
to 40 μm

Middle zone
to 500 μm

Deep zone
>500 μm

Pericellular
region (≤2 μm)

Territorial
region (≤9 μm)

Interterritorial
region

Subchondral bone

C

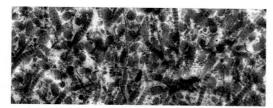

FIGURE 1–4. Transmission electron micrograph of articular cartilage in which the collagen II fibrils are clearly defined by their 760-Å periodicity. All the remaining materials are matrix glycoproteins. (Courtesy of D. R. DiBona, Ph.D., Massachusetts General Hospital.)

functioning as an aid to diffusion, a regulator of transport, and a mechanism for adhesion.

FIBER-ASSOCIATED COLLAGENS.

Type IX. These are shorter molecules than are fibrillar collagens and have fewer triple-helical regions. At "hinge" regions there are attachment sites for proteoglycans. These fibrils may help determine the spatial organization of proteoglycans and collagen within cartilage.

Degradation of Collagens

The enzymes that degrade collagen are be discussed in full in later chapters where the degradation of cartilage by invasive rheumatoid synovium is presented. The sequence of collagenolysis in mammalian tissues is as follows:

- Active collagenase (Fig. 1–8) attaches to individual triple-helical molecules approximately three fourths of the way from the amino-terminal end of the molecule and cleaves through all three polypeptide helical chains.
- The two fragments that are produced (historically named TC^A and TC^B) denature at temperatures above 32°C (Fig. 1–9).
- TC^A and TC^B lose helical structure, uncoil to gelatin, and either are degraded by extracellular proteases (e.g., stromelysin, gelatinase) or are endocytosed and degraded within phagolysosomes (Fig. 1–10). Details of collagen degradation are presented in Chapter 12.

Matrix Glycoproteins. More than 30 "matrix glycoproteins" have been characterized. They range from molecules such as hyaluronan, constructed of nonsulfated repeating disaccharides (glucuronic acid and *N*-acetylgalactosamine) without any covalent links to protein, to SPARC (a *se*creted *p*rotein *a*cidic *r*ich in *c*ysteine, also called osteonectin), a small protein with only a few saccharide side chains. In a broad definition,[11] these matrix glycoproteins include all extracellular noncollagenous components of connective tissue, and include the proteoglycans, hyaluronan and its receptors (CD44), fibronectin, and integrins and their variants. Functionally, they account for cellular adhesives (e.g., cell adhesion molecules, fibronectin, integrins); filtration (e.g., laminin, perlecan, entactin, and SPARC—all components of basement membrane); receptor activity (e.g., syndecan, betaglycan, transferrin receptor, glypican); and signaling activity for developmental events (e.g., hyaluronate and fibronectin).

It is very likely that, as research into the structure, function, and regulation of matrix evolves, the importance of these glycoproteins in determining the ways in which cells are organized and how growth and remodeling occur in both physiologic and pathologic states will expand remarkably. This applies particularly to the *cell surface matrix* that is formed of cellular receptors and matrix ligands. This cell surface matrix can be directly or indirectly visualized on cells, is several microns thick, and is fluid in composition.[12]

Basement membrane, for example, can be considered as a cell surface molecular coat. Its function[11] is to protect the cell surface, to govern the filtration of molecules while partitioning cells from one another. In synovium (see Chapter 9), there is no defined basement membrane that separates one group of cells from another, such as that separating renal epithelial cells from mesangial cells. Nevertheless, all the components of basement membrane (i.e., type IV collagen, laminin, perlecan, and entactin) are present in synovium *except* for entactin (N. Zvaifler, personal communication). As a result, the **"basement membrane" in synovium has no definite morphology, but is diffusely and amor-**

FIGURE 1–3. *A,* Zones of articular cartilage showing apparent random organization of collagen fibrils. (From Mow, V. C., et al: *In* Nordin, M., and Frankel, V. H. [eds.]: Basic Biomechanics of the Musculoskeletal System, 2nd ed. Philadelphia, Lea & Febiger, 1989. Used by permission.) *B,* Three-dimensional view of collagen plates in articular cartilage illustrating how the appearance of the collagen changes from "arcades" to random to plates, depending upon the orientation of the section. (From Jeffery, A. K., et al: Three-dimensional collagen architecture in bovine articular cartilage. J. Bone Joint Surg. Br. 73:795, 1991. Used by permission.) *C,* Diagrammatic representation of the zones and regions of bovine articular cartilage. (From Poole, A. R., Pidoux, I., Reiner, A., et al: An immuno-electron microscope study of the organization of proteoglycan monomer, link protein, and collagen in the matrix of articular cartilage. J. Cell Biol. 93:921, 1982. Used by copyright permission of The Rockefeller University Press.)

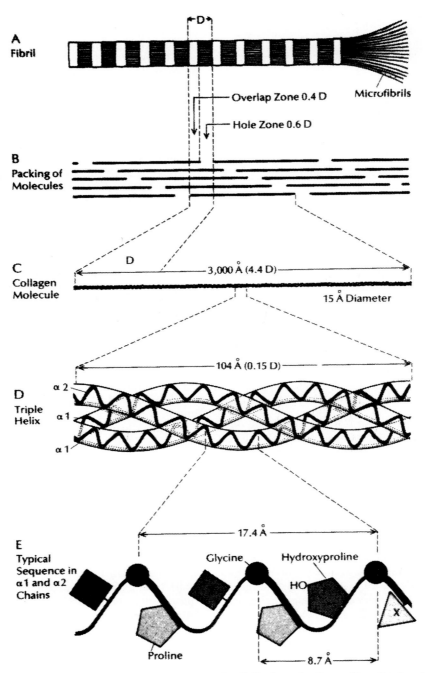

FIGURE 1–5. Schematic representation of the structure of a fibril of type I collagen. (From Prockop, D. J., and Guzman, N. A.: Collagen diseases and the biosynthesis of collagen. Hosp. Pract. 12[12]:61, 1977. Used by permission. © 1977, The McGraw-Hill Companies, Inc. Illustration by Bunji Tagawa.)

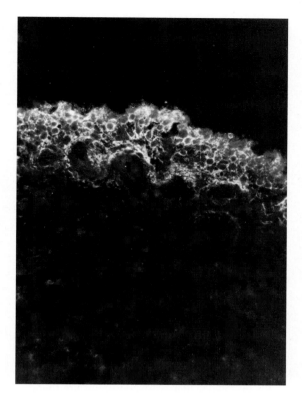

FIGURE 1–6. Using immunofluorescence microscopy, type VI collagen can be seen around the lining cells of rheumatoid synovium but not in sublining areas where the cells are faintly outlined. (× 140) (Courtesy of Dr. Y. Okada, Kanazawa University, Japan.)

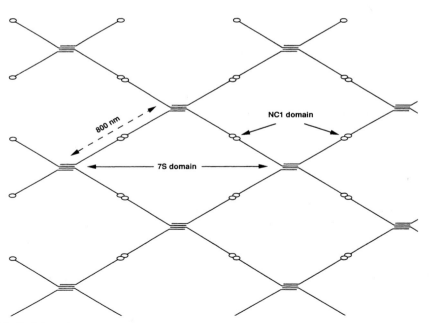

FIGURE 1–7. Schematic representation of the network-like structures formed by the assembly of type IV collagen in basement membranes. The NC1 domains are the globular extensions at the carboxyl terminus of the molecule. The 7S domains are noncollagenous domains at the amino terminus of the protein. (From Williams, C. J., Vandenberg, P., and Prockop, D. J.: Collagen and elastin. *In* Kelley, W. N., Harris, E. D. Jr., Ruddy, S., and Sledge, C. B. [eds.]: Textbook of Rheumatology, 4th ed., Vol. 1. Philadelphia, W. B. Saunders, 1993, p. 25. Used by permission.)

Fibril

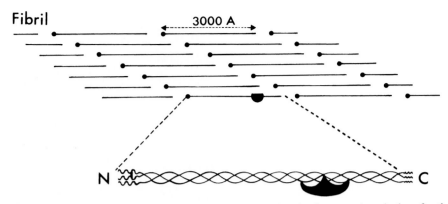

FIGURE 1–8. Active collagenase attaches to individual triple-helical molecules approximately three fourths of the way from the amino-terminal end of the collagen molecule and cleaves through all three polypeptide helical chains.

phously spread among the synovial lining cells. It renders the same functions to these cells as do the well-defined basement membranes of other tissues.

Articular cartilage contains one of the most important "supermolecules" in biology: the massive complex of hyaluronan, aggrecan, and link protein that provides the resiliency of cartilage and that plays a major role in nutrient diffusion (Fig. 1–11).

Several major matrix glycoproteins are found in the soft tissue components of joints (and destroyed in rheumatoid arthritis).

HYALURONAN. This repeating disaccharide (see earlier) occupies an enormous domain with its powerful polyanionic charge. Making a "superaggregate" in cartilage with aggregan and link protein (Fig. 1–12), this is the major noncollagenous component of cartilage. It is responsible for soft tissue lubrication between synovial layers in joints.

AGGRECAN. This is the major proteoglycan of cartilage. The long protein core (350 nm) binds to hyaluronan at its amino-terminal end (Fig. 1–11). Side chains of glycosaminoglycans (GAGs) are either chondroitin sulfate or keratan sulfate. The negative charges on polysaccharide side chains contribute to the charge domain of the superaggregate. When cartilage is compressed, these negative charges resist being forced together and push back the matrix to its original volume when pressure is released. The osmotic properties of aggrecan aid in this resistance to compression as well.

BETAGLYCAN. This molecule is a receptor for transforming growth factor β (TGFβ) on cells and, in its soluble form as a proteoglycan in matrix, enhances the activity of TGFβ.

BIGLYCAN AND DECORIN. These small glycoproteins have chondroitin sulfate and dermatan sulfate GAG side chains, bind growth factors such as TGFβ,[13] and have a regulatory function in the rate and architecture of matrix construction. They bind types I and II collagen and may regulate the size of collagen fibrils as they form in tissues.

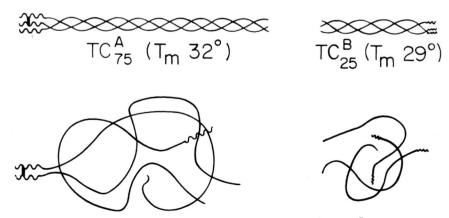

FIGURE 1–9. The two fragments that are produced (historically named TC^A and TC^B) denature at temperatures above 32°C.

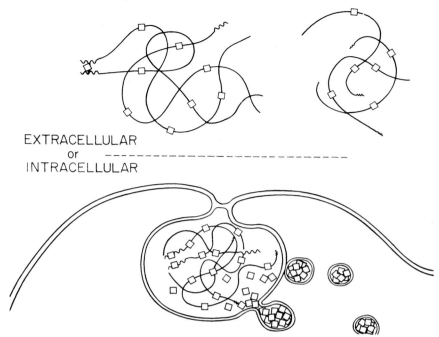

EXTRACELLULAR
or
INTRACELLULAR

FIGURE 1–10. The collagen fragments lose helical structure and uncoil to gelatin, and are either degraded by extracellular proteases or endocytosed and degraded within phagolysosomes. Open squares represent proteases capable of degrading denatured collagen (gelatin fragments).

CARTILAGE MATRIX PROTEIN. This protein is found in nonarticular cartilage and has structural homologies with several other proteins, including complement factor B, α chains of integrins, and globular domains of type VI collagen.

FIBRONECTIN. This is a multifunctional glycoprotein of two 200-kDa polypeptides. It serves as an adhesive to cells (through the arginine-glycine–aspartic acid [RGD] sequence common to adhesive proteins), a cell surface matrix protein, and a fluid-phase blood element serving as an opsonin and cell attractant during the immune and fibrotic response during rheumatoid synovitis.

PERLECAN. This is the major keratan sulfate proteoglycan of basement membrane, interacting with laminin and type IV collagen and having a major link with endothelial cells in blood vessels.

SPARC. This protein is also called osteonectin. As a matrix component in basement membrane and a component of endothelial cells, it has wide distribution. Damage to endothelium results in release of SPARC, and it creates rounding of these cells, producing gaps in the endothelium with exposure to basement membrane.

MATRIX REGULATORS. Recent data have provided an appreciation of the active physical and functional role that matrix components have in regulating cellular activity. For instance, TGFβ, a potent inducer of structural protein synthesis, binds to decorin[14] and may be down-regulated by this interaction.[13] Another example is hyaluronan. It is the first matrix component for which a cellular receptor has been identified; it is a ligand for the lymphocyte-homing receptor, CD44, and may play a role in the clustering of these cells within synovium.

Cells and Tissues in the Joint

Chondrocytes

Chondrocytes, which are relatively isolated one from one another amid cartilage matrix components, occupy less than 2 per cent of the total cartilage volume[15] yet are exclusively responsible for the maintenance of a normal cartilage matrix. They are not polarized, but rather direct secretion of gene products in all directions from the lacunae in which they are embedded. They have the capacity to produce matrix components (e.g., collagens type II, IX, and XI and proteoglycans), as well as the enzymes capable of destroying the matrix (e.g., matrix metalloproteases) and a variety of cytokines, in response to activating stimuli.

In response to sustained inflammation, chondrocytes proliferate; clusters become prominent, and

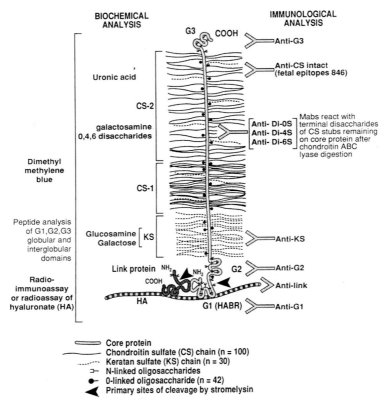

BIOCHEMICAL
ANALYSIS

IMMUNOLOGICAL
ANALYSIS

Globular domains G1, G2, and G3 are indicated

FIGURE 1–11. This diagram illustrates one small segment, often repeated, in the "supermolecule" formed as many aggrecan subunits of proteoglycan combine with link protein to unite with sites on hyaluronan (hyaluronate). Hundreds of these aggrecan molecules springing off hyaluronan form a "bottle brush" megamolecular complex with strong negative charge occupying an enormous domain within cartilage. The references to monoclonal antibodies (Mabs; e.g., anti-Di-0S) and various assays (e.g., "peptide analysis...") noted in the figure indicate the many ways in which components of this complex can be identified. (From Poole, A. R., Mort, J. S., and Roughley, P. J.: Methods for evaluating mechanisms of cartilage breakdown. *In* Woessner, J. F. Jr., and Hawell, D. S. [eds.] Joint Cartilage Degradation. New York, Marcel Dekker, 1992, p. 235. Used by permission.)

the balance between chondrocyte production of matrix components and degradative enzymes is shifted toward destruction.

Synovium

Synovium lines all parts of the inside of joints except for articular and meniscal cartilage, and small bare areas of bone between cartilage and synovial insertions into subchondral bone (Fig. 1–13). Because synovium is derived from mesenchymal tissue, no epithelial cells are present and there is no formal basement membrane underlying synovial lining cells, although many components of basement membrane (e.g., type IV collagen) can be demonstrated by immunohistologic techniques around synovial lining cells (N. Zvaifler, personal communication). The normal lining of synovial cells is only two to four cells deep. Below these lining cells there are scattered fibroblasts and loose areolar tissue that blends into the thickly collagenous joint capsule. Despite the continuum from lining to capsule, anatomists have artificially separated the tissue into (1) synovial lining or intima, (2) subsynovial tissue, and (3) joint capsule.

Synovium is highly vascularized with a large capillary bed found close to the intima. The capillaries have gaps (pores?) between endothelial cells that may facilitate passive diffusion in both directions. The interendothelial cell gaps increase during inflammation. The joint is highly innervated by sensory neurons and neurons responsible for definition and detection of joint motion and location. Nerve endings are rich in the capsule, but there are relatively few in the synovium itself.

Synovial lining cells have two principal func-

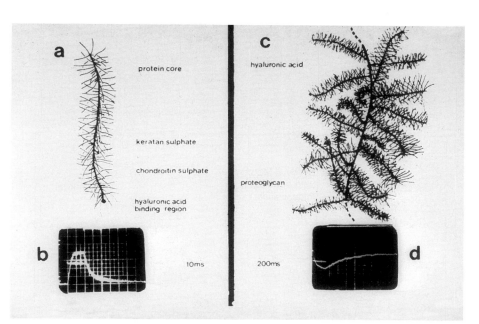

FIGURE 1–12. Artistic rendering of the "bottle brush" organization of the supermolecule formed by multiple aggrecan subunits bound by link protein to a core of hyaluronan.

tions: **synthesis** of proteins, GAGs, glycoproteins, enzymes, and growth factors, and **phagocytosis/ endocytosis.** Type A cells (Fig. 1–14*A*) have a macrophage-like appearance, with multiple cell processes, residual bodies, and lysosomes. They express surface human leukocyte antigen type DR (HLA-DR) antigens and Fc receptors. Type B cells (Fig. 1–14*B*), forming the majority of normal synovium, are marked by their prominent rough endoplasmic reticulum and are similar in appearance to fibroblasts. Some of these cells also have HLA-DR surface antigens but express no other monocyte-lineage surface antigens.[16] Other cells (type C) have mixed anatomy and, possibly, mixed function.

It is likely that lining cells can modulate function by differential gene expression in response to varied stimuli (e.g., growth factors or cytokines). For example, in severe inflammatory states, cells without a highly developed endoplasmic reticulum are rarely found[17]; conversely, synovial "fibroblasts" in culture can aggressively phagocytose particulate matter, similar to macrophages.[18] The process of ingestion of degraded red blood cells after hemarthrosis is sufficient to induce biosynthesis of collagenase and other metalloproteases in synovial cells.[19] This induction of a proliferative synovitis by blood is a prominent factor in hemophilia, and is a major reason for aspirating blood from these joints or from joints containing blood after trauma. **The lesson is that synovial lining cells function in accord with the activating stimuli in their environment. If debris is present, they phagocytose it; if growth factors and inflammatory cytokines are present, they proliferate and produce proteases or matrix components.**

Type I collagen is the predominant structural protein in synovium (as it is in ligaments and tendons); type VI collagen is present in the lining layers. Its function may be to help adherence of synovial lining cells in the absence of basement membranes in this tissue.[20]

Synovial Fluid

When synovial cells that resemble generic fibroblasts by electron microscopic analysis are placed in tissue cultures, they generate significant quantities of **hyaluronan** (hyaluronic acid), unlike other soft tissue fibroblasts. Normal synovial fluid is a mixture of hyaluronan, other proteins produced by synovial cells, including **lubricin** (a "bearing" lubricant glycoprotein for cartilage surfaces), and a plasma ultrafiltrate of low protein concentration that diffuses through synovial capillaries. In normal joints, this viscous fluid coats the synovium and cartilage, enhancing diffusion of nutrients into cartilage, but does not collect in a measurable volume. In response to any trauma or inflammation, however, increased synovial vascularity and permeability produces significant amounts of intra-articular

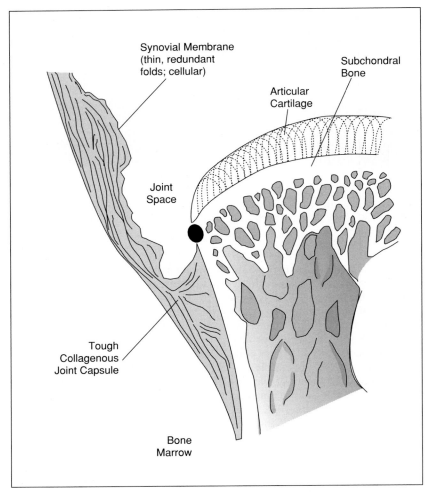

FIGURE 1–13. The black circle represents the only part within a joint that is not surfaced either by synovium or articular cartilage. Such intermittently placed areas of ''bare bone'' may be particularly vulnerable to early erosion by proliferative synovitis. They are particularly prominent in the metacarpophalangeal and proximal interphalangeal joints. (From Harris, E. D. Jr.: Synovial inflammation in rheumatoid arthritis. Hosp. Pract. 21:71, 1986. Used by permission. © 1986, The McGraw-Hill Companies. Illustration by Robert Margulies.)

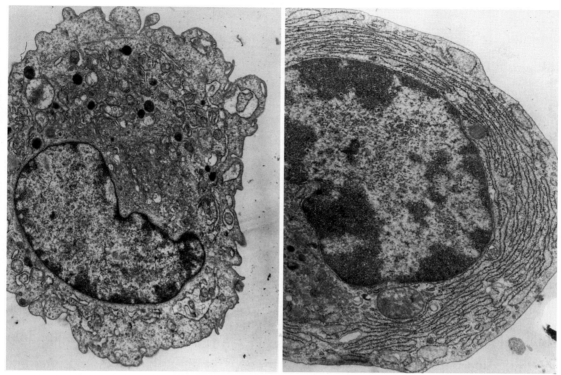

A

B

FIGURE 1–14. The large differences in function between type A cells (*A*) and type B cells (*B*) in the synovial lining are implied strongly by their morphology in these electron photomicrographs. The type A cell has multiple cytoplasmic processes and abundant granules, vacuoles, and dense bodies, consistent with its function as a scavenging macrophage. The type B cell has an extensive network of rough endoplasmic reticulum and a well-developed Golgi apparatus, consistent with a cell primarily involved in biosynthesis of products destined for secretion from cells. (Courtesy of D. Charles Faulkner, Dartmouth-Hitchcock Medical Center.)

fluid quickly. In chronic inflammation, immuno-globulins secreted by B lymphocytes and plasma cells in the subsynovial lining areas increase the protein (and immunoglobulin) concentrations in the synovial fluid. Because of their large molecular sizes, fibrinogen, α_2-macroglobulin, and immuno-globulin M are essentially excluded from normal synovial fluid; within inflamed joints, however, they are found in significant amounts.

The concentration of glucose in noninflamed synovial fluid is similar to that of plasma, but it actually decreases in chronic inflammation. Although increased glucose utilization by synovial fluid and lining cells may be partly responsible for this reduction, the major factor appears to be impaired delivery/diffusion into the joint fluid.[21]

Although synovial lining cells ingest debris and cells from synovial fluid, and the lymphatic system enhances removal of macromolecules,[22] the synovial fluid is more aptly viewed as a "sink" for both solute and cells. In "normal" synovial fluid (usually obtained from patients who have had mild trauma to a knee joint), there are fewer than 200 cells/mm[3], and most of these are resting mononuclear cells and synoviocysts shed from the lining.

Bone

In adults, bone has been formed and the architecture is complete. The predominant cellular activity in mature bone is *remodeling*, a five-step process (Fig. 1–15). The first step is *activation*, with the exposure of a mineral surface enabling osteoclasts to resorb a certain quantity of bone. Osteoblasts then spread into the area, reversing the process and replacing the osteoclasts. Then the *formation* phase begins. This takes several months and is followed by a phase of *quiescence*. The margins of this bone structural unit are visible on histologic sections and are known as cement lines. It is the balance between resorption and formation as well as the rate of remodeling that is affected by both rheumatoid arthritis and glucocorticoids used in its treatment. One structural fact that has great importance for the

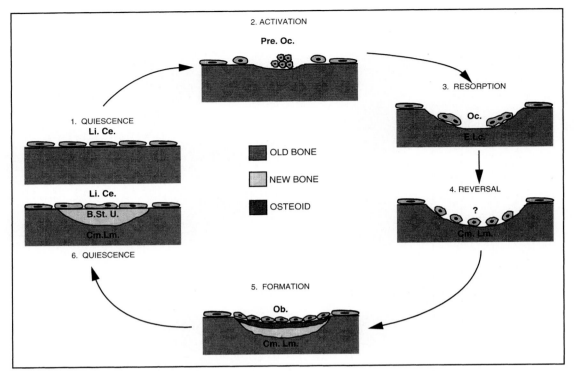

FIGURE 1–15. Illustration of the remodeling cycle in mature bone. Li. Ce., lining cell; Pre. Oc., osteoclast precursor; Oc., osteoclast; Ob., osteoblast; B. St. U., bone structural unit. (From Parfitt, A. M.: Morphometry of bone resorption: introduction and overview. Bone 14:435, 1993. Used by permission.)

function of cartilage is that, in adults, the subchondral bone blocks all vascular connection or communication by diffusion between cartilage and bone marrow.

REFERENCES

1. Bland, J., and Eddy, W.: Hemiplegia and rheumatoid hemiarthritis. Arthritis Rheum. 11:72, 1968.
2. Glick, E. N.: Asymmetrical rheumatoid arthritis after poliomyelitis. Br. Med. J. 3:26, 1967.
3. Cooke, T. D., Hurd, E. R., Jasin, H. E., et al.: Identification of immunoglobulins and complement in rheumatoid articular collagenous tissues. Arthritis Rheum. 18:541, 1975.
4. Jasin, H. E.: Autoantibody specificities of immune complexes sequestered in articular cartilage of patients with rheumatoid arthritis and osteoarthritis. Arthritis Rheum. 28:241, 1985.
5. Rowley, M., Tait, B., Mackay, I. R., et al.: Collagen antibodies in rheumatoid arthritis: significance of antibodies to denatured collagen and their association with HLA-DR4. Arthritis Rheum. 29:174, 1986.
6. Terato, K., Shimozuru, Y., Katayama, K., et al.: Specificity of antibodies to type II collagen in rheumatoid arthritis. Arthritis Rheum. 33:1493, 1990.
7. Trentham, D. E., Townes, A. S., and Kang, A. H.: Autoimmunity to type II collagen: an experimental model of arthritis. J. Exp. Med. 146:857, 1977.
8. Stuart, J. M., Cremer, M. A., Townes, A. S., et al.: Type II collagen-induced arthritis in rats: transfer with serum. J. Exp. Med. 155:1, 1982.
9. Trentham, D. E., Dynesius, R. A., and David, J. R.: Passive transfer by cells of type II collagen-induced arthritis in rats. J. Clin. Invest. 62:359, 1978.
10. Sledge, C. B.: Biology of the joint. In Kelley, W. N., Harris, E. D. Jr., Ruddy, S., and Sledge, C. B. (eds.): Textbook of Rheumatology, 4th ed., Vol. 1. Philadelphia, W. B. Saunders, 1994, pp. 1–21.
11. Trelstad, R. L., and Kemp, P. D.: Matrix glycoproteins and proteoglycans. In Kelley, W. N., Harris, E. D. Jr., Ruddy, S., and Sledge, C. B. (eds.): Textbook of Rheumatology, 4th ed., Vol. 1. Philadelphia, W. B. Saunders, 1994, pp. 35–57.
12. Lee, G. M., Johnstone, B., Jacobson, K., et al.: The dynamic structure of the pericellular matrix on living cells. J. Cell. Biol. 123:1899, 1993.
13. Yamaguchi, Y., Mann, D. M., and Ruoslahti, E.: Negative regulation of transforming growth factor-beta by the proteoglycan decorin. Nature 346:281, 1990.
14. Ruoslahti, E., and Yamaguchi, Y.: Proteoglycans as modulators of growth factor activities. Cell 64:867, 1991.
15. Stockwell, R. A., and Meachim, G.: The chondrocytes. In Freeman, M. A. R. (eds.): Adult Articular Cartilage. London, Pitman Medical, 1979, pp. 69–145.
16. Burmester, G. R., Dimitriu-Bona, A., Waters, S. J., et al.: Identification of three major synovial lining cell populations by monoclonal antibodies directed to Ia antigens and antigens associated with monocytes/macrophages and fibroblasts. Scand. J. Immunol. 17:69, 1983.
17. Roy, S., Ghadially, F. N., and Crane, W. A. I.: Synovial

membrane in traumatic effusion: ultrastructure and auto-radiography with tritiated leucine. Ann. Rheum. Dis. 25: 259, 1966.

18. Werb, Z., and Reynolds, J. J.: Stimulation by endocytosis of the secretion of collagenase and neutral proteinases from rabbit synovial fibroblasts. J. Exp. Med. 140:1482, 1976.

This important paper represented the first concrete evidence that collagenase was a protein synthesized de novo by fibroblasts and not an artifact of organ culture. It also was the first paper to report induction of biosynthesis of collagenase by fibroblasts in response to certain stimuli—in this case, tiny latex particles. This concept, and the methodology used to describe it, made possible subsequent studies of metalloprotenase biosynthesis and activation and cytokine induction of destructive matrix proteases.

19. Mainardi, C. L., Levine, P. H., Werb, Z., et al.: Proliferative synovitis in hemophilia: report of a case with biochemical and morphologic observations. Arthritis Rheum. 21:137, 1978.

20. Okada, Y., Naka, K., Minamoto, T., et al.: Localization of type VI collagen in the lining cell layer of normal and rheumatoid synovium. Lab. Invest. 63:647, 1990.

21. Ropes, M. W., Muller, A. F., and Bauer, W.: The entrance of glucose and other sugars into joints. Arthritis Rheum. 3:496, 1960.

22. Brown, D. L., Cooper, A. G., and Bluestone, R.: Exchange of IgM and albumin between plasma and synovial fluid in rheumatoid arthritis. Ann. Rheum. Dis. 29:644, 1969.

SECTION II

PREDISPOSITION, PREDILECTION, AND CAUSATION OF RHEUMATOID ARTHRITIS

Because the cause of rheumatoid arthritis is not known, much research has been invested in sorting out the factors that patients with the disease have in common. These epidemiologic studies are extremely difficult to do, but have been very useful in giving investigators crucial links in understanding the disease. Most useful has been the research in immunogenetic epidemiology that has evolved in the past decade. Linked to immunogenetics and a number of factors in the environment that may contribute to rheumatoid arthritis are the candidates for direct or indirect causation of the disease. The results of immunogenetics studies have overshadowed findings on environmental, hormonal, and other commonalities, but all will be relevant research topics until the final details about the cause have been determined.

2

History and Epidemiology of Rheumatoid Arthritis: How Long Has It Affected Us, and Who Is at Risk?

The cause of rheumatoid arthritis is not known. Therefore, analysis of what types of individuals are susceptible to acquiring rheumatoid arthritis may give us clues as to *why* it occurs. In addition, being able to identify *when* the disease first was manifest in human populations would yield useful information about possible environmental factors related to its development then and now.

FIRST APPEARANCE OF RHEUMATOID ARTHRITIS

The question of when rheumatoid arthritis first appeared is not a trivial one. If its origins were in antiquity, pathogenesis could be linked more closely to the composition and function of human immune responses to multiple antigens. Conversely, if the disease was not present significantly before its description in 1800,[1] the search for a principal cause of the disease should be focused on one or several infectious agents that could have evolved.

Skeletal remains are of minimal help; unlike osteoarthritis, the eburnation and osteophytes of which have been identified in remains from antiquity, erosions of bone found in such remains that are typical of rheumatoid arthritis could also have been caused by tophaceous gout or a direct infection. Recognizing these limitations, paleopathologic studies have found bone erosions in thousands of Native American skeletons dating from as far back as 6,500 years ago in a circumscribed area of the upper west part of the Mississippi basin.[2] This supports hypotheses that rheumatoid arthritis began with geographic limitations and suggests major environmental factors in pathogenesis in a susceptible population.

Another interesting approach has been the analysis of paintings. Presumably, if artists were faithful to their models' anatomy, paintings of rheumatoid joints would have been done quite by accident. Portrayal of deformities consistent with rheumatoid arthritis have been found by trained eyes in several paintings:

The Temptation of St. Anthony, Dutch-Flemish School (circa 1450)[3]

The Donators, Jan Gossaert (1525)[4]

Avignon Pieta, Flemish School (1470)[5]

The Painter's Family, Jacob Jordaen (1620–1650)[4]

The problem here is obvious; many illnesses, including Parkinson's disease, peripheral neuropathy, leprosy, or trauma, could have been responsible for the same changes in appearance of joints that were captured on canvas.

It is enjoyable work, this sleuthing among paintings and bones. However, it has failed to determine convincing dates for the first appearance of rheumatoid arthritis.

INCIDENCE AND PREVALENCE OF RHEUMATOID ARTHRITIS

It seems reasonable to accept the premise that rheumatoid arthritis has been more prevalent during the past 300 years than previously, perhaps in part due to longer life spans of the populations at risk. A logical follow-up question is: Are there data to suggest relatively recent changes in incidence or prevalence of the disease?

Most epidemiologic studies have shown a prevalence of rheumatoid arthritis of about 1 per cent

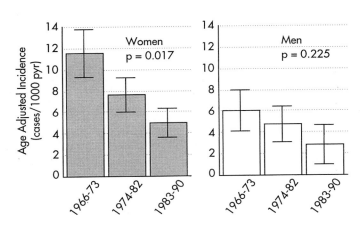

FIGURE 2–1. Mean age-adjusted incidence of rheumatoid arthritis in male and female Pima Indians during three consecutive time periods between 1966 and 1990. *P* values represent significance of the linear trend after controlling for age in men and for age, use of estrogens or oral contraceptives, and pregnancy in women. (From Jacobsson, L. T. H., Hanson, R. L., Knowler, W. C., et al: Decreasing incidence and prevalence of rheumatoid arthritis in Pima Indians over a twenty-five-year period. Arthritis Rheum. 37: 1158, 1994. Used by permission.)

in Caucasian populations.[1,6] Nevertheless, a trend toward a lower incidence than expected from historical surveys is notable from some studies. In Rochester, Minnesota—an area carefully and often surveyed by the Mayo Clinic—there was estimated to be a 50 per cent decline in the incidence of rheumatoid arthritis among women from 1950 to 1974.[7] Similar declines have been noted in the United Kingdom.[8,9] In England, the prevalence of rheumatoid factor declined from 63 per cent in women with definite rheumatoid arthritis in 1960 to 25 per cent in 1992, implying that the severity of the disease has decreased as well. In a second evaluation of a well-studied subpopulation, Pima Indians shown to have a high incidence of rheumatoid arthritis in 1966 had a 55 to 60 per cent decline in incidence in 1990[10] (Fig. 2–1).

A major problem in studies of incidence or prevalence of rheumatoid arthritis is in methodology used "then" and now. The American College of Rheumatology (ACR) criteria for rheumatoid arthritis, first developed in 1958,[11] had a classification of "probable" rheumatoid arthritis that would include patients who very likely had another disease. For example, in Sudbury, Massachusetts,[12] of 78 individuals diagnosed by ACR criteria as having "probable" rheumatoid arthritis, only 11 could be classified as having either "probable" or "definite" rheumatoid arthritis 3 to 5 years later. The remainder had either become well again or gone on to manifest a different disease. Another problem has been pooling men and women together in survey statistics; the fourfold higher frequency in women makes it essential that the sexes be separated in these types of studies.

Given the different classification criteria, differences in health care–seeking behavior, and methods for case identification, it is interesting that the **incidence** of rheumatoid arthritis in a central Massachusetts population between 1987 and 1990 was

similar to that found in Rochester, Minnesota, between 1950 and 1974: 22:100,000 in men and 60:100,000 in women, with a marked increase in women older than 60 years of age.[13] In contrast, in a study of British subjects, rheumatoid arthritis was found to have a **prevalence** of 1.2 per cent in women age 45 to 64 years between 1990 and 1992 compared with 2.5 per cent between 1958 and 1960.[9] The incidence of rheumatoid arthritis increased with age, with a marked increase in women older than 50.

The contrasts in data make it difficult to draw firm conclusions about possible changes in numbers of patients developing rheumatoid arthritis each year, but it is reasonable to continue using a 1 per cent prevalence rate in most populations until other solid information to the contrary is available. Similarly, it is advisable not to make too much of differences in reported incidence or severity in various subpopulations unless the necessary immunogenetic studies in these groups reveal *HLA-DRB1* sequences that are not expected from clinical manifestations.

One confounding factor that will affect every study of current years compared to data collected many years ago is that all populations are aging. People live longer. Also, because the incidence of disease rises markedly in older women, the prevalence in population groups is likely to increase, or not decrease, even though the age distribution within the population changes markedly.

Rheumatoid Arthritis in Siblings

There is a higher likelihood, of course, that genetic material will be shared among siblings more than among unrelated individuals. Nevertheless, variability in sibling concordance was one of the reasons that genetic links were defined as late as they were in this disease. There are some useful data from studies of twins and other siblings, however. Firm data are published showing that there is an increased disease concordance in monozygotic, as compared with dizygotic, twins.[14,15] These studies give firm support to a genetic influence in the disease, because both identical and fraternal twins in these studies had been exposed to the same environmental influences. It has been more challenging to determine the influence of non-twin sibship on aquisition of rheumatoid arthritis. Jones and colleagues approached this by studying the prevalence of rheumatoid arthritis in both 518 first-degree relatives of 207 well-defined, unselected incidence cases of rheumatoid arthritis and 414 first-degree relatives of 180 local controls.[16] The controls were either friends of the patients matched for gender and age and living within the same area, or persons similarly matched for gender and age chosen from a roster of the patients' general practitioners. The risk ratio of having rheumatoid arthritis for a first-degree relative of a rheumatoid patient compared with controls was 1.6 (7.7 cases/1,000 compared with 4.8 : 1,000). This is not an important familial risk. In another study of 190 female and 50 male same-sexed sibships in which the proband had classical or definite rheumatoid arthritis,[17] sibship concordance rates were consistently higher when probands had severe disease, a factor not accounted for by age or disease duration. **These data are consistent with a multifactorial threshold model of rheumatoid arthritis in which an accumulation of the influence of several genetic and environmental factors must be focused in the same individual in order for the disease to be manifest.** Future studies may be able to evaluate effects on genetic expression, such as imprinting or X-chromosome inactivation in women.

POSSIBLE PREDISPOSING FACTORS (OTHER THAN IMMUNOGENETIC ONES)

As described in Chapter 3, the shared epitope or susceptibility cassette on *HLA-DRB1* chains has appeared at a higher frequency in most populations that have an excess over expected prevalence of rheumatoid arthritis. However, because it is probable that rheumatoid arthritis is of polygenic determination, it is not surprising that other biologic and environmental factors have been linked with rheumatoid arthritis. The Mayo Clinic studies have linked the HLA-DR shared epitope with severity as well as with susceptibility to rheumatoid arthritis. Other influences on patients can be looked at in the same fashion.

Education Level

Epidemiologists have focused on higher levels of education as having a possible beneficial effect on rheumatoid arthritis. This is not surprising because rheumatoid arthritis is one of several chronic diseases in which the patient can have a major role in determining outcome through "self-help." Attention to detail in taking medication; careful, regular, and prescribed exercises; and safe work habits are all likely to have a beneficial effect on outcome. Precedent is plentiful; previous studies have found that years of schooling correlate with work disability status, employment in hazardous jobs, smoking habits, blood pressure, body mass index, and mortality.[18] Initial studies[19] in rheumatoid arthritis discovered that increased mortality and morbidity were associated with lower formal education in 75 patients followed over 9 years. Follow-up data in more than 2,000 patients[18] found a marginal contribution of schooling for men in the disability index after controlling for occupation and income, but no such change for women. One study of young women with rheumatoid arthritis from the Netherlands showed that patients with rheumatoid arthritis who had low and medium levels of education had more initial joint erosions and poorer functional scores compared with those with high levels of education, even though the symptoms had been present for the same length of time in all three groups.[20]

Lifestyle Habits

Although cigarette smoking and alcohol consumption are appropriately considered public health problems, one study by an experienced group in Holland has reported a low relative risk for developing rheumatoid arthritis in those who smoke cigarettes (at least one per day) and drink alcohol (at least once drink per day).[21] Benefits from these habits were independent of each other and also independent of oral contraceptive use (see later). However, this was a retrospective study, and emphasizes the difficulty in disentangling cause from effect in this type of clinical research. Taking advantage of the usefulness of discordant twin pair studies in allowing adjustment for confounding effects of both genetic and other social factors, a recent nationwide study demonstrated that cigarette smoking increases the risk of rheumatoid arthritis.[22] As expected, most of the monozygotic and dizygotic pairs discordant for rheumatoid arthritis were concordant for smoking history. In the smoking-discordant pairs, however, substantially more monozygotic pairs in which the twin with rheumatoid arthritis smoked while the twin without rheumatoid arthritis was a nonsmoker (11 pairs) were found, compared with the rheumatoid arthritis non-smoker/non–rheumatoid arthritis smoker pairs (2 pairs). The odds ratio (similar to relative risk) between smoking and rheumatoid arthritis in the monozygotic pairs was 12.0 and in the dizygotic pairs was 2.5. These data support a role for smoking in disease susceptibility.

Other Diagnoses

It is probable that individuals with very mild disease might escape diagnosis because insufficient criteria have been met or another diagnosis (e.g., fibromyalgia, depression, palindromic rheumatism) was made. It would follow, then, that the apparent prevalence of rheumatoid arthritis in a cohort that included numerous individuals with mild disease would be less than that in groups with fewer mildly affected patients. This is particularly apparent when considering effects of sex, pregnancy, and oral contraceptives on incidence or severity.

Sex and Sex Hormones

Rheumatoid arthritis, along with many diseases associated with self-injury by the host's immune system, is more common in women than in men.[23] Estrogens generally have a stimulatory effect upon the immune system; they inhibit T-suppressor function and facilitate T-helper cell maturation.[24] Estrogen receptors are present in rheumatoid synovium on macrophage-like synoviocytes and CD8[+]/CD29[+] CD4RO[+] (memory) T cells. In established rheumatoid arthritis, the increased concentration of estradiol present during the postovulatory phase of menstrual cycles is associated with worsening of rheumatic symptoms. None of these factors definitively explains the increased frequency of rheumatoid arthritis in women, but the associations are intriguing.

In a study of whether gender affects the pattern of disease (Schmidt et al., Abstract 816), 51 men and 50 women were examined. The following data emerged:

- Age of onset and seropositivity were equal
- Erosive disease developed earlier in men
- Rheumatoid lung was 10 times (27 per cent) more common in men
- Sicca syndrome was more common in women (14 per cent)
- Forty-nine per cent of men carried two disease-associated alleles, whereas only 29 per cent of women carried two.

These data are compatible with a hypothesis that rheumatoid arthritis exhibits a lower penetrance in men.

Women and Rheumatoid Arthritis

Several studies have focused on aspects of female gender relevant to rheumatoid arthritis.

Age of Menarche. In discordant sibling studies, a slight delay in menarche was observed in those women with the disease.[25]

Pregnancy. Many studies have documented the remission in symptoms that accompanies pregnancy, particularly during the first trimester, since the first description of this effect by Hench in 1938.[26] The benefit is short lived, however, and during the postpartum period activity of the disease recurs and it is often more active than before.

Also interesting are data that focus on whether or not pregnancy or nulliparity affects the risk of developing rheumatoid arthritis. The most recent studies that do not use flawed methodology of earlier work can be summarized as follows:

- There is a decreased risk of rheumatoid arthritis for women who *have ever been* pregnant. The earlier the first pregnancy, the lower the risk. Adverse outcome of pregnancy does not affect the decrease in risk, and the protective effects are independent of oral contraceptive use or a family history of rheumatoid arthritis.[27] **These data could indicate either that nulliparity is a risk factor for development of the disease or that parity is protective against rheumatoid arthritis.**
- Focusing on the narrow time period during pregnancy and shortly after childbirth, data have indicated that there is a slight reduction of the onset of rheumatoid arthritis during pregnancy and an increase in risk of developing symptoms of rheumatoid arthritis during the first 3 months or more postpartum.[28]
- There appears to be no difference in adverse outcomes of pregnancy (including spontaneous abortions and stillbirths) in women who later developed rheumatoid arthritis.[29] In contrast, a group of 176 women with rheumatoid arthritis and at least one child were compared with a similar group of porous women without rheumatoid arthritis. Having more than three children increased the risk of developing severe disease by a factor of 4.8.[30]

Recent information has linked differences in maternal-fetal HLA antigens with remission of rheumatoid arthritis during pregnancy.[31] Maternal-fetal disparities for HLA-DRB1, -DQA, and -DQB were found in 26 of 34 pregnancies (76 per cent) in women whose rheumatoid arthritis went into remission or improved during pregnancy, versus a 25 per cent disparity (3 of 12) in those whose rheumatoid arthritis remained active. **It is possible that in instances of a maternal-fetal HLA mismatch, blocking antibodies to class II major histocompatibility complex antigens could evolve and inhibit the activation of T-cell clones essential for induction of synovitis.** Alternatively, because it is known that HLA molecules can present self-peptides derived from other HLA molecules, presentation to T cells of fetal HLA peptides could be beneficial for a woman during pregnancy,[32] because they compete for open grooves in HLA molecules with the purported arthritogenic peptides. Of course, the brief remission during pregnancy may have little to do with antigen presentation to T cells; rather, it may be related to events further downstream in the pathophysiologic cascade of this disease. In this vein, there are reasons to believe that there is an increased production of Th2 cytokines during pregnancy.[33] As is discussed in Chapter 5, there are two subclasses of helper T cells, Th1 and Th2. The Th1 cells generate interleukin-2 and interferon γ, lymphokines believed to enhance autoimmune disease, while Th2 cells down-regulate Th1 cell expression. In line with this concept is the use of alloantibodies against class II HLA peptides eluted from placentas and used in Europe for treatment of rheumatoid arthritis.[34]

Breast-Feeding. Although numbers of patients are small, there may be a correlation of breast-feeding with the development of rheumatoid arthritis.[35] This predilection appears to be limited to only the first postpartum period, not subsequent ones. The possible association with elevated prolactin levels is intriguing but without solid foundation. Another, more recent study[30] of rheumatoid and control women who had one or more children suggested that breast-feeding did not increase the risk of developing rheumatoid arthritis. In the same patients, duration of breast-feeding was significantly related to severe rheumatoid arthritis but, when adjusted for age and parity, a history of lactation before disease onset did not alter the course of the disease.

Use of Oral Contraceptives. Few families of drugs have been scrutinized as much as oral contraceptives for possible injurious effects upon women who have taken them for long periods of time. The small but real risks of inducing hypocoagulability, possible associations with breast cancer or other malignancies, and a possible protective effect against coronary events are well known.

The data associating rheumatoid arthritis and oral contraceptives are conflicting in detail and interpretation. A report in 1978 showed protection of oral contraceptives against developing rheumatoid arthritis.[36] These European studies have been countered by case studies in North America that have failed to confirm any protection from rheumatoid arthritis of prior or current use of oral contraceptives.[37]

Several possibilities have been advanced to explain these conflicting data. One is that the incidence and prevalence of rheumatoid arthritis have changed in some subpopulations. In a large group of women (23,000 who were using oral contraceptives and the same number who never had used them), the risk ratio between current users and never-users of developing rheumatoid arthritis in the 1968 to 1974 period was significantly reduced (0.49), whereas that between former users and never-users was 0.84. Between 1981 and 1987, however, the former-users group had only statistically insignificant reduction in their risk for rheumatoid arthritis[38] because the frequency in never-users dropped, perhaps reflecting a general decrease in rheumatoid arthritis in the general population.

The other hypothesis put forth to explain the discrepancy between European and North American data is that European studies were, for the most part conducted among hospitalized patients, whereas the studies in the United States were on outpatients. This has been supported by meta-analysis[39] of published data and by a prospective Dutch study.[40] One conclusion reached is that oral contraceptives may protect women from developing more severe disease. This is supported by a study[30] of women with rheumatoid arthritis and at least one child. Comparison of rheumatoid women according to severity of disease showed that oral contraceptive use before the onset of rheumatoid arthritis was significantly less in patients with severe disease (44 per cent use in mild rheumatoid arthritis versus 21 per cent use in severe disease). The risk of severe rheumatoid arthritis was more diminished in those who took oral contraceptives for longer periods than in those who took them for less than 5 years. Figure 2–2 graphically summarizes the relative risks of *developing* rheumatoid arthritis during a hypothetical life span for a woman.

Estrogen Replacement Therapy. Use of estrogen replacement in the postmenopausal state has never been associated with a protective effect on the development of rheumatoid arthritis,[41] but may have a protective effect on the course of rheumatoid arthritis, similar to that provided by oral contraceptives.

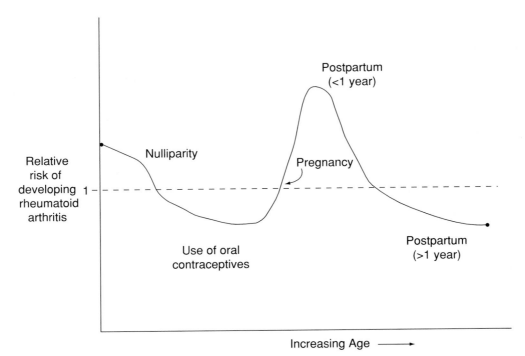

FIGURE 2–2. Semi-quantitative portrait of the relative risk that a woman may have for developing rheumatoid arthritis compared with the general population of women at the same age. (Data compiled by Carin Dugowson, University of Washington.)

Sex Hormones and Immunologic Responses. Because there clearly are no useful therapeutic guidelines found in these data, the hope has been that they will unlock understanding of pathophysiology of rheumatoid arthritis. One hypothesis is that fecundity and oral contraceptives could induce clones of arthritis-protective T cells or exert another suppressor effect upon joint inflammation. More likely is the possibility that estrogens and prolactin leave immunosuppression effects not yet deciphered by investigators in the field. The need for further research in immunoendocrinology is clear.

Effect of Other Hormones

A hypothesis has been presented that **lower androgen concentrations** must be considered as a major predisposing factor for rheumatoid arthritis. Unfortunately, there seems to be little that can be done to test this hypothesis further. It is based primarily upon data that both men and women with rheumatoid arthritis have lower mean androgen concentrations than do controls.

REFERENCES

1. Short, C. L.: The antiquity of rheumatoid arthritis. Arthritis Rheum. 17:193, 1974.

2. Rothschild, B. M., Turner, K. R., and DeLuca, M. A.: Symmetrical erosive peripheral polyarthritis in the late Archaic period of Alabama. Science 241:1498, 1988.
3. Dequeker, J., and Rico, H.: Rheumatoid arthritis-like deformities in an early 16th-century painting of the Flemish-Dutch school. JAMA 268:249, 1992.
4. Dequeker, J.: Arthritis in Flemish paintings (1400–1700). Br. Med. J. 1:1203, 1977.
5. Dequeker, J.: Paleopathology of rheumatism in paintings. Paper presented at the Symposium on Human Paleopathology: Current Synthesis and Future Options, Zagreb, Yugoslavia, July 24–31, 1988.
6. Fraser, K. J.: Anglo-French contribution to the recognition of rheumatoid arthritis. Ann. Rheum. Dis. 41:335, 1982.
7. Linos, A., Worthington, J. W., O'Fallon, W. M., et al.: The epidemiology of rheumatoid arthritis in Rochester, Minnesota: a study of incidence, prevalence and mortality. Am. J. Epidemiol. 111:87, 1980.
8. Silman, A. J.: Has the incidence of rheumatoid arthritis declined in the United Kingdom? Br. J. Rheumatol. 27:77, 1988.
9. Spector, T. D., Hart, D. J., and Powell, R. J.: Prevalence of rheumatoid arthritis and rheumatoid factor in women: evidence for a secular decline. Ann. Rheum. Dis. 52:254, 1993.

A total of 1,003 women ages 45 to 64 from a group of general practitioners in East London were examined for rheumatoid arthritis during 1990–1992. Twelve had definite rheumatoid arthritis, a prevalence of 1.1 per cent, and three had a positive test for rheumatoid factor. This is in marked contrast to a study in Northern England between 1960 and 1968 in which a prevalence of 2.5 per cent and 63 per cent positivity for rheumatoid factor were observed.

10. Jacobsson, L. T. H., Hanson, R. L., Knowler, W. C., et al.: Decreasing incidence and prevalence of rheumatoid arthritis in Pima Indians over a twenty-five-year period. Arthritis Rheum. 37:1158, 1994.

In 2,894 subjects, 78 incident cases of rheumatoid arthritis were identified. The age-adjusted incidence between 1966 and 1990 declined by 55 per cent in men and 57 per cent in women. Age-adjusted prevalence for active disease decreased by 29 per cent in men and 40 per cent in women. A possible explanation is the treatment of more patients with second-line drugs; however, even with these drugs, complete remission is rare. The data were controlled for use of oral contraceptives.

11. Ropes, M. W., Bennett, G. A., Cobb, S., et al.: 1958 revision of diagnostic criteria for rheumatoid arthritis. Bull. Rheum. Dis. 9:175, 1958.
12. O'Sullivan, J. B., and Cathcart, E. S.: The prevalence of rheumatoid arthritis: follow-up evaluation of the effect of criteria on rates in Sudbury, Massachusetts. Ann. Intern. Med. 76:753, 1972.
13. Chan, K.-W. A., Felson, D. T., Yood, R. A., et al.: Incidence of rheumatoid arthritis in central Massachusetts. Arthritis Rheum. 36:1691, 1993.
14. Aho, K., Koskenvuo, M., Tuominen, J., and Kaprio, J.: Occurrence of rheumatoid arthritis in a nationwide series of twins. J. Rheumatol. 13:899, 1986.
15. Silman, A. J., MacGregor, A. J., Thomson, W., et al.: Twin concordance rates for rheumatoid arthritis: a nationwide study. Br. J. Rheumatol. 32:903, 1993.
16. Jones, M. A., Silman, A. J., Whiting, S., et al.: Occurrence of rheumatoid arthritis is not increased in the first degree relatives of a population based inception cohort of inflammatory polyarthritis. Ann. Rheum. Dis. 55:89, 1996.
17. Deighton, C. M., Roberts, D. F., and Walker, D. J.: Effect of disease severity on rheumatoid arthritis concordance in same sexed siblings. Ann. Rheum. Dis. 51:943, 1992.
18. Leigh, J. P., and Fries, J. F.: Education level and rheumatoid arthritis: evidence from five data centers. J. Rheumatol. 18:24, 1991.
19. Pincus, T., and Callahan, L. F.: Formal education as a marker for increased mortality and morbidity in rheumatoid arthritis. J. Chronic. Dis. 38:973, 1985.
20. Vlieland, T. P. M. V., Buitenhuis, N. A., van Zeben, D., et al.: Sociodemographic factors and the outcome of rheumatoid arthritis in young women. Ann. Rheum. Dis. 53:803, 1994.
21. Hazes, J. M. W., Dijkmans, B. A. C., Vandenbroucke, J. P., et al.: Lifestyle and the risk of rheumatoid arthritis: cigarette smoking and alcohol consumption. Ann. Rheum. Dis. 49:980, 1990.
22. Silman, A. J., Newman, J., and MacGregor, A. J.: Cigarette smoking increases the risk of rheumatoid arthritis. Arthritis Rheum. 39:732, 1996.
23. Beeson, P. B.: Age and sex associations of 40 autoimmune diseases. Am. J. Med. 96:457, 1994.
24. Ahmed, S. A., Dauphinee, M. J., and Talal, N.: Effects of short-term administration of sex hormones on normal and autoimmune mice. J. Immunol. 134:204, 1985.
25. Deighton, C. M., Sykes, H., and Walker, D. J.: Rheumatoid arthritis, HLA identity, and age at menarche. Ann. Rheum. Dis. 52:322, 1993.
26. Hench, P. S.: The ameliorating effect of pregnancy on chronic atrophic (infectious rheumatoid) arthritis, fibrositis, and intermittent hydrarthrosis. Proc. Mayo Clin. 13:161, 1938.
27. Hazes, J. M. W., Dijkmans, B. A. C., Vandenbroucke, J. P., et al.: Pregnancy and the risk of developing rheumatoid arthritis. Arthritis Rheum. 33:1770, 1990.
28. Silman, A., Kay, A., and Brennan, P.: Timing of pregnancy in relation to the onset of rheumatoid arthritis. Arthritis Rheum. 35:152, 1992.
29. Nelson, J. L., Voigt, L. F., Koepsell, T. D., et al.: Pregnancy outcome in women with rheumatoid arthritis before disease onset. J. Rheumatol. 19:18, 1992.
30. Jorgensen, C., Picot, M. C., Bologna, C., and Sany, J.: Oral contraception, parity, breast feeding, and severity of rheumatoid arthritis. Ann. Rheum. Dis. 55:94, 1996.
31. Nelson, J. L., Hughes, K. A., Smith, A. G., et al.: Maternal-fetal disparity in HLA class II alloantigens and the pregnancy-induced amelioration of rheumatoid arthritis. N. Engl. J. Med. 329:466, 1993.
32. Nelson, J. L.: Maternal–fetal immunology and autoimmune disease. Arthritis Rheum. 39:191, 1996.
33. Wegman, T. G., Lin, H., Builbert, L., Mosmann, T. R.: Bidirectional cytokine interactions in the maternal-fetal relationship: is successful pregnancy a TH2 phenomenon? Immunol. Today 14:353–356, 1993.
34. Moynier, M., Cosso, B., Brochier, J., et al.: Identification of class II HLA alloantibodies in placenta-eluted gamma globulins used for treating rheumatoid arthritis. Arthritis Rheum. 30:375, 1987.
35. Brennan, P., and Silman, A.: Breast feeding and the onset of rheumatoid arthritis. Arthritis Rheum. 37:808, 1994.
36. Wingrave, S. J., and Kay, C. R.: Reduction in incidence of rheumatoid arthritis associated with oral contraceptives. Lancet 1:569, 1978.
37. Linos, A., Worthington, J. W., O'Fallon, W. M., et al.: Case-control study of rheumatoid arthritis and prior use of oral contraceptives. Lancet 1:1938, 1985.
38. Hannaford, P. C., Kay, C. R., and Hirsch, S.: Oral contraceptives and rheumatoid arthritis: new data from the Royal College of General Practitioners' oral contraception study. Ann. Rheum. Dis. 49:744, 1990.
39. Spector, T. D., and Hochberg, M. C.: The protective effect of the oral contraceptive pill on rheumatoid arthritis: an overview of the analytic epidemiological studies using meta-analysis. J. Clin. Epidemiol. 43:1221, 1990.
40. van Zeben, D., Hazes, J. M. W., Vandenbroucke, J. P., et al.: Diminished incidence of severe rheumatoid arthritis associated with oral contraceptive use. Arthritis Rheum. 33:1462, 1990.
41. Carette, S., Marcoux, S., and Gingras, S.: Postmenopausal hormones and the incidence of rheumatoid arthritis. J. Rheumatol. 16:911, 1989.

3

Immunogenetics

Several years ago, with the discovery that a majority of northern European and American patients with rheumatoid arthritis carried a "shared epitope" on one or both class II major histocompatibility complex (MHC) *HLA-DR* β-chains, it was reasonable to surmise that eventually it would be proven that this epitope was both necessary and sufficient in an individual for rheumatoid arthritis to develop. This has proven not to be realistic. In many populations (e.g., African-Americans), the shared epitope is minimally associated with rheumatoid arthritis. In addition, there are suggestions that another component of the MHC, DQ, may have an immunogenetic influence. At this time it is a reasonable estimate that no more than half of rheumatoid arthritis patients worldwide share this special epitope in the MHC. Nevertheless, this epitope, the conserved amino acid sequence in the third hypervariable region of the *DRB1* allele, when combined with a positive test for rheumatoid factor, allows prediction that the individual with rheumatoid arthritis is more than 13-fold at risk for developing radiographically apparent bone erosions in joints within one year.[1]

Although it has been appreciated for many years that there were strong heritable influences in the determination of which individuals developed rheumatoid arthritis, it also was appreciated that, if genetic factors were involved, they were multifactorial and complex. Thus, when Astorga and Williams[2] reported that lymphocytes from 14 of 22 different patients with rheumatoid arthritis in mixed lymphocyte cultures did not activate each other, in contrast to lymphocytes from controls that readily activated each other, there was no sudden appreciation that genetics was involved in the mechanism. The authors astutely noted, however, that their findings were "a new and potentially exciting lead . . . towards understanding the pathogenesis of rheumatoid arthritis."

Building on these data, an acceptable paradigm for immunogenetic influence in rheumatoid arthritis was generated in 1976 when Stastny[3] found that 68 per cent of patients with rheumatoid arthritis but only 12 per cent of controls shared mixed lymphocyte culture type HLA-Dw4. This established a genetic basis for the phenomenon observed by Astorga and Williams.

Before detailing recent studies on the composition of *DRB1* β-chains, it is important to put HLA-DR into context with the other components of the MHC.

Dendritic Cells—Potent Presentors of Antigen in Rheumatoid Synovium

These antigen-presenting cells (APCs) have spindly cell processes, low density in most tissues, great motility, and a potent ability to present antigen to T cells.[4] The dendritic cells become differentiated and mature by action of cytokines such as granulocyte-macrophage colony-stimulating factor (GM-CSF) and tumor necrosis factor alpha that up-regulate expression of MHC class II molecules and the co-stimulatory molecules B7-1 and B7-2 (Thomas et al., Abstract 378). Rheumatoid synovium is enriched with dendritic cells that probably arrive from the circulation through postcapillary venules. Presentation by dendritic cells enhances the immunogenicity of peptides 100-fold.

It is possible that these dendritic cells, stimulated to differentiate by synovial cytokines, can present *self*-peptides from within to autoreactive T cells that somehow escaped intact from the thymus to the periphery (see Chapter 5). If one postulates that the initial production of cytokines could be stimulated in the synovium by nonspecific events such as trauma or a viral infection, it follows that an immune response *not* dependent on an exogenous antigen could be initiated by the dendritic cells presenting self-peptides.

THE MAJOR HISTOCOMPATIBILITY COMPLEX

The MHC is a cluster of genes that encode HLA molecules on chromosome 6 in humans. The MHC has allelic diversity but little or no somatic diversity. Because the immunogenetic associations of the MHC with rheumatoid arthritis have been linked to class II molecules (DR and DQ), the emphasis here is on class II. There are many similarities, however, as well as important differences, between class I and class II MHC molecules.

The class I molecules are responsible for surveillance against intracellular viruses or other somatic alterations. The class II molecules have three main varieties: HLA-DR, HLA-DQ, and HLA-DP. These are encoded by different loci (Fig. 3–1). An-

other newly recognized MHC glycoprotein, CD1, appears capable of presenting lipid/lipoprotein molecules (e.g., bacterial membranes) to T cells.

CD8[+] (suppressor) T cells are governed by MHC class I (HLA-A, -B, and -C) molecules. CD4[+] (helper) T cells have antigen presented by MHC class II molecules. It is the HLA-D region, approximately 1,000 kb long, that has been associated with rheumatoid arthritis. In humans it codes for the class II molecules as well as genes involved in antigen processing (e.g., proteosome and peptide transporter genes). The MHC class II molecules have an antigen-binding groove (Fig. 3–2) formed by a floor of β-pleated sheet conformation and sides formed by α-helices. The ends of the floor or groove are open sufficiently so that it is possible for a relatively large polypeptide to bind to the MHC and then be clipped to a peptide of less than

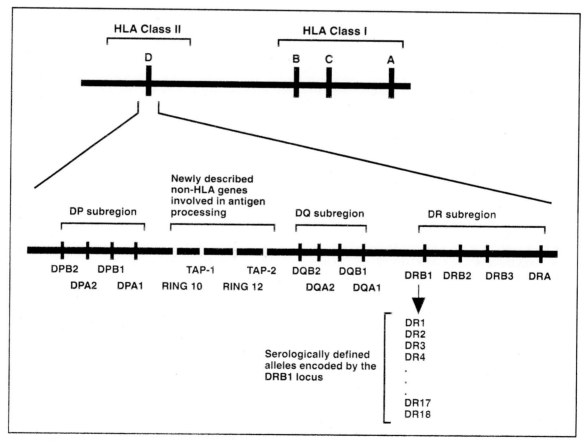

FIGURE 3–1. Partial schematic view of the HLA genes located in the MHC on chromosome 6. The "newly described" non-HLA genes (*RING 10* and *12*) may be involved in producing 9-amino-acid peptides that result from processing of antigen. Transporter genes (*TAP-1* and *TAP-2*) help deliver peptides to the HLA molecules for binding and presentation to T cells. (From Gregerson, P. K.: HLA and rheumatoid arthritis: insights into pathogenesis and implications for clinical practice. Cliniguide Rheumatol. 2[2]:3, 1992. Used by permission.)

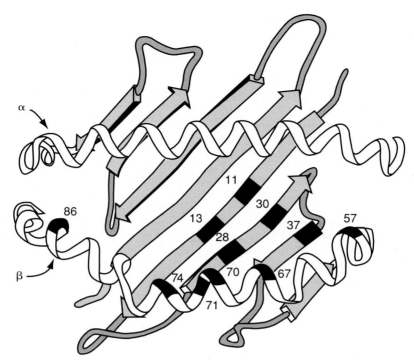

FIGURE 3–2. This structural ribbon diagram of an HLA class II molecule is viewed from the top and is based on early crystallographic evidence. Amino acids that vary widely among alleles are designated by dark regions and numbers. Those on the ''floor'' of the molecule probably bind antigen alone; those on the ''wall (see Fig. 3–3) present a combination of antigen and β chain to T cells. (From Gregerson, P. K.: HLA and rheumatoid arthritis: insights into pathogenesis and implications for clinical practice. Cliniguide Rheumatol. 2[2]:3, 1992. Used by permission.) Using hemagglutinin peptides, the crystal structure of HLA-DR4 Dw4 and HLADR1 have recently been defined and compared; the same peptide binds to both DR molecules.[26]

25 residues before the class II peptide complex is transported to the cell surface.

The class I MHC DR and DQ molecules are formed of two transmembrane-anchored proteins. These are constitutively expressed by B cells and dendritic cells (APCs) and are induced by cytokines (e.g., interferon γ and GM-CSF) on macrophages and on some mesenchymal cells.

Synthesis of class II MHC proteins and the binding of antigens to them occurs through the following steps:

1. Both α- and β-chains of class II proteins are synthesized in the endoplasmic reticulum of cells along with another protein, the *invariant chain*. A portion of the invariant chain, named CLIP, effectively protects the antigen-binding groove of the newly synthesized class II molecules so that intracellular peptides cannot bind to it.

2. The α/β invariant chain complex is transported to the Golgi apparatus, then to the *trans*-Golgi network, and finally to an endosomal/lysosomal compartment known as the ''MHC class II compartment.''

3. In the MHC class II compartment two crucial events occur:

   a. The CLIP and other portions of the invariant chain are removed, perhaps with the help of another MHC-encoded dimer protein DM, which has homologies with the α- and β-chains of DR.

   b. Removal of CLIP permits binding in the groove of antigens that were internalized at the plasma membrane and delivered to the MHC class II compartment. Portions of the peptide not bound in the groove are removed.

4. The complex of class II peptide is transported to the cell surface for presentation to CD4$^+$ T cells. It is a testable hypothesis that individual differences in DM proteins or the invariant chains can determine susceptibility to rheumatoid arthritis.

It is important to emphasize that the conformation of the clipped antigenic peptide bound in the class II molecule groove does not resemble its conformation in the native protein from which it originated, and it is the highly struc-

TABLE 3–1. Crucial Amino Acid Sequence in *DRB1* Shared Epitope

RESIDUE NUMBER	AMINO ACID	SINGLE LETTER CODE FOR AMINO ACID
67	Leucine	L
70	Glutamine	Q
71	Lysine	K
72	Arginine	R
74	Alanine	A

tured and specific conformation of the peptide *and* MHC that is recognized by the T cells.

THE SHARED EPITOPE HYPOTHESIS

Concurrent studies of human B-cell alloantigens (now recognized as the MHC class II molecules) enabled development of serologic reagents that were used to identify Dw4 specificity in patients with rheumatoid arthritis.[5] Subsequently, DNA sequencing technology linked with the polymerase chain reaction (PCR) has allowed amplification of small bits of DNA obtained from blood samples of individuals. This has enabled investigators to map susceptibility for acquisition or severity of rheumatoid arthritis to a sequence motif in the third hypervariable region of the DR β-chain gene (*DRB1*). This region has been named the "shared epitope" or "susceptibility cassette."

The crucial amino acid sequences in this region are listed in Table 3–1, and a schematic representation of where they appear on the class II MHC molecule is portrayed in Figure 3–3. Comparative sequence studies of *DRB1* alleles that are associated or not associated with rheumatoid arthritis are shown in Table 3–2. It should be mentioned that allele-specific oligotyping has identified at least 19 different allelic variants of HLA-DR4.

The data indicate that the *DRB1* sequences with neutral or positive charges are fit to bind a negatively charged peptide side chain on antigens, whereas sequences with an acidic residue (e.g., glutamic acid or aspartic acid) do not readily bind the same antigens. Thus, arthritogenic antigens are likely to be negatively charged. In other immune diseases (e.g., type I diabetes mellitus), disease-related polymorphisms also frequently involve similar charge polymorphisms on bound peptides.

As shown in Figure 3–3, residues 67 to 74 in the α-helix are believed to be positioned high in the saddle-like structure of the DR protein, pointing "up" to the T-cell receptor (TCR) that putatively descends to dock upon it. Current thought holds that it is likely that the importance of this shared epitope is related to the way in which the HLA-DR–antigen complex is presented to T cells, rather than to binding of a specific antigen in the DR molecule groove. This is supported by the fact that, in the "pocket" in which antigen peptides bind on the floor of the class II HLA molecule, there are large variations in amino acid sequences among *HLA* alleles that share the shared epitope. **The inference is that the shared epitope does not restrict the precise structure of antigens selected for presentation to T cells, but rather the conformation of the antigen–DR complex that the TCR "sees."** Other data supporting this hypothesis are that some T-cell clones recognize the same antigenic peptides, but in the context of different HLA-DR molecules.

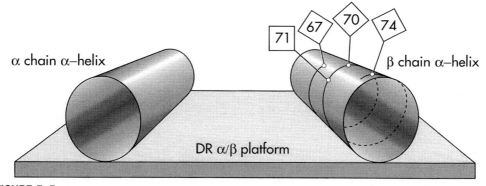

FIGURE 3–3. Schematic view of HLA-DR α- and β-chain polymorphic domains. The shared epitope region is flagged to illustrate its potential for interactions with T cells. As noted in the text, the shared epitope probably does not restrict the precise structure of antigens selected for presentation to T cells but rather restricts an antigen–DR complex conformation that the TCR "sees." (Adapted from Nepom, G. T.: Reverse immunogenetics: investigations of HLA-associated disease based on the structural and genetic identification of candidate susceptibility genes. Prog. Immunol. 7:808, 1989. Used by permission.)

TABLE 3–2. *DRB1* Allele Sequence Association with Rheumatoid Arthritis (RA)

ALLELE	THIRD DIVERSITY REGION SEQUENCES*				ASSOCIATION WITH RA
	67	70	71	74	
*DRB1*0101* (Dw1)	L	Q	R	A	Yes
*DRB1*0401* (Dw4)	L	Q	K	A	Yes
*DRB1*0402* (Dw10)	I	D	E	A	No
*DRB1*0403* (Dw13)	L	Q	R	E	No
*DRB1*0404* (Dw14)	L	Q	R	A	Yes

* L, leucine; Q, glutamine; R, arginine; A, alanine; K, lysine; I, isoleucine; D, aspartic acid; E, glutamic acid.

The impact on peptide binding of differences in amino acid sequences in the floor or peptide-binding region of the *DRB1* allele–encoded proteins has been studied intensively. The *DRB1* β-chains can be viewed as a grouping of five polymorphic "pockets" that accommodate side chains of bound peptides. One of these, identified as the p4 pocket, has the greatest effects on peptide binding specificity in *DRB1*. In particular, negatively charged residues on peptides confer this specificity, while perhaps preventing binding to *DRB1* β-chains not associated with rheumatoid arthritis.[6] **Thus, for the T cell, it is probably not relevant which peptide is presented in the susceptibility epitope; this recognition is likely to be peptide dependent but not peptide specific.** The susceptibility epitope itself may be bound in the rheumatoid pocket of DR molecules, and because there are at least several exogenous proteins that contain the same sequence of amino acids found in the susceptibility epitope (e.g., *dnaJ* heat shock protein in bacteria, surface glycoproteins of Epstein-Barr virus), cross-reactivity could activate T cells. The complementarity-determining region 2 loop on the TCRs interacts with the peptide–class II allele; it is probable that many (five, six, or more?) T-cell clones can bind various peptides in this groove.

When considering T-cell activation in rheumatoid synovium, it should be recognized that, in addition to the presence of dendritic cells that are highly effective in presenting antigen, and macrophages that generate co-stimulatory factors, it has been shown that type B rheumatoid synoviocytes that resemble fibroblasts more than macrophages are potent accessory cells for T-cell responses to bacterial superantigens.[7] It is intriguing to note that, in these experiments, cell-to-cell contact between the synoviocytes and T cells was essential for activation of the latter, and that MHC class II molecules were only weakly expressed on the synovial cells. Are the antigens presented to lymphocytes by a non-MHC mechanism? More data are necessary to effectively test this hypothesis.

Population Variance in Rheumatoid Arthritis–Associated Alleles

The emerging immunogenetic data have subsequently been linked with various subpopulations in which the prevalence of rheumatoid arthritis is similar to or different from general populations. Although the dominance of Dw4 alleles in northern European/North American Caucasians is a definite one, other *DRB1* genes assume dominance in populations in which Dw4 is not common. In many of these groups, the dominant *DRB1* gene contains the shared epitope for susceptibility/severity, a finding that validates the hypothesis that this sequence is important, although not necessarily sufficient, for development of rheumatoid arthritis in a given individual. Some interesting tribal and ethnic associations with rheumatoid arthritis and *DRB1* chain sequences have been discovered:

• Israeli Jews with *DRB1*0101* (Dw1) have a 5.4 relative risk of developing rheumatoid arthritis. A similar risk is present in British Indian subpopulations. The shared epitope is found in these *DRB1* chains.

• Yakima Indians of the Pacific Northwest have an extremely high frequency of rheumatoid arthritis, but very few in the population have *DR4* haplotypes. *DR6* is very common in these native tribes. The *DR6* (HLA-Dw16) allele *DRB1*1402* that is found in 83 per cent of the Yakima with rheumatoid arthritis contains the shared epitope sequence.[8] Because it is likely that this Dw16 gene is ancestral in Yakima Indians, the possibility exists that rheumatoid arthritis was present in ancient tribes, in contrast to its probable relatively recent appearance in northern Europeans.

- In Alaskan Tlingit tribes, *HLA-DR4* is found less frequently in rheumatoid patients because the predominant *DR4* allele in Tlingits is *DRB1*0403* (Dw13.1), which does not express the shared epitope. Ninety-one per cent of rheumatoid Tlingits have *DRB1*1402*, similar to the Yakima people.

- In Korean patients with rheumatoid arthritis, a phenotype frequency of HLA-DR4 of 60 per cent versus 31 per cent in controls has been demonstrated.[9] Forty-two of 57 *DR4*+ patients possessed *DRB1*O405*. *0405* in this population was strongly associated with rheumatoid arthritis (44 per cent of patients, 12 per cent of controls). Fifty-two of the 57 *DR4*+ patients carried one of the susceptibility epitopes (e.g., QRRAA or QKRAA).

- Other populations with *HLA-DR* genes skewed away from *DR4* have higher frequencies of the shared epitope in other *DRB1* alleles in rheumatoid patients. Examples include Polynesians,[10] Japanese,[11] Israeli Jews,[12] and Greeks.[13,14]

Data from other subgroups of populations indicate that the shared epitope hypothesis is not the whole story, and that susceptibility/severity for rheumatoid arthritis is polygenic. In a Spanish population up to one third of patients carrying a diagnosis of rheumatoid arthritis do not share the shared epitope in the third hypervariable region sequence in their *DRB1* genes. The same applies to certain groups of African-Americans as well.[15] In another cohort of African-Americans, neither rheumatoid factor, *HLA-DR4*, nor the shared epitope was associated with disease severity. Forty patients (54 per cent of the total) were shared epitope positive and 34 (46 per cent of the total) were shared epitope negative (Jonas et al., Abstract 246). These differences in the immunogenetics of rheumatoid arthritis could be explained in several ways: (1) there is another, as yet unappreciated *HLA*-associated gene responsible for rheumatoid arthritis in these populations (e.g., the DM proteins involved in construction of DR within cells); (2) these patients developed rheumatoid arthritis independently of genetic "help" from the susceptibility/severity epitope on the *DRB1* alleles; or (3) in populations in which there are relatively few individuals with *HLA* sequences containing the susceptibility epitope, there is an insufficient density of the susceptibility epitope to override or dominate environmental influences. The last of these three alternatives is the most attractive.

Black Caribbeans have a cumulative prevalence of rheumatoid arthritis of 3:1,000, whereas Caucasians in Manchester, England have a cumulative prevalence of 8:1,000.[16] These data, added to the HLA studies of African-Americans,[15] form an interesting puzzle. Is the decreased prevalence in Black Caribbeans related to the presence or absence of an as yet unknown environmental factor compared with inner-city Manchester inhabitants, or is there a sufficient decrease in expression of the "shared epitope" on *HLA-DRB1* β-chains to result in decreased numbers of the population who are susceptible to developing clinical rheumatoid arthritis? Another alternative is that there is another more powerful genotype that enhances susceptibility and severity in black populations, such as the regions of immunoglobulin chains that encode enhancer regions for immunoglobulin (and possibly rheumatoid factor) synthesis (see later).

One potential influence that adds to the complexity of immunogenetics in rheumatoid arthritis are that "protective" phenotypes of *HLA-DR* have been identified. These are reported to have a higher frequency in healthy controls than in rheumatoid patients in the same populations.[17] It is hypothesized that these haplotypes may incite a vigorous immune response that clears arthritogenic antigens from the body, that the "protective" DR peptides are presented as self-antigens (perhaps by DQ) and interfere with normal T-cell responses, or that these *DR* genes induce sufficient suppressor T cells to keep the inflammatory response in check.

In accord with this, one of the alleles of class II MHC *DR* that is not associated with rheumatoid arthritis is DR2. A human *DRB1*1502-DR2* transgene was introduced into a mouse that ordinarily is genetically susceptible to collagen-induced arthritis. These transgenic mice were resistant to arthritis and had decreased anti-collagen antibodies and proliferative responses (Gonzalez-Gay et al., Abstract 937).

Risk Ratios for Rheumatoid Arthritis Associated with *DRB1* Alleles

Despite the variations in prevalence of both rheumatoid arthritis and the shared epitope on *DRB1* genes in some subgroups described earlier, the presence of the shared epitope remains an important determinant of this disease in many populations. The upper limit of risk ratios for *HLA* genes associ-

TABLE 3–3. Risk Ratio for Rheumatoid Arthritis (RA) for Various *HLA* Genes

HLA CLASS II GENE	RISK RATIO OF DEVELOPING RA
Dw4 (*DRB1*0401*)	1:35
Dw14 (*DRB1*0404*)	1:20
Dw1 (*DRB1*0101*)	1:80
Dw4 *or* Dw14	1:35
Dw4, Dw14, *or* Dw1	1:46
Dw4 *and* Dw14	1:7
Other	1:580

From Nepom, G. T., and Nepom, B. S.: Prediction of susceptibility to rheumatoid arthritis by human leukocyte antigen genotyping. Rheum. Dis. Clin. North Am. 18:785, 1992. Used by permission.

ated with rheumatoid arthritis in Caucasian patients, assuming a prevalence of rheumatoid arthritis in this population of 1 per cent, have been calculated by Nepom and Nepom[18] (Table 3–3).

The synergism of Dw4 and Dw14 implies that portions of the *DRB1* chain other than the shared epitope may be additionally important in effective presentation of antigens to reactive T cells, or that the effect of positive selection on T-cell repertoire selection during fetal thymic development by the two *HLA* genes is also important. As one might expect, there are differences between the **sensitivity** and **specificity** of having one allele or another.

For example, homozygosity for *DRB1*04* is highly specific for rheumatoid arthritis, but it is an insensitive determinant because so few individuals in the general population are homozygous for these alleles. In contrast, sensitivity is increased if only one of all of the shared epitopes is considered in calculations, but the specificity diminishes.

DRB1 *Genes and Severity of Rheumatoid Arthritis*

In order to explore the potential effects of *HLA* genes on the severity, progression rate, or extra-articular involvement of rheumatoid arthritis, availability of both DNA sequencing by PCR expansion and precise clinical data on study patients is essential. Weyand and colleagues at the Mayo Clinic have both of these capabilities. This has enabled them to address numerous immunogenetic and clinical questions. For example, do *HLA* genotypes in severely affected patients differ from those in patients with mild disease? From data in Figure 3–4, it is apparent that homozygosity for the shared epitope is more common in patients with rheumatoid vasculitis or erosive arthritis, and is virtually never found in patients without extra-articular complications or rheumatoid nodules. Weyand and colleagues also examined whether seronegative rheumatoid arthritis differs immunogenetically from seropositive disease. This analysis required using patients who had had the disease for a minimum of 5 years with repeated negative tests for rheumatoid

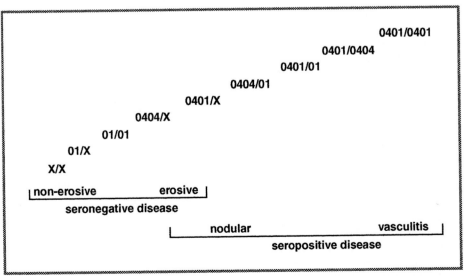

FIGURE 3–4. Proposed hierarchy of *HLA-DRB1* alleles in determining disease severity in seronegative and seropositive rheumatoid arthritis. The model implies that distinct *HLA-DRB1* alleles differ in their impact on the disease process. 0404 represents the group of alleles including *B1*0404*, **0405*, and **0408*. (Data from Weyand et al.[14,15].)

TABLE 3-4. *HLA-DR* Allele Frequency in Rheumatoid Arthritis Patients

	FREQUENCY (%)	
HLA-DR ALLELES	RHEUMATOID FACTOR NEGATIVE (60 PATIENTS)	RHEUMATOID FACTOR POSITIVE (142 PATIENTS)
B1*0101	42	23
B1*0403	23	18
B1*0401	35	91
B1*0404	2	4

Data from Weyland et al.[14]

factor and no family history for spondyloarthropathies.[19] Results of the allele typing in patients are shown in Table 3-4.

Taken together (considering all available data), 68 per cent of all seronegative patients carried the shared epitope, as did 97 per cent of seropositive patients. When focus was put on the 71st residue of the third hypervariable region of *DRB1*, 65 per cent of seropositive patients had *lysine* in position

71 and 57 per cent had *arginine*. Lysine at position 71 was rarely seen in seronegative patients. It is becoming clear that amino acid position 71 in the *HLA-DRB1* gene has a unique and important role, although the significance of this for understanding TCR recognition or antigen binding is not known.

In this group of patients, clinical heterogeneity correlated with genetic heterogeneity. Those who developed erosions early in the course of their disease frequently typed *HLA-DRB1*04*, whereas those with a benign course and few if any erosions typed *HLA-DRB1*01*, or lacked a rheumatoid arthritis–linked haplotype (Fig. 3–5).

Another way of interpreting these data is that the *DRB1* allele markers are inherited in a recessive mode, not an additive or dominant mode. This view is supported by a recent study of the genotypic distribution of shared epitope *DRB1* alleles in 309 rheumatoid patients and 283 control subjects[21]; a definite tendency was found for these *DRB1* alleles to be represented in rheumatoid arthritis genotypes in pairs, not singly. If we can assume that each *DRB1* susceptibility allele predisposes to different clinical manifestations, inheritance of two such alleles would increase the likelihood that rheumatoid

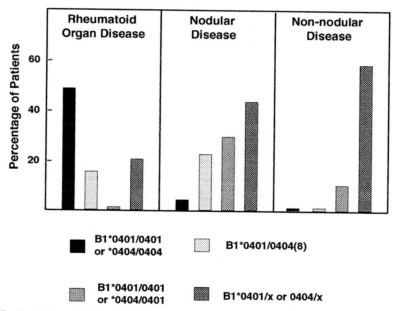

FIGURE 3–5. Correlation of allelic combinations at the *HLA-DRB1* locus with disease severity in rheumatoid arthritis. A total of 102 patients with rheumatoid arthritis were grouped into subset according to their extra-articular disease manifestations. Thirty-seven patients had erosive disease without extra-articular manifestations; most of these patients combined an *HLA-DRB1*04* variant with a disease-nonassociated *HLA-DRB1* allele. Patients with nodular disease but no major organ involvement (*n* = 43) were frequently homozygous for the disease-associated sequence polymorphism, by combining either two *HLA-DRB1*0* variants or one *HLA-DRB1*04* variant with *HLA-DRB1*0101*. Patients with major organ involvement were predominantly homozygous for an *HLA-DRB1*04* allele. (From Weyand, C. M., and Goronzy, J. J.: Functional domains on HLA-DR molecules: implications for the linkage of HLA-DR genes to different autoimmune diseases. Clin. Immunol. Immunopathol. 70:94, 1994. Used by permission.)

arthritis would be expressed; the clinical presentations among those with different genotypes would differ.

HLA-DR Alleles and Their Numbers

HLA-DR molecules have amino acid sequences that differ primarily in the β-chain that is encoded for by the *HLA-DRB1* gene. The variants have limited sequence polymorphism in the third hypervariable region of the *DRB1* gene. Because a new nomenclature has replaced the old for *HLA-DR* alleles, both are listed in Table 3–5.[20]

TABLE 3–5. Nomenclature for *HLA-DR* Alleles

OLD NOMENCLATURE (HLA ALLELES)	NEW NOMENCLATURE (*HLA-DRB1* ALLELES)
DR1	*0101
DR4, Dw4	*0401
DR4, Dw14	*0404 *0408
DR4, Dw15	*0405
DRw14, Dw16	*1402
DR4, Dw10	*0402
DR2	*1501, *1502, *1601, *1602
DR3	*0301, *0302
DR5	*1101, *1104, *1201, *1202
DR7	*0701, *0702
DRw8	*0801, *0803
DR9	*0901
DRw10	*1001
DRw13	*1301, *1304
DRw14, Dw9	*1401

From Weyand, C. M., Hicok, K. C., Conn, D. L., et al.: The influence of HLA-DRB1 genes on disease severity in rheumatoid arthritis. Ann. Intern. Med. 117:801, 1992. Used by permission.

A Role for HLA-DQ in Rheumatoid Arthritis?

There is linkage disequilibrium between certain *DQ* alleles and the *DR* alleles associated with rheumatoid arthritis. Experiments have been done that express human class II MHC *DQ* and *DR* genes in mice using transgenic technology, with subsequent scrutiny of susceptibility to collagen-induced arthritis in these mice. Certain *DQ8* alleles fostered arthritis, whereas implantation of *DQ6* alleles produced mice resistant to collagen-induced arthritis. Most intriguing is that the DQ8 molecules presented *DRB1* hypervariable segment peptides *only*

from haplotypes associated with resistance to rheumatoid arthritis. (Nabozny, et al., Abstract 206).

The data were interpreted to imply that *DQ* polymorphism determined susceptibility to arthritis by presenting MHC peptides associated with resistance to rheumatoid arthritis to T cells in such a way (high-affinity binding) that negative selection (T-cell deletion) would occur. In contrast, MHC peptides from *DRB* chains containing the shared epitope would be presented by *DQ* and have weak TCR binding, leading to positive selection. This would enable an immune response to "mimicking" peptides (e.g., those from heat shock proteins, Epstein-Barr virus, or type II collagen; see Chapter 4) to initiate an inflammatory synovitis.

Genetic Susceptibility to Rheumatoid Arthritis is Linked a TCR α (A) Locus

Painstaking mapping of polymorphism in the variable region of the α-chain of the TCR has identified one gene family (*TCRAV5*) that was associated with *DR4+* patients with rheumatoid arthritis but not with normal controls. (So et al., Abstract 204). It is possible that certain TCR genes produce proteins that enhance acceptance of peptides presented by APCs in association with the shared epitope on *DRB* chains. The data suggest that the susceptibility epitope in *DRB1* molecules is a self-peptide that shapes the T-cell repertoire and influences the predisposition to rheumatoid arthritis only in those carrying the predisposing *DQ* alleles.[22]

Summary

The shared epitope that appears as a cassette in many *DRB1* β-chains is important more for severity than susceptibility of rheumatoid arthritis, and probably exerts its influence through presentation of multiple different antigen peptides (including self-peptides, even HLA antigen peptides) to several TCRs.

Heritable Factors in Immunoglobulin Structure and Rheumatoid Arthritis

Although sharp focus has been placed on the immunogenetics of *HLA* class II haplotypes in determining inheritance patterns for rheumatoid arthritis, the clinical appearance of rheumatoid arthritis is consistent with involvement of several genes. One of these may be a sequence of amino acids near the constant segment of immunoglobulin Cκ.[25]

Immunogenetics of Giant Cell Arteritis: A Contrast with Rheumatoid Arthritis

There is a fascinating contrast in the HLA-DR association of giant cell arteritis (GCA) and rheumatoid arthritis.[23,24] The GCA patients share a sequence motif in *DRB1* that spans amino acids 28 to 31, mapping near the antigen-binding sites that are on the floor of the DR molecular complex rather than in the antigen-presenting site/TCR-binding area where the shared epitope for rheumatoid arthritis is found. This implies that there is more likely to be a specific antigen bound in GCA than in rheumatoid arthritis.

Equally interesting in this light are data by Weyand et al.[19] showing that, of 835 patients with biopsy-proven GCA, only 3 had rheumatoid arthritis, and 22 were *expected* to develop it. Both GCA and rheumatoid arthritis patients have more *DRB1*0401* than do controls, yet both diseases occur in the same individual less often than expected. This emphasizes the different functions for different portions of the HLA-DR molecules and possible competition between them.

This sequence, about 30/kb long, could be the kappa enhancer that would interact with *trans*-activating factors that increase the initiation of transcription. Homozygosity for the $\beta3$ or $C\kappa$ genotype for this segment confers a relative risk for rheumatoid arthritis of 2.2, and in the *DR4−* subgroup of rheumatoid patients the relative risk is 3.9.

The studies on the differences in galactosylation of rheumatoid factors in normal subjects and rheumatoid arthritis patients are discussed in Chapter 6.

REFERENCES

1. Gough, A. K., Lilley, J., Eyre, S., et al.: Generalized bone loss in patients with early rheumatoid arthritis occurs early and relates to disease activity. Lancet 334:23, 1994.
2. Astorga, G. P., and Williams, J. R. C.: Altered reactivity in mixed lymphocyte culture of lymphocytes from patients with rheumatoid arthritis. Arthritis Rheum. 12:547, 1969.
3. Stastny, P.: Mixed lymphocyte culture in rheumatoid arthritis. J. Clin. Invest. 57:1148, 1976.
4. Steinman, R. M.: The dendritic cell system and its role in immunogenicity. Annu. Rev. Immunol. 9:271, 1991.
5. Winchester, R. J.: B-lymphocyte allo-antigens, cellular expression, and disease significance with special reference to rheumatoid arthritis. Arthritis Rheum. 20:159, 1977.
6. Woulfe, S. L., Bono, C. P., Zacheis, M. L., et al.: Negatively charged residues interacting with the p4 pocket confer binding specificity to DRB1*0401. Arthritis Rheum. 38:1744, 1995.
7. Tsai, C., Diaz, L. A. Jr., Singer, N. G., et al.: Responsiveness of human T lymphocytes to bacterial superantigens presented by cultured rheumatoid arthritis synoviocytes. Arthritis Rheum. 39:125, 1996.
8. Willkens, R. F., Nepom, G. T., Marks, C. R., et al.: Association of HLA-Dw1 with rheumatoid arthritis in Yakima Indians: further evidence for the "shared epitope" hypothesis. Arthritis Rheum. 34:43, 1991.
9. Kim, H.-Y., Kim, T.-G., Park, S.-H., et al.: Predominance of HLA-DRB1*0405 in Korean patients with rheumatoid arthritis. Ann. Rheum. Dis. 54:988, 1995.
10. Tan, P. L. J., Farmiloe, S., Roberts, M., et al.: HLA-DR4 subtypes in New Zealand Polynesians. Arthritis Rheum. 36:15, 1993.

Although Dw4 and Dw15 were similar among Polynesian controls (7.6 and 4.6 per cent, respectively), only Dw15 was significantly associated with rheumatoid arthritis implying that the Polynesian T-cell repertoire contributing to rheumatoid arthritis may differ from that in Caucasians.

11. Tsuchiya, K., Nishimura, Y., and Sasazuki, T.: Contribution of genetic factors to RA. Nippon Rinsho 50:438, 1992.
12. de Vries, N., Ronningen, K. S., Tilanus, M. G., et al.: HLA-DR1 and rheumatoid arthritis in Israeli Jews: sequencing reveals that DRB1*0102 is the predominant HLA-DR1 subtype. Tissue Antigens 41:26, 1993.
13. Boki, K. A., Drosos, A. A., Tzioufas, A. G., et al.: Examination of HLA-DR4 as a severity marker for rheumatoid arthritis in Greek patients. Ann. Rheum. Dis. 52:517, 1993.
14. Boki, K. A., Panayi, G. S., Vaughan, R. W., et al.: HLA class II sequence polymorphisms and susceptibility to rheumatoid arthritis in Greeks. Arthritis Rheum. 35:749, 1992.
15. McDaniel, D. O., Alarcon, G. S., Pratt, P. W., et al.: Most African-American patients with rheumatoid arthritis do not have the rheumatoid antigenic determinant. Ann. Intern. Med. 123:181, 1995.

This is a cross-sectional study of 86 African-American patients with rheumatoid arthritis and 88 healthy African-Americans. The seropositive patients had an increased frequency of *HLA-DRB1*O4* alleles (27.3 per cent) compared with only 13.1 per cent of controls, but other *HLA-DRB1* alleles were similar in both groups. Most of both the seropositive and seronegative patients were *HLA-DR4* negative.

16. MacGregor, A. J., Riste, L. K., Hazes, J. M., et al.: Low prevalence of rheumatoid arthritis in Black-Carribeans compared with Whites in inner city Manchester. Ann. Rheum. Dis. 53:293, 1994.
17. Larsen, B. A., Alderdice, C. A., Hawkins, D., et al.: Protective HLA-DR phenotypes in rheumatoid arthritis. J Rheumatol. 16:455, 1989.

A total of 115 patients from Newfoundland and 134 from Saskatchewan were studied along with healthy controls. Four "protective" phenotypes (HLA-DR1, DR5; DR2; DR2, DR3; and DR3, DR7) were found.

18. Nepom, G. T., and Nepom, B. S.: Prediction of susceptibility to rheumatoid arthritis by human leukocyte antigen genotyping. Rheum. Dis. Clin. North Am. 18:785, 1992.
19. Weyand, C. M., McCarthy, T. G., and Goronzy, J. J.: Correlation between disease phenotype and genetic heterogeneity in rheumatoid arthritis. J. Clin. Invest. 95:2120, 1995.

The "shared epitope" can be integrated into at least eight different *HLA-DRB1* genes: *B1*0101, *0102,*

*0401, *0404, *0405, *0408, *1402, and *1001. It spans the amino acids 70 to 74 position in the third hypervariable region. In this study, 142 Caucasian patients who were rheumatoid factor positive (RF+), 60 RF-negative (RF−) patients, and 81 normal individuals were studied. *HLA-DRB1* genotyping was determined by PCR and oligonucleotide hybridization. Analysis of the amino acids 71 to 74 motif showed that 65 per cent of RF+ patients had a lysine residue in position 71. In contrast, RF− usually type positive for an arginine residue at position 71. Analysis of patients with early erosive disease showed that all patients expressed disease-linked *HLA-DRB1* alleles; two thirds typed positive for *04 and 41 per cent for *01. The *04 allele was present in only 11 per cent in the subset with nonerosive, less aggressive disease. It is possible that position 71 in *HLA-DRB1* plays a major role in the induction of autoantibody production.

20. Weyand, C. M., Hicok, K. C., Conn, D. L., et al.: The influence of HLA-DRB1 genes on disease severity in rheumatoid arthritis. Ann. Intern. Med. 117:801, 1992.

A total of 132 patients with seropositive erosive rheumatoid arthritis were genotyped for *HLA-DRB1* alleles. Only 4 of 102 were negative for all disease-associated *HLA-DRB1* alleles. Erosive rheumatoid arthritis was linked to the presence of *HLA-DRB1*0401* and *0404. Eleven patients were negative for *HLA-DRB1*0401* and *0404*; none had rheumatoid nodules or other extra-articular manifestations. Thus, the second *HLA-DRB1* allele in *HLA-DR4*−positive patients correlates with disease severity.

21. Evans, T. I., Han, J., Singh, R., and Moxley, G.: The genotypic distribution of shared-epitope DRB1 alleles suggests a recessive mode of inheritance of the rheumatoid arthritis disease-susceptibility gene. Arthritis Rheum. 38: 1754, 1995.

22. Zanelli, E., Krco, C. J., Baisch, J. M., et al.: Immune response of HLA-DQ8 transgenic mice to HLA-DRB1 HV3 peptides correlates with predisposition to rheumatoid arthritis. Proc. Natl. Acad. Sci. U.S.A., 93:1814, 1995.

23. Weyand, C. M., Hicok, K. C., Hunder, G. G., et al.: The HLA-DRB1 locus as a genetic component in giant cell arteritis: mapping of a disease-linked sequence motif to the antigen binding site of the HLA-DR molecule. J. Clin. Invest. 90:2355, 1992.

Forty per cent of patients were negative for *B1*0401* and *0404/8*. This indicates that the contribution of *HLA-DR* in GCA is probably not related to a unique function of the *DRB1*04* allele. GCA patients shared a sequence motif spanning amino acid 28 to 31 of *HLA-DRB1*, mapped near the antigen-binding site of *HLA*, rather than the rheumatoid arthritis area in the α-helical loop surrounding the antigen-binding groove.

24. Weyand, C. M., and Goronzy, J. J.: Functional domains on HLA-DR molecules: implications for the linkage of HLA-DR genes to different autoimmune diseases. Clin. Immunol. Immunopathol. 70:91, 1994.

Based on the *HLA-DRB1*04* association with both rheumatoid arthritis and GCA, the authors review data to support their hypothesis that HLA-DR molecules in rheumatoid arthritis patients are involved in determination of the potentially pathogenic repertoire of TCR specificities (Fig. 3–5).

25. Moxley, G.: Variable-constant segment genotype of immunoglobulin kappa is associated with increased risk for rheumatoid arthritis. Arthritis Rheum. 35:19, 1992.

26. Woulfe, W. C., Stallings, A. M., Stevens, R., et al.: Crystal Structure of Rheumatoid Arthritis Associated HLA-DR4 Dw4 Molecule. St. Louis, G. D. Searle & Co.

SECTION III

ACTIVATION OF THE IMMUNE SYSTEM IN RHEUMATOID ARTHRITIS

The data are mounting to support the hypothesis that rheumatoid synovitis is an antigen-driven disease. Lymphocytes found in synovium resemble very little the naive ones found in the circulation. The synovial T cells are terminally differentiated memory cells that are irreversibly committed to the activated state. The unanswered question is: Which antigen is driving these cells to proliferate? The answer can be found only by analysis of the T-cell receptor of very early disease before polyclonal expansion to multiple antigens and superantigens begins. Finding such patients and having access to their synovium or synovial fluid is very difficult.

B lymphocytes come into play later in the process. Helped by T cells and by cytokines, as well as by specific antigen binding, B cells in rheumatoid arthritis have a high frequency of rheumatoid factor production. Production of higher affinity, monoreactive rheumatoid factor by these cells often is a result of somatic mutations in the germline genes. The result is an apparent antigen-driven immune response with activation of both cellular and humoral immune pathways.

4

Is There One Cause of Rheumatoid Arthritis?

Could there be a single cause of rheumatoid arthritis, a discreet and defined antigen that has been overlooked despite use of increasingly sophisticated probes by multiple talented investigators? Is there a single infectious agent that is the primary cause of rheumatoid arthritis in the same way that group A streptococci cause pharyngitis and, by autoimmune mechanisms, rheumatic fever? The answer to these questions is probably "no." Odds are building to support the theory that rheumatoid arthritis is generated by a tight intermeshing of pathogenic pathways in a genetically susceptible host in whom a cascade of immunologic pathways are triggered by an initial immune response to an antigen, but probably not the same antigen in all patients.

Why, then, do some individuals develop rheumatoid arthritis late, others early in life, and others not at all, even when all have a very similar immunogenetic system? How much does it take to start these cascades, and when, if ever, does the process develop a cyclic automaticity and become self-sustaining?

The discussion that follows is not an exhaustive review of the studies that have attempted to identify one or another cause of rheumatoid arthritis, but rather an attempt to focus on evidence that provides useful approaches to defining mechanisms that may underlie the development of inflammatory and proliferative synovitis. A basic assumption is that, in every patient who develops rheumatoid arthritis, an immune system necessary for initiating and sustaining the process is present and dictated by immunogenetics, as discussed in Chapter 3.

The leading candidates for a triggering stimulus in this disease are infection, cross-reactive immunity, and autoimmunity. They clearly would be integrated with immunogenetic factors, both established and as yet unknown (Fig. 4–1).

INFECTIOUS AGENTS OR THEIR COMPONENTS

In consideration of these possibilities, it is useful to accept the fact that no infectious agent has been cultured from synovial tissue, synovial fluid, or blood with reproducibility sufficient to be relevant to causation, although many enthusiastic studies have been reported[1] (Table 4–1). Sera from patients with active rheumatoid arthritis have been reported to have higher than normal titers against *Proteus mirabilis*,[2,3] and enterobacteria have been linked to inflammatory joint disease in the same way that they have to reactive arthritis.[4] The data on *Proteus* antibodies are particularly intriguing because of the apparent specificity of these antibodies; antibody titers correlated with C-reactive protein, the acute-phase reactant, in the patients studied.[3]

Using tests for reactivity of lymphocytes from rheumatoid patients to antigens from infectious agents, sporadic associations have been noted in about 15 per cent of cases studied in one laboratory,[5] and are summarized as follows:

1. Rubella antigen elicited responses in five cases, and in three cases rubella virus was isolated.[6]

2. In one of six patients whose lymphocytes reacted to adenovirus, adenoviral nucleotide sequences were found in the synovium.[7]

3. In eight cases, synovial lymphocytes responded to cytomegalovirus antigen on two or more occasions.[8]

It is indeed possible that these agents were responsible for chronic synovitis in these small subsets of patients. Equally likely, however is that the patients had rheumatoid arthritis but that it was caused by an unrelated immune response, with an accessory immune response to one or another of these infectious agents. If any of these agents is involved in causation, it is likely to be through an epitope that stimulates an immune response triggering recognition by molecular mimicry of autologous proteins.

The data on *P. mirabilis* are an example of how thinking about infectious agents has moved from considering them as direct causative agents to regarding them as immunogens that cross-react with relevant host antigens. One study has shown a mo-

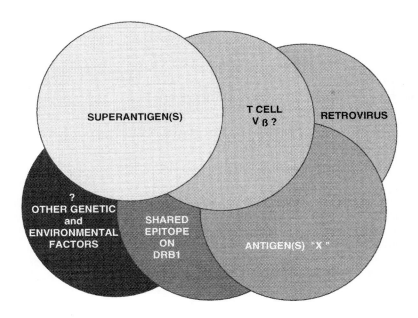

FIGURE 4–1. These overlapping circles are meant to imply multiple possible interactions among host and environmental factors that may summate into sustained polyarthritis. It should be noted that the circles labeled Superantigen(s) and Antigen(s) "X" include both exogenous and host factors, including bacterial heat shock proteins (e.g., dnaJ) collagen type II, immunoglobulin G, Epstein-Barr viral proteins.

lecular similarity between two sequences of *P. mirabilis*, HLA-DR4 antigens and collagen type I α1 chains.[9] Rheumatoid patients had significantly higher immunoglobulin (Ig) G antibody titers against *Proteus* urease than did control patients or

TABLE 4–1. Evidence That Rheumatoid Arthritis (RA) Is Caused by Infection*

- Treatment with sulfasalazine (Azulfidine) causes improvement or remission in 30% of pts
- Increased ab. to and increased culture of *Clostridial* species from stool in RA (70% vs. 45%)
- Elevated antibodies to a commonly shared bacterial cell wall peptidoglycan occur in RA
- Increased ab. to *Proteus mirabilis* in RA
- *Proteus* surface antigens cross-react with DR4
- RA synovial fluid lymphocytes proliferate after stimulation with bacterial HSP-65K
- RA sera contain elevated antibody titers to bacterial HSP-65K
- Post-rubella arthritis can become chronic and resemble RA, and live *Rubella* virus has been occasionally isolated from RA synovia
- Epstein-Barr virus antigens (EBV-gp110, EBNA-5) cross-react with DR-w4, DR-w14, DR-1, and type II collagen molecules
- Bacterial peptidoglycan, lipopolysaccharide, and staphylococcal Protein A experimentally induce anti-IgG (rheum. factor) in vivo and in vitro

From Smiley, J. D., and Hoffman, W. L.: Southwestern Internal Medicine Conference: The role of infections in the rheumatic diseases: molecular mimicry between bacterial and human stress proteins? Am. J. Med. Sci. 301:138, 1991. Used by permission.

* pts, patients; ab., antibodies; rheum., rheumatoid.

those with ankylosing spondylitis. To firm up these data, absorption studies will be essential to blot out the specific urease and be sure that the cross-reactivity is eliminated as well. These findings are consistent with a variation of the hypothesis of cross-reaction of bacterial immunogens with components of the immune response or connective tissue. It is of interest that, in patients treated with a vegetarian diet who improved in response to this intervention, there was a concomitant decrease in anti-*Proteus* antibodies, but not in antibody titers against *Escherichia coli*.[10] Although intriguing, these data may be best explained by the possibility that some component of the rheumatoid process boosts titers of antibodies against certain *Proteus* proteins.

Human parvovirus B19 has been implicated as a causative agent in rheumatoid arthritis. In a recent study to determine whether B19 persists in patients with rheumatoid arthritis, synovial fluid or peripheral blood cells from 61 patients with early rheumatoid arthritis and fluid or tissue from 28 patients with advanced rheumatoid arthritis were studied for B19 genome fragments using PCR.[11] B19-specific gene sequences were found in samples from two patients who fulfilled the criteria for rheumatoid arthritis. It remains possible that in certain immunogenetically susceptible individuals, parvovirus B19 triggers an autoimmune response.

Although, as mentioned, no infectious agent has been routinely cultured from rheumatoid tissue, there is much interest in some components of them as triggering agents, particularly **heat shock proteins** (HSPs).

Heat Shock (Stress) Proteins and Rheumatoid Arthritis

Expression of the proteins that are coded by heat shock genes—perhaps better named "stress proteins"—is induced in all cells by different environmental assaults, such as oxidative injury, infection with pathogens, and increases in temperature. The human homologue (HSP 60) has a 40 to 50 per cent sequence homology with a mycobacterial 65-kDa HSP, and examples of such conservation across species are very common. Because of the high degree of homology and the strong antigenicity of HSPs, antibodies formed against HSPs of one species often react with HSPs from other species.[12,13] In humans, four families of HSPs have been identified that are separated one from the other by molecular weights: 90 to 100, 70, 65, and 20 kDa. Ubiquitin, a 76-amino-acid protein (7 to 8 kDa), is also an HSP.

The function of HSPs appears to be in stabilizing the structure or function of other proteins. For example, the HSP 70 family of stress proteins are ATP-dependent "molecular chaperones" that correct abnormalities in newly formed glycoprotein conformation and help assemble protein subunits into complete and functional molecules. HSP 90, found in cytoplasm, is part of steroid hormone receptors, including estrogen receptors.[14] Ubiquitin, among other duties, marks cytosolic proteins for degradation when they cannot be repaired.

A role for HSPs in rheumatic diseases is supported by several pieces of evidence. In another disease, ankylosing spondylitis, about half of patients studied have antibodies against a 63-kDa HSP, but no antibodies are found in any controls or patients with other rheumatic diseases.[15,16]

A fascinating link between HSPs and rheumatoid arthritis was revealed by the finding that the arthritogenic component of *Mycobacterium tuberculosis* used with Freund's adjuvant to produce arthritis in rats was a 65-kDa HSP.[17] Building on these data, a series of experiments led investigators toward a possible major role for HSPs in rheumatoid arthritis. In one study, a T-cell clone autoreactive for a determinant on the *M. tuberculosis* HSP 65 produced arthritis when it was transferred into heavily irradiated syngeneic rats. Prior immunization with pure HSP 65 antigen protected against arthritis. Rats sensitized to *M. tuberculosis* and then challenged intra-articularly with recombinant HSP 65 developed arthritis, whereas those challenged in the same way with a 10-kDa HSP from *M. tuberculosis* did not.[18]

In another study, T-cell clones reactive against *M. tuberculosis* HSP 65 were activated by an antigen from the proteoglycan core protein in articular cartilage.[19] The arthritogenic segment of HSP 65 was found to be a nine-amino-acid sequence that had structural mimicry to a cartilage-derived proteoglycan epitope.

Finally, in studies of rheumatoid patients, lymphocytes from peripheral blood and synovial fluid of patients with rheumatoid arthritis were activated by both the *mtb* HSP 65 and cartilage proteoglycans.[20,21] Monoclonal antibodies to the 65-kDa mycobacterial antigen labeled synovial tissue sections from rats with adjuvant arthritis and from patients with either rheumatoid arthritis or osteoarthritis, but not normal tissues.[22] The lack of specificity of the antibody reaction was confirmed by studies of synovial fluid lymphocytes, stimulation of which was found in excess of peripheral blood mononuclear cells from both rheumatoid patients and patients with reactive arthritis.[23] In immunohistochemical studies, strong reactivity of anti–HSP 65 was found in sections of the cartilage-pannus junction in rheumatoid arthritis and in rheumatoid nodules.[24] In other studies of cross-reactivity, populations of mycobacteria-specific T-cell clones from synovial tissue and fluid were able to lyse macrophages pulsed with bacillus Calmette-Guérin. This cytotoxicity was, for the most part, restricted by HLA-DR4. Several clones were TCR γ/δ^+. B lymphocytes isolated from rheumatoid synovial tissue and transformed by Epstein-Barr virus (EBV) produce antibody against HSP 73, a member of the HSP 70 human stress protein family.[25]

Although none of these observations serves to definitively link the cause of rheumatoid inflammation to an infection with mycobacteria or HSPs from another microbial source, they strengthen possibilities that HSPs (stress proteins) accumulating at sites of local inflammation within a joint could trigger autoreactive T cells that subsequently could amplify the synovial immune response as well as being potentially cytotoxic. The fact that reactive lymphocytes are "memory" cells and that synovial and synovial fluid T cells are more reactive than peripheral blood cells may indicate an intrasynovial T-cell activation of lymphocytes by bacterial or viral HSPs that then can cross-react with host tissues (e.g., epitopes on proteoglycans or type II collagen).

The mycobacterial antigen most frequently employed in studies of cellular reactivity to *M. tuberculosis* is an acetone-precipitable fraction (named AP-MT) that contains the particularly reactive HSP 65. It is of interest that AP-MT can rapidly induce expression of proliferating cell nuclear antigen in human cells, a protein that has a role in DNA repair and against which antibodies are formed in some patients with systemic lupus erythematosus.

An intriguing hypothesis links the stimulatory effects of estrogens on stress protein expression and the predilection of women to develop rheumatoid arthritis,[26] particularly since a protein (p29) believed to be closely associated with the estrogen receptor has been found in inflammatory synovitis[27] and estrogen-binding sites were identified on macrophage-like synoviocytes and on memory T lymphocytes in rheumatoid synovium.[28]

Among foreign antigens that have similar amino acid sequences to the third hypervariable region of *HLA-DR4,* which contains the "susceptibility epitope" (discussed in Chapter 3), are **EBV gp110** and the *E. coli* HSP **dnaJ**[29]:

PEPTIDES	RESIDUES
HLA-DRB1*0401	K D L L E **Q K R A A** V D T Y C
EBV gp110	E Q N Q E **Q K R A A** Q R A A G
E. coli dnaJ	V L T D S **Q K R A A** Y D Q T G

The dnaJ HSP has the following qualities:

• It forms a particulate complex with other DNA samples.
• It is conserved in evolution; there are several human homologues.
• It is strongly antigenic.
• It is involved in polypeptide binding.

A highly specific antibody to dnaJ was produced and used for immunofluorescent studies of human B lymphoblasts. The antibody stained cells expressing *DRB1*0401* (Dw4), but not cells expressing other *DRB1* alleles. The next step was to look at T-lymphocyte proliferation in the presence of dnaJ. Lymphocytes from peripheral blood of untreated patients with rheumatoid arthritis during the first 6 months of their disease had a fivefold greater activation response ([³H] thymidine uptake) than did cells from control patients. Interestingly, this proliferative response was not seen in patients with longstanding disease who had been treated with various regimens.[30]

The epitope recognized by the T cells was on the 15-amino-acid amino-terminal fragment of the expressed dnaJ, and it contained QKRAA (i.e., the shared epitope). No difference in humoral immunity (defined by IgG response) to the complete dnaJ antigen was found between rheumatoid patients and controls, but, again, the rheumatoid patients did have IgG responses directed against the dnaJ fragment containing the shared epitope.

In interpretation of these data, Dennis Carson has proposed the following sequence for the development of rheumatoid arthritis (Fig. 4–2):

• Through positive selection, individuals with the HLA susceptibility epitope (QKRAA) develop a T-cell repertoire skewed toward dnaJ.
• B-cell somatic mutations could then facilitate antigen capture and presentation, leading to an actual, rather than potential, immune response against the ubiquitous dnaJ.
• Because of repeated antigenic exposure to dnaJ, antigen-antibody complexes would become available for monocyte precursors of synovial macrophages, initiating a delayed hypersensitivity reaction. Non-rheumatoid patients without the shared epitope would not be so sensitive (immunologically) to dnaJ, and non-rheumatoid patients *with* the shared epitope in *DRB1* chains may have an immune response restricted only to the gut, where the body first contacts *E. coli* antigens.
• Secondary events would amplify the initial responses in these immunogenetically susceptible persons:
    — IgG rheumatoid factor would be generated.
    — Cartilage destruction and an amplified synovitis would result in release of previously sequestered antigens (e.g., autologous HSPs, collagen type II, IP[39], and proteoglycans).
    — The cyclic automaticity of the synovitis would lead to selection of aggressive synovial fibroblast proliferation, excessive cytokine release, and irreversible joint destruction.

It could follow[30] that, in patients with early rheumatoid arthritis, a combination of immunotherapy and antibiotics to clear the gut of organisms with dnaJ HSPs so that the sustained immune activation could be interrupted might ameliorate the disease. A point of emphasis must be that the sequence outlined above could be applicable to any molecule, peptide, or glycoprotein that could generate an immune response in an immunogenetically susceptible host.

Viruses and Rheumatoid Arthritis

The **Epstein-Barr virus** has been associated for many years with rheumatoid arthritis. In 1975, Alspaugh and Tan described an antibody in the sera of rheumatoid patients that reacted with an antigen (EBV nuclear antigen[31]) extracted from a lymphoblastic cell line carrying EBV.[32] Although these antibodies are found after the disease has begun, rather

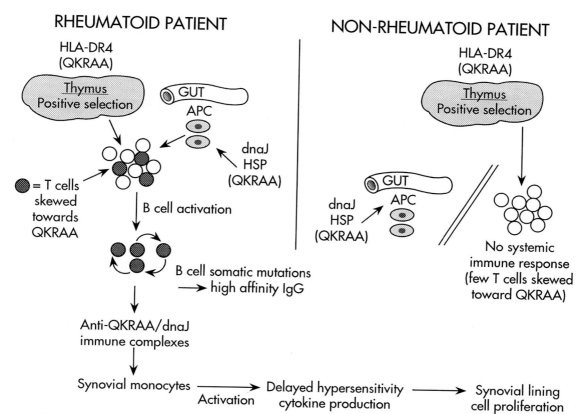

FIGURE 4–2. Some individuals with genetic expression of the shared epitope on *HLA-DR β*-chains develop rheumatoid arthritis, whereas others do not. The hypothesis sketched here has been developed by Dennis Carson and exploits the potential for involvement of common bacterial HSPs such as *E. coli* dnaJ that would be picked up and processed by QKRAA-containing antigen-presenting cells (APC) in the gut. Patients with the shared epitope destined to develop rheumatoid arthritis would, through positive selection in the thymus, produce a T-cell response skewed toward QKRAA. Then, by cross-reactivity with QKRAA sequences in the *E. coli* dnaJ HSP, an immune response would be generated. In those individuals with B cells that have somatic mutations sufficient to generate high-affinity antibodies to QKRAA, the anti-QKRAA–dnaJ complexes would be sufficient to activate synovial monocytes and synovial lining cell proliferation. In individuals without sufficient T cells skewed toward QKRAA, or without B cells capable of producing high-affinity anti-QKRAA antibodies, the immune response would be insufficient to produce synovitis.

than preceding it,[33] there are more than a few reasons to continue to explore this association:

- The EBV receptor on B lymphocytes is the complement receptor type 2.[34] This provides ready entry of the virus to these immunocytes.
- EBV is a polyclonal activator of B lymphocytes, enhancing production of many immunoglobulins, including rheumatoid factor.[35]
- Rheumatoid patients have increased numbers of EBV-infected B cells in the peripheral blood compared with non-rheumatoid controls.
- There is a defective suppression by EBV-specific T lymphocytes of infected B cells.[36]
- Purified antibodies from rheumatoid arthritis patients that are directed against EBV internal repeat sequences containing only Gly-Ala react also

with a human intracellular protein, cytokeratin,[37] to homologous epitopes on denatured collagen type II, and to actin.[38]

However, EBV DNA is present in the cells of rheumatoid patients in no greater frequency than in patients with other arthropathies.[39] This suggests that the major way by which EBV could contribute to rheumatoid arthritis would be by amplification mechanisms. In a sequence of data similar to that reported earlier with dnaJ HSPs, the possibility of molecular mimicry between EBV viral glycoprotein gp110 and the *HLA-DRB1* chains has been raised. Patients with previous EBV infections have serum antibodies that recognize peptides from both EBV surface glycoprotein (gp110) and HLA-Dw4.[40] It is reasonable to hypothesize that reactivation of EBV immunity in a patient with potentially

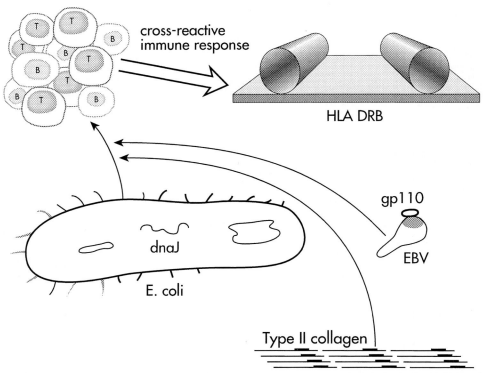

FIGURE 4–3. The concept of cross-reactivity among exogenous proteins (e.g., sequences on the gp110 surface glycoprotein of EBV, the dnaJ HSP of *E. coli*), segments of endogenous proteins (e.g., collagen), and the shared epitope on *HLA-DRB1* β-chains may produce sufficient augmentation of the immune response to any one of these to produce a self-sustaining synovitis.

reversible synovitis initiated by another antigen could—with polyclonal B-cell activation and production of antibodies that cross-react with *HLA* alleles, collagen, or other host proteins—alter the inflammatory response sufficiently to make it self-sustaining (Fig. 4–3).

Retroviruses must also remain in the running as active candidates for a causative or amplifying role in rheumatoid arthritis. Retroviruses are RNA viruses. They use a specialized enzyme, **reverse transcriptase**, that copies viral RNA to proviral DNA, which subsequently is integrated into the genomic DNA of the host. Three families of retroviruses cause illnesses in animals and humans:

Oncornaviruses are the oncogenic family, causing leukemia in cats; included in this family are human T-cell lymphotropic virus types 1 and 2 (HTLV-1 and HTLV-2).

The *lentiviruses* include human immunodeficiency virus types 1 and 2 (HIV-1 and HIV-2), the caprine arthritis encephalitis virus (CAEV), and ovine maedi-visna viruses that cause an arthritis in domesticated animals.

The *spumaviruses* are probably nonpathogenic.

Endogenous retroviruses exist. Up to 10 per cent of the genomes of all organisms—including humans—contain these codons, some of which are capable of directing the expression of viral proteins.[41] It is hypothesized that they could encode endogenous superantigens, immunosuppressive proteins, growth factors, or proteins that activate expression of otherwise quiescent genetic material.

Gay and his colleagues[42] argue that a retrovirus could initiate rheumatoid arthritis through T-cell–independent mechanisms. The hypothesis is that retrovirus infection could trigger transactivator gene expression, enabling cytokine production, and at the same time essentially transform mesenchymal cells, leading to expression of oncogene products and subsequent synovial cell proliferation with metalloprotease production resulting in tissue destruction (Fig. 4–4).

In animals, the lentiviruses do cause arthritis. CAEV affects goats and the visna virus affects sheep; in sheep, the pre- or subclinical disease is remarkable for synovial collections of CD8[+] and γδ cells, although increased numbers of CD4[+] subsets are found in synovia from clinically arthritic sheep.[43] Before dismissing these models as differ-

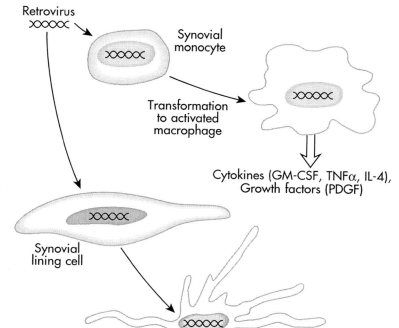

FIGURE 4–4. A hypothesis of retroviral initiation of rheumatoid arthritis by mechanisms independent of T cells focusing upon transformation of both monocytes to activated macrophages and synovial lining cells to dendritic cells secondary to retroviral infection.[42] Data supporting and opposing this possibility are outlined in the text.

ent from rheumatoid arthritis, in which CD4+ cells predominate in the established disease, it is worth remembering that studies of lymphocyte subsets in preclinical rheumatoid arthritis have never been done!

Is there any association between the lentivirus HIV-1 and rheumatoid arthritis? Probably only an inverse correlation exists, and for good reason. The amplification of cellular immunity necessary for development of rheumatoid arthritis is diminished and eventually obliterated by the acquired immunodeficiency syndrome (AIDS) virus as CD4+ cells, including naïve ones, are killed off. There have been reports of synovitis persisting in individuals after manifestations of AIDS appear, but their preexisting autoimmune diseases have not been typical for classical rheumatoid arthritis.[44]

The oncornavirus HTLV-1 is the etiologic agent of adult T-cell leukemia/lymphoma, but also is associated with a proliferative synovitis that accompanies HTLV-1–associated myelopathy or tropical spastic paraparesis. In addition, patients with chronic inflammatory arthropathy in Japan have a high prevalence of high titers of antibodies against HTLV-1. Two recent studies suggest that HTLV-

1 infection is a risk factor for rheumatoid arthritis. In a study from Nagasaki City, the seroprevalence of HTLV-1 in 19,796 normal female blood donors was 4.2 per cent, and that in 113 rheumatoid women was 20.4 per cent.[45] On Tsushima, an island northwest of Kyushu, the main island of Japan, seropositivity (confirmed by documenting proviral DNA in peripheral lymphocytes) was established in 26 per cent of 7,087 inhabitants, whereas 37 per cent of 111 patients (both men and women) were seropositive for HTLV-1. A corrected odds ratio for arthritis in HTLV-1 carriers was only 1.66. Interestingly, the HTLV carrier patients tended to have a milder form of synovitis.[46] It probably would be appropriate to consider HTLV-1 not as a causative agent, but as another mild predisposing factor. There are no data to indicate that the infection itself is sufficient for development of the disease.

It has been known for several years that HTLV-1–transformed T cells produce a multitude of cytokines, but recently it has been shown that HTLV-1 can infect human synovial fibroblasts, leading to their excess proliferation and production of cytokines such as GM-CSF.[47] Synovial cell clones have been established from patients with polyarthritis who have anti–HTLV antibodies. These clones express the *tax* transactivator gene encoded by HTLV-1 and appear to have a high capacity for proliferation.[47,48] By activating both T lymphocytes and synovial cells, and perhaps by contributing a superantigen from its own proteins, a retrovirus has all the machinery needed to generate a chronic inflammatory and proliferative synovitis.

Retroviral-like particles have been photographed in synovial fluid cells of rheumatoid patients[49]; in addition, using immunofluorescent techniques, reactivity in rheumatoid synovial tissues, but not osteoarthritic or psoriatic synovium, with monoclonal antibodies to the p19 and p24 HTLV antigens has been demonstrated.[50] Patients whose synovial tissues were immunoreactive by immunofluorescence were seronegative to HTLV-1 antigens as determined by enzyme-linked immunosorbent assay (ELISA) and immunoblotting.

As with any immunochemical reagents, the possibility that the antibodies are cross-reactive with a self-protein or another exogenous protein has not been ruled out. Accordingly, attempts to specifically demonstrate HTLV-1 have used the highly sensitive polymerase chain reaction. In contrast to the data from Japan reported above, the data showed no evidence of DNA for either a lentivirus or an HTLV-like virus at or above a concentration of 1 infected cell per 20,000 blood leukocytes or 250,000 synovial cells from 27 patients with rheumatoid arthritis.[51] In another study using PCR, and with adequate controls, antibodies with retroviral proteins were found in sera from a minority of patients with rheumatoid arthritis, but also in polymyositis and systemic lupus erythematosus.[52]

In light of the striking similarities of the rheumatoid synovial lining cell to a cell transformed by a virus, the search for retroviruses is being pursued. The next step will be using the reverse transcription PCR using broad-spectrum oligonucleotide retroviral primers, a technique that may add an increase in both sensitivity and specificity.[53]

AUTOIMMUNITY

Ever since rheumatoid factor, the antibody against **gamma globulin**, was first associated with the disease, hypotheses have been tested that autoimmunity not only was associated with rheumatoid arthritis but was its cause as well. Data that implicate immunity to IgG have been tantalizing at times, such as when it was demonstrated that one mouse monoclonal antibody reacted with 50 per cent of rheumatoid factors from unrelated individuals.[54] However, as reviewed in Chapter 6, close analysis

of sequences of rheumatoid factors from rheumatoid patients indicate more that the rheumatoid factor response is an antigen-driven one, and is driven by antigens other than IgG.

One difference between normal and rheumatoid patients remains to be placed into a proper context: IgG in rheumatoid patients appears to have a decreased amount of galactosyl residues, perhaps related to a decreased B-cell galactosyltransferase activity.[55] Could this post-translational alteration in IgG make it immunogenic, and therefore a direct cause of rheumatoid arthritis, or at least an amplifier of nonspecific inflammation sufficient to generate a full-blown synovitis?

Immunity against **type II collagen** found in cartilage is another possible cause or amplifier of rheumatoid arthritis. Interest in this segment of autoimmunity was triggered by the evidence that experimental arthritis in rats and mice that is tightly restricted by the MHC can be caused by injections of type II collagen. The arthritis can then be passively transferred by IgG fractions containing anticollagen antibodies or by transfer of lymphocytes from affected animals.[56,57] One study even demonstrated that, if mice were immunized with immune complexes of collagen type II/anti–collagen type II, clones could be isolated that produced rheumatoid factors directed against the idiotype of anti–collagen II.[58]

In rheumatoid arthritis, the ''cart or horse'' quandary persists: Is type II collagen intrinsic to the pathogenesis, or rather a powerful adjunctive amplifier of an immune response set into action by another antigen? Some of the data that define this quandary are

- Antibodies to native type II collagen are present in sera or synovial fluids of up to 25 per cent of patients with rheumatoid arthritis.[59]
- Purified anticollagen antibodies from sera of patients with rheumatoid arthritis have the capability—when bound to cartilage—to activate complement.[60]
- Anticollagen antibodies from patients with relapsing polychondritis recognize a different epitope(s) than do anti-collagen antibodies from rheumatoid patients.[58]
- Antibodies to native type II collagen have been found in sera from patients with rheumatoid arthritis of less than 6 months' duration, well before any detectable radiologic evidence of damage to cartilage was observed.[61]
- Anti–type II collagen antibodies were produced by B cells or plasma cells from synovial fluid of 16 of 31 patients with rheumatoid arthritis but not by cells from peripheral blood in these pa-

tients; the IgG anticollagen II–reactive cells were found exclusively in patients with *HLA-DR4*.[62]

- The possibility that EBV and type II collagen could synergize in causing synovitis is suggested by the fact that EBV shares an epitope with type II collagen (see earlier discussion on dnaJ).[63] It is plausible that, after an EBV infection or activation of latent infection, antibodies against a component of the organism could cross-react not only with *HLA-DRB1* β-chains but also with epitopes on type II collagen.

Collagen and Therapy for Rheumatoid Arthritis

Whether or not immunity to type II collagen is a primary cause of rheumatoid arthritis, the finding of anti–collagen II antibodies opens the door to immune therapy. Vaccinations by type II collagen–reactive T lymphocytes is a reasonable strategy for the future. Attempts to develop anergy to type II collagen in rheumatoid patients have led to trials of oral tolerance that are reviewed in Chapter 31. The study of collagen as an oral toleragen is not based on assumptions that autoimmunity to type II collagen is the principal or initial cause of rheumatoid arthritis, but rather that, as a secondary immunogen, it plays a major role in amplification and persistence of the synovitis.

Autoimmunity against Other Matrix Components

A purified domain of the cartilage proteoglycan **aggrecan** can alone induce a polyarthritis and spondylitis in certain strains of mice.[64] Interestingly, it was only after the keratan sulfate chains associated with this domain were removed by proteases that the residual proteoglycan generated an erosive polyarthritis. It also is reported that immunity to **cartilage link protein** can induce an erosive polyarthritis in the same BALB/c mice.[65] During destruction of cartilage in rheumatoid arthritis, these proteoglycan side chains are stripped by various enzymes, perhaps exposing these same epitopes and leading to an autoimmune (or cross-reactive) immune response.

At the very least, it is probable that any or all of the agents or self-proteins discussed here could contribute a substantial secondary immune response through cross-reactivity. This would lead to substantial amplification of what may have been, in another individual, a transient synovitis marked by a little stiffness in the morning that went away as quickly as it had come on.

REFERENCES

1. Smiley, J. D., and Hoffman, W. L.: Southwestern Internal Medicine Conference: The role of infections in the rheumatic diseases: molecular mimicry between bacterial and human stress proteins? Am. J. Med. Sci. 301:138, 1991.

   This review summarizes evidence for infectious causes of many "autoimmune" processes, including rheumatic fever. Table 4–1 (see text) lists evidence for an infectious cause of rheumatoid arthritis; references for specific observations in the table are found in this paper.

2. Ebringer, A.: Rheumatoid arthritis as an infectious disease [Letter]. Br. M. J. 303:524, 1991.

3. Deighton, C. M., Gray, J., and Bint, A. J.: Specificity of the Proteus antibody response in rheumatoid arthritis. Ann. Rheum. Dis. 51:1206, 1992.

   Sera from 146 patients with rheumatoid arthritis were screened for multiple antibodies. The only antibodies found to be significantly increased in rheumatoid arthritis patients with active disease were those against *Proteus mirabilis*.

4. Maki-Ikla, O, Viljanen, M. K., Tiitinen, S., et al.: Antibodies to arthritis-associated microbes in inflammatory joint diseases. Rheumatol. Int. 10:231, 1991.

5. Ford, D. K.: Synovial lymphocytes can indicate specific microbiologic causes of rheumatoid arthritis. Arthritis Rheum. 10:1351, 1993.

6. Chantler, J. K., da Roza, D. M., Bonnie, M. E., et al.: Sequential studies on synovial lymphocyte stimulation by rubella antigen, and rubella virus isolation in an adult with persistent arthritis. Ann. Rheum. Dis. 44:564, 1985.

7. Ford, D. K., Stein, H. B., Schulzer, M., et al.: Lymphocytes from the site of disease suggest adenovirus is one cause of persistent or recurrent inflammatory arthritis. J. Rheumatol. 20:310, 1993.

8. Ford, D. K., da Roza, D. M., Schulzer, M., et al.: Persistent synovial lymphocyte responses to cytomegalovirus antigen in some patients with rheumatoid arthritis. Arthritis Rheum. 30:700, 1987.

9. Wilson, C., Ebringer, A., Ahmadi, K., et al.: Shared amino acid sequences between major histocompatibility complex class II glycoproteins, type α1 collagen and *Proteus mirabilis* in rheumatoid arthritis. Ann. Rheum. Dis. 54: 221, 1995.

10. Kjeldsen-Kragh, J., Rashid, T., Dybwad, A., et al.: Decrease in anti-*Proteus mirabilis* but not anti-*Escherichia coli* antibody levels in rheumatoid arthritis patients treated with fasting and a one year vegetarian diet. Ann. Rheum. Dis. 54:221, 1995.

11. Nikkari, S., Roivainen, A., Hannonen, P., et al.: Persistence of parvovirus B19 in synovial fluid and bone marrow. Ann. Rheum. Dis. 54:597, 1995.

12. Harboe, M., and Quayle, A. J.: Heat shock proteins: friend and foe? Clin. Exp. Immunol. 86:2, 1991.

13. Winrow, V. R., McLean, L., Morris, C. J., et al.: The heat shock protein response and its role in inflammatory disease. Ann. Rheum. Dis. 49:128, 1990.

14. Catelli, M. G., Binart, N., Jung-Testas, N., et al.: The common 90 kD protein component of non-transformed '8S' steroid receptors is a heat shock protein. EMBO J. 4: 3131, 1985.

15. Lakomek, H.-J., Will, H., Zech, M., et al.: A new serologic marker in ankylosing spondylitis. Arthritis Rheum. 27: 961, 1984.

16. Brand, S. R., McIntosh, D. P., and Bernstein, R. M.: Antibody to a 63 kD protein in ankylosing spondylitis [Abstract]. Br. J. Rheumatol. 28(suppl. 1):5, 1989.

17. van Eden, W., Thole, J. E., van der Zee, R., et al.: Cloning of the mycobacterial epitope recognized by T lymphocytes in adjuvant arthritis. Nature 331:171, 1988.

18. Warrow, V. R., Ragno, S., Morris, C. J., et al.: Arthritogenic potential of the 65 kDa stress protein—an experimental model. Ann. Rheum. Dis. 53:197, 1994.

19. Van Eden, W., Holoshitz, J., Nevo, Z., et al.: Arthritis induced by a T lymphocyte clone that responds to *Mycobacterium tuberculosis* and to cartilage proteoglycans. Proc. Natl. Acad. Sci. U.S.A. 82:5117, 1985.

20. Bahr, G. M., Rook, G. A. W., Al-Saffar, M., et al.: An analysis of antibody levels to mycobacteria in relation to HLA type: evidence for non-HLA-linked high levels of antibody to the 65 kD heat shock protein of *M. tuberculosis* in rheumatoid arthritis. Clin. Exp. Immunol. 74:211, 1988.

21. Holoshitz, J., Klajman, A., Druker, I., et al.: T lymphocytes of rheumatoid arthritis patients show augmented reactivity to a fraction of mycobacteria cross-reactive with cartilage. Lancet 2:305, 1986.

22. de Graeff-Meeder, E. R., Voorhorst, M., van Eden, W., et al.: Antibodies to the mycobacterial 65-kd heat shock protein are reactive with synovial tissue of adjuvant arthritic rats and patients with rheumatoid arthritis and osteoarthritis. Am. J. Pathol. 137:1013, 1990.

23. Res, P. C. M., Schaar, C. G., Beedveld, F. C., et al.: Synovial fluid T-cell reactivity against 65 kD heat-shock protein of mycobacteria in early chronic arthritis. Lancet 2:278, 1988.

24. Karlsson-Parra, A., Söderström, K., Ferm, M., et al.: Presence of human 65 kD heat shock protein (HSP) in inflamed joints and subcutaneous nodules of RA patients. Scand. I. Immunol. 31:283, 1990.

25. Burmester, G. R., Altstidl, U., Kalden, J. R., et al.: Stimulatory response towards the 65 kDa heat shock protein and other mycobacterial antigens in patients with rheumatoid arthritis. J. Rheumatol. 18:171, 1991.

26. da Silva, J. A. P.: Heat shock proteins: the missing link between hormonal and reproductive factors and rheumatoid arthritis? Ann. Rheum. Dis. 50:735, 1991.

27. Clay, K., Foly, A. D., and Hall, N. D.: The expression of estrogen receptor and p29 antigen in rheumatoid arthritis. Arthritis Rheum. 37:S314, 1994.

28. Cutolo, M., Accaido, S., Villoggio, B., et al.: Presence of estrogen-binding sites on macrophage-like synoviocytes and CD8$^+$ CD29$^+$, CD45RO$^+$ T lymphocytes in normal and rheumatoid synovium. Arthritis Rheum. 36:1087, 1993.

29. Winchester, R., Dwyer, E., and Rose, S.: The genetic basis of rheumatoid arthritis: the shared epitope hypothesis. Rheum. Dis. Clin. North Am. 18:761, 1992.

30. Albani, S., Keystone, E. C., Ollier, W. E. R., et al.: Positive selection in autoimmunity: abnormal immune responses to a bacterial dnaJ antigenic determinant in patients with early rheumatoid arthritis. (in press).

31. Alspaugh, M. A., Henle, G., Lennette, E. T., et al.: Elevated levels of antibodies to Epstein-Barr virus antigens in sera and synovial fluids of patients with rheumatoid arthritis. J. Clin. Invest. 67:1134, 1981.

32. Alspaugh, M. A., and Tan, E. M.: Antibodies to cellular antigens in Sjögren's syndrome. J. Clin. Invest. 55:1067, 1975.

33. Silverman, S. L., and Schumacher, H. R.: Antibodies to Epstein-Barr viral antigens in early rheumatoid arthritis. Arthritis Rheum. 24:1465, 1981.

34. Fingeroth, J. D., Weis, J. J., Tedder, T. F., et al.: Epstein-Barr virus receptor of human B lymphocytes is the C3d receptor CR2. Proc. Natl. Acad. Sci. U.S.A. 81:4510, 1984.

35. Slaughter, L., Carson, D. A., Jensen, F. C., et al.: *In vitro* effects of Epstein-Barr virus on peripheral blood mononuclear cells from patients with rheumatoid arthritis and normal subjects. J. Exp. Med. 148:1429, 1978.

36. Yaq, Q. Y., Rickinson, A. B., Gaston, J. S. H., et al.: Disturbance of the Epstein-Barr virus-host balance in rheumatoid arthritis patients: a quantitative study. Clin. Exp. Immunol. 64:302, 1986.

37. Baboonian, C., Halliday, D., Venables, P. J. W., et al.: Antibodies in rheumatoid arthritis react specifically with the glycine/alanine repeat sequence of Epstein-Barr nuclear antigen-1. Rheumatol. Int. 9:161, 1989.

38. Baboonian, C., Venables, P. J. W., Williams, D. G., et al.: Cross reaction of antibodies to a glycine/alanine repeat sequence of Epstein-Barr virus nuclear antigen-1 with collagen, cytokeratin, and actin. Ann. Rheum. Dis. 50:772, 1991.

39. Zhang, L., Nikkari, S., and Skurnik, M.: Detection of herpes viruses by polymerase chain reaction in lymphocytes from patients with rheumatoid arthritis. Arthritis Rheum. 36:1080, 1993.

40. Roudier, J., Petersen, J., Rhodes, G. H., et al.: Susceptibility to rheumatoid arthritis maps to a T-cell epitope shared by the HLA-Dw4 DRB1 chain and the Epstein-Barr virus glycoprotein gp110. Proc. Natl. Acad. Sci. U.S.A. 86:5104, 1989.

41. Wilder, R. L.: Hypothesis for retroviral causation of rheumatoid arthritis. Curr. Opin. Rheumatol. 6:295, 1994.

42. Gay, S., Gay, and Koopman, W. J.: Molecular and cellular mechanisms of joint destruction in rheumatoid arthritis: two cellular mechanisms explain joint destruction? Ann. Rheum. Dis. 52:S39, 1993.

43. Anderson, A. A., Harkiss, G. D., and Watt, N. J.: Quantitative analysis of immunohistological changes in the synovial membrane of sheep infected with Maedi-Visna virus. Clin. Immunol. Immunopathol. 72:1, 1994.

44. Kerr, L. D., and Spiera, H.: The coexistence of active classic rheumatoid arthritis and AIDS. J. Rheumatol. 18:1739, 1991.

45. Eguchi, K., Origuchi, T., Takashima, H, et al.: High seroprevalence of anti-HTLV-I antibody in rheumatoid arthritis. Arthritis Rheum. 39:463, 1996.

46. Motokawa, S., Hasunuma, T., Tajima, K., et al.: High prevalence of arthropathy in HTLV-I carriers on a Japanese island. Ann. Rheum. Dis. 55:193, 1996.

47. Sakai, M., Eguchi, K., Terada, K., et al.: Infection of human synovial cells by human T cell lymphotropic virus type I: proliferation and granulocyte/macrophage colony-stimulating factor production by synovial cells. J. Clin. Invest. 92:1957, 1993.

   HTLV-1 produces a gene product, Tax (trans-regulatory protein). Tax increases transcription of viral and cellular genes by exploiting two host transcription factor channels. One is the multifunctional transcription factor NF-κB that activates numerous cellular promoters, including promoters of interleukin-2 and interleukin-2 receptor (Lenardo, M. J., and Baltimore, D.: NF-κB: a pleiotropic mediator of inducible and tissue-specific gene control. Cell 58:227, 1989.) Another is the cAMP-responsive element binding protein.

48. Nakajima, T., Aono, H., Hasunuma, T., et al.: Overgrowth of human synovial cells driven by the human T cell leukemia virus type I genus. J. Clin. Invest. 92:186, 1993.

49. Stransky, G., Vernon, J., Aicher, W. K., et al.: Virus-like

particles in synovial fluids from patients with rheumatoid arthritis. Br. J. Rheumatol. 22:1044, 1993.

50. Ziegler, B., Gay, R. E., Guo-Quiang, H., et al.: Immunohistochemical localization of HTLV-1 P19 and P23-related antigens in synovial joints of patients with rheumatoid arthritis. Am. J. Pathol. 135:1, 1989.

51. di Giovine, F. S., Bally, S., Bootman, J., et al.: Absence of lentiviral and human T cell leukemia viral sequences in patients with rheumatoid arthritis. Arthritis Rheum. 37: 349, 1994.

52. Nelson, P. N., Lever, A. M. L., Bruckner, F. E., et al.: Polymerase chain reaction fails to incriminate exogenous retroviruses HTLV-1 and HIV-1 in rheumatological diseases although a minority of sera cross react with retroviral antigens. Ann. Rheum. Dis. 53:749, 1994.

53. Nelson, P. N.: Retroviruses in rheumatic diseases. Ann. Rheum. Dis. 54:441, 1995.

54. Carson, D. A., and Fong, S.: A common idiotope on human rheumatoid factors identified by a hybridoma antibody. Mol. Immunol. 20:1081, 1983.

55. Axford, J. S., Lydyard, P. M., Isenberg, D. A., et al.: Reduced B-cell galactosyltransferase activity in rheumatoid arthritis. Lancet 2:1486, 1987.

56. Stuart, J. M., Cremer, M. A., Townes, A. S., et al.: Type II collagen-induced arthritis in rats: transfer with serum. J. Exp. Med. 155:1, 1982.

57. Trentham, D. E., Dynesius, R. A., and David, J. R.: Passive transfer by cells of type II collagen-induced arthritis in rats. J. Clin. Invest. 62:359, 1978.

58. Holmdahl, R., Nordling, C., Rubin, K., et al.: Generation of monoclonal rheumatoid factors after immunization with collagen II-anti-collagen immune complexes: an anti-idiotype antibody to anti-collagen II is also a rheumatoid factor. Scand. J. Immunol. 24:197, 1986.

59. Terato, K., Shimozuru, Y., Katayama, K., et al.: Specificity of antibodies to type II collagen in rheumatoid arthritis. Arthritis Rheum. 33:1493, 1990.

60. Watson, W. C., Cremer, M. A., Wooley, P. H., et al.: Assessment of the potential pathogenicity of type II collagen autoantibodies in patients with rheumatoid arthritis. Arthritis Rheum. 29:1316, 1986.

61. Cook, A. D., Rowley, M. J., Stockman, A., et al.: Specificity of antibodies to type II collagen in early rheumatoid arthritis. J. Rheumatol. 21:1186, 1994.

In 16 patients, 10 had antibodies to native type II collagen and 6 did not. Sequential assays remained true to the initial measurements: Those who had antibodies initially continued to have the same titers, and those who did not have anti-collagen antibodies never developed them. There were no differences in the two groups in the initial clinical evaluation. For the most part, these antibodies were IgG; only one patient had an IgM antibody. The authors suggest that "the presence of an established and persisting IgG antibody response to type II collagen in early RA before cartilage destruction is evident points to a subset of RA, perhaps equivalent to the collagen induced model in animals, in which this immune response is intrinsic to pathogenesis."

62. Ronnelid, J., Lysholm, J., Engstrom-Laurent, A., et al.: Local anti-type II collagen antibody production in rheumatoid arthritis synovial fluid. Arthritis Rheum. 37:1023, 1994.

63. Birkenfeld, P., Haratz, N., Klein, G., et al.: Cross-reactivity between the EBNA-1 p. 107 peptide, collagen, and keratin: implications for the pathogenesis of rheumatoid arthritis. Clin. Immunol. Immunopathol. 54:14, 1990.

64. Leroux, J. Y., Pole, A. R., Webber, C., et al.: Characterization of proteoglycan-reactive T cell lines and hybridomas from mice with proteoglycan-induced arthritis. J. Immunol. 148:2090, 1992.

65. Poole, A. R., and Dieppe, P.: Biological markers in rheumatoid arthritis. Semin. Arthritis Rheum. 23:17, 1994.

5

T Lymphocytes

It is apparent that lymphocytes must share the leading role in pathogenesis of rheumatoid arthritis with macrophages and synovial lining cells. Nevertheless, the importance of these cells in initiation and sustenance of rheumatoid arthritis must be emphasized. As with all other studies of this disease, it is useful to go back to the pathology. There one sees T lymphocytes and dendritic cells/macrophages around tiny blood vessels (Fig. 5–1). More important, good data indicate that, although the majority of T lymphocytes transmigrate through the endothelium in a nonactivated state, within the synovium they become activated as they move into groups further from blood vessels. The evidence for activation of lymphocytes once they are within the synovium is strong evidence for an antigen-driven immune response occurring in the joint,[1,2] and this becomes a central dogma in this disease. It is supported by the finding in rheumatoid synovium of an excess of activated dendritic cells capable of presenting antigen to T cells.[3] In response to activated T cells, there also is polyclonal activation of B cells, particularly those primed to produce rheumatoid factor.

The T-cell system is a superbly adaptable and flexible one. Similar to B cells, T lymphocytes use products of *rag* genes to somatically rearrange variable (V), diversity (D), and joining (J) elements to create as many as 10^{11} different clones, each with a distinct TCR capable of recognizing a specific peptide in the context of a MHC class I or II molecule and co-stimulatory proteins. As is described in more detail subsequently, when a peptide binds to the TCR with appropriate affinity, clonal proliferation expands the cell population and they become "memory" cells. During this process, cytokines of the activated T cells activate macrophages and induce differentiation of B cells. Once activated, T-cell clones expand. Then a major portion of them die by apoptosis and a variable portion remain as memory cells. A quantitative change in the expansion, death, or memory phases will determine whether immunity (or autoimmunity) is long or short lived.

THE T–CELL RECEPTOR

The TCR is composed of two disulfide-linked polymorphic chains, α and β, or γ and δ. The enormous diversity in receptor structure present in each individual is made possible by recombination during somatic rearrangement of the germline-encoded V, D, and J segments with a constant (C) region. The complementarity-determining regions (CDR1, 2, and 3) interact with the MHC-antigen complex (Fig. 5–2). These CDR domains are hypervariable in composition; it is modification in the CDR regions of TCRs that affects the recognition of their ligand-MHC-antigen complexes, resulting in either enhanced or decreased recognition. Specific MHC-peptide complexes can select for TCR CDR regions that optimally fit their own conformation. CDR1 and 2 regions interact with the α-helices of the MHC molecule, the CDR3 region interacts with the antigen presented in the pleomorphic peptide-binding groove by the MHC, and the CDR4 region, which is highly conserved among V_β gene families, is believed to be where superantigens bind.

Depending on the exact composition of the antigen presented to T cells, there is variable activation of these cells. For example, changing one amino acid residue in an antigenic peptide can result in a T cell producing interleukin (IL)-4 but not undergoing clonal expansion, or becoming cytotoxic while releasing no lymphokines, or actually becoming anergic. This variation in the ability of one receptor to vary the qualitative nature of the activation response adds one more layer to the enormous diversity and specificity of the T-cell response.

DEVELOPMENT OF THE IMMUNE RESPONSE IN THE RHEUMATOID JOINT

Before going into more detail regarding attempts to identify specific clones of T cells that are relatively specific for patients with rheumatoid arthritis, it is useful to review evidence that implicates

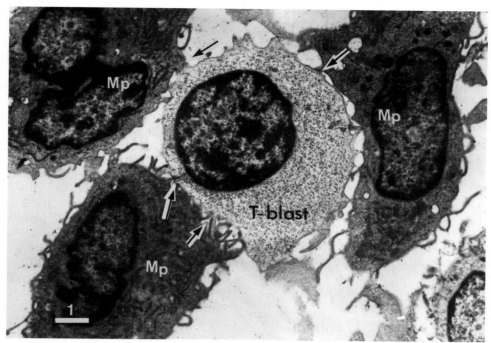

FIGURE 5–1. Electron photomicrograph of cells in rheumatoid synovium. The center cell with speckled cytoplasm represents a lymphocyte. Contacts with macrophages (Mp) are shown by arrows. (Courtesy of Dr. Morris Ziff, University of Texas Southwestern Medical College, Dallas, Tx.)

the T lymphocytes in disease presentation. Even a casual examination of the histopathology of rheumatoid synovium makes clear the involvement of lymphocytes in this process (Fig. 5–3). The earliest of synovial biopsies, taken shortly after symptoms begin but before any diagnosis can be made, show diffuse perivascular collections of lymphocytes.[4] As the synovitis consolidates, lymphocytes appear to aggregate around the synovial capillaries below the lining cells. Most of these appear to carry the CD4 surface markers of T-helper/inducer cells, whereas T cells further out toward the joint capsule have more equal ratios of CD4$^+$ and CD8$^+$ (suppressor) cells.[5]

T lymphocytes in synovium are often closely associated with dendritic cells or macrophages bearing HLA-DR surface markers (Fig. 5–1). Dendritic cells are potent APCs that take up, sequester, and present antigen to T cells via class II MHC in the primary and secondary immune responses. Using immunofluorescent cell sorting, the numbers of dendritic cell precursors in synovium can be compared with those in peripheral blood.[3] They have been found to be enriched in rheumatoid synovium and synovial fluid. Functionally, these dendritic cells are stimulated even further by the cytokines GM-CSF and tumor necrosis factor α (TNFα), and express large amounts of adhesion molecules.

T-Cell Subsets in the Rheumatoid Joint

Isoforms of the leukocyte common antigen have been used for several years to divide CD4$^+$ T lymphocytes into subpopulations based upon their degree of activation (see Correlations of Surface Antigens and Functions in Subsets of T Cells, in the box on page 54)

Primed T cells are called to migrate from peripheral blood. This process is directed by a combined effect of expression of adhesion molecules on both endothelial cells and T cells and chemoattractants within the inflamed joints (see Chapter 7).[1,2,7] Within the circulation, there is sufficient cytokine activity to prime certain T lymphocytes to enable them to slow, bind, and then transmigrate through endothelium into the synovium. The majority of T cells in the synovium are CD4$^+$ cells.

It is apparent that certain subsets of the CD$^+$ CD45RO$^+$ T cells have an intrinsic capability for migration through endothelium. They brightly express CD44 (Brezinschek, et al., Abstract 205) and β_1-integrin. CD44 is a ligand for hyaluronan, which is produced by synovial lining cells and remains in the tissue as well as being a major component of synovial fluid. This may explain why lymphocytes are found in *both* the tissue and fluid, whereas neutrophils—which have no ligand for synovial com-

---

Correlations of Surface Antigens and Functions in Subsets of T Cells

The use of the fluorescence-activated cell sorter has enabled investigators to tag surface markers of cells and separate them cleanly from other nonlabeled cells. Monoclonal antibodies used to bind to cell surface glycoproteins can be tagged with either fluorescein isothiocyanate (green) or phycoerythrin (red) labels. Some antigens and the functions subsequently identified for them (or in cell populations negative for them) include

CD4$^+$: this antigen works with the TCR to receive antigen presented by MHC class II molecules; CD4$^+$ cells are functionally either Th1 or Th2 cells (Fig. 5–5).

CD8$^+$: this antigen, in concert with the TCR, receives antigen presented by class I MHC molecules on APCs

CD69$^+$: cells expressing this antigen are in a phase of early activation

CD45RO$^+$: cells with reactivity to recall antigens; primed or memory T cells producing IL-2 and IFNγ

CD45RA$^+$: unprimed or naive cells; they produce IL-2 but no IL-4 or IFNγ

CD45RO$^+$/CD45RB^{bright}: early memory T cells

CD45RO$^+$/CD45RB^{dim}: terminally differentiated memory cells with an enhanced capacity to provide help for B cells

CD27$^+$: this antigen is related to the TNF receptor and may make cells more responsive to activation and receptor-mediated apoptosis

CD27$^-$: CD4$^+$/CD45RA$^-$/CD27$^-$ cells brightly express β_1-integrins (very late antigen 4 and 5), which enable binding to mesenchymal cells in synovium; they have an enhanced migratory capability (reviewed in Chapter 7)

CD4$^+$/CD45RA$^-$/CD45RO$^+$/CD45RB^{dim}/CD27 $-$: these cells are most effective at B cell help, and have a capacity to produce IL-4 as well as IFNγ; this implies the presence of Th1 and Th2 cells in this subpopulation

CD44$^+$: cells expressing this antigen can bind to hyaluronate within connective tissue

CD8$^+$/FcR$^+$/IL-2R$^+$/CD28$^-$: these cells have functional capabilities of suppressor cells, capable of inducing anergy in CD4$^+$ antigen-responsive clones. They have a Th2 phenotype, producing little IFNγ but much IL-4

---

ponents—migrate on through to the synovial fluid, attracted by the chemotactic substances there.

These activated T cells with the capability to migrate use some of the same surface antigens for migration as for co-stimulation with APCs. For example the interaction of leukocyte function antigen (LFA)-1 with intercellular adhesion molecule (ICAM)-1 probably has a key role in transendothelial migration of T cells,[8] and the initial binding of T cells to endothelium may be mediated by vascular cell adhesive molecule (VCAM)-1–very late antigen (VLA)-4 interactions.

The CD4$^+$, CD45RB^{dim} cells are enriched within rheumatoid synovial fluid and synovium.[9] They also express CD27 only weakly; the CD27 molecule is a member of the TNF receptor superfamily, a class of structurally related molecules involved in cell activation and receptor-mediated apoptosis.[10] Loss of the CD27 surface expression has been implicated as a final step in the cascade of CD4$^+$ memory T-cell differentiation into antigen-primed T cells with the capacity to migrate into areas of inflammation, such as rheumatoid synovium.[9] **It can be inferred that these migratory CD45RB^{dim}, CD27$^-$, memory T cells so prominent in rheumatoid tissue, have differentiated in response to recurrent stimulation by arthritogenic peptides.**

Among the CD4$^+$ cells are subsets of helper-inducer and suppressor-inducer cells. There are many more of the CD8$^+$ suppressor cells in synovial fluid than in synovial tissue.[11,12] However—and this caveat applies to all qualitative studies of synovial fluid that attempt to extrapolate to synovial tissue—the differences in localization of certain cells between these two compartments may be explained in part by differential expression of adhesion proteins on both matrix proteins and the transmigrating cells. A cell type that is bound with high affinity by matrix receptors or other cellular receptors within the synovium is unlikely to be present in significant numbers in the synovial fluid. Because activated T cells have been observed to transcribe significantly more gene message for TCRs,[13] as well as more ''activating'' cytokines, than do ''naive'' cells, it is likely that the activated cells are very receptive to presentation of antigen by the appropriate APCs.

Suppressor Cells in Rheumatoid Arthritis

There continues to be a great deal of skepticism about T-suppressor cells, their characterization, or their importance in human disease. Part of the problem has been in the extrapolation of results from murine hybridoma systems to humans.

One model that has support from data in humans is *clonal anergy* (see ref 14). It is based on the need for co-stimulation; if an antigen is presented by cells in an MHC-restricted form but without co-stimulatory factors, clonal anergy or apoptosis in responding cells is produced.[15]

Experiments with cells from lepromatous leprosy, in which there is a striking immunologic unresponsiveness to *Mycobacterium leprae*, are relevant in studies of suppressor T cells (sT cells)[16] (see Correlations of Surface Antigens and Functions in Subsets of T Cells, earlier). These sT cells are not cytotoxic[17] and induce a state of anergy in CD4 antigen-responsive clones. Sufficient co-stimulation is present but negated. It appears that this suppressor subset of human T-cell clones produces relatively small amounts of interferon (IFN)γ but substantial IL-4; this cytokine down-regulates antigen-specific T-cell activation.[18] IL-10 and TGFβ also can mediate T-cell suppression in mouse models and could be involved in human disease. In situations such as these it may be that the Th2 cell is the elusive "T-suppressor cell."

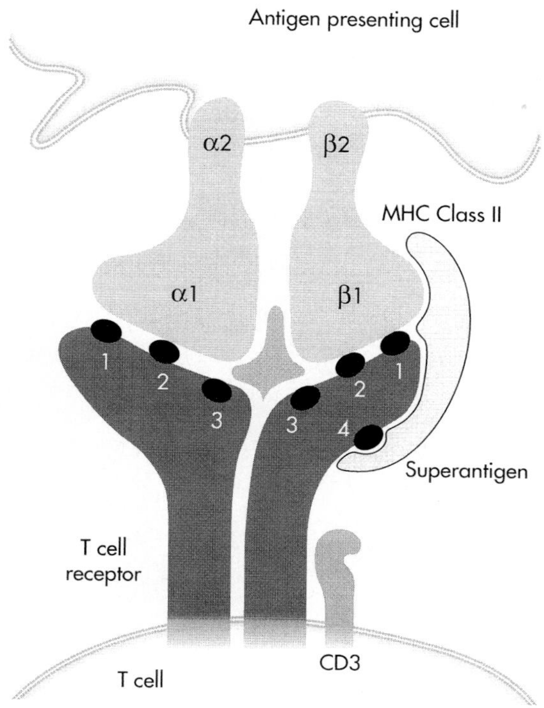

Antigen presenting cell

FIGURE 5–2. Schematic representation of the interaction of the TCR with the class II MHC-peptide complex, or the interaction of a superantigen with the TCR and MHC. The dark ovals represent the domains of hypervariability called complementarity-determining regions. CDR3 is a principal reactor with antigen peptides, whereas CDR4, with amino acid sequences highly conserved between particular TCR V_β gene families, is probably the target of superantigen binding (see ref. 68). (Modified from Struyk, L., Hawes, G. E., and Chatila, M. K.: T cell receptors in rheumatoid arthritis. Arthritis Rheum. 38:577, 1995. Used by permission.)

Th1 and Th2 Cells

Within the subset of CD4$^+$ cells there are at least two species: Th1 and Th2 cells. It is assumed that the same types of subsets are present in humans. **Th1 cells** secrete IL-2 and IFNγ, which stimulate cellular immunity and are responsible for delayed hypersensitivity. IFNγ induces B cells to switch their Ig isotype to IgG1, promoting phagocytosis by activating complement and binding to Fc receptors on macrophages. In turn, after being activated by tissue macrophages, Th1 cells express TNFα and IL-12. IL-12 enhances development of Th1 cells, whereas IL-4 and IL-10 inhibit their proliferation. IL-12 curtails IL-4 production by naive stimulated CD4 cells. IFNγ and IL-12 combine to produce autocrine positive feedback to increase IFNγ, resulting in increased macrophage activation. IL-2, produced by Th1 cells, feeds back locally to induce more proliferation and activation of Th1 cells (Fig.

5–5). A dominance of Th1 over Th2 cytokine-producing cells has been reported in rheumatoid synovial fluids (Dolhain, et al., Abstract 492).

Th2 cells are induced by IL-4, produce the cytokines IL-4, IL-5, IL-6, and IL-10, and inhibit monocyte function. IL-12 and IFNγ inhibit development of Th2 cells. Primarily through the cytokines that they produce, Th2 cells provide help to B cells in expressing immunoglobulins, particularly IgE. IL-10, a major Th2 cytokine, also induces expression of Bcl-2 in cells; this protein helps prevent apoptosis, or programmed cell death. IL-10 inhibits protease production and proinflammatory cytokine production by a variety of cells.

Co-stimulatory molecules (see Fig. 5–7) expressed by macrophages, other APCs, and lymphocytes can affect the Th1/Th2 balance. Thus, antibodies against the co-stimulatory molecule B7-1 prevent development of allergic encephalitis (a

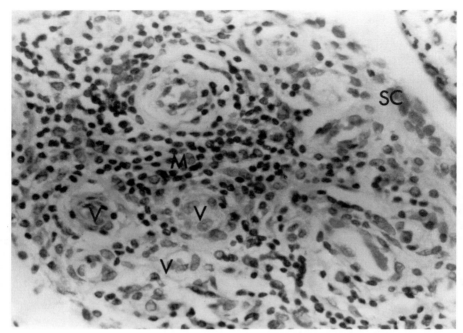

FIGURE 5–3. Mononuclear cells (M), predominantly lymphocytes, are beginning to accumulate in the extravascular space around small postcapillary venules (V). The endothelium, tall and activated, can be shown to have adhesion molecules that slow, then bind ligands on these lymphocytes. The lymphocytes then migrate through the endothelium and bind to matrix proteins and fibroblasts. These perivascular collections are distinctly separated from synovial lining cells (SC). The lymphocytes have become ''fixed'' in the perivascular tissue, perhaps by very late antigen-4 binding to a ligand, such as intracellular adhesion molecule-1.

model for multiple sclerosis) in mice, diminish production of IFNγ, and enhance secretion of IL-10. In contrast, anti–B7-2 accelerates development of allergic encephalitis in mice. Both B7-1 and B7-2 must be present and interacting with their counter-receptors on T cells if T cells are to proliferate at all, rather than becoming anergic.

It is a reasonable hypothesis that rheumatoid arthritis is a disease driven by Th1 CD4⁺ lymphocytes. In addition to finding Th1-producing cells in

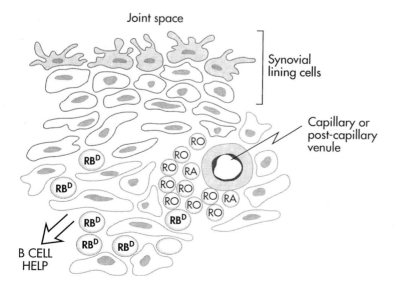

FIGURE 5–4. Relatively few naive CD4⁺ T cells (CD45RA⁺ cells), labeled ''RA,'' bind to endothelial cells and transmigrate into the synovium. Most synovial T cells have a ''memory'' phenotype (CD45RO⁺), labeled ''RO.'' CD45RA⁺ cells produce high levels of IL-2 but no IL-4 or IFNγ; CD45RO⁺ cells produce all three. The CD45RB^{dim} cells (''RB^D'') are mature memory cells, are believed to evolve from CD45RO⁺ cells, and have an important role in initiating B-cell help.[1,7] It is also likely that CD45RA⁺ cells may undergo activation/maturation within the synovium and acquire the CD45RO phenotype.[2]

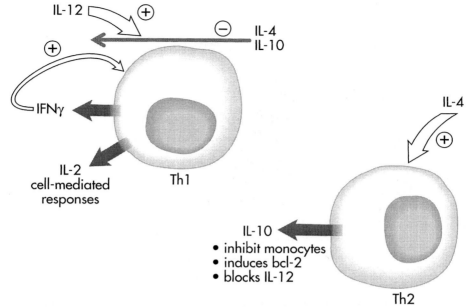

FIGURE 5–5. Th1 and Th2 cells have different phenotypic expression and are activated differently. IL-12 initiates expansion of the Th1 population, whereas IL-10 and IL-4 both suppress it. The Th1 cell is believed to dominate diseases characterized as examples of delayed hypersensitivity (e.g., rheumatoid arthritis). Th2 cells respond by expansion and activation to IL-4. They generate IL-10. These cells presumably mediate allergic reactions.

synovial fluid of rheumatoid patients, mRNA from peripheral blood mononuclear cells appears to be skewed toward Th1-linked cytokines (e.g., IL-2, IFNγ) rather than IL-4, a Th2-linked cytokine (Schulze-Koops, et al., Abstract 825) (Fig. 5–6). Conversely, because patients with severe allergies have much IgE production with a presumed up-regulation of Th2 cells, it is an unproved—yet testable—hypothesis that patients with allergies might have a diminished frequency of autoimmune diseases. In considering the pathogenesis of AIDS, an imbalance in favor of Th2 cells could accelerate premature death of Th1 cells.

The phenotype of the majority of T cells in rheumatoid synovium has been described previously. The dominating characteristic is a T cell with markers of a "helper" cell that is terminally differentiated, suggesting prolonged exposure to an antigen(s) in the tissue. However, there are other types of lymphocytes in the rheumatoid lesion. Each contributes its own characteristics to the immunologic mixture.

Cytolytic T Cells

Cytolytic T cells have the capacity to express products damaging to other cells. Two of these are granzyme A and perforin.

- *Granzyme A* is a protease that degrades target cell DNA.

- *Perforin* is a "molecular drill" that punches pores (20 nm) in cell membranes sufficient to destroy their integrity.

Using in situ hybridization, both CD4[+] and CD8[+] cells in rheumatoid synovial fluids were found to express granzyme A and perforin. Only cells from patients with severe active disease expressed these molecules; cells from immunosuppressed patients did not,[19] nor did cells from osteoarthritic synovial fluid. The target cells of cytolysis are not known, and the contribution that these cells may make to rheumatoid synovitis is not known.

Emphasizing the heterogeneity, and therefore the possible cross-talk, among cells found in synovium are data showing that cells with **natural killer (NK) cell** phenotypes[20] were almost three times more common in peripheral blood from rheumatoid patients compared with controls, and were twofold higher in synovial fluid than peripheral blood. There is a direct correlation of the NK cells with duration of disease, although not with activity of inflammation. The NK cells are in part activated by and proliferate in response to IL-12 generated by macrophages.

T-Cell Receptor $\gamma\delta$ Cells

One other subset of T cells must be considered in sorting out the roles for lymphocytes in rheumatoid

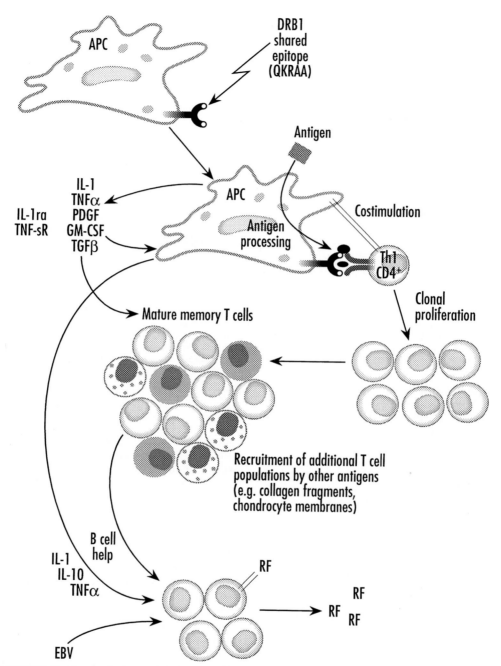

FIGURE 5–6. The complex interaction of an antigen (or superantigen) with a dendritic cell (e.g., B cell), its processing, and subsequent presentation to Th1 CD4$^+$ cells along with co-stimulatory molecular interaction leads to clonal proliferation of antigen-specific as well as additional clones of T cells that become involved much as innocent bystanders of the immune process. Macrophages and fibroblasts, including APCs, generate cytokines (and inhibitors of cytokines) that accelerate the T-cell response and help proliferation of B cells (including those programmed to synthesize rheumatoid factor [RF]). Epstein-Barr virus (EBV), although perhaps not involved in initiation of the immune process, can accelerate polyclonal B-cell proliferation.

arthritis: the TCR $\gamma\delta$ cell group. The γ and δ chains replace the α and β chains in the TCR. Morphologically, these $\gamma\delta$ T cells often resemble large granular lymphocytes.[12] Without α or β polypeptides, they do not have clear MHC restriction but can be activated by superantigens. Dendritic cells (APCs) alone, but not monocytes, can activate these T cells without antigen; however, such activation is highly dependent on the presence of the accessory molecule CD28 as well as molecules such as CD2 and CD11a that mediate cell-cell adhesion.[21] CD28 molecules are expressed on nearly all CD4+ T cells, the majority of CD8+ T cells, and about half of circulating $\gamma\delta$ T cells. The counter-receptor for CD28 on dendritic cells, activated B cells, or activated monocytes is the B7-1 (CD80) molecule. Dependency for activation by T cells on the expression of CD28 is about twofold greater for $\gamma\delta$ cells than for α/β cells.

$\gamma\delta$ T cells could have a primary role, or one only of amplification of the immune response in this rheumatoid arthritis. They represent 5 to 20 per cent of synovial T cells in this disease.[22] Although $\gamma\delta$ T cells are lower in frequency in blood of rheumatoid arthritis patients compared with controls, they are increased in synovial membranes[23,24] and utilize an unusual (and not yet characterized) clonotype receptor.[24] There are data to suggest that they migrate through capillary endothelium better than the α/β cells (see Chapter 7).

Which of these lymphocyte populations is the principle driver of the rheumatoid synovitis? Most bets should be on the CD4+ helper/inducer with α/β receptor configuration that binds in a heterotrimeric configuration with an antigen or superantigen and the DR alleles carrying the shared epitope. The activation of the T-cell clones that follows leads to an expanded immune response to ''bystander'' antigens, superantigens reactive with $\gamma\delta$ cells, cytokine production, B-cell activation, and sustained inflammation.

Importance of T Cells in Initiation and Sustenance of Rheumatoid Synovitis

It is illogical to allocate to a single cell type the responsibility for rheumatoid arthritis. Macrophages, with their vigorous production of cytokines easily identified in rheumatoid synovium, certainly are involved.[25] Similarly, the argument can be made appropriately that synovial lining cells proliferating to form a bulky pannus that becomes a factory producing destructive proteases and cytokines are the principal cause of cartilage destruction.[26]

Lymphocytes do not produce as many potent growth factors and enzymes as do macrophages and synovial cells, but it is likely that without them rheumatoid arthritis would not be initiated. Some experiments in humans and in nature confirm this:

- Individuals with rheumatoid arthritis who contract AIDS have virtually complete remission of their arthritis.
- Patients with rheumatoid arthritis given therapy directed against lymphocytes, ranging from thoracic duct drainage to specific antibodies against T cell membrane proteins, have had alleviation—albeit partial and transient—of symptoms (see Chapter 32).
- Thymectomy in chickens (leaving B cells intact but abolishing T cells) inhibits development of experimental arthritis.[27]
- Functional T cells are essential for initiation of collagen-induced arthritis.[28]
- T cells in rheumatoid synovium show evidence of activation and terminal differentiation into memory cells (see earlier).
- The association of rheumatoid arthritis with particular *HLA-DR* alleles implies that MHC class II–restricted T cells are involved in pathogenesis.

Despite this compilation of evidence, it has remained a difficult challenge to identify antigen-specific T cells in rheumatoid disease.[29] First of all, the antigen is not known, and in diseases such as leprosy and leishmaniasis, in which the causative antigens are both known and characterized, less than 2 per cent of lymphocytes in skin lesions are antigen specific. Buried amid many reactive but bystander lymphocytes in each rheumatoid patient is possibly a clone of lymphocytes reactive to a primary antigen in that patient, but finding it (see later) will be difficult if not impossible.

It is highly likely that identification and obliteration of T cells reactive with the primal causative agent in rheumatoid arthritis could be effective therapy. For this reason, and because identification of the specific reactive T cells would permit identification of the antigen they bind, the quest for clonally reactive CD4+ cells in rheumatoid synovium continues.

Essential Co-stimulation during T-Cell Activation

Co-stimulation during T-cell activation is essential for clonal proliferation.[30] This statement is generated by evidence that engagement of the TCR of naive resting cells with their ligand in the absence

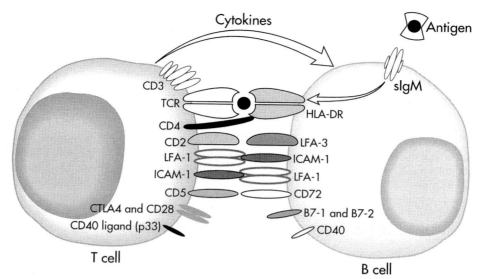

FIGURE 5–7. Graphic representation of the numerous molecules that must be considered ''co-stimulatory'' in the activation of T cells by an APC, in this case a B cell. Without effective links of these molecules, T cells are not activated by antigen. Each is important in its own right for other reasons, some of which are detailed in other portions of the text. (Modified from Lipsky, P. E., Davis, L. S., Meek, K., and Wacholtz, M. C.: T cells and B cells. *In* Kelley, W. N., Harris, E. D. Jr., Ruddy, S. and Sledge, C. B. [eds.]: Textbook of Rheumatology, 4th ed., Vol. 1. Philadelphia, W. B. Saunders, 1993, pp. 108–154. Used by permission.)

of a co-stimulatory signal leads to T cell tolerance and cell death by apoptosis rather than to proliferation.[31] T-cell activation within the joint requires at least two signals: (1) the interaction of the TCR with antigen presented by the MHC, and (2) interaction of accessory molecules on the APCs and lymphocytes. Presentation of antigen to T cells by APCs without co-stimulation results in anergy. The data indicate that numerous molecules on the surfaces of APCs and lymphocytes are essential for full activation of T cells and production of IL-2 and its receptor.[30,32] Important co-stimulatory molecules are listed here and illustrated in Figure 5–7. It must be emphasized that numerous cytokines, including IL-1, IL-6, IL-8, and IL-12, have co-stimulatory roles in lymphocyte activation. In addition, the activation system has significant redundancy; several co-stimulatory molecules can accomplish the same tasks. Having stated this, it nevertheless remains likely that the B7/CD28/CTLA–4 molecules are the major co-stimulatory factors essential for proliferation of T cells.

- **B7-1 (CD80), B7-2 (CD86), CD28, and CTLA–4:** B7-1 and B7–2, expressed on B cells, monocytes, and dendritic cells, are counter-receptors for CD28 and its structural homologue CTLA–4 on T lymphocytes. B7-1 is expressed on activated, not resting, cells, whereas B7-2 is expressed on some resting cells. As mentioned

earlier, B7-1 may enhance Th1 CD4$^+$ lymphocyte development, whereas B7-2 may diminish Th1 cell maturation, perhaps by enhancing Th2 cell development. B7-2 is the earlier expressed and dominant influence on preventing anergy after antigen presentation to T cells.

Interesting work has been done on the CD28 molecule and its possible role in rheumatoid arthritis through generating immune dysregulation. CD28 is expressed on the majority of CD4$^+$ T cells and on about half of the CD8$^+$ cells in humans. In patients with active rheumatoid arthritis, there are diminished numbers of CD28$^+$CD8$^+$ T cells in the circulation, suggesting that these cytotoxic cells have homed to the inflamed joint.[33] Immunohistochemical studies show macrophage-like cells positive for B7-2 surrounding CD28$^+$ cells in lymphoid aggregates in rheumatoid synovium.[34] B7-1 and B7-2 bind with CTLA-4, a surface glycoprotein on T cells that is a close relative of CD28. However, CTLA-4 is not a functional alternative to CD28. Using antibody against CTLA-4, it has been shown that this molecule has opposing effects to CD28.[35] There is dynamic competition between CD28 and CTLA-4. It may be that when low levels of B7 are expressed on APCs, the inhibitory effect of CTLA-4 is dominant, whereas at higher levels of B7 expression by dendritic cells or activated B cells, the co-stimulation by CD28 becomes dominant.

- **LFA-3:** This molecule binds to the CD2 receptor on T cells and augments specific signaling through the TCR-associated antigen CD2.
- **ICAM-1 (CD-54) and ICAM-2:** These molecules are counter-receptors for LFA-1 (CD11b/CD18) and CD43.
- **VCAM–1:** This inducible adhesion molecule found on endothelial cells binds to the VLA-4 receptor on T cells.
- **αVβ3:** This integrin (the vitronectin receptor) functions as a co-stimulatory molecule for IL-4 production in γ/δ T cells.
- **CD40:** This molecule and its counter receptor co-stimulate B cell, macrophage, endothelial cell, and T cell activation. Expressed transiently on T and B cells, it may help CD28-B7 in overcoming inhibitory forces of CTLA-4 on T-cell activation and clonal expression.
- **CD44:** Expression of this receptor is markedly increased on synovial fluid T lymphocytes of rheumatoid patients relative to their peripheral blood T cells.[36] Because CD44 is a receptor for hyaluronan, and because hyaluronan is a major component of synovial fluid, this may implicate CD44 as a ''homing'' receptor for lymphocytes.

Synovial fluid has been considered the mirror of what is happening in the synovium. Supporting this concept is the finding of an increased expression of the accessory molecule B7-1 on mononuclear cells in synovial fluid of rheumatoid patients compared with cells in their peripheral blood.[37] These data raise the possibility that the synovial fluid may be generating its own immune response system in rheumatoid arthritis. For example, B cells, which comprise only 1 to 5 per cent of most synovial fluid samples, nevertheless are very capable of capturing antigens on surface immunoglobulins for presentation to T cells. B cells expressing high-affinity surface immunoglobulin specific for self-immunoglobulin (rheumatoid factor) are present in rheumatoid synovial fluids[38] and may actively present these self-peptides to autoreactive T cells in the synovial fluid. Unknown is whether T cells activated within the synovial fluid can re-enter the synovium to join the organized cellular immune response there.

The absence of co-stimulating molecules on APCs also leads to unresponsiveness of T cells to subsequent stimulation and possible apoptosis. However, it is likely that activated T cells in rheumatoid synovium can receive co-stimulatory signals from bystander cells that have not presented antigen.[39] Similarly, because some activated T cells can proliferate in response to B7 in the absence of

a TCR ligand,[40] a self-sustaining cycle of T-cell proliferation in the absence of a specific antigen could be generated in the rheumatoid synovium. Simultaneous ligation of CD5 and CD28 by use of a monoclonal antibody induced T-cell activation in the absence of TCR/CD3 occupancy,[41] and, in a converse experiment, synovial fluid T-cell proliferation was inhibited by anti-CD5 antibodies.[42,43] Addition of rheumatoid synovial fluid to T cells being stimulated with IL-2 markedly enhanced T-cell proliferation, a phenomenon that suggests a process of co-stimulation.[44]

As an index of the activated state of T cells in rheumatoid synovium, it has been observed that 30 per cent of T cells in these tissues react with anti-B7 monoclonal antibody, as did a significant number of synovial fluid T cells. The importance of these data is that they suggest that purified synovial fluid T cells could function as APCs and co-stimulators of other resting T cells. This could be considered autocrine stimulation,[45] and possibly could bypass antigenic stimulation.

Cellular Mechanisms of Anergy

Without co-stimulation, few T cells can be activated sufficiently to begin clonal expansion and IL-2 production; this is the state of anergy. The direct cause of anergy is failure of the transcription factor activator protein 1 (AP-1) to activate the IL-2 gene. By working backward from this step, it has been found that there is failure of activation of the Ras signaling pathway[46] upon T cell stimulation. Ras is a product of the *ras* oncogene and is widely used to control growth and differentiation in many cells. Without Ras expression, mitogen activation of protein kinases (ERK-1 and ERK-2) and $p21^{ras}$ do not occur. This effectively blocks both the direct TCR/CD3 pathway and the co-stimulatory CD28 pathway. Both must be turned on to activate *fas* and *jun*, leading to generation of AP-1.

THE PROGRAMMED DEATH OF CELLS: APOPTOSIS

Were it not for programmed death of cells (apoptosis), regulation of many functions in our bodies would be in disarray. In synovium, for example, lining cells would expand the joint space. Unregulated chondrocyte proliferation would generate osteoarthritis-like excrescences even in chil-

TABLE 5–1. Key Differences Between Apoptosis and Necrosis

	NECROSIS	APOPTOSIS
Induction	Pathologic	Physiologic or pathologic
Cell appearance	Swollen	Shrunken
New RNA/protein synthesis	No	Frequent
Release of nucleosomes	No	Yes
Inflammation	Usual	No

From Elkon, K. B.: Defects in apoptosis as a cause of systemic autoimmunity. Cliniguide Rheum. Dis. 4(3):1, 1994. Used by permission.

dren, and inflammation in the joint, once started, would never stop until pus accumulated in the synovial fluid and mononuclear infiltrates in the synovium resembled plasmacytomas. In other tissues and the bone marrow, serious defects in apoptosis can lead to immortality in clones of cells and be manifested as malignancy.

The Process of Apoptosis in Lymphocytes

Before analyzing apoptosis, it is important to underscore the differences between *apoptosis* and *necrosis* of cells. These are summarized in Table 5–1.

Necrosis ends by the cell membrane becoming permeable. Water flows into the cytoplasm, causing irreversible swelling. It usually accompanies inflammation or ischemia, and after a necrotic death the fragments of cell nuclei are often visible. In contrast, the apoptotic cell is shrunken, with condensed nuclei. Neighboring cells phagocytose the dead or dying cell and no residual is apparent in normal tissues. There is no accompanying inflammation.[47]

Numerous molecules within and exterior to the cell influence survival of the cell. Cytokines such as IL-1, IL-2, IL-4, and growth factors enhance survival. Viral infections, including EBV, can generate proteins that interfere with apoptosis.[48] The CD40 ligand that is transiently expressed on T cells binds to CD40R on B cells and activates differentiation, including expression of *bcl-2*, a mitochondrial proto-oncogene that promotes B cell survival (Fig. 5–8). The *bcl-2* gene product may work by repressing oxygen free radical formation and intracellular oxidation,[49] thereby protecting cells from suicide. The gene product also blocks cell death caused by gamma irradiation. IL-10 appears to induce *Bcl-2* expression.

In contrast, apoptosis is encouraged or accelerated by external stimuli that cause excessive DNA strand breaks (e.g., ionizing radiation, toxic oxygen radicals, and alkylating agents). High doses of glu-

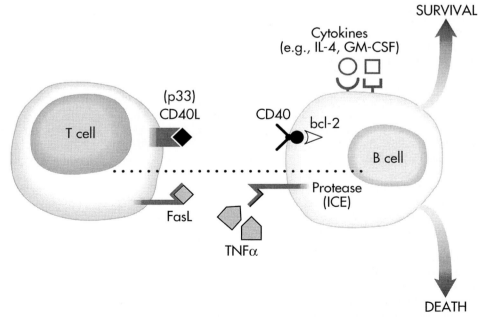

FIGURE 5–8. Apoptosis or survival of a cell is governed by numerous molecules within and outside cells. In the example portrayed here, the binding of CD40 and its ligand (CD40L/p33) induces expression of *bcl-2*, a proto-oncogene that promotes cell survival. In contrast, if the cell surface Fas receptor is activated by Fas ligand similar to TNFx, IL-1–converting enzyme (ICE) is expressed, leading to apoptosis.

cocorticoids cause a rapid lysis by apoptosis in lymphocytes.

A cell-surface receptor named Fas, a member of the TNF/CD40/nerve growth factor type I plasma membrane receptor family, is an apoptosis polypeptide, and studies in the MRL *lpr/lpr* mouse have indicated that a mutation in Fas is responsible for the lymphoproliferative aspects of this diseased animal[50] (see later). A protein homologous to TNFα (FasL) is a ligand for the Fas receptor. This Fas ligand is a type II transmembrane protein. Fas/FasL binding may be important in the action of cytolytic T cells on their targets. Interestingly, three children have been described who have lymphoproliferative disorders and autoimmunity associated with a deletion in the gene encoding Fas.[51] Fas-mediated apoptosis was defective in their T cells, and their cells proliferated without regulation or programmed cell death.

A very specific example of apoptotic deletion is idiopathic CD4$^+$ lymphocytopenia. In this condition, not associated with HIV infection, the following abnormalities have been reported[52]:

- Accelerated programmed cell death was associated with T cell receptor cross-linking.
- There was enhanced expression of Fas and Fas ligand in unstimulated CD4$^+$ cell populations.
- Apoptosis was suppressed by inhibitors (e.g., tamoxifen) of calcium-dependent endonucleases and proteases.

In a transgenic animal model for rheumatoid arthritis (HTLV-1 *tax*), it has been shown that anti-Fas, which activated the Fas receptor, induced apoptosis in synovium and a remission of paw swelling (Fujisawa, et al., Abstract 1328). Also, a homologue of the proto-oncogene *bcl-2* encodes IL-1β–converting enzyme (ICE), which functions to catalyze generation of active IL-1β from its inactive proform. ICE also provokes apoptosis in a counter-regulatory mode from *bcl-2*.[47,53,54]

Central Regulation of Lymphocyte Development

In the thymus, the fate of maturing T lymphocytes can take one of three courses (Fig. 5–9)[47]:

1. Negative selection: Self-reactive T cells bind with high affinity to self-antigens . . . and are promptly induced to die.
2. Default death: Those "neglected" cells that do not bind to antigen disappear by an apoptotic default pathway.
3. Positive selection: For thymocytes that bind with low affinity to self-antigens, death is spared.

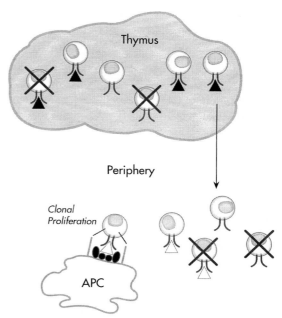

FIGURE 5–9. Regulation of T-cell development in the thymus and in the periphery. In the thymus, three fates await developing T cells: (1) they bind with high affinity to self-antigens, a process that induces apoptosis; (2) they do not bind antigen and become apoptotic by default; or (3) they bind with low affinity to self-antigens and migrate to the periphery. In the circulation, similar opportunities await: (1) neglected cells die; (2) cells presented with antigen but with insufficient co-stimulation become apoptotic (true anergy); and (3) T cells presented with antigen and co-stimulatory molecules proliferate in response to IL-2. (Adapted from Elkon, K.B. Defects in apoptosis as a cause of systemic autoimmunity. Cliniguide Rheum. Dis. 4[3]:1, 1994. Used by permission.)

They are rescued from apoptosis and migrate to the peripheral circulation and lymph nodes.

Peripheral Regulation of Lymphocytes

After emerging from the thymus, T lymphocytes circulate for several days, even weeks. Then they have one of several fates:

1. Default death of resting cells: Neglected cells, ones that are not activated by antigen or superantigen, undergo an apoptotic death.
2. Apoptosis of activated cells: These are activated cells that have a limited life, undergoing apoptosis because the death signals overwhelm the survival ones, particularly if they are not retriggered by antigen or if co-stimulatory factors and cytokines are not present. This apoptotic death helps minimize the risk of binding of self-antigens and

subsequent autoimmunity. Fas is highly expressed on activated peripheral lymphocytes.

3. Clonal proliferation: After initial activation—if antigen, cytokines such as IL-2, and costimulatory factors such as CD28/CTLA-4 and B7-1 are all present—the particular clones of lymphocytes proliferate, expand, and initiate an immune response with activation of B cells.

The Relevance of Apoptosis to Rheumatoid Arthritis

The MRL *lpr/lpr* mouse strain has a defect in the extracellular domain of the *fas* gene that leads to a defect in apoptosis, allowing T cells to become autoimmune (Fig. 5–10). The gene defect produces an insertion of an extra 180 base pairs that is homologous with a retroviral transposon.[50,55] The phenotype of the affected mice is one of lymphoproliferation of T cells, arthritis, autoantibody formation, and vasculitis. These animals lose neonatal tolerance to superantigens such as staphylococcal enterotoxin B, a phenomenon mediated by TNFα.[56,57] A leading hypothesis is that, because of the defect in apoptosis, a small number of self-reactive T cells escape from the thymus of *lpr/lpr* mice, expand in the periphery, and become pathologically self-reactive.[58]

In several cleverly designed experiments, a DNA construct was formed of the normal *fas* gene plus a *CD2* minigene that has a tropism for T cells. The construct was injected into *lpr/lpr* embryos. Subse-

quently, normal Fas could be demonstrated in T cells of the lymph nodes and thymus. These "genetically corrected" mice developed no adenopathy, anti-DNA, kidney disease, or synovitis with lining cell hyperplasia, indicating the abnormal *fas* gene caused this autoimmune disease with arthritis.[58]

There is no evidence that abnormal *fas* is responsible for manifestations of rheumatoid arthritis, but the possibility that a cytokine similar to TNFα may be the ligand for the Fas receptor indicates that anti-TNF therapies may have major effects upon immune cell development as well as on other cytokine formation and protease production. In addition, in animals, protection from Fas-mediated apoptosis has been brought about in cell lines by a soluble form of the Fas molecule,[59] presumably by competitive inhibition.

Apoptotic death of rheumatoid synovial cells in culture has been demonstrated.[60] *c-fos*, one of the proto-oncogenes involved in induction of apoptosis, is activated in rheumatoid synovial cells and has been implicated in the induction of metalloproteases by these cells. An unusual overexpression of p53, a tumor suppressor gene, has been demonstrated in rheumatoid synovium.[61a] This could be in response to excessive DNA damage, or be associated with diminished or defective apoptosis.[61a]

NATURE OF ANTIGENS PRESENTED TO T CELLS

Data are accumulating that the contribution of disease-linked HLA-DR molecules is associated with their role in helping to form the TCR repertoire in addition to their role as primary determinants of which (or how) antigenic peptides will be presented to T cells by HLA class II molecules.[61] Thus there is good logic in comparing synovial and peripheral TCR repertoires in rheumatoid arthritis patients in search of dominant clonotypes that would specifically bind an arthritogenic peptide of a certain conformation.

While searching for antigens that could trigger rheumatoid arthritis, it is first essential to know the limits of molecular size of possible peptides that can be presented by HLA-DR molecules. The size can vary between 13 and 25 amino acid residues,[62] and these can be derived from endogenously produced proteins such as those of the MHC itself as well as exogenous ones.[63] Given this variability, contrasted with the precise regulation of TCR binding by the MHC, it is likely that the shared epitope on *DRB1* chains exerts its major effects by controlling binding of the MHC-antigen complex to the TCR. The TCR must recognize a specific confor-

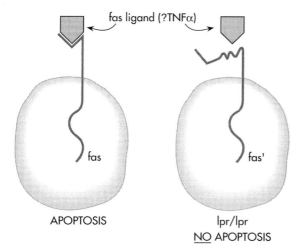

fas ligand (?TNFα)

fas

fas'

APOPTOSIS

lpr/lpr
NO APOPTOSIS

FIGURE 5–10. The genetic lesion of the MRL *lpr/lpr* mouse is one that results in insertion of an extra 180 bp in the extracellular Fas receptor. This prevents it from binding ligand, and apoptosis does not occur to an extent sufficient to regulate proliferation of lymphocytes.

mation formed by both the class II MHC molecule and the antigen, not just the antigen alone.

Of the total number of MHC molecules presented on the surface of an APC, only 0.1 per cent need be complexed with antigen in order for T-cell stimulation to occur.[63,64] However, because homozygosity for certain DR molecules does select for disease severity and extra-articular manifestations in rheumatoid arthritis,[61] the density of the MHC molecules on the APCs must have some importance.

Superantigens

Another type of antigen presented by the class II MHC molecules on APCs are referred to as superantigens. Superantigens are bacterial, viral, or retroviral proteins that can activate (or delete) a large number of T-cell clones.[65] All superantigens have a similar structure. In contrast to the classical antigen recognition during which a peptide processed intracellularly is presented to T cells by MHC molecules, with help from CD4 or CD8 and other co-stimulatory molecules, superantigens are unprocessed, larger molecules that cross-link the

CDR4 region of the V_β chain of the TCR with an edge of the α chain of MHC class II molecules at a site external to the antigen-binding groove of the MHC molecules (Fig. 5–11). There is evidence that association of a superantigen with the MHC class II proteins precludes the T cell from recognizing or binding to an antigen that may already be bound in the polymorphic peptide binding groove of the MHC. One superantigen may actually bridge across two class II molecules, essentially cross-linking them. Whereas in the classical MHC-restricted T-cell response, 1 in 100,000 T cells can be activated by one particular antigen-MHC complex, superantigens can activate as many as 1 in 10 T cells.[66,67] This promiscuous capability is possible because the superantigen interacts with the CDR4 of several different TCR V_β chains, thereby amplifying greatly the opportunities for binding. Most superantigens bind two or three different V_β chains in different TCRs.

In addition, it appears that there is no requirement for accessory molecules on the T cell for foreign superantigen stimulation, unlike T-cell recog-

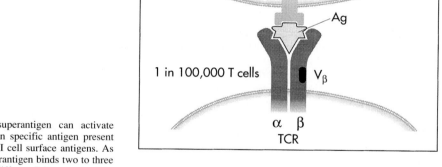

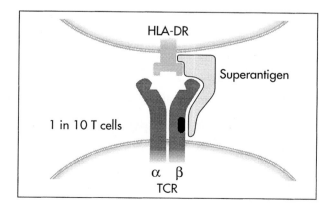

FIGURE 5–11. A single superantigen can activate 10,000-fold more T cells than specific antigen present in context of the HLA class II cell surface antigens. As described in the text, the superantigen binds two to three different V_β chains in several different TCR outside of the tightly fitted TCR-MHC link. Another factor in enhancing superantigen activation power is that the superantigens have little if any need for co-stimulatory molecule interactions.[59,60]

nition of conventional antigen-MHC complexes. A major effect of this stimulation of multiple T-cell clones is induction of large quantities of cytokines such as TNFα that produce the clinical syndromes of toxic shock and food poisoning in acute situations. It is speculated that if superantigens are involved in rheumatoid arthritis, their numbers (and therefore their clinical impact) would lead to a sustained and chronic rather than an acute clinical picture.

The most studied of foreign superantigens are staphylococcal and streptococcal enterotoxins. These are small basic proteins ranging in size from 25 to 30 kDa. They have a strong binding affinity for the MHC class II molecules (in the nanomolar range). Other known and characterized superantigens include proteins found in *Mycoplasma arthritidis, Yersinia pseudotuberculosis*, mouse mammary tumor virus, and *Mycobacterium tuberculosis*. Even small mutations in superantigens, such as the staphylococcal endotoxin B, destroy their capacity to induce cytokine production and clinical disease. When ingested by mouth, the superantigens appear to gain access to the bloodstream by transcytosis, absorption within clathrin-coated pits in intestinal epithelium through a facilitated (receptor-mediated?) process.

Depending on the amount of superantigen, the duration of its persistence in tissues, and its affinity for TCRs, these elements can have effects of clonal expansion or cytotoxicity, or deletion and anergy. It is common that following superantigen stimulation a number of T-cell clones expand and then undergo apoptosis and decline in numbers.[68]

The discovery of these superantigens that can induce polyclonal antibody responses and activate many different T cells, possibly including autoreactive ones, has potential relevance for understanding early events in pathogenesis of autoimmune diseases. One hypothesis is that a microbe with components that have composition (and perhaps conformational similarities) close to those of certain host protein sequences could infect a person and activate host cells with sufficient power to break tolerance to a crucial autoantigen. A more appealing alternative is that the superantigen need not be a molecular mimic, but, by its capability to activate many clones of T cells expressing millions of different antigen specificities, autoreactive cells might be activated.

Superantigens in Rheumatoid Arthritis?

Data supporting the association of superantigens and rheumatoid arthritis are meager. It is intriguing, however, that synovial fibroblasts (type B cells) from rheumatoid synovium, in the presence of IFNγ (which can induce MHC class II proteins in these cells), can present staphylococcal superantigen to T cells. This adds another cell type to those others (e.g., dendritic cells and macrophages) that can present antigen to immunocytes in the potpourri of inflammatory synovitis.[69]

T-CELL SELECTION AND BIAS IN RHEUMATOID ARTHRITIS

Because the TCR repertoire is determined by particular V_β elements, it has been logical to search for restricted use of V_β genes in the TCRs of rheumatoid patients. Crucial to understanding the pathogenesis of rheumatoid arthritis is determining whether activated synovial T cells are polyclonal (perhaps activated by a superantigen) or oligoclonal (expanded in response to a specific antigen). The evidence is strong that there are clonally expanded T cells in rheumatoid arthritis. A controversy, however, lies in whether it is a nonspecific polyclonal or monoclonal/oligoclonal specific activation. Newer technology may help us resolve this problem. Using a sequence enrichment nuclease[70] that eliminates infrequent DNA sequences from a population of cells, T-cell clonal expansion can be demonstrated in both synovial fluid and peripheral blood from rheumatoid arthritis.

There have been numerous problems facing investigators looking for possible T-cell clonal selection in rheumatoid arthritis. One is that activated T cells, in the absence of sufficient coactivating factors, may be deleted through apoptosis not long after being activated. Another is that the techniques used by some investigators for sufficient expansion of T cells in vitro to assay them for V_β elements may induce selective artifacts; the cells that expand in response to anti-CD3 or IL-2, for instance, may not be the relevant T cells for rheumatoid arthritis. A third is that, unless cells from tissue fluid in very early rheumatoid arthritis are examined, the expanded populations of T cells may represent a secondary and nonspecific expansion rather than a primary one.

A number of reports have shown little or no TCR polymorphism (i.e., no dominant clones) in patients with rheumatoid arthritis.[71–75] Other studies have focused upon DNA sequence analysis of CDR3 regions of the V_β chains because of the increasing suggestions from many data that T cells recognize antigen not as antigen alone but as a complex with the MHC. These investigations have provided evidence for selective expansion of synovial T lymphocytes in rheumatoid arthritis. The data are summarized by one paper as follows:

> Although the specific target antigens involved in rheumatoid arthritis have yet to be identified, the specific clonal and/or oligoclonal outgrowth of T lymphocytes and shared amino acid distribution patterns in the CDR3 regions of multiple TCR rearrangements in individual patients suggest that there is a specific response to antigens present at the site of inflammation. These observations suggest that the disease is antigen driven and that a focus on the CDR3 region of the TCR can provide a means for selective analysis of antigen-reactive T cells in the joint.[76]

It is appropriate to review the data showing that T cells reactive with the disease-associated HLA-DR structure are *not* selected at random. In one study that stimulated much work by others,[77] $V_\beta14^+$ T cells were found to be over-represented in synovial fluid but decreased in peripheral blood. The inference was that a superantigen activated $V_\beta14^+$ cells, and then all except those cells responding to a specific antigen within the joint were deleted. These data have not been confirmed in another study, but the hypothesis is a reasonable one.[78]

Others[79] have found that TCR V_β elements were limited; as many as 43 per cent of T-cell clones from four patients expressed $V_\beta6$, and DNA analysis indicated that only a few members of the $V_\beta6$ gene family were used. In other work from the same center (J. J. Goronzy, unpublished data, 1995), identical T-cell clones were prominent in synovium and peripheral blood from the same patients. The V_β elements varied; however, $V_\beta3.3$ and $V_\beta17$ were more often found. Some studies have shown an association between HLA-DR4 and $V_\beta8$ TCR genes,[80] but in relatively small numbers. In another study, a slight decrease in $V_\beta13.2$ in peripheral blood compared with synovial cells was found, and an increased usage in synovial T cells was demonstrated for $V_\beta14$, $V_\beta6$, and $V_\beta15$.[64]

In one of the only studies indicating a uniform clonal prominence in all rheumatoid patients, $V_\beta17^+$ T cells were increased in the peripheral blood and synovial fluid of rheumatoid patients (analyzed by monoclonal antibodies to the V_β chains).[81] It is intriguing that $V_\beta17$, $V_\beta3$, and $V_\beta14$, each found to be increased in one or more studies of lymphocytes from rheumatoid patients, are all members of subgroup IV of lymphocytes, based on sequence homologies in an area (CDR4) thought to have a major role in binding of superantigens.

Twin studies should be able to provide information about V_β gene usage. One monozygotic twin study[82] has shown that there was a marked similarity in the TCR V_β gene repertoires between identical twins, whether or not they were concordant or discordant for rheumatoid arthritis. In contrast, T lymphocytes of the γ/δ subclass have TCR V_γ repertoires that are extremely diverse, even in twins who were concordant for rheumatoid arthritis.[83] If we can assume that the functional TCR V_γ repertoire is determined by (1) inherited gene segments of the TCR, (2) the TCR recombination patterns, and (3) positive and negative selection, V_γ chains all should be identical in monozygotic twins. Because they are not, post-thymic selection in the environment for TCR V_γ must be dictated by factors not under strict genetic control.

A possible explanation for these conflicting data is as follows. Very early in the synovitis of rheumatoid arthritis, there is indeed a restricted clonal proliferation of lymphocytes with specific TCR construction dictated by the V_β chains. After initiating the immune response, however, nonspecific recruitment of T cells occurs, and activation of multiple clones by superantigens may occur. In addition, cells activated without sufficient co-stimulatory factors may undergo apoptosis. In the ensuing proliferative cellular response, the instigator T cells are diluted out or die away, and thus remain essentially anonymous.

Future studies of TCR specificity in rheumatoid arthritis, therefore, must focus on patients with early disease; the T-cell repertoire found later may be significantly different. In one attempt to do this, freshly isolated T cells from inflamed (but not end-stage) synovial fluids of seven patients with rheumatoid arthritis were analyzed without expansion in vitro and found to have consistent increases of $V_\beta2$ and $V_\beta6$ usage in CD4$^+$ cells compared with peripheral blood, and decreased use of $V_\beta13.1$ and $V_\beta13.2$.[84] This work supports the hypothesis that some type of antigen selection process occurs in those synovia within the CD4$^+$, MHC class II–restricted T-cell population. If there were indications that one or another antigen were ''arthritogenic'' in humans, they could be tested for their ability to induce in vitro a V_β bias similar to that found in vivo.

The evidence that, over a period of 1 year, the frequencies of clonally expanded $V_\beta17^+$ CD4$^+$ T cells fluctuated widely, and that there were independent variations in the frequencies of two distinct clonotypes in the same patient, indicates that mechanisms other than stimulation by a single arthritogenic antigen were driving proliferation of these clones, although the data do not rule out the possibility that the process was triggered initially by one antigen.[85]

One of the most recent studies on this topic involved eight patients whose synovial fluid was aspirated within the first year of symptoms and who later developed unequivocal rheumatoid arthritis.[86] Only one patient had received nonsteroidal anti-inflammatory drugs; none had been given gold, D-penicillamine, methotrexate, or corticosteroids. Of the seven patients in whom HLA-DRB analysis was done, five carried either the *HLA-DR1* or *HLA-DR4* haplotype. TCR V_α and V_β of all cells in the fluid were amplified by reverse transcriptase–PCR, and those products were identified by using oligonucleotide probes. TCR $V_\alpha 17$ gene elements were preferentially used in seven of the eight patients. V_β usage was more heterogeneous. These data indicate that in early stages of rheumatoid arthritis an oligoclonal or even monoclonal T-cell population is found in affected joints. The authors of the study closed their discussion with the following reasonable hypothesis:

Therefore, our data clearly support the idea of an antigen-driven immune response. Whether this antigen is a conventional antigen or a superantigen has yet to be determined. It is tempting to speculate that during a primary immune response to an as-yet-unknown antigen, the TCR $V_\alpha 17$ T cell population was activated, and that in the course of this immune response, cytokines such as IL-8 and monocyte chemotactic protein were released, and induced the accumulation and activation of inflammatory cells in the affected joints. Destruction of cartilage by enzymes and oxygen radicals, released by activated granulocytes and macrophages, then led to the exposure of a variety of formerly hidden antigens or epitopes in the immune system, which resulted in a secondary polyclonal T cell immune response to these antigens. Whether TCR $V_\alpha 17$ T cells from the oligoclonal primary immune response also contribute to the perpetuation of disease has yet to be clarified.

T-Cell Receptor CDR3 Analyses

In addition to study of V region usage, it is possible now to focus study on the CDR3 region, which interacts directly with the peptide presented in the MHC groove. A number of sequence determinations of the CDR3 region in lymphocytes from rheumatoid patients reveal strong evidence for selective expansion of synovial T cells.[76,87] This is additional support for the hypothesis that the disease is antigen driven, and that analyses of the CDR3 regions can help define target antigens in rheumatoid arthritis.[76]

Exploitation of T-Cell Receptor V_β Bias for Therapy

Later in this book (see Chapter 32), the possible and actual strategies for specific immunotherapy

for rheumatoid arthritis are discussed in detail. There are several observations from in vitro studies, however, that should stimulate continued search for T-cell clones stimulated early in the disease as well as the antigen(s) that trigger rheumatoid arthritis in order to develop antigen-specific immunomodulation. With what is known already about the shared epitope in the MHC, it has been demonstrated that "blocking" peptides for *HLA-DRB1*04* and *-DRB1*01* inhibit antigen-specific responses in multiclonal lymphocyte populations in both rheumatoid and control patients.[88] In a particularly intriguing study that has therapeutic implications,[89] it was shown that, when antigen complexed to HLA-DR1–bearing cells is presented to specific T cells, the antagonism of T-cell activation is two orders of magnitude more sensitive than by blockade of the MHC alone. Why? Probably because, whereas successful MHC blockade requires occupation of virtually 100 per cent of the DR molecules, less than 1 percent of MHC-analogue peptides are needed to block TCR activation.

Another useful approach will be to eliminate or inactivate T cells with selected CDR3 regions using peptide vaccination to elicit anti-idiotype immune responses, or by use of CDR3-based antisense oligonucleotides.

INTERLEUKIN–2 AND ITS RECEPTOR IN RHEUMATOID ARTHRITIS

Rheumatoid synovial T cells have a relative deficiency in IL-2 production and in their ability to suppress B-cell growth.[90] They appear to have partial anergy. Although they effectively provide B cell help, they have lost the capacity to down-regulate B-cell responses and they produce relatively little IL-2 or IFNγ.[91] The phenotype for these cells is CD45RB[dim], that of terminally differentiated T cells. It is possible that inhibitory factors found in the synovium (e.g., prostaglandin E_2, TGFβ)[15] contribute to their developing this differentiated state.

In this context, it is interesting that soluble IL-2 receptors (IL-2Rs) are significantly elevated in synovial fluid compared with serum levels.[92] The inference can be made that IL-2 production by the aggregate of T cells in rheumatoid synovium may be increased, whereas production measured on a per-cell basis is markedly decreased.

It is well known that when T lymphocytes are activated by stimulation of the TCR leading to clonal proliferation, the same and neighboring cells also express increased numbers of copies of the

IL-2R. Recently, genetically engineered mice have been produced that lack a functional IL-2R. These animals have increased numbers of B cells and plasma cells with increased IgG and IgE production and autoantibody formation. Depletion of CD4+ cells from these animals appeared to rescue the B-cell overdrive. Antigen-specific immune responses in these cells could not be elicited.[93] These data make it clear that, in addition to its role as a mediator of activation signals, the IL-2R has a central role in regulating T cells, and that an insufficient number of IL-2Rs on T cells could lead to autoimmune responses. There is no human model, of course, for IL-2R deficiency, but depletion of this receptor could enhance autoantibody formation.

CD8+ T cells normally do not make significant amounts of IL-2. In planning immune therapeutic strategies in rheumatoid arthritis, molecules such as B7-1/B7-2 could be introduced into synovium. Co-stimulated CD8+ cells might make enough IL-2 on their own to become fully activated and expand.[32] However, provision of additional co-stimulation might lead to proliferation of unwanted autoreactive clones of Th1 lymphocytes.

The weight of evidence suggests that biased V_β gene family utilization can be observed in different compartments (i.e., peripheral blood, synovial tissue, synovial fluid) of rheumatoid patients using unselected or expanded T cells. Although no known superantigen could account for enhancement or depletion of the particular V_β gene products that have been recorded, the collective data do support the hypothesis that a specific antigen or superantigen could be driving the activated T-cell response in the rheumatoid patients.

REFERENCES

1. Cush, J. J., Pietschmann, P., Oppenheimer-Marks, N., et al.: The intrinsic migratory capacity of memory T cells contributes to their accumulation in rheumatoid synovium. Arthritis Rheum. 35:1434, 1992.

   Synovial T cells are rich in CD4+ T cells bearing a "memory" phenotype: (CD45RO+, CD29bright) and increased density of adhesion molecules. In this study, T cells exhibiting a capacity for transendothelial migration were analyzed to determine phenotypes to compare with those found in synovium. T lymphocytes were added to endothelial cells cultured on collagen gel; nonadherent, bound, and migrating cells were recovered. In contrast to peripheral blood lymphocytes, rheumatoid arthritis synovial lymphocytes (CD45RA−) had decreased ($p < .05$) CD3 and L-selectin markers and increased CD29, CD11abright CD3+, HLA-DR+ markers. Naive CD4+ T cells (expressing CD45RA) bound poorly to endothelial cells and did not transmigrate. The poor expression of L-selectin by migratory cells is interesting; this molecule—important for trafficking of lymphocytes to lymph nodes—has no apparent role in migration of cells into synovium. These data support the premise that migratory capacity resulting from differentiation or activation status contributes to the accumulation of cells in the rheumatoid synovium.

2. Koch, A. E., Robinson, P. G., Radosevich, J. A., et al.: Distribution of CD45RA and CD45RO T-lymphocyte subsets in rheumatoid arthritis synovial tissue. J. Clin. Immunol. 10:192, 1990.

3. Thomas, R., Davis, L. S., and Lipsky, P. E.: Rheumatoid synovium is enriched in mature antigen-presenting dendritic cells. J. Immunol. 152:2613, 1994.

   Dendritic cells are potent APCs that take up, sequester, and present antigen to T cells in the primary and secondary immune responses. Using immunofluorescent cell sorting, populations of cells were separated from peripheral blood and rheumatoid synovium and fluid using the myeloid marker CD33 and the monocyte marker CD14 as follows:

   CD33+ CD14dim—dendritic cell precursors

   CD33+ CD14+—monocytes

   CD33− CD14−—B cells

   cD33+ CD14dim cells were enriched two- to fourfold in rheumatoid synovium and three- to eightfold in rheumatoid synovial fluid in the non–T cell population. In addition, the synovial fluid dendritic cell precursors, which did not phagocytose sheep red blood cells (in contrast to monocytes), more rapidly assumed a dendritic appearance in cell culture and were potent stimulators of autologous T cells. The dendritic cells expressed large amounts of adhesion molecules (i.e., ICAM-1 [CD54], LFA-3 [CD58], and B7 [BB1]). GM-CSF and TNFα enhanced dendritic cell stimulatory function. The data are consistent with the hypothesis that dendritic cells migrate to synovium from peripheral blood, and differentiate to potent APCs, perhaps after exposure to local cytokines or arthritogenic peptides.

4. Schumacher, H. R., and Kitridou, R. C.: Synovitis of recent onset: a clinicopathological study during the first month of disease. Arthritis Rheum. 15:465, 1972.

5. Kurosaka, M., and Ziff, M.: Immunoelectron microscopic study of the distribution of T cell subsets in rheumatoid synovium. J. Exp. Med. 158:1191, 1983.

6. Steinman, R. M.: The dendritic cell system and its role in immunogenicity. Annu. Rev. Immunol. 9:271, 1991.

7. Matthews, N., Emery, P., Pilling, D., et al.: Subpopulations of primed T helper cells in rheumatoid arthritis. Arthritis Rheum. 36:603, 1993.

   Primed T cells can be divided into two populations. CD4+ CD45RA+ cells produce high levels of IL-2 but no IL-4 or IFNγ, whereas primed CD45RO+ cells produce all three cytokines. The CD45 isoform subset in rheumatoid synovium was dominated by a highly selected population of cells (CD45RBdim), probably primed through many cycles of activation.

8. Oppenheimer-Marks, N., Davis, L. S., Bogue, D. T., et al.: Differential utilization of ICAM-1 and VCAM–1 during the adhesion and transendothelial migration of human T lymphocytes. J. Immunol. 147:2913, 1991.

9. Kohem, C. L., Brezinschek, R. I., Wisbey, H., et al.: Enrichment of differentiated CD45RBdim, CD27− memory T cells in the peripheral blood, synovial fluid, and synovial tissue of patients with rheumatoid arthritis. Arthritis Rheum. 39:844, 1996.

10. Camerini, D., Walz, G., Loenen, W. A., et al.: The T cell activation antigen CD27 is a member of the nerve growth factor/tumor necrosis factor receptor gene family. I. Immunol. 147:3165, 1991.

11. Pitzalis, C., Kingsley, G., Murphy, J., et al.: Abnormal distribution of the helper-inducer and suppressor-inducer T-lymphocyte subsets in the rheumatoid joint. Clin. Immunol. Immunopathol. 45:252, 1987.

12. Ferrini, S., Zarcone, D., Viale, M., et al.: Morphologic and functional characterization of human peripheral blood T cells expressing the T cell receptor γ/δ. Eur. J. Immunol. 19:1183, 1989.

13. Kohsaka, H., Chen, P. P., Taniguchi, A., et al.: Divergent T cell receptor γ repertoires in rheumatoid arthritis monozygotic twins. Arthritis Rheum. 36:213, 1993.

   This study was designed to discern how independent of genetic factors, rheumatoid arthritis changes the TCR Vγ repertoire. Activated cells (8 to 10 per cent of total) (HLA-DR$^+$) transcribed at least six times more TCR γ gene message than did DR$^-$ T cells without an associated increased frequency of TCR V$_\gamma$ genes.

14. Schwartz, R. H.: Acquisition of immunologic self-tolerance. Cell 57:1073, 1989.

15. Sambhara, S. R., and Miller, R. G.: Programmed cell death of T cells signaled by the T cell receptor and the $\alpha 3$ domain. Science 252:1424, 1991.

16. Bloom, B. R., Modlin, R. L., and Salgame, P.: Stigma variations: observations on suppressor T cells and leprosy. Annu. Rev. Immunol. 10:453, 1992.

17. Salgame, P., Modlin, R., and Bloom, B. R.: On the mechanism of human T cell suppression. Int. Immunol. 1:121, 1989.

18. Salgame, P. R., Abrams, J. S., Clayberger, C., et al.: Differing lymphokine profiles of functional subsets of human CD4 and CD8 T-cell clones. Science 254:279, 1991.

19. Griffiths, G. M., Alpert, S., Lambert, E., et al.: Perforin and granzyme A expression identifying cytolytic lymphocytes in rheumatoid arthritis. Proc. Natl. Acad. Sci. U.S.A. 89:549, 1992.

20. d'Angeac, A. P., Monier, S., Jorgensen, C., et al.: Increased percentage of CD3$^+$, CD57$^+$ lymphocytes in patients with rheumatoid arthritis. Arthritis Rheum. 36:608, 1993.

   CD57 (HNK1) is a 100-kDa glycoprotein found on NK cell membranes and small granular T cells. In peripheral blood of 26 rheumatoid arthritis patients, the percentage of CD3$^+$ cells that were also CD57$^+$ was 22 $\pm$ 3, compared with 8 $\pm$ 1 in controls. Most of the CD3$^+$ CD57$^+$ cells expressed the CD8 molecule and almost no HLA-DR; they were CD45RA$^+$ (resting cells) (80 per cent), and 85 $\pm$ 3 per cent expressed TCR α/β. Levels of CD3$^+$ CD57$^+$ cells were twofold higher in synovial fluid than in peripheral blood. Although there was no correlation of CD3$^+$ CD57$^+$ cells and parameters of inflammation, there was a strong link to the duration of disease.

21. Takamizawa, M., Fagnoni, F., Mehta-Damai, A., et al.: Cellular and molecular basis of human $\gamma\delta$ T cell activation: role of accessory molecules in alloactivation. J. Clin. Invest. 95:296, 1995.

22. Shen, Y., Li, S., Quayle, A. J., et al.: TCR gamma/delta$^+$ cell subsets in the synovial membranes of patients with rheumatoid arthritis and juvenile rheumatoid arthritis. Scand. J. Immunol. 36:533, 1992.

   Synovial membranes from 11 patients with rheumatoid arthritis were examined using immunohistochemical techniques for the numbers of TCR γ/δ^+ cells. Five of 11 had 5 to 10 per cent cells and 5 others had 10 to 20 per cent.

23. Smith, M. D., Bröker, B., Moretta, L., et al.: T$\gamma\delta$ cells and their subsets in blood and synovial tissue from rheumatoid arthritis patients. Scand. J. Immunol. 32:585, 1990.

24. Andreu, J. L., Trujillo, A., Alonso, J. M., et al.: Selective expansion of T cells bearing the γ/δ receptor and expressing an unusual repertoire in the synovial membrane of patients with rheumatoid arthritis. Arthritis Rheum. 34:808, 1991.

25. Firestein, G. S., and Zvaifler, N. J.: How important are T cells in chronic rheumatoid synovitis? Arthritis Rheum. 33:768, 1990.

26. Harris, E. D. Jr.: Etiology and pathogenesis of rheumatoid arthritis. In Kelley, W. N., Harris, E. D. Jr., Ruddy, S., and Sledge, C. B. (eds.): Textbook of Rheumatology, 4th ed., Vol. 1. Philadelphia, W. B. Saunders, 1993, pp. 833–873.

27. Dumonde, D. C., Jones, E. H., Kelly, R. H., et al.: Experimental models of rheumatoid inflammation. In Glynn, L. E., and Schlumberger, H. D. (eds.): Experimental Models of Chronic Inflammatory Diseases. Berlin, Springer-Verlag, 1977, pp. 127–138.

28. Klareskog, L., Holmdahl, R., Larsson, E., et al.: Role of T lymphocytes in collagen II induced arthritis in rats. Clin. Exp. Immunol. 51:117, 1983.

29. Panayi, G. S., Lanchbury, J. S., and Kingsley, G. H.: The importance of the T cell in initiating and maintaining the chronic synovitis of rheumatoid arthritis. Arthritis Rheum. 35:729, 1992.

30. Liu, Y., and Linsley, P. S.: Costimulation of T-cell growth. Curr. Opin. Immunol. 4:265, 1992.

31. Goronzy, J. J., and Weyand, C. M.: Interplay of T lymphocytes and HLA-DR molecules in rheumatoid arthritis. Curr. Opin. Rheumatol. 5:169, 1993.

   The hypothesis supported here by data from the Mayo Clinic is that multiple factors modulate the repertoire of T cells recruited to synovium. Adhesion molecules that attract phenotypically selected T cells with a wide spectrum of specificities, and B-cell activation of different T-cell specificities, are among these factors.

32. Schwartz, R. H.: Costimulation of T lymphocytes: the role of CD28, CTLA−4, and B7/BB1 in interleukin-2 production and immunotherapy. Cell 71:1065, 1992.

33. Sfikakis, P. P., Zografou, A., Viglis, V., et al.: CD28 expression on T cell subsets in vivo and CD28-mediated T cell response in vitro in patients with rheumatoid arthritis. Arthritis Rheum. 38:649, 1995.

34. Liu, M. F., Kohsaka, H., Sakurai, H., et al.: The presence of costimulatory molecules CD86 and CD28 in rheumatoid arthritis synovium. Arthritis Rheum. 39:110, 1996.

35. Krummel, M. F., and Allison, J. P.: CD28 and CTLA−4 have opposing effects on the response of T cells to stimulation. J. Exp. Med. 182:459, 1995.

36. Kelleher, D., Murphy, A., Hall, N., et al.: Expression of CD44 on rheumatoid synovial fluid lymphocytes. Ann. Rheum. Dis. 54:566, 1995.

37. Ranheim, E. A., and Kipps, T. J.: Elevated expression of CD80 (B7/BB1) and other accessory molecules on synovial fluid mononuclear cell subsets in rheumatoid arthritis. Arthritis Rheum. 37:1637, 1994.

38. Olee, T., Lu, E. W., Huang, D. F., et al.: Genetic analysis of self-associating immunoglobulin G rheumatoid factors from two rheumatoid synovia implicates an antigen-driven response. J. Exp. Med. 175:831, 1992.

39. Jenkins, M. K., Ashwell, J. D., and Schwartz, R. H.: Allogeneic non-T spleen cells restore the responsiveness of normal T cell clones stimulated with antigen and chemically

modified antigen-presenting cells. J. Immunol. 140:3324, 1988.

40. Linsley, P. S., Brady, W., Grosmaire, L., et al.: Binding of the B cell activation antigen B7 to CD28 costimulates T cell proliferation and IL-2 mRNA accumulation. J. Exp. Med. 173:721, 1991.

41. Verwilghen, J., Vandenberghe, P., Wallays, G., et al.: Simultaneous ligation of CD5 and CD28 on resting T lymphocytes induces T cell activation in the absence of T cell receptor/CD3 occupancy. J. Immunol. 150:835, 1993.

42. Verwilghen, J., Kingsley, G. H., Ceuppens, J. L., et al.: Inhibition of synovial fluid T cell proliferation by anti-CD5 monoclonal antibodies. Arthritis Rheum. 35:1445, 1992.

43. Lasky, H. P., Bauer, K., and Pope, R. M.: Increased helper inducer and decreased suppressor inducer phenotypes in the rheumatoid joint. Arthritis Rheum. 31:52, 1988.

44. Hain, N., Alsalameh, S., Bertling, W. M., et al.: Stimulation of rheumatoid synovial and blood T cells and lines by synovial fluid and interleukin-2: characterization of clones and recognition of a co-stimulatory effect. Rheumatol. Int. 10:203, 1990.

45. Verwilghen, J., Lovis, R., de Boer, M., et al.: The expression of functional B7 and CTLA4 on rheumatoid synovial T cells. J. Immunol. 153:1378, 1994.

46. Fields, P. E., Gajewski, T. F., and Fitch, F. W.: Blocked Ras activation in anergic CD4+ T cells. Science 271:1276, 1996.

47. Elkon, K. B.: Defects in apoptosis as a cause of systemic autoimmunity. Cliniguide Rheum. Dis. 4(3):1, 1994.

48. Henderson, S., Huen, D., Rowe, M., et al.: Epstein-Barr virus-coded BHRF−1 protein, a viral homologue of Bcl-2, protects human B cells from programmed cell death. Proc. Natl. Acad. Sci. U.S.A. 90:8479, 1993.

49. Hockenberry, D. M., Oltvai, Z. N., Yin, X. M., et al.: *Bcl-2* functions in an anti-oxidant pathway to prevent apoptosis. Cell 75:241, 1993.

50. Watanabe-Fukunaga, R., Brannan, C. I., Copeland, N. G., et al.: Lymphoproliferation disorder in mice explained by defects in *Fas* antigen that mediates apoptosis. Nature 356:314, 1992.

51. Rieux-Laucat, F., Le Deist, F., Hivroz, C., et al.: Mutations in *Fas* associated with human lymphoproliferative syndrome and autoimmunity. Science 268:1347, 1995.

52. Laurence, J., Mitra, D., Steiner, M., et al.: Apoptotic depletion of CD4 + T cells in idiopathic CD4 + T lymphocytopenia. J. Clin. Invest. 97:672, 1996.

53. Miura, M., Zhu, H., Rotello, R., et al.: Induction of apoptosis in fibroblasts by IL-1 converting enzyme, a mammalian homolog of the *C. elegans* cell death gene ced-3. Cell 75:653, 1993.

54. Carson, D. A., and Tan, E. M.: Apoptosis in rheumatic disease. Bull. Rheum. Dis. 44:13, 1995.

55. Wu, J., Zhou, T., He, J., et al.: Autoimmune disease in mice due to integration of an endogenous retrovirus in an apoptosis gene. J. Exp. Med. 178:461, 1993.

56. Zhou, T., Bluethmann, H., Zhang, J., et al.: Defective maintenance of T cell tolerance to a superantigen in MRL-*lpr/lpr* mice. J. Exp. Med. 176:1063, 1992.

57. Miethke, T., Wahl, C., Heeg, K., et al.: T cell-mediated lethal shock triggered in mice by the superantigen staphylococcal enterotoxin B: critical role of tumor necrosis factor. J. Exp. Med. 175:91, 1992.

58. Mountz, J. D., Zhou, T., Long, R. E., et al.: T cell influence on superantigen-induced arthritis in MRL-*lpr/lpr* mice. Arthritis Rheum. 37:113, 1994.

59. Cheng, J., Zhou, T., Liu, C., et al.: Protection from *Fas*-mediated apoptosis by a soluble form of the *Fas* molecule. Science 263:1759, 1994.

60. Nakajima, T., Aono, H., Hasunuma, T., et al.: Apoptosis and functional *Fas* antigen in rheumatoid arthritis synoviocytes. Arthritis Rheum. 38:485, 1995.

61. Weyand, C. M., Xie, C., and Goronzy, J. J.: Homozygosity for the HLA-DRB1 allele selects for extra-articular manifestations in rheumatoid arthritis. J. Clin. Invest. 89:2033, 1992.

This is an immunogenetic study of 81 patients with seropositive rheumatoid arthritis and different patterns of disease manifestation. Patients with erosive disease and no extra-articular involvement predominantly combined *HLA-DRB1*04* with disease-nonassociated *HLA-DRB1* alleles. Patients with nodular disease were frequently homozygous for the disease-associated epitope. Most were either typed *HLA-DRB1*04/01* heterozygous or *HLA-DRB1*0401/0404* heterozygous. Patients with major organ involvement were predominantly homozygous for the *HLA-DRB1*0401* allele. This study suggests that homozygosity is important in shaping disease manifestations and establishes the concept that MHC density is of critical importance in the pathogenesis of rheumatoid arthritis. The authors raise the hypothesis that the pathogenetic role of HLA density may relate to the function of polymorphic HLA structures in determining HLA-TCR interaction and selecting the TCR repertoire. A critical role of MHC density that may influence the thymic selection of the pathogenesis of rheumatoid arthritis is hypothesized.

61a. Firestein, G. S., Nguyen, K., Aupperle, K., et al.: p53 overexpression in rheumatoid arthritis synovial tissue. Arthritis Rheum. 39:S118, 1996.

62. Chicz, R. M., Urban, R. G., Lane, W. S., et al.: Predominant naturally processed peptides bound to HLA-DR1 are derived from MHC-related molecules and are heterogeneous in size. Nature 358:764, 1992.

Peptides naturally bound to the HLA-DR1 molecule have a length of 13 to 25 amino acid residues. Of 20 sequenced DR1-bound peptides, 16 were derived from the self-proteins HLA-A2 and the class II−associated invariant chain. Peptides were truncated at both the amino and carboxyl terminals. Alignment of the peptides bound to HLA-DR1 and the sequence of 35 known HLA-DR1−binding peptides revealed a putative motif. The authors hypothesize that this sequence motif, which includes three key amino acids within a sequence of 10 amino acids, defines allele specificity of peptide binding.

63. Weiss, S., and Bogen, B.: MHC class II-restricted presentation of intracellular antigen. Cell 64:767, 1991.

64. Steinman, R. M.: The dendritic cell system and its role in immunogenicity. Annu. Rev. Immunol. 9:271, 1991.

65. Herman, A., Kappler, J. W., and Marrack, P.: Superantigens: mechanism of T-cell stimulation and role in immune responses. Annu. Rev. Immunol. 9:745, 1991.

66. Acha-Orbea, H.: Bacterial and viral superantigens: roles in autoimmunity? Ann. Rheum. Dis. 52:56, 1993.

67. Marrack, P., and Kappler, I.: The staphylococcal enterotoxins and their relatives. Science 248:705, 1990.

68. White, J., Herman, A., Pullen, A. K. M., et al.: The Vβ-specific superantigen staphylococcal enterotoxin B: stimulation of mature T cells and clonal deletion in neonatal mice. Cell 56:27, 1989.

69. Tsai, C., Diaz, L. A., Mitra, R., et al.: Rheumatoid fibroblast-like synoviocytes can support T cell responses to staphylococcal superantigens. Arthritis Rheum. 37:S313, 1994.

70. González-Quintial, R., Baccalà, R., Pope, R. M., and Theofilopoulos, A. N.: Identification of clonally expanded T

cells in rheumatoid arthritis using a sequence enrichment nuclease assay. J. Clin. Invest. 97:1335, 1996.

71. Lunardi, C., Ibberson, M., Zeminian, S., et al.: Lack of association of T cell receptor Vβ8 polymorphism with rheumatoid arthritis in United Kingdom and Italian white patients. Ann. Rheum. Dis. 53:341, 1994.

In this study, 81 northern Italian and 29 British patients were compared against control populations. No associations between V$_\beta$8 and DR4 were found.

72. de Vries, N., Prinsen, C. F. M., Mensink, E. B. J. M., et al.: A T cell receptor β chain variable region polymorphism associated with radiographic progression in rheumatoid arthritis. Ann. Rheum. Dis. 52:327, 1993.

A total of 110 controls and 118 patients were typed for a segment of the TCR V$_\beta$8 gene. No differences were found between the groups. A significant association of this allele (assayed by Southern blot technique using the Bam HI 2.0-kb restriction fragment) with less radiographic progression of disease over 3 years was found.

73. Pile, K., Wordsworth, P., Lioté, F., et al.: Analysis of a T-cell receptor Vβ segment implicated in susceptibility to rheumatoid arthritis: Vβ2 germline polymorphism does not encode susceptibility. Ann. Rheum. Dis. 52:891, 1993.

The germline variation of V$_\beta$2.1, reported by others to be more common in rheumatoid patients, was examined in 136 patients with erosive rheumatoid arthritis and in 150 healthy individuals. No significant differences between the patients with rheumatoid arthritis and controls were found in the expression of the TCR V$_\beta$23.1 allele.

74. Wallin, J., Hillert, J., Olerup, O., et al.: Association of rheumatoid arthritis with a dominant DR1/Dw4/Dw14 sequence motif, but not with T cell receptor β chain gene alleles or haplotypes. Arthritis Rheum. 34:1416, 1991.

Although the expected associations of DR1, DwR, and Dw14 alleles in rheumatoid and Felty's syndrome patients were found, there was no difference in TCR β-chain haplotypes from normal controls. In particular, no V$_\beta$8 and V$_\beta$11 haplotype frequencies were found. The data did not support the notion of an influence of TCR β germline allotypes on rheumatoid arthritis susceptibility.

75. Van Laar, J. M., Miltenburg, A. M. M., Verdonk, M. J. A., et al.: Lack of T cell oligoclonality in enzyme-digested synovial tissue and in synovial fluid in most patients with rheumatoid arthritis. Clin. Exp. Immunol. 83:352, 1991.

T-cell populations from synovial tissue and peripheral blood of rheumatoid arthritis patients and from peripheral blood of healthy donors were studied for TCR β-chain gene rearrangements. No oligoclonal T-cell response was observed; dominant rearrangements were found in T cells of only 2 of 18 patients. Interpreting these data in light of other results suggesting an oligoclonal response in rheumatoid arthritis cells focuses on techniques. When cell populations are grown out from tissue by adding T-cell growth factors, oligoclonality may occur as an in vitro artifact.

76. Struyk, L., Hawes, G. E., and Chatila, M. K.: T cell receptors in rheumatoid arthritis. Arthritis Rheum. 38:577, 1995.

77. Paliard, X., West, S. G., Lafferty, J. A., et al.: Evidence for the effects of a superantigen in rheumatoid arthritis. Science 253:325, 1991.

78. Jenkins, R. N., Nikaein, A., Zimmermann, A., et al.: T cell receptor Vβ gene bias in rheumatoid arthritis. J. Clin. Immunol. 92:2688, 1993.

79. Weyand, C. M., Oppitz, U., Hicok, K., et al.: Selection of T cell receptor Vβ elements by HLA-DR determinants predisposing to rheumatoid arthritis. Arthritis Rheum. 35:990, 1992.

Data from this study suggest that T cells reactive with the disease-associated HLA-DR structure are *not* selected at random. TCR V$_\beta$ gene segments in T-cell clones selected for their specificity to the disease-associated epitope in the *HLA-DRB1* chains were analyzed. TCR V$_\beta$ elements specific for the disease-associated determinant were limited. Twenty-five to 43 per cent of T-cell clones analyzed expressed V$_\beta$6 from all four responding individuals. In addition, DNA analysis after amplification indicated that only a few members of the V$_\beta$6 family of genes were utilized. Conclusions were that the HLA determinants are crucial for TCR interaction with the TCR-peptide complex, and that the HLA-DR disease-associated determinants influence the T-cell repertoire rather than selective binding of an arthritogenic peptide.

80. Gao, X., Ball, E. J., Dombransky, L., et al.: Class II human leukocyte antigen genes and T cell receptor polymorphisms in patients with rheumatoid arthritis. Am. J. Med. 85(suppl. 6A):14, 1988.

These studies showed an association between HLA-DR4 and a 2-kb polymorphic restriction fragment of Bam HI–digested DNA, using a TCR Vβ8 probe.

81. Zagon, G., Tumang, J. R., Li, Y., et al.: Increased frequency of Vβ17-positive T cells in patients with rheumatoid arthritis. Arthritis Rheum. 37:1431, 1994.

82. Kohsaka, H., Taniguchi, A., Chen, P. P., et al.: The expressed T cell receptor V gene repertoire of rheumatoid arthritis monozygotic twins: rapid analysis by anchored polymerase chain reaction and enzyme-linked immunosorbent assay. Eur. J. Immunol. 23:1895, 1993.

Using a combination of anchored PCR techniques and ELISAs, these studies assessed peripheral blood TCR V gene frequencies in nine sets of identical twins; twins normal, concordant, or discordant for rheumatoid arthritis were studied. There was a marked similarity in the TCR V$_\beta$ gene repertoires between identical twins (compared to unrelated subjects) whether or not they were concordant or discordant for rheumatoid arthritis. The methodology involved capture of biotinylated PCR products on steptavidin and subsequent addition of labeled V gene family–specific primer that could be detected, if bound, by chromogenes. It still is possible, however, that specific changes in V$_\beta$ gene repertoires exist only in inflamed synovia, not in peripheral blood T cells.

83. Kohsaka, H., Chen, P. P., Taniguchi, A., et al.: Divergent T cell receptor gamma repertoires in rheumatoid arthritis monozygotic twins. Arthritis Rheum. 36:213, 1995.

84. Cooper, S. M., Roessner, K. D., Naito-Hoopes, M., et al.: Increased usage of Vβ2 and Vβ6 in rheumatoid synovial fluid T cells. Arthritis Rheum. 37:1627, 1994.

85. Goronzy, J. J., Bartz-Bazzanella, P., Hu, W., et al.: Dominant clonotypes in the repertoire of peripheral CD4$^+$ T cells in rheumatoid arthritis. J. Clin. Invest. 94:2068, 1994.

86. Fischer, D. -C., Opalka, B., Hoffmann, A., et al.: Limited heterogeneity of rearranged T cell receptor V$_\alpha$ and V$_\beta$ transcripts in synovial fluid T cells in early stages of rheumatoid arthritis. Arthritis Rheum. 39:454, 1996.

87. Ikeda, Y., Masuko, K., Nakai, Y., et al.: High frequencies of identical T cell clonotypes in synovial tissues of rheumatoid arthritis patients suggest the occurrence of common antigen-driven immune responses. Arthritis Rheum. 39:446, 1996.

88. Skinner, M. A., Watson, L., Geursen, A., et al.: Lymphocyte responses to DR1/4 restricted peptides in rheumatoid arthritis. Ann. Rheum. Dis. 53:171, 1993.
89. De Magistris, M. T., Alexander, J., Coggenshall, M., et al.: Antigen analog-major histocompatibility complexes act as antagonists of the T cell receptor. Cell 68:625, 1992.
90. Cush, J. J., and Lipsky, P. E.: Phenotypic analysis of synovial tissue and peripheral blood lymphocytes isolated from patients with rheumatoid arthritis. Arthritis Rheum. 31:1230, 1988.
91. Thomas, R., McIlraith, M., Davis, L. S., et al.: Rheumatoid synovium is enriched in CD45RB^{dim} mature memory T cells that are potent helpers for B cell differentiation. Arthritis Rheum. 35:1455, 1992.
92. Rubin, L. A., and Nelson, D. L.: The soluble interleukin-2 receptor: biology, function, and clinical application. Ann. Intern. Med. 113:619, 1990.

This review of IL-2R describes the quantitation by ELISAs of soluble IL-2 in normal individuals and those with various diseases. IL-2R has two subunits. The α (p55 or Tac) and β (p70/75) subunits each bind IL-2 at relatively low affinity. Together, they bind IL-2 with high affinity. Tac is expressed after T cell activation but before lymphocyte proliferation. In rheumatoid arthritis, synovial fluid soluble IL-2R levels are significantly elevated when compared with serum levels and may be useful in serial measurements.

93. Suzuki, H., Kundig, T. M., and Furlonger, C.: Deregulated T cell activation and autoimmunity in mice lacking interleukin-2 receptor beta. Science 268:1472, 1995.
94. Thomas, R., and Lipsky, P. E.: Presentation of self peptides by dendritic cells: possible implications for the pathogenesis of rheumatoid arthritis. Arthritis Rheum. 39:183, 1996.

6

B Lymphocytes and Rheumatoid Factor

Rheumatoid factor, the cells that synthesize it, and rheumatoid arthritis have been linked since 1947, when a technician who had rheumatoid arthritis discovered that her own serum agglutinated excessively. Her supervisor, Dr. Harry Rose, and Dr. Charles Ragan, his colleague and a rheumatologist at Columbia-Presbyterian Hospital, pursued the possibility that the agglutination had something to do with rheumatoid arthritis. A good argument can be made that it was this finding and the discovery of the LE cell phenomenon in 1945 by Hargraves that were the principal factors in the maturation and development of academic rheumatology.

Drs. Rose and Ragan and their colleagues[1] developed the sheep cell agglutination test. The agglutinins were complexes of IgM and IgG. These rheumatoid factors were found later to be autoantibodies directed against multiple antigenic determinants on the Fc fragment of IgG (Fig. 6–1). Using advanced techniques, including radioimmunoassay and ELISA, precise measurement of rheumatoid factor in the IgM, IgG, and IgA classes of immunoglobulin can be made.

THE DIAGNOSTIC SIGNIFICANCE OF RHEUMATOID FACTOR

It is well known that patients with rheumatoid arthritis who have a persistently positive test for rheumatoid factor within 3 years of onset of the disease will have[2]

- more radiologic abnormalities
- more disease activity
- more extra-articular manifestations
- worse functional ability
- a need for more second-line drug treatment

How much of this increased severity of disease is a direct effect of the presence of rheumatoid factor, and how much is a development associated with

rheumatoid factor but not caused by it? In rheumatoid patients, raised levels of IgA rheumatoid factor are associated with more aggressive disease, certainly in comparison with patients who have an isolated increase in IgM rheumatoid factor.[3]

Although very high titers of rheumatoid factor are found virtually only in patients with very active rheumatoid arthritis, lower—but significant—titers are found in the aging population and in a number of other viral, parasitic, and chronic bacterial infections, neoplasms, rheumatic diseases, and hyperglobulinemic states[4] (Table 6–1).

In a cohort of 8,287 outpatients with various rheumatic diseases, the specificity of 1:80 titers of the latex fixation test were as follows[5]:

In rheumatoid arthritis patients: 78%

Against noninflammatory rheumatic diseases: 98%

Against noninflammatory plus inflammatory rheumatic diseases: 97%

Despite the association of rheumatoid factor with a worse prognosis in patients with rheumatoid arthritis, it is probable that the risk of morbidity or future disease associated with seropositivity in an otherwise healthy individual is less than 5 per cent.[7] We would be well served to have a test for rheumatoid factor that is more specific for rheumatoid arthritis. One such test has been reported (see annotated ref. 6) but awaits confirmation and a practical means for an inexpensive assay.

In a large Finnish population, there was a fourfold higher incidence of significant titers of rheumatoid factor in current smokers than in those who had never smoked, but no difference in the prevalence of rheumatoid arthritis.[9] Another opposing study has been published (see Chapter 2) in which a positive correlation between ever-smokers and rheumatoid arthritis has been found. In general, rheumatoid patients appear to smoke less than their peers without joint disease.[8]

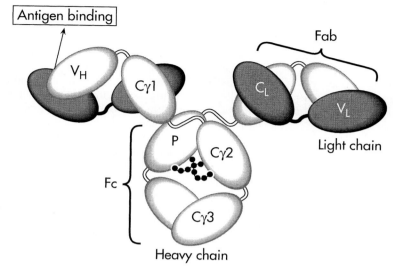

FIGURE 6–1. Schematic diagram of an IgG molecule. The antigen-binding sites are formed by the juxtaposition of V_L and V_H domains in the Fab region. The amino termini of the chains are here, whereas the carboxyl termini are found on the Fc ends of the molecule. The *hinge* regions with flexible conformations are between $C\gamma1$ and $C\gamma2$. Heavy chains form interchain disulfide bonds in the region near the carboxyl terminus of the hinge. Fc receptor and complement-binding sites are located on the Fc portion, as are sites that bind rheumatoid factors. Oligosaccharides that provide variability in the degree of glycosylation of the molecules are designated by the dotted chains. These oligosaccharides form a bridge that separates the two $C\gamma2$ domains of the heavy chains. (Modified from Axford, J. S., Lydyard, P. M., Isenberg, D. A., et al.: Reduced B-cell galactosyltransferase activity in rheumatoid arthritis. Lancet 2:1486, 1987. Used by permission. Copyright by The Lancet Ltd., 1987.)

PRODUCTION OF RHEUMATOID FACTOR

Rheumatoid factor–positive B cells are abundant within rheumatoid synovial tissues.[10] They appear to substantially amplify the synovial immune response. It is instructive to follow through the sequences leading to production of rheumatoid factor, and to its effects within joints after being synthesized and released (see the box on page 76).

T-Cell Help

As detailed in Chapter 5, within the synovial space a high percentage of the T cells present are terminally differentiated and possibly focused on B-cell help. Many of these synovial and synovial

TABLE 6–1. Diseases Commonly Associated with Rheumatoid Factor

CATEGORY	DISEASES
Rheumatic diseases	Rheumatoid arthritis, systemic lupus erythematosus, scleroderma, mixed connective tissue diseases, Sjögren's syndrome
Viral infections	AIDS, mononucleosis, hepatitis, influenza, and many others; after vaccination (may yield falsely elevated titers of antiviral antibodies)
Parasitic infections	Trypanosomiasis, kala-azar, malaria, schistosomiasis, filariasis, and others
Chronic bacterial infections	Tuberculosis, leprosy, yaws, syphilis, brucellosis, subacute bacterial endocarditis, salmonellosis
Neoplasms	After irradiation or chemotherapy
Other hyperglobulinemic states	Hypergammaglobulinemic purpura, cryoglobulinemia, chronic liver disease, sarcoid, other chronic pulmonary diseases

From Carson, D. A.: Rheumatoid factor. *In* Kelley, W. N., Harris, E. D. Jr., Ruddy, S., and Sledge, C. B. (eds.): Textbook of Rheumatology, 4th ed., Vol. 1. Philadelphia, W. B. Saunders, 1993, pp. 155–163. Used by permission.

B Cell Development

B cells, the lymphocytes responsible for production of rheumatoid factor, are selected in a two-step process: the first occurs early in the central lymphoid organs and the second, an antigen-driven process, occurs in mature B cells in the germinal centers.[11] In humans there are relatively few genes encoding for the variable regions of the heavy (H) and light (L) chains, but this is compensated for by a greater length of CDR3 which is of primary importance in antigen binding. In the bone marrow, B cells mature from pro-B cells through to immunoglobulin-producing cells. Those with faulty gene rearrangement are deleted by apoptosis. In germinal centers somatic mutations of V_H and V_L genes begin in B cells in the center (known as centrocytes). The centrocytes begin migrating toward the periperal light zones of the germinal centers. If surface Ig (Ig) does not interact with antigen in this area, the cell is at high risk for apoptotic death. Antigen binding plus interaction with CD40 on the B cell surface with its ligand (CD40L or p33) produced by T cells assure survival. Germinal center formation is impeded by IFNγ and IL-2; it is enhanced by IL-4 and IL-6. IL-10 may be essential for induction of spontaneous production of IgM rheumatoid factor by B cells capable of this.[12] High levels of IL-10 have been demonstrated in blood and synovium of rheumatoid patients.[13]

---

fluid T cells are mature memory cells and have a CD45RB^{dim} phenotype.

These mature memory cells do not produce many lymphokines (e.g., IL-2, IFNγ), nor do they proliferate, but they strongly influence B-cell activation. Because T lymphocytes reactive with autologous IgG have not been detected in rheumatoid arthritis patients, it seems likely that certain T cells react with an antigen in an immune complex that is bound and processed by rheumatoid factor precursor B lymphocytes; these B cells then proliferate in response to the T-cell help.[14] In addition, or alternatively, nonspecific T-cell help may trigger the rheumatoid factor precursor cells to divide. The work showing that the gp110 glycoprotein of EBV and the dnaJ HSP of some *Escherichia coli* strains have sequence similarities with the ''shared epitope'' on *HLA-DRB1* chains (see Chapters 3 and 5) may have relevance here. Immune complexes with these ex-

ogenous or host peptides could stimulate rheumatoid factor precursor cells sufficiently so that some helper T cells restricted by autologous class II MHC sequences could in turn be activated, and autoimmunity would develop.

During stimulation of rheumatoid factor–producing B cells, there is continuing somatic mutation in immunoglobulin genes that leads to production of rheumatoid factors with increasing binding affinity for IgG. If sufficiently high binding affinity is reached through ongoing somatic mutation, intermittent exposure to small amounts of any antigen-antibody complex would progressively boost rheumatoid factor synthesis.[14]

Molecular Contacts in T Cell–B Cell Interaction

When activated T cells and B cells come into contact, there are multiple molecules on the surfaces of each that have a role in binding and reciprocal activation in collaboration. Many of these have been described in Chapter 5. Membrane-associated IgG enables the B cell to recognize specific antigens, bind them, internalize and partially degrade them, and present the antigen in the context of class II MHC to CD4$^+$ T-helper cells in association with co-stimulatory factors. Once the T cells are activated in this process, subsequent B-cell stimulation is not MHC restricted, and the result may be polyclonal B-cell activation.[15]

Of the many bimolecular interactions between the cells, the ones that largely account for inducing synthesis of immunoglobulins by B cells are the reciprocal locking of (1) LFA-1 to ICAM-1, and (2) CD40 with its ligand, also known as p33, on T cells. Interestingly, the presence of IL-4 around the CD40/p33 linkage generates a predominance of production of IgE by the B cell, whereas IL-2 facilitates IgG and IgM production (see the box on page 77).

Cytokine Help

Several cytokines with potential to help activate B lymphocytes have been found in synovium and synovial fluid or rheumatoid patients. These include IL-1, TNFα, and IL-6. Recently, IL-10 production has been shown to be dramatically increased by peripheral blood mononuclear cells from patients with rheumatoid arthritis and in Sjögren's syndrome.[18] IL-10 is a potent activator of B lymphocytes, inducing both their proliferation and immunoglobulin production. In addition, IL-10 induces *bcl-2* expression in these cells, (see Chapter 5) which may protect them from programmed cell death.[19] The mechanism for the increased produc-

---

Ig Class Switching and the Hyper-IgM Syndrome

IgM is the first class of antibodies to appear in an immune response. As the process evolves, immunoglobulin class switching produces other isotypes: IgG, IgA, and IgE. The orderly sequence of immunoglobulin class switching involves effective collaboration between B cells and helper CD4[+] T cells. B cell–T cell contact is needed to induce the T cell to express a ligand (also known as p33) for CD40 expressed on B cells. This leads to expression of B7-1/B7-2 on the B cell. The counter-receptor for B7 is CD28 on the T cell. Formation of these molecular links (including presentation of antigen to the TCR) leads to secretion of IL-2, IL-4, and other lymphokines by the fully activated T cell[16] (see Fig. 6–2) and to IgG production by the B cells.

Children with the hyper-IgM syndrome cannot perform immunoglobulin class switching. They have elevated amounts of IgM in serum but no IgG or IgA. Their X-linked defect is a failure of their T cells to express CD40 ligand because of numerous mutations and deletions in the CD40 ligand gene.[17]

CD40 is expressed not only by B cells but also by dendritic cells and monocytes, and therefore may have a role in regulating antigen presentation as well as immunoglobulin class switching.

---

tion of IL-10 is not known, but it is intriguing that both EBV and retroviruses have the capability to induce its expression in monocyte cultures. IL-10 levels are elevated in rheumatoid arthritis[13] and have a major involvement in the induction of autoreactive B cells.

Monocyte Help

Taken together, many data suggest that both rheumatoid arthritis patients and normal individuals share a pool of B cells that produce rheumatoid factor after activation by T-helper cells in the presence of superantigen and, in rheumatoid patients, by T-helper cells alone.[7] The inference from this is that B cells in rheumatoid patients may be chronically exposed to stimuli with superantigen capabilities. Accordingly, it has been shown that cells of monocyte (CD14[+]) lineage induced by the growth factor GM-CSF from bone marrow of rheumatoid patients enhanced rheumatoid factor production by

CD4[+] cell–stimulated normal B cells in the absence of added antigen. The same type of CD14[+] cell from marrow of osteoarthritic patients did not affect rheumatoid factor production.[20] The inference is that a different (abnormal?) bone marrow cell destined to be a monocyte, in the presence of growth factors, can effect a major increase in rheumatoid factor production by B cells in these patients.

CD5[+] B Lymphocytes

CD5[+] B lymphocytes are associated with autoimmunity and are reported to be elevated to as much as 40 per cent of the B-cell population in some patients with rheumatoid arthritis. Normal individuals have up to 20 per cent CD5[+] cells in peripheral blood,[21] whereas this surface glycoprotein is expressed on all mature T lymphocytes. In studies of rheumatoid arthritis B cells in culture, the expression of CD5 and IgM rheumatoid factor was downregulated by the addition of recombinant IL-4, but not by IL-1, IL-2, IL-5, or IL-6.[22]

CD5[+] cells produce rheumatoid factor when feeder cells are added and when they are activated by EBV.[21] The possibility that these cells were presenting autoantigens to T cells or secreting high-affinity autoantibodies led investigators to trials of anti-CD5 in rheumatoid arthritis[23] (see Chapter 32). The results showed that anti-CD5 showed minimal efficacy of short duration.

CD8[+] T cells are reported to be increased in peripheral blood or rheumatoid patients in proportion to levels of serum IgM. Because CD8[+] cells from these patients appeared to act as suppressors of rheumatoid factor production, a case can be made that CD8[+] cells may be responding to down-regulate the immunologic abnormalities of rheumatoid arthritis, albeit unsuccessfully.[3]

Receptors for Immunoglobulin G

Many circulating and fixed tissue cells have receptors for the constant region (the Fc portion) of IgG. These are designated Fc receptors. They do not bind IgA or IgM. A major function of Fc receptors is to bind and help clear immune complexes from tissues and the circulation. During this receptor-ligand association, however, the cells are activated. When IgG in complex with another IgG molecule, IgM, or an antigen binds to the Fc receptors on a phagocyte, oxidative bursts are triggered, as are release of cellular granule contents and other components of activation.[24] In more obvious ''immune complex'' diseases such as systemic lupus erythematosus, the binding and saturation of Fc re-

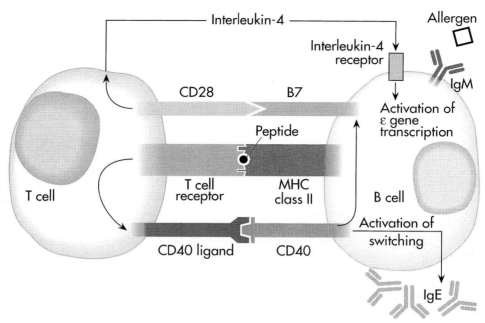

FIGURE 6–2. Representation of factors involved in one type of immunoglobulin class switching. B cell–T cell contact induces expression on T cells of CD40 ligand (p33) and B7-1. With ligand-receptor interaction in certain cells, IL-4 is produced by T cells that facilitates expression of the ε gene in B cells that enables construction of IgE. Other T cells produce IL-2 that helps facilitate IgG synthesis. The X-linked defect in T-cell production of CD40 ligand blocks immunoglobulin class switching that is essential for normal immunity. (Modified from Geha, R. S., and Rosen, F. S.: The genetic basis of immunoglobulin-class switching. N. Engl. J. Med. 330:1008, 1994. Used by permission.)

ceptors may have pathogenic significance. For rheumatoid arthritis, the potential for exploiting Fc receptors either for understanding the disease process or for treatment has not been developed.

The cell-surface antigen **CD23** is the low-affinity receptor for the Fc portion of IgE. It is present on B cells as well as T cells and monocytes. Soluble CD23 can be measured in biologic fluids. The percentage of B cells expressing CD23 and serum levels of soluble CD23 are increased in patients with rheumatoid arthritis.[25] IL-4 is a potent inducer of soluble CD23 by peripheral blood mononuclear cells. In these same cultures of cells, the increased secretion of soluble CD23 induced by IL-4 was associated with an inhibitory effect of IL-4 on immunoglobulin production, a phenomenon more pronounced in cultures of rheumatoid cells than in control cell cultures.

ANTIBODY DIVERSITY— SOMATIC RECOMBINATION OF GERMLINE GENES

Each person has approximately 10 million different antibody molecules, about a million more than there are genes in the human genome. This diversity is made possible by juxtaposition through somatic recombination of various gene segments to make a functional antibody. The diversity is a function of the number of different gene segments available for recombination; there are 150 V_H, 30 D_H, and 6 J_H gene segments. Thus, from V-D-J combinations alone there are about 27,000 possible combinations to generate a heavy chain variable region exon. Any heavy chain can pair with any light chain.[26,27] Despite this system, the recombination is not random; some recombinations are more common than others, but the reasons for this are not deciphered.

Immunoglobulins can resemble germline sequences or can undergo somatic rearrangement. Somatic mutations add to diversity. In addition, during the maturation of an antibody response, mutated antibodies that have a higher antigen-binding activity are selectively expanded by a T-cell–mediated process. Autoantibody genes undergo somatic rearrangement much more commonly than other antibodies. Because of somatic mutations, identical twins do not have the same B-cell immunity. Perhaps this is the reason that there is such weak concordance for rheumatoid arthritis among identical

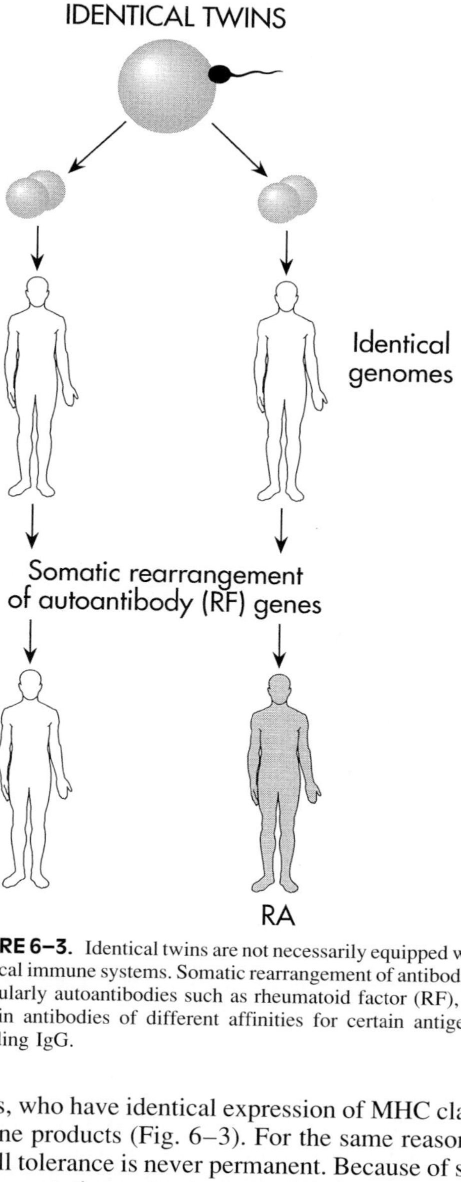

IDENTICAL TWINS

Identical genomes

Somatic rearrangement of autoantibody (RF) genes

RA

FIGURE 6–3. Identical twins are not necessarily equipped with identical immune systems. Somatic rearrangement of antibodies, particularly autoantibodies such as rheumatoid factor (RF), results in antibodies of different affinities for certain antigens, including IgG.

twins, who have identical expression of MHC class II gene products (Fig. 6–3). For the same reasons, B-cell tolerance is never permanent. Because of somatic mutations, the immunoglobulins produced constantly change in response to contact with different antigens.

Synovial plasma cell samples from rheumatoid patients have exhibited increased proportions of clones with unusual lengths of the CDR3 regions that form the center of the antigen-binding site on κ light chains.[28] Enrichment of the repertoire for B lymphocytes expressing κ light chains with unusual CDR3 lengths can potentially expand the diversity of antigens recognized by over 1000-fold. These long CDR3 regions could encode autoantibodies, leading to amplification of the immune response in this disease.

Biased Selection of B Cells for Activation and Expansion in Rheumatoid Arthritis

Study of cloned B cells from rheumatoid synovium indicates that the cells that are producing IgM rheumatoid factor in rheumatoid arthritis have a different utilization of V gene segments for both the heavy and light chains than is found in IgM rheumatoid factor in other diseases and older normal persons. Data for heavy chain gene segment use are outlined in Table 6–2, which shows that the gene segment $V_H III$ is overutilized. There is a similar over-representation at the molecular level for light chains. In one study, of 20 monospecific rheumatoid factors from rheumatoid arthritis patients, 13 have κ light chains and 8 of the 13 are encoded by $V_\kappa III$.[27] Despite these selection biases in patients, it is important to emphasize that the possible gene repertoire for encoding rheumatoid factor is large, includes multiple genes and gene combinations through somatic mutation not found in malignancy-associated rheumatoid factors, and is not restricted to genes used in the fetal antibody repertoire.[29]

In addition to this qualitative difference in gene segments chosen for expression in rheumatoid factor, there are data showing that the "natural" rheumatoid factor expressing B lymphocyte subpopulations is hyperactive in rheumatoid arthritic twins, whether or not rheumatoid arthritis has developed in both siblings. This could be the result of inherited abnormalities in regulation of immunoglobulin V region gene segments in pre-B cells, a situation that could generate signals to activate autoreactive T cells, leading in turn to high-affinity rheumatoid factor production, formation of immune complexes, activation of complement, and amplified disease.[30]

Can germline genes generate rheumatoid factor specificity, or is rheumatoid factor a product of genes altered by somatic mutation and, therefore, an antigen-driven phenomenon?

The first molecular structure of rheumatoid factor from rheumatoid synovial B cells displayed a nearly exact germline configuration throughout its

TABLE 6–2. Utilization of Heavy Chain Gene Segment

	RHEUMATOID ARTHRITIS	OTHER ILLNESSES
$V_H I$	10%	40%
$V_H III$	75%	30%

Data from Thompson et al.[26]

entire heavy chain, and thus represented an example of an autoantibody encoded by one of the V_H gene segments from the preimmune fetal repertoire.[31] However, in another study, the molecular structures of two clonally related antibodies with rheumatoid factor activity from one patient were determined. One rheumatoid factor was close to a germline configuration. The other showed evidence for somatic mutations and had a 100-fold higher affinity for IgG than the rheumatoid factor structured closer to the germline sequence. This "affinity maturation" is a somatic pathway to having rheumatoid factor with a higher affinity for IgG,[32] and we must assume that it is occurring continuously in patients with an activated immune response.

Similarly, the light chain of immunoglobulins from a rheumatoid factor–positive patient with rheumatoid arthritis has revealed κ-chain transcripts in IgM rheumatoid factor enriched for two V_κ gene segments that often are associated with self-reactive antibodies; in addition, there were frequent somatic mutations in the classic antigen-binding site. Several of these unique sequences from the V_κIII gene segments were found in synovial cells but not in peripheral blood lymphocytes or spleen of the patient.[33] These findings support the hypothesis that these synovium-derived B cells and plasma cells are the product of antigen-driven selection,[31] and that in synovium there is expansion of a limited set of B-cell clones bearing evidence of antigen selection.[33] What is this antigen? We do not know.

IgG rheumatoid factors also have varied genetic origins. In three IgG rheumatoid factors derived from synovial fluid of two rheumatoid arthritis patients, two of the three had substantial somatic mutations in their V regions, whereas one IgG rheumatoid factor had only one mutation in each V region. The latter observation suggests that potentially pathogenic rheumatoid factors in rheumatoid arthritis patients arise from natural autoantibodies, and conversion (class switching) to IgG rheumatoid factors only requires a few somatic mutations.[34]

There are quantitative as well as qualitative differences in the immunoglobulins expressed in rheumatoid synovium compared to peripheral blood. On average, IgM rheumatoid factor–producing precursor B cells are 15-fold higher in synovial fluid than in peripheral blood of seropositive rheumatoid arthritis patients, but not in seronegative patients.[10] The inference is that rheumatoid factor–producing B cells preferentially "home" to sites of inflammation in seropositive patients (Fig. 6–4).

Of course, antibodies to immunoglobulins are not the only antibodies produced in rheumatoid synovial tissue. Yet it is interesting that there are relatively few proteins (most of which are not identified yet) against which antibodies are directed.[35]

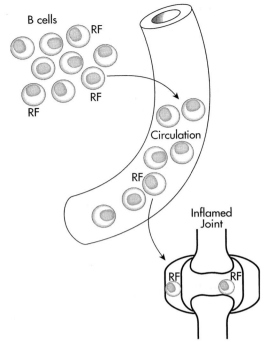

FIGURE 6–4. IgM rheumatoid factor (RF)–producing B cells are selectively increased in synovial fluid compared with peripheral blood of rheumatoid patients who are seropositive. It can be inferred, therefore, that B cells primed to produce rheumatoid factor somehow preferentially home to inflamed joints.[10]

The Significance of Monoreactive and Polyreactive Rheumatoid Factors

Studies of monoclonal rheumatoid factor–secreting cell clones using EBV-infected B lymphocytes has enabled investigators to define two types of rheumatoid factor, monoreactive and polyreactive.[36] *Polyreactive* rheumatoid factor has a low affinity ($K_d \sim 10^{-4}$ to 10^{-5} mol/l) for human IgG Fc and binds to many different antigens (e.g., single-stranded DNA, insulin, tetanus toxoid, type II collagen, β_2 microglobulin).[37] *Monoreactive* rheumatoid factor has a much higher affinity ($K_d \sim 10^{-7}$ mol/l) for human Ig Fc and does not effectively bind any other antigens. It is a threefold more effective activator of complement in a reaction with IgG Fc.[36]

The relevance to studies of rheumatoid arthritis is as follows:

- Monoreactive rheumatoid factor could be obtained from B lymphocytes of patients with rheumatoid arthritis but not from healthy subjects.[38] Polyreactive rheumatoid factor could be obtained from both normal and rheumatoid individuals.

- The V_H genes of monoreactive high-affinity rheumatoid factor show somatic point mutations in their segment sequences, indicating that their production has been driven by antigen.[39] In contrast, the V_H genes of polyreactive rheumatoid factor were in the germline configuration.[39]

A working hypothesis can be that rheumatoid patients generate monoreactive high-affinity rheumatoid factors that are stimulated to form by antigen, perhaps a primary and persistent one, and possibly by selected autoreactive T cells. Somatic mutations in V_H and V_L genes may increase rheumatoid factor binding affinity. These rheumatoid factors form tight complexes with IgG that have a strong capability to activate complement and enhance inflammation. Polyreactive rheumatoid factors are generated as a secondary response and, through reactivity with epitopes on molecules such as type II collagen, may enhance inflammation and focus it in and around cartilage.

TRIGGERS OF RHEUMATOID FACTOR BIOSYNTHESIS

There is a dissociation between cells expressing surface rheumatoid factor and circulating rheumatoid factor. In normal people, B lymphocytes with rheumatoid factor on cell surfaces are common, despite the absence of rheumatoid factor in the circulation (see ref. 4 for review and details). This is particularly true in the very young. In normal adults, rheumatoid factor synthesis and release into the blood is initiated by at least three environmental factors: anamnestic immune responses, polyclonal B-cell activation,[40] and bacterial superantigens.

Emphasis on superantigens is appropriate; these substances (e.g., staphylococcal enterotoxin) bind to nonpolymorphic portions of the TCR and link multiple clones of T cells to rheumatoid factor expressed on multiple B cells, leading to polyclonal B-cell activation (see Chapter 5). One superantigen, staphylococcal enterotoxin D (SED), but not other bacterial superantigens, can induce IgM, IgG, and especially rheumatoid factor production in B cells from both rheumatoid arthritis patients and normal individuals.[41] The evidence suggests that SED preferentially stimulates rheumatoid factor–positive B lymphocytes after it cross-links HLA class II molecules and the TCR on those T cells sharing a binding site for superantigens on the outer surface of

the TCR V_β element. As many as 14 per cent of peripheral blood B cells secrete IgM and IgG in SED-driven cultures, and one third of these responsive cells, previously anergic, produce rheumatoid factor. Vaughan has suggested that the superantigen SED provides an additional bonding between T cells and rheumatoid factor–expressing B cells to overcome a poorly anergized state for B cells, initiating their production of rheumatoid factor[42] (Fig. 6–5).

Another staphylococcal antigen, enterotoxin B (SEB), has been studied and implicated in the pathophysiology of rheumatoid arthritis. Levels of IgM SEB antibodies are significantly elevated in sera of rheumatoid patients over those of normal subjects.[43] No TCR V_β bias was found in these studies, but the possibility exists that excessive response to SEB could perturb the immune system to generate a broad proliferation of T-cell clones to autologous antigens.

RHEUMATOID FACTOR IN LYMPHOPROLIFERATIVE STATES

There are major differences between rheumatoid factors in rheumatoid arthritis and those found in lymphoproliferative diseases, and some cases of Sjögren's syndrome, as shown in Table 6–3. This heterogeneity suggests that production of rheumatoid factor in rheumatoid arthritis is a result of a T-cell response driven by antigen.

EFFECTS OF RHEUMATOID FACTOR UPON THE IMMUNE RESPONSE

Rheumatoid factor–producing B cells in normal adults are found in the mantle zones of lymphoid tissue.[14] The function of this rheumatoid factor, which is not secreted into the circulation, is probably to bind and process antigens trapped in circulating immune complexes. Experiments with transgenic mice expressing the IgM heavy chain and κ light chain genes coding for a human IgM rheumatoid factor reveal striking similarities to findings in patients: rheumatoid factor transgene-expressing B cells localize to B-cell follicles and the mantle zone regions of secondary follicles in the spleen, and their function in this nonrheumatoid state appears to be one of antigen presentation and regulation of immune responses to antibody-bound nonself- (and possibly self-) antigens.[44] There was

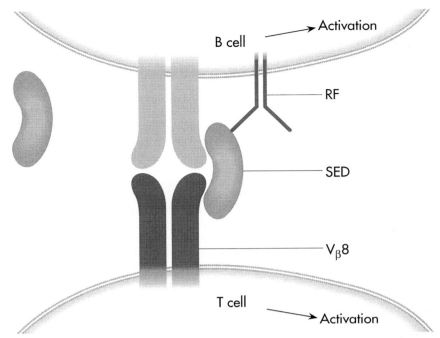

FIGURE 6–5. The hypothesis advanced by Vaughan[42] is that superantigens such as staphylococcal endotoxin D (SED) can boost activation of rheumatoid factor (RF)–expressing B cells by additional bonding with the B cell–T cell–rheumatoid factor complex.

TABLE 6–3. Comparison of Rheumatoid Factors in Lymphoproliferative and Autoimmune Diseases

TYPE OF DISEASE	CHARACTERISTICS
Lymphoproliferative	Restricted genes, cross-reactive idiotypes
	Limited or no somatic mutations
	Low affinity
	Mainly IgM
Autoimmune	Many genes, private idiotypes
	Multiple somatic mutations
	Higher affinity
	All immunoglobulin classes

From Carson, D. A.: Rheumatoid factor. *In* Kelley, W. N., Harris, E. D. Jr., Ruddy, S., and Sledge, C. B. (eds.): Textbook of Rheumatology, 4th ed., Vol. 1. Philadelphia, W. B. Saunders, 1993, pp. 155–163. Used by permission.

an enhanced IgM rheumatoid factor expression when the human rheumatoid factor genes with intrinsically increased levels of autoimmunity were transposed into mice.[44] These observations may be the reason that individuals who have autoantibodies in the premorbid state (e.g., first-degree relatives of patients with rheumatoid arthritis) are at a greater risk for developing clinical symptoms of autoim-

munity. It has been suggested that, because autoantibodies can focus antigen on APCs, this might inhibit degradation of the antigen and permit an immune response to develop against it.[45]

Immunoglobulin G Rheumatoid Factor—Self-Association into Immune Complexes in Rheumatoid Arthritis

Another important property of rheumatoid factor is to aggregate antigen into complexes sufficiently large to be immunogenic and to activate complement (Fig. 6–6). A single IgM rheumatoid factor

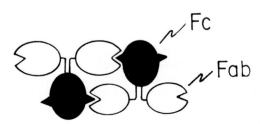

FIGURE 6–6. Diagram of two IgG molecules that have self-associated. One can appreciate that this complex of two IgG molecules can grow by accretion to a large aggregate, almost particulate in size. (Redrawn from presentations by Dr. Mart Mannik, University of Washington.)

molecule and a single IgG have a low association constant and are relatively benign. However, if rheumatoid factor comes into contact with polymeric IgG, then the association constant is tighter.

Hybridomas from rheumatoid synovium produce IgG rheumatoid factors that self-associate to form immune complexes.[46] These self-associated IgG complexes bind to IgM rheumatoid factor as much as 1 million times more effectively than does monomeric IgG. They are effective activators of complement and are phagocytosed by neutrophils, causing their activation.[47]

Immune Complexes in Rheumatoid Arthritis

Immune complexes in rheumatoid arthritis have been identified in the circulation, synovial fluid, synovial tissue, phagocytic cells in the synovial cells in the synovial lining cells, and articular cartilage. Those immunoglobulins in articular cartilage[48] are particularly interesting because circumstantial evidence supports the hypothesis that deposits of aggregated immune complexes in the superficial layers of articular cartilage act as chemoattractants for the invasive and destructive pannus that moves centripetally over and into the cartilage. Characteristics of these cartilage-bound immunoglobulins include the following:

- Immunofluorescent histopathology reveals a granular pattern of superficial immunoglobulin in articular cartilage characteristic of immune complexes and not found when cartilage is stained for other proteins (e.g., serum albumin), nor seen in similar preparations of cartilage from osteoarthritis.[49]

- Extraction of cartilage with guanidine yields much more IgG than does extraction with neutral buffer, implying that the complexes may be covalently bound to cartilage matrix. Further studies showed that there are disulfide bonds between the IgG and cartilage GAGs.[50]

- Within the immunoglobulin complexes in articular cartilage in rheumatoid arthritis, there are antibodies against native and denatured type II (cartilage) collagen as well as IgM and IgG rheumatoid factors.[51] More antibodies against type II collagen bind to neutrophil elastase–treated cartilage, a process that mimics what is present in the inflamed joint, than to "unharmed" cartilage.[52]

- Immune complexes are absent under areas in cartilage actively being invaded by pannus, suggesting that they had been phagocytosed by cells in the tissue that had been drawn from the periphery across the cartilage.[53]

GALACTOSYLATION OF IMMUNOGLOBULINS—ITS RELEVANCE TO RHEUMATOID FACTOR

Since 1976, it has been known that IgG from rheumatoid patients had fewer galactose residues at certain sites in the $C\gamma2$ region, resulting in oligosaccharides terminating in *N*-acetylglucosamine.[54] This reduced galactosylation may be caused by a demonstrated deficiency in B-lymphocyte galactosyltransferase activity in patients with rheumatoid arthritis.[55] The question has been: Does the agalactosyl IgG have functional effects for inducing rheumatoid factor production and immune complex formation? One study has determined that patients with early synovitis who have the lowest galactose concentrations of IgG are more likely to progress to definite rheumatoid arthritis than are those with normal glycosylation,[56] and that immune complex concentrations in blood of rheumatoid patients are strongly associated with agalactosyl IgG.[57]

Agalactosyl monosaccharide (Gal[0]) sequences increase with age in normal subjects from a mean prevalence of around 25 per cent at age 50 to near 50 per cent at age 85.[58] Although increased Gal(0) is seen in pulmonary tuberculosis and Crohn's disease, it is not seen in other inflammatory states (including bacterial infections) in which acute-phase reactants are elevated. Pregnant women with rheumatoid arthritis enjoying a remission in their disease have low levels of Gal(0), but after parturition, when their disease relapses, Gal(0) levels rise.[59]

Data to suggest that Gal(0) levels may be useful in predicting the course of rheumatoid arthritis are reviewed in Chapter 24. At this time, however, no data are available to implicate decreased galactosylation in IgG as a causative factor of the disease.

REFERENCES

1. Rose, H. M., Ragan, C., Pearce, E., et al.: Differential agglutination of normal and sensitized sheep erythrocytes by sera of patients with rheumatoid arthritis. Proc. Soc. Exp. Biol. Med. 68:1, 1948.
2. van Zeben, D., Hazes, J. M. W., Zwinderman, A. H., et al.: Clinical significance of rheumatoid factors in early rheumatoid arthritis: results of a follow up study. Ann. Rheum. Dis. 51:1029, 1992.
3. Jonsson, T., and Valdimarsson, H.: Clinical significance of rheumatoid factor isotypes in seropositive arthritis. Rheumatol. Int. 12:111, 1992.
4. Carson, D. A.: Rheumatoid factor. *In* Kelley, W. N., Harris, E. D. Jr., Ruddy, S., and Sledge, C. B. (eds.): Textbook of Rheumatology, 4th ed., Vol. 1. Philadelphia, W. B. Saunders, 1993, pp. 155–163.
5. Wolfe, F., Cathey, M. A., and Roberts, F. K.: The Latex test

revisited: rheumatoid factor testing in 8,287 rheumatic disease patients. Arthritis Rheum. 34:951, 1991.

6. Noritake, D. T., Colburn, K. K., Chan, G., et al.: Rheumatoid factors specific for active rheumatoid arthritis. Ann. Rheum. Dis. 49:910, 1990.

The assay developed was an ELISA to measure rheumatoid factors in human serum that bind a cross-reactive determinant shared on human and other mammalian IgG. In assays of 108 samples of sera from patients with rheumatoid arthritis, 231 samples of sera from patients with other connective tissue diseases, and samples of sera from 365 diverse normal subjects or patients sick with unrelated diseases, 99 per cent specificity was found, although the test was not particularly sensitive: only 37 of the 108 rheumatoid arthritis samples were positive at a titer that maintained the specificity. This test might have more relevance for the biology of rheumatoid factor than as a diagnostic tool.

7. He, X., Goronzy, J. J., and Weyand, C. M.: The repertoire of rheumatoid factor-producing B cells in normal subjects and patients with rheumatoid arthritis. Arthritis Rheum. 36:1061, 1993.

8. Hazes, J. M. W., Dijkmans, B. A. C., Vandenbroucke, J. P., et al.: Lifestyle and the risk of rheumatoid arthritis: cigarette smoking and alcohol consumption. Ann. Rheum. Dis. 49:980, 1990.

9. Tuomi, T., Heliövaara, M., Palosuo, T., et al.: Smoking, lung function, and rheumatoid factors. Ann. Rheum. Dis. 49:753, 1989.

10. Moynier, M., Abderrazik, M., Didry, C., et al.: The B cell repertoire in rheumatoid arthritis. III. Preferential homing of rheumatoid factor-producing B cell precursors in the synovial fluid. Arthritis Rheum. 35:49, 1992.

11. Caligaris-Cappio, F., and Ferrarini, M.: B cells and their fate in health and disease. Immunol. Today 17:206, 1996.

12. Perez, L., Orte, J., and Brevia, J. A.: Terminal differentiation of spontaneous rheumatoid factor-secreting B cells from rheumatoid arthritis patients depends on endogenous interleukin-10. Arthritis Rheum. 38:1771, 1995.

13. Cush, J. J., Splawski, J. B., Thomas, R., et al.: Elevated interleukin-10 levels in patients with rheumatoid arthritis. Arthritis Rheum. 38:96, 1995.

14. Carson, D. A., Chen, P. P., and Kipps, T. J.: New roles for rheumatoid factor. J. Clin. Invest. 87:379, 1991.

15. Lipsky, P. E., Davis, L. S., Meek, K., and Wacholtz, M. C.: T cells and B cells. In Kelley, W. N., Harris, E. H. Jr., Ruddy, S., and Sledge, C. B., (eds.): Textbook of Rheumatology, 4th ed., Vol. 1. Philadelphia, W. B. Saunders, 1993, pp. 108–154.

16. Geha, R. S., and Rosen, F. S.: The genetic basis of immunoglobulin-class switching. N. Engl. J. Med. 330:1008, 1994.

17. Allen, R. C., Armitage, J. R., Conley, M. E., et al.: CD40 ligand gene defects responsible for X-linked hyper-IgM syndrome. Science 259:990, 1993.

18. Lorente, L., Richaud-Patin, Y., Fior, R., et al.: In vivo production of interleukin-10 by non-T cells in rheumatoid arthritis, Sjögren's syndrome, and systemic lupus erythematosus. Arthritis Rheum. 37:1647, 1994.

19. Levy, Y., and Brouet, I.-C.: Interleukin-10 prevents spontaneous death of germinal center B cells by induction of the bcl-2 protein. J. Clin. Invest. 93:424, 1994.

20. Hirohata, S., Yanagida, T., Koda, M., et al.: Selective induction of IgM rheumatoid factors by CD14⁺ monocyte-lineage cells generated from bone marrow of patients with rheumatoid arthritis. Arthritis Rheum. 38:384, 1995.

21. Plater-Zyberk, C., and Maini, R. N.: Phenotypic and func-

22. Kiddaka, T., Kitani, A., Hara, M., et al.: IL-4 down-regulates the surface expression of CD5 on B cells and inhibits spontaneous immunoglobulin and IgM–rheumatoid factor production in patients with rheumatoid arthritis. Clin. Exp. Immunol. 89:223, 1992.

23. Plater-Zyberk, C., Brown, C. M. S., Andrew E. M., et al.: CD5⁺ B in rheumatoid arthritis. Ann. N. Y. Acad. Sci. 651:540, 1992.

24. Kimberly, R. P., Salmon, J. E., and Edberg, J. C.: Receptors for immunoglobulin G: molecular diversity and implications for disease. Arthritis Rheum. 38:306, 1995.

25. Chomarat, P., Briolay, J., Banchereau, J., et al.: Increased production of soluble CD23 in rheumatoid arthritis, and its regulation by interleukin-4. Arthritis Rheum. 36:234, 1993.

26. Thompson, K. M., Randen, I., Natvig, J. B., et al.: Human monoclonal rheumatoid factors derived from the polyclonal repertoire of rheumatoid synovial tissue: incidence of cross-reactive idiotypes and expression of V_H and V_K subgroups. Eur. J. Immunol. 20:863, 1990.

27. Sasso, E. H.: Immunoglobulin V region genes in rheumatoid arthritis. Rheum. Dis. Clin. North Am. 18:809, 1992.

28. Bridges, S. L. Jr., Lee, S. K., Johnson, M. L., et al.: Somatic mutation and CDR3 lengths of immunoglobulin kappa light chains expressed in patients with rheumatoid arthritis and in normal individuals. J. Clin. Invest. 96:831, 1995.

29. Youngblood, K., Fruchter, L., Ding, G., et al.: Rheumatoid factors from the peripheral blood of two patients with rheumatoid arthritis are genetically heterogeneous and somatically mutated. J. Clin. Invest. 93:852, 1994.

30. Mageed, R. A., Vencovsky, J., and Maini, R. N.: Rheumatoid factors and germline genes in rheumatoid arthritis: evidence of an intrinsic B-lymphocyte defect? Br. J. Rheumatol. 33:104, 1994.

31. Pascual, V., Randen, I., Thompson, K., et al.: The complete nucleotide sequences of the heavy chain variable regions of six monospecific rheumatoid factors derived from Epstein-Barr virus-transformed B cells isolated from the synovial tissue of patients with rheumatoid arthritis. J. Clin. Invest. 86:1320, 1990.

32. Randen, I., Brown, D., Thompson, K. M., et al.: Clonally related IgM rheumatoid factors undergo affinity maturation in the rheumatoid synovial tissue. J. Immunol. 148:3296, 1992.

33. Lee, S. K., Bridges, S. L. Jr., Kirkham, P. M., et al.: Evidence of antigen receptor-influenced oligoclonal B lymphocyte expansion in the synovium of a patient with long-standing rheumatoid arthritis. J. Clin. Invest. 93:361, 1994.

34. Deftos, M., Olee, T., Carson, D. A., et al.: Defining the genetic origins of three rheumatoid synovium-derived IgG rheumatoid factors. J. Clin. Invest. 93:2545, 1994.

35. Lafyatis, R., Flipo, R. M., Duquesnoy, B., et al.: Antibodies in rheumatoid synovial fluids bind to a restricted series of protein antigens in rheumatoid synovial tissue. Arthritis Rheum. 35:1016, 1992.

36. Sato, Y., Sato, R., Watanabe, H., et al.: Complement activating properties of monoreactive and polyreactive IgM rheumatoid factors. Ann. Rheum. Dis. 52:795, 1993.

37. Williams, R. C., Malone, C. C., and Harley, J. B.: Rheumatoid factors from patients with rheumatoid arthritis react with tryptophan 60 and 95, lysine 58, and arginine 97, on human B2 microglobulin. Arthritis Rheum. 36:916, 1993.

38. Burastero, S. E., Casali, P., Wilder, R. L., et al.: Monoreac-

tive high affinity and polyreactive low affinity rheumatoid factors are produced by CD5$^+$ B cells from patients with rheumatoid arthritis. J. Exp. Med. 168:1979, 1988.

39. Harindranath, N., Goldfarb, I. S., Ikematsu, H., et al.: Complete sequence of the genes encoding the V_H and V_L regions of low- and high-affinity monoclonal IgM and IgA$_1$ rheumatoid factors produced by CD5$^+$ B cells from rheumatoid arthritis patients. Int. Immunol. 3:865, 1991.

40. Slaughter, L., Carson, D. A., Jensen, F. C., et al.: In vitro effects of Epstein-Barr virus on peripheral blood mononuclear cells from patients with rheumatoid arthritis and normal subjects. J. Exp. Med. 148:1429, 1978.

41. He, X., Goronzy, J., and Weyand, C.: Selective induction of rheumatoid factors by superantigens and human helper T cells. J. Clin. Invest. 89:673, 1992.

42. Vaughan, J. H.: Pathogenetic concepts and origins of rheumatoid factor in rheumatoid arthritis. Arthritis Rheum. 36:1, 1993.

43. Origuchi, T., Eguchi, K., Kawabe, Y., et al.: Increased levels of serum IgM antibody to staphylococcal enterotoxin B in patients with rheumatoid arthritis. Ann. Rheum. Dis. 54:713, 1995.

44. Tighe, H., Chen, P. P., Tucker, R., et al.: Function of B cells expressing a human immunoglobulin M rheumatoid factor autoantibody in transgenic mice. J. Exp. Med. 177:109, 1993.

The following information expands on that in the text about the transgenic mice expressing rheumatoid factor genes:

- High levels of surface IgM rheumatoid factor expression are not accompanied by high levels of rheumatoid factor secretion.

- Anti-human IgM stimulates the mouse cells expressing human IgM to proliferate.

- The transgenic rheumatoid factor B cells are highly efficient APCs for immune complexes.

- By breeding the transgene onto strains of mice prone to autoimmunity (i.e., the *lpr/lpr* genes of MRL mice), human IgM rheumatoid factor secretion increased more than 200-fold.

45. Carson, D. A.: Genetic factors in the etiology and pathogenesis of autoimmunity. FASEB J. 6:2800, 1992.

46. Lu, E. W., Deftos, M., Tighe, H., et al.: Generation and characterization of two monoclonal self-associating IgG rheumatoid factors from a rheumatoid synovium. Arthritis Rheum. 35:101, 1992.

47. Mannik, M., Nardella, F. A., and Sasso, E. H.: Rheumatoid factors in immune complexes of patients with rheumatoid arthritis. Springer Semin. Immunopathol. 10:215, 1988.

48. Cooke, T. D., Hurd, E. R., Jasin, H. E., et al.: Identification of immunoglobulins and complement in rheumatoid articular collagenous tissues. Arthritis Rheum. 18:541, 1975.

49. Vetto, A. A., Mannik, M., Zatarain-Rios, E., et al.: Immune deposits in articular cartilage of patients with rheumatoid arthritis have a granular pattern not seen in osteoarthritis. Rheumatol. Int. 10:13, 1990.

50. Trujillo, P. E., and Mannik, M.: IgG is bound by antigen-antibody bonds and some IgG and albumin are bound by intermolecular disulfide bonds to cartilage in rheumatoid arthritis and osteoarthritis. Rheumatol. Int. 11:225, 1992.

51. Jasin, H. E.: Autoantibody specificities of immune complexes sequestered in articular cartilage of patients with rheumatoid arthritis and osteoarthritis. Arthritis Rheum. 28:241, 1985.

52. Jasin, H. E., and Taurog, J. D.: Mechanisms of disruption of the articular cartilage surface in inflammation: neutrophil elastase increases availability of collagen type II epitopes for binding with antibody on the surface of articular cartilage. J. Clin. Invest. 87:1531, 1991.

53. Shiozawa, S., Jasin, H. E., and Ziff, M.: Absence of immunoglobulins in rheumatoid cartilage-pannus junctions. Arthritis Rheum. 23:816, 1980.

54. Mullinax, F., Hymes, A. J., and Mullinax, G. L.: Molecular site and enzymatic origin of IgG galactose deficiency in rheumatoid arthritis and SLE. Arthritis Rheum. 19:813, 1976.

55. Axford, J. S., Lydyard, P. M., Isenberg, D. A., et al.: Reduced B-cell galactosyltransferase activity in rheumatoid arthritis. Lancet 2:1486, 1987.

56. Young, A., Sumar, N., Bodman, K., et al.: Agalactosyl IgG: an aid to differential diagnosis in early synovitis. Arthritis Rheum. 34:1425, 1991.

57. Bond, A., Kerr, M. A., and Hay, F. C.: Distinct oligosaccharide content of rheumatoid arthritis-derived immune complexes. Arthritis Rheum. 38:744, 1995.

58. Rahman, A., and Isenberg, D.: Does it take sugar? A clinical role for measuring the glycosylation of IgG. Ann. Rheum. Dis. 54:689, 1995.

59. Rook, G. A. W., Steele, J., Brealey, R., et al.: Changes in IgG glycoform levels are associated with remission of arthritis during pregnancy. J. Autoimmun. 4:779, 1991.

SECTION IV

VASCULAR AND SYNOVIAL CELL COMPONENTS OF INFLAMMATION AND PROLIFERATION IN RHEUMATOID ARTHRITIS

The immune response of lymphocytes and antigen-presenting cells must have a physical context in which to develop. This context is the synovium, packed with increasing numbers of new blood vessels and an elaborate system of adhesion molecules in a milieu of multiple types of cells and cytokines. In the fluid phase, multiple inflammatory pathways are activated, contributing heavily to the growing process that leads to loss of cartilage. In this section, many of these supporting arms of the inflammatory and proliferative response in the joints of rheumatoid patients are discussed.

Early in the rheumatoid process, angiogenic stimuli lead to the development of a new and extensive capillary network. Cytokines drive this development, and it is cytokines that lead to the appearance of endothelial cells of adhesion molecules to which circulating leukocytes adhere and then slide between into the synovium. Within the synovium, a heterogeneous array of mesenchymal and inflammatory cells exchange messenger molecules, continue proliferating, and produce the proteases capable of destroying all joint tissues.

7

Leukocyte Translocation from Blood to Synovium

In order for rheumatoid synovitis to develop, cells must move from the bone marrow and lymphoid tissues through synovial blood vessels and into the synovium. In order for synovium to proliferate from a lining layer several cells thick into the abundant and luxurious fleshy mass that can be felt on examination, an enormous new network of small blood vessels must form in the inflamed tissue. In order for the cells to translocate, a complex system of adhesion molecules, homing receptors, and chemoattractants must be organized that arrests leukocyte flow through the capillaries and drags them by a chemical gradient into the synovium, fixing them there to respond to the immunologic challenge (Fig. 7–1).

When considering the mature rheumatoid synovium, two important questions arise when one views the large number of "immigrant" cells, principally lymphocytes and macrophages, and the complex network of new capillaries and connecting vascular channels that have transported the cells to the tissue:

1. How do new blood vessels grow within synovium?
2. How do circulating cells reach the synovium?

Accordingly, this discussion is presented in two sections, one to consider the forces driving angiogenesis in the synovium, and another to consider the relative involvement of different adhesion molecules in leukocyte traffic into and within the inflamed synovium.

ENHANCEMENT AND CONTROL OF ANGIOGENESIS IN RHEUMATOID SYNOVIUM

The term "angiogenesis-dependent disease" has been applied to rheumatoid arthritis.[1] The inference is that, without extensive growth of new blood vessels, proliferative synovitis could not be maintained. After seeing the large mass of highly vascular synovium removed from joints at the time of synovectomy or arthroplasty, this seems abundantly clear. In this sense, as in many others, rheumatoid arthritis resembles a localized malignancy. A highly vascularized synovium is essential to sustain vigorous growth of synovial tissue and to provide sustenance for the "immigrant" cells from the circulation drawn to the joint by chemoattractants generated within the synovium and joint space. Indeed, a rough correlation between angiogenic activity estimated by histologic examination and synovial hyperplasia and synovial infiltration by inflammatory cells has been made.[2]

However, rheumatoid synovium frequently demands more of its blood supply than that supply can provide; this is exacerbated when high pressure from excessive joint fluid actually tamponades capillary flow (reviewed in Chapter 13). Even the most luxuriously vascularized synovium can become ischemic, acidotic, and dependent upon anaerobic glycolysis for energy.

The cells determining angiogenesis are the specialized endothelial cells. Whereas fibroblasts can be thought of as "round" in the sense that they are not polarized, nor do they send cytokines in one direction and have receptors projecting in another, endothelial cells have a polarized phenotype. It can be demonstrated that endothelial cells have vectorial secretion, similar to osteoclasts or epithelium in the gut. Endothelial cells secrete collagen, fibronectin, and metalloproteases in a basal direction, not apically.[3] This functional polarity doubtless contributes to the precision and complexity of the angiogenic process.

The angiogenic response is a precise and reproducible one, identical in all tissues[4,4a] (Fig. 7–2).[1] In rheumatoid synovium, this response is directed by many different stimuli, most of them cytokines produced by one of the many cells in the heterogeneous synovitis.

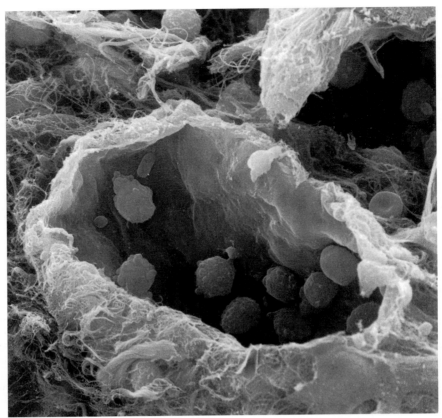

FIGURE 7–1. In this scanning electron photomicrograph, polymorphonuclear leukocytes are found bound to endothelial cells before they transmigrate through into the extracellular matrix. (Courtesy of M. J. Karnovsky and G. B. Ryan, Harvard Medical School.) (×4,000) (From Harris, E. D. Jr.: Pathogenesis of rheumatoid arthritis. *In* Kelley, W. N., Harris, E. D. Jr., Ruddy, S., and Sledge, C. B. [eds.]: Textbook of Rheumatology, 2nd ed. Philadelphia, W. B. Saunders, 1985, p. 891. Used by permission.)

Cytokines That Enhance Development of Angiogenesis in Rheumatoid Arthritis

In considering these data, it is important not to rely on in vitro assays for endothelial cell proliferation. Neither proliferation nor migration of endothelial cells in response to cytokines in vitro is equivalent to angiogenesis. Formation of true new capillaries is a complex and tightly controlled process, as demonstrated by Figure 7–2.[1] For example, types I and III collagens enhance both mitogenesis and migration of endothelial cells, but types IV and V collagens inhibit these functions in various assays. However, there are no data to suggest that any of these matrix macromolecules do more than facilitate new capillary growth once this process is triggered by the proper signals.

Heparin-Binding Growth Factors (HBGFs). These polypeptides (15 to 17 kDa) are members either of an acidic (anionic) or a basic (cationic) family and are precursors of fibroblast growth factors. HBGF-2, the basic form, is found bound to extracellular matrix components.[5] The acidic form, HBGF-1, is found within synovial mononuclear cells, and its amount has been measured to be in proportion to the inflammatory response gauged by mononuclear cell infiltration.[6] HBGF-1 also induces synthesis of both plasminogen activator and collagenase by endothelial cells.[7] So potent is basic FGF (or HBGF-2) that its capability of inducing angiogenesis has led to its use in accelerating healing of peptic ulcers. Orally administered HBGF-2 has been demonstrated to heal gastric ulcers caused by nonsteroidal anti-inflammatory drugs.[8]

Macrophage Angiogenic Factor. In populations of macrophages from rheumatoid synovium, there is one (F3, corresponding to a fraction of cells eluting at a certain density on Percoll gradients) that has strong angiogenic activity.[9] These F3 macro-

1) Activation of endothelial cells

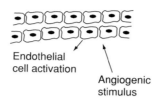

Endothelial
cell activation

Angiogenic
stimulus

2) Secretion of proteases to degrade
basement membrane and tissue
matrix

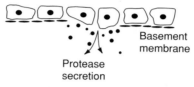

Basement
membrane

Protease
secretion

3) Formation of capillary sprout

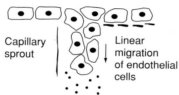

Capillary
sprout

Linear
migration
of endothelial
cells

4) Growth of capillary sprout

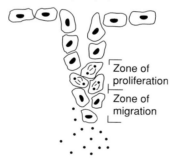

Zone of
proliferation

Zone of
migration

5) Lumenation of sprout
and synthesis of new basement
membrane

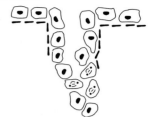

6) Two sprouts link to form capillary
loop

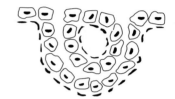

7) Development of second
generation capillary sprouts

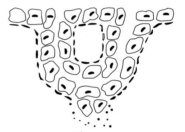

FIGURE 7–2. The seven-step sequence of angiogenesis that is continuous and repeated time and time again as new blood vessels develop. (From Colville-Nash, P. R., and Scott, D. L.: Angiogenesis and rheumatoid arthritis: pathogenic and therapeutic implications. Ann. Rheum. Dis. 51:919, 1992. Used by permission.)

phages are mature, expressing Fc receptor, complement receptor type 3 (CR3), and HLA-DR and staining for esterase activity. They bind avidly to fibronectin-coated collagen gels. The data suggest that IL-8 and TNFα account for a large proportion of the macrophage-derived angiogenic activity.[10]

Vascular Endothelial Growth Factor (VEGF). This substance increases vascular permeability, expressing potency comparable with histamine or bradykinin. It also is a chemoattractant for monocytes. Rheumatoid synovial lining cells and macrophages express this polypeptide, but normal synovial cells do not.[11] VEGF accounts for a large portion of the vascular migration and proliferation activity in rheumatoid arthritis synovial fluid and supernatants of synovial tissue cultures.[11] VEGF also induces synthesis and release of metalloprotease I (interstitial collagenase), the only enzyme that can initiate degradation of the interstitial collagens (types I, II, and III).[12]

Prostaglandins. Both prostaglandin (PG) E_1 and E_2 appear to be angiogenic both in vivo and in ex vivo models.[13] This is particularly interesting because the net effect in most systems is for PGE_1 to be anti-inflammatory, in contrast to the phlogistic PGE_2.

Endothelial-cell stimulating angiogenic factor. This low-molecular-weight substance is similar to the tumor angiogenic factor isolated by Folkman and his colleagues; it is present in approximately 15 per cent of rheumatoid synovial fluids.[14] It has the unusual quality of being able to dissociate complexes of metalloproteases and tissue inhibitor of metalloproteases (TIMP).[15]

Interleukin-8. This 8-kDa polypeptide is best known for its chemotactic capability, but in a rabbit corneal pocket model can induce neovascularization.[16] Angiogenic activity present in conditioned medium of rheumatoid synovial tissue could be blocked equally well by antibodies to IL-8 and TNFα.[10]

Another angiogenic factor, **gliostatin/platelet-derived endothelial cell growth factor,** has been isolated and purified from rheumatoid synovial fluids.[17] This protein promotes proliferation and chemotactic migration of endothelial cells, resulting in angiogenesis, while inhibiting proliferation of synovial lining cells. Immunohistochemical stains revealed that this angiogenic factor is found in, and perhaps produced by, the type B (fibroblast-like) synovial lining cells.

Natural Substances That Diminish Angiogenesis in Rheumatoid Synovitis

Interferon γ. This lymphokine induces a down-regulation of angiogenesis, perhaps by decreasing the number of receptors for endothelial cell growth factors.[18]

Transforming Growth Factor β. As a reparative cytokine, TGFβ increases macrophage numbers in inflammatory sites but down-regulates their activity; it induces collagen production.[19] It appears to antagonize the effects of other growth factors that stimulate endothelial cell proliferation, but in intact systems may enhance angiogenesis. This attests to the multiple facets and complexity of this cytokine, depending into which context it is released.

Interleukin-1β. IL-1β has a negative effect on angiogenesis, inhibiting proliferation of endothelial cells.[20] This is one of the few antiproliferative actions of this cytokine.

Platelet Factor 4. This component of α-granules of platelets has immunodulatory activity and is angiostatic through its ability to specifically inhibit endothelial cell proliferation.[21]

Thrombospondin. This matrix glycoprotein regulates certain aspects of the coagulation process as well as down-regulating angiogenesis. It has been demonstrated in the macrophages and blood vessels of rheumatoid synovium.[22]

Intact Cartilage. One of the most interesting qualities of cartilage is its capability, mediated by low-molecular-weight substances, of resisting invasion by blood vessels.[4] Untested to date is the hypothesis that, early in the rheumatoid process, the loss of proteoglycans caused by proteases from neutrophils and from activated chondrocytes also results in depletion of the substances that protect cartilage from vascular invasion, thereby facilitating infiltration of the destructive pannus.

Present and Potential Therapeutic Modalities To Prevent Angiogenesis

Many of the therapeutic agents used in rheumatoid arthritis can inhibit neovascularization or diminish endothelial cell proliferation or migration in various assay systems. Among them are certain steroid compounds, methotrexate, sulfasalazine, gold compounds, D-penicillamine, and chloroquine.[1,23,24] Whether or not this activity of these drugs has relevance to their therapeutic effects in rheumatoid arthritis is not known.

Although heparin alone can stimulate endothelial cell proliferation in some systems, heparin and certain steroid compounds are potent inhibitors of angiogenesis. One of these inhibitors is a cyclic complex of a modified heparin component, β-cyclodextrin tetradecasulfate, given with an angiostatic steroid such as tetrahydrocortisol.[25]

Minocycline has been reported to be an effective adjunct in treatment of rheumatoid arthritis (see Chapter 34). In addition to having inhibitory effects upon metalloproteases, it is a locally effective inhibitor of angiogenesis and may potentiate the effects of other inhibitors.[26] Two of these inhibitors are the compound AGM-1470 and the micotubule-stabilizing agent taxol. AGM-1470 inhibits fibroblast growth factor–induced stimulation of endothelial cell migration, endothelial cell proliferation, and capillary tube formation that results in effective suppression of new blood vessel formation. Taxol interferes with normal microtubule function in cell mitosis, migration, chemotaxis, and intracellular transport. Used in combination, AGM-1470 and Taxol significantly reduced clinical arthritis in rats induced by injections of type II collagen.[27]

The potential for using protease inhibitors to restrain angiogenesis is intriguing. Metalloproteases are undoubtedly involved in formation of new vessels.[28] Inhibitors of these enzymes are being developed, but the problem is delivery. How can potent compounds be delivered to the joint without the need for polyarticular injection? Are there ways to devise drug delivery systems that can target inflamed joints, even if they must be given by intravenous injection? Most of these angiogenesis inhibitors have low toxicity, and their potential for treatment of rheumatoid or arthritis deserves significant study.

LEUKOCYTE–ENDOTHELIAL CELL INTERACTIONS AND ADHESIVE MOLECULES ON ENDOTHELIAL CELLS AND LEUKOCYTES

Multiple molecules are a part of the sequence that leads to leukocyte slowing in capillaries, binding to endothelial cells, and then emigration from the circulation into the extravascular tissues. The process can be best described as a "reversible adhesion cascade" (see Fig. 7–4 later in this section). It is an active process mediated by glycoproteins variably expressed on the surfaces of both the leukocytes and the endothelial cells. This is a complex process, made so by the sequential activation and expression of many different molecules, depending on the site and intensity of inflammation in the synovium.

The molecules known to be involved in the leukocyte–endothelial cell interaction are listed in Table 7–1.[29] The footnote to the table gives a glossary for understanding of eponyms and abbreviations. Table 7–2 gives details of molecules involved in lymphocyte–endothelial cell recognition and lymphocyte homing.[30] Readers in this field must accept an enormous redundancy of names given to the same molecules. Soon, it is hoped, there will be one name, and no more, agreed upon for each gene product. Until that happens, a glos-

TABLE 7–1. Adhesion Molecules Involved in Leukocyte Traffic in Inflammation*

MOLECULE	SYNONYMS	LIGANDS	EXPRESSION
Selectins			
L-selectin	LAM-1, MEL-14 antigen	PNAd, other	N, E, M, L subsets
P-selectin	GMP-140	Sialyl-Lewis X	Platelets, EC
E-selectin	ELAM-1	Sialyl-Lewis X, CLA	EC
Integrins			
$\alpha_L\beta_2$	LFA-1; CD11a/CD18	ICAM-1, -2, and -3	N, E, M, L
$\alpha_M\beta_2$	CR3 (Mac-1); CD11b/CD18	ICAM-1, other	N, E, M, NK
$\alpha_X\beta_2$	p150,95; CD11c/CD18	Fibrinogen, other	N, E, M, L subsets
$\alpha_4\beta_1$	VLA-4, CD49d/CD29	VCAM-1, fibronectin	M, E, NK, L
$\alpha_4\beta_7$		MAdCAM-1, VCAM-1, fibronectin, Peyer's patch	M, E, NK, L
$\alpha_5\beta_1$	VLA-5	RGD sequences	E, L, platelets
Immunoglobulin superfamily			
ICAM-1	CD54	$\alpha_L\beta_2$, (LFA-1), $\alpha_M\beta_2$	EC, leukocytes, other (inducible)
ICAM-2	CD102	$\alpha_L\beta_2$	EC, leukocytes, other (constituitive)
ICAM-3	CD50	$\alpha_L\beta_2$	Leukocytes, ?EC
VCAM-1	CD106	$\alpha_4\beta_1$ (VLA-4), ($\alpha_4\beta_7$)	EC, other
MAdCAM-1		$\alpha_4\beta_7$	EC (mucosal)
PECAM-1	CD31	CD31, other	EC, leukocytes
Other			
CD44		Hyaluronan, other	Leukocytes, EC, other
VAP-1		?	EC

From Haskard, D. O.: Cell adhesion molecules in rheumatoid arthritis. Curr. Opin. Rheumatol. 7:229, 1995. Used by permission.

* Key: E, eosinophils; EC, endothelial cells; ELAM-1, endothelial leukocyte adhesion molecule-1; GMP-140, granular membrane protein 140; ICAM, intercellular adhesion molecule; L, lymphocytes; LAM-1 leukocyte adhesion molecule-1; LFA-1, leukocyte function associated antigen-1; M, monocytes-macrophages; Mac-1, macrophage antigen-1; MAdCAM-1, mucosal addressin cell adhesion molecule-1; N, neutrophils; NK, natural killer cells; PECAM-1, platelet–endothelial cell adhesion molecule-1; PNAd, peripheral lymph node addressin; VAP-1, vascular adhesion protein-1; VCAM-1, vascular cell adhesion molecule-1; CLA, cutaneous lymphocyte antigen.

TABLE 7–2. Molecules Involved in Lymphocyte–Endothelial Cell Recognition and Lymphocyte Homing

MOLECULAR FAMILY	PROPOSED PRIMARY FUNCTION IN LYMPHOCYTE HOMING
A. Selectin LECAM-1 (L-selectin, Mel-14, LAM-1 Ags)	The prototypic primary ''activation-independent'' homing receptor. On lymphocytes, serves as the peripheral lymph node homing receptor; recognizes sialylated oligosaccharide determinants on the peripheral lymph node vascular addressin (PNAd).
ELAM-1 (E-selectin)	Inflammation-induced endothelial adhesion molecule which in the setting of chronic inflammation is selectively expressed in the skin (i.e., is a skin vascular addressin). Recognizes the cutaneous lymphocyte antigen, CLA.
B. Oligosaccharide Ligands for Selectins Peripheral node addressin (PNAd)	Selectively expressed on peripheral lymph node HEV; contains the sialylated carbohydrate ligand for LECAM-1. Appears to be inducible late in the course of chronic inflammation in many tertiary sites.
CLA (cutaneous lymphocyte antigen)	Skin lymphocyte homing receptor: Sialylated oligosaccharide ligand for ELAM-1, expressed on a skin-associated subset of memory T cells.
C. Integrin $\beta2$ class (CD18), LFA-1 ($\alpha_L\beta_2$)	Recognizes ICAM-1, -2, and probably other ligands on endothelium. Likely serves as an activation-dependent ''secondary'' adhesion molecule involved in adhesion strengthening and diapedesis in many sites.
$\alpha4$ class (CD49d), VLA-4 ($\alpha4\beta1$)	VCAM-1 is one known endothelial ligand. Also recognizes fibronectin. Currently thought to participate in lymphocyte homing to sites of chronic inflammation, perhaps as an activation-dependent adhesion molecule analogous to LFA-1. May also participate in binding Peyer's patch-HEV.
$\alpha4\beta$p; $\alpha4\beta7$	Participates in binding to Peyer's patch-HEV but HEV ligand is unknown. *In vivo* function and distribution are not well characterized at present.
D. Ig Superfamily ICAM-1, -2	Endothelial ligands for LFA-1; ICAM-1 is upregulated with inflammation, but ICAM-2 is constitutively expressed on EC.
VCAM-1	Endothelial ligand for $\alpha_4\beta_1$. Inflammation induced. *In vivo* distribution is incompletely characterized, but expression is heterogeneous, suggesting the possibility of tissue-selective function.
E. Proteoglycan/Cartilage-Link Protein CD44 (HCAM, Pgp-1)	Binds hyaluronate, collagen type VI, and the mucosal addressin, but the physiologic significance of each of these ligand interactions in relationship to lymphocyte-EC binding is unknown. Likely serves as a general adhesion molecule involved in adhesion strengthening, signal transduction, and/or cytoskeletal anchoring.
F. Other Mucosal addressin (MAd)	Endothelial adhesion molecule selectively expressed on mucosal HEV and lamina propria vessels. Binds mucosa-homing lymphoid subsets through interaction with an uncharacterized lymphocyte receptor.
HEBFpp	80-kDa lymphocyte cell surface receptor defined in the rat that is involved in Peyer's patch-HEV binding. Its roles *in vivo* and cellular distribution are poorly characterized, but it remains a potential candidate for a MAd receptor.

From Picker, L. J., and Butcher, E. C.: Physiological and molecular mechanisms of lymphocyte homing. Annu. Rev. Immunol. 10:561, 1992. Used by permission from the Annual Review of Immunology, © 1992 by Annual Reviews Inc.

sary such as Table 7–1 will be a useful reference. In addition to redundancy of names, there is also a redundancy in the molecules themselves. There appear to be ''backup'' adhesion molecules; more than one molecule is expressed that has functions similar to others.

Types of Adhesive Molecules

The different groups of adhesion molecules can be classified as follows: integrins, selectins, immunoglobulin superfamily adhesive molecules, and others.

Integrins

Integrins are a superfamily of transmembrane glycoproteins. They mediate cell-cell as well as cell-matrix interactions. As can be seen in Table 7–1, the integrins are found on the circulating cells destined to leave vessels and enter the tissues. They are diverse.

The β_1 integrin VLA family is involved primarily in adhesion of cells to other cells and to the extracellular matrix. Cells that express VLA (e.g., lymphocytes) will have an affinity for fibronectin and other matrix proteins, including collagen, laminin, and entactin, in the subsynovial tissues and remain there. In contrast, cells that do not express VLA (e.g., neutrophils) pass on into the joint space. VLA-4 is of particular relevance to rheumatoid arthritis because it helps mediate lymphocyte-monocyte-eosinophil interaction with endothelium as well as the extracellular matrix.[31] VLA-4–VCAM-1 interconnections are probably involved in accumulation of CD8+ memory T cells at sites of inflammation.[32]

Entactin is a basement membrane component that "laces" type IV collagen, laminin, and proteoglycans into the structural element that is basement membrane, serving as a "glue" amid complexes of matrix and cells. Entactin promotes leukocyte cell adhesion and chemotaxis through an RGD sequence found in this and other matrix molecules that bind integrins.[33]

With special relevance for arthritis, chondrocytes can attach to many cartilage and bone proteins, a process mediated by β_1 and β_3 integrins[34] on the chondrocyte cell membranes.

The β_2 subfamily of three integrins is found on neutrophils, eosinophils, monocytes, and lymphocytes. The family of β_2 integrins comprises several homologous heterodimers. The principal ones are complement receptors CR3 (CD11b/18, macrophage antigen 1 [Mac-1]) and CR4 (CD11c/18, p150,95) and LFA-1 (CD11a/18). Some may recognize a large variety of substance. For example CR3 binds to complement component iC3b, ICAM-1, fibrinogen, factor X, and certain bacteria. Their function, after ligand binding, is to mediate transmembrane chemical signaling. Their ligands are given in Table 7–1 (see also refs. 9 and 35). These adhesion molecules are examples of those that become "stickier" when cells are activated, presumably through a conformational change. Two different adhesion molecules on different leukocytes may have the same ligand. For example, the ligand for both leukocyte Mac-1, or CR3, and LFA-1 on endothelial cells is ICAM-1.[36]

The biologic importance of these integrins is demonstrated by the finding of a group of patients whose neutrophils are deficient in their capacity for normal chemotaxis and phagocytosis; neutrophils did not accumulate in infected or necrotic lesions and were missing CD11a/18, CD11b/18, and CD11c/18, the β_2 integrins.[37] Monocytes from these patients, however, migrate very well by relying on VLA-4.[38]

Selectins

Structural details of these molecules are shown in Figure 7–3.[39] The three known members of the family (and their aliases) are

L-selectin (Leu-8, Ly-22, LAM-1, MEL-14)
P-selectin (CD-62, PADGEM, GMP-140)
E-selectin (ELAM-1)

The selectins bind to carbohydrate moieties on glycoproteins via their lectin domains.

L-selectin, expressed on most circulating leukocytes, mediates the first step of leukocyte translocation, the "rolling" of neutrophils along capillary walls.[40]

P-selectin, found on endothelium and platelets, also helps in mediation of "rolling" and stopping of neutrophils on activated (i.e., tall) endothelium. It is mobilized rapidly to the surface of endothelial cells, where it is stored in Weibel-Palade bodies following stimulation by thrombin or other mediators.[39] P-selectin associated with the synovial microvasculature appears to initiate shear-resistant adhesion of monocytes and stabilizes bonds formed by other selectins and integrins.[41] P-selectin may be the endothelial adhesion molecule most responsible for the recruitment of monocytes to synovium.

In contrast to P-selectin, *E-selectin* is found only on endothelium, and is expressed after the endothelial cells are activated by cytokines (IL-1, TNFα, and substance P).[42] E-selectin appears on the membranes of tall endothelial cells of rheumatoid synovial capillaries, and is the only selectin known to function as a vascular addressin for T lymphocytes. Therapy with gold salts reduces expression of E-selectin by these cells.[43]

Immunoglobulin Superfamily Adhesive Molecules

This third family of adhesive molecules is characterized by immunoglobulin homology regions consisting of disulfide-bridged loops that primarily resemble heavy chains. Four members have been characterized in detail:

Intercellular adhesion molecule-1
Intercellular adhesion molecule-2
Vascular cell adhesion molecule-2

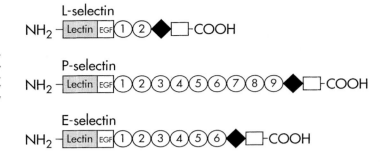

FIGURE 7–3. Structures of L-, P-, and E-selections. (From Bevilacqua, M. P., and Nelson, R. M.: Selectins. J. Clin. Invest. 91:379, 1993. Used by copyright permission of The Society for Clinical Investigation, 1993.)

Platelet–endothelial cell adhesion molecule (PECAM), also known as CD31 **ICAM-1,** the better studied of the ICAMs, serves a ligand to LFA-1 (CD11a/18) on leukocytes, and to some viruses as well. **VCAM-1,** like E-selectin and ICAM-1, is expressed after activation of endothelium by cytokines such as IL-1 and TNFα. VCAM-1 binds with VLA-4, also known as $\alpha_4\beta_1$, the integrin that is expressed on lymphocytes, mononuclear cells, and eosinophils but not neutrophils. Evidence is mounting that this VCAM-1–VLA-4 adhesive interaction may be the predominant one in fostering migration and adherence of leukocytes to inflamed synovium. **PECAM** (CD31) is found on endothelial cells, platelets, and leukocytes.[44] It may be required for transmigration of neutrophils across endothelial monolayers; antibodies against it inhibit neutrophil accumulation in experimental models of inflammation.[45]

Other Molecules Involved in Adhesion

CD44 is a transmembrane protein expressed on many cells, including leukocytes and endothelial cells. It has sequence homology with the red blood cell Lutheran antigen system and to cartilage link protein. It binds to fibronectin, collagen, and hyaluronate in the extracellular matrix.[46] CD44 may be one of the central molecules of T-lymphocyte adhesion and activation, and a mediator of cytokine release from monocytes.[47] The excessive expression of CD44 in rheumatoid synovial tissues may facilitate fixation of chronic inflammatory cells within inflamed joints.[38,48]

The Adhesion Cascade

The apparent redundancy of this plethora of adhesive molecules is better understood by a review of the "adhesion cascade" (Fig. 7–4).

Step 1: Leukocyte Rolling . . . Primary Adhesion

As leukocytes traverse vessels, many of them roll along the endothelial surface much more slowly than cells zipping along in the main current. This is made possible by **L-selectin** on lymphocytes or neutrophils, which forms a loose, transient, and reversible link with carbohydrate moieties on the endothelial cell surfaces. In a way, this phenomenon can be considered as an opportunity for the cells to sample the environment for activating factors that would arrest them at one particular segment of endothelium.

Step 2: Activation

In response to stimuli such as endotoxin or cytokines such as IL-1, IL-6, IFNγ, TNFα, and platelet-activating factor,[49] the capillary and postcapillary venule endothelium is volume expanded, becoming full, columnar, and tall. This activated state is associated with induction of expression of more adhesion molecules on both endothelial cells, particularly **E-selectin, P-selectin,** and the immunoglobulin-like **ICAM-1** and **VCAM-1.** It has been demonstrated that IFNγ is synergistic with TNFα in enhancing ICAM-1 surface expression on endothelial cells.[50] On neutrophils, the rolling is followed by activation of β_2 integrins, which promote attachment.

Step 3: Activation-Dependent Sticking

Although stable even under the shear stress of capillary and venule blood flow, this binding—similar to the other steps in the cascade—is reversible if endothelial activation ceases or if chemoattractants below the endothelium do not draw the attached cells into the extravascular space. Multiple adhesion pairs are active at this step (Table 7–3). Rolling neutrophils attach with greater efficiency to P-selectin than to E-selectin.[51]

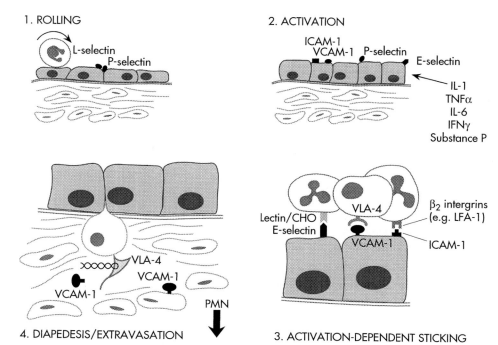

FIGURE 7–4. The sequence of adhesion within blood vessels of leukocytes, based on suggestions by Cronstein[36,86] and Butcher.[52] The four steps are described in the text. It is clear that there is redundancy built into this process; whereas certain receptor-ligand interactions are illustrated here, numerous others are engaged as well. The important point is realizing that until diapedesis, each bonding is reversible. Similarly, it appears that numerous cytokines can activate the endothelium to express selectins, VCAM-1, ICAM-1, and other endothelial adhesion molecules. Note: The blocks in steps 1 and 2 are drawn at one-quarter scale of the blocks in steps 3 and 4. Definition of abbreviations is given in Table 7–1. PMN, polymorphonuclear leukocytes.

Step 4: Diapedesis/Extravasation

This final process is dependent upon the presence of a chemoattractant gradient between the extravascular/extracellular space and the venules and capillaries. It is apparent that some cytoattractants are specific for lymphocytes, whereas others attract polymorphonuclear leukocytes or eosinophils. There must be a mechanism for detaching cells sufficiently from the endothelium to allow them to migrate without slipping back into the circulation. Neutrophils appear to use **LFA-1** for both

TABLE 7–3. Adhesion Pairs Active in Step 3 of Adhesion Cascade

LEUKOCYTE (NEUTROPHIL AND LYMPHOCYTE)	ENDOTHELIUM
L-selectin	CHO moiety
CHO moiety	E-selectin
CHO moiety	P-selectin
VLA-4	VCAM-1
β_2 integrins (LFA-1, CRT3)	ICAM-1

stabilized adhesion and transendothelial migration.[52] The transendothelial migration of T cells bound to endothelial cells involves LFA-1 and **ICAM-1**.[53] The cytokine **IL-8** may usefully inhibit adhesion, allowing transmigration[54] as may homing receptor molecules shed from leukocytes[55] and nitric oxide. In addition to the chemokine IL-8, other chemokines, including monocyte chemoattractant protein 1 (MCP-1), macrophage inflammatory protein (MIP) 1α, and β epithelial neutrophil activating protein (ENA) 78, are chemoattractants for neutrophils in rheumatoid arthritis (reviewed in ref. 56).

Although neutrophils and lymphocytes use many of the same mechanisms to adhere and transmigrate through the same areas of endothelial surfaces, their final destinations within the joints of rheumatoid patients differ strikingly. As mentioned earlier, it is rare to find polymorphonuclear leukocytes in the synovium, but they are abundant within the synovial fluid. Although perhaps 1 billion neutrophils may enter a large inflamed joint in rheumatoid arthritis each day,[57] they traverse the synovium and enter the synovial fluid so quickly as to be rarely seen in the synovium. In contrast, lymphocytes can dominate the cell population in some rheumatoid synovial samples, although they are found in reasonable numbers in synovial fluid as well. There are two logical explanations for this difference in localization: either (1) the chemoattractants in synovial fluid for neutrophils (e.g., C5a, leukotriene B_4, platelet-activating factor, IL-8) are so powerful as to overcome adhesive attraction of cells or matrix in the synovium, or (2) the adhesive forces for lymphocytes in synovium are sufficient to prevent many or most of them from migrating far from the vessels they have just left. Support for the latter possibility comes from the observations that VCAM-1, the ligand for VLA-4 that is expressed so abundantly on memory T cells, is found in high density in the synovial lining.[58] The expression of VLA-4 is increased on rheumatoid synovial and synovial fluid T lymphocytes compared either to control cells or peripheral blood cells from rheumatoid patients.[59] Thus VCAM-1 could fix the T cells in the lining, and the neutrophils that do not express VLA-4 could be drawn through to chemoattractants within the joint fluid. In addition, lymphocytes with migratory capabilities express CD44, a ligand for hyaluronan, which is present in synovium as well as synovial fluid (Brezinschek et al., Abstract 205).

Homing of Lymphocytes to the Synovium in Rheumatoid Arthritis

The assumption must be made that certain lymphocytes have "homing receptors" that guide them to "addressins" on endothelial cells of venules and capillaries in joints, enabling the early inflammation of rheumatoid arthritis to be focused there. Indeed, this is a subcategory of one of the major and basic unanswered questions about rheumatoid arthritis: Why, since the pathogenic mechanisms of inflammation in rheumatoid arthritis are so similar to chronic diseases in other tissues, does the primary inflammation occur within the synovium and not other organs? The **integrin $\alpha_4\beta_7$** on certain lymphocytes leads them to the gut and Peyer's patches. In rheumatoid patients there is a 6 to 12-fold higher expression of $\alpha_4\beta_7$ on synovial lymphocytes than is found in peripheral blood and synovial fluid lymphocytes, respectively.[60] These data suggest that $\alpha_4\beta_7$ may be involved in retention of lymphocytes within synovial tissue, although it is not known when (in the circulation or in the synovium?) this molecule is expressed so abundantly.

The **$\alpha_4\beta_1$ integrin/VLA-4** is a counter-receptor for a 25-amino-acid sequence (**CS1**) on an alternatively spliced species of fibronectin. This CS1 is selectively expressed within rheumatoid but not normal synovium, and its expression is limited to rheumatoid synovial vasculature and intimal lining cells.[61] It is reasonable to speculate that T-cell attachment may be mediated by the integrin VLA-4 on lymphocytes interacting with a CS1 counter-receptor on tall (activated) synovial endothelial cells. As mentioned, $\alpha_4\beta_1$/VLA-4 also binds to VCAM-1 that has been found in rheumatoid synovial vasculature[62] and to fibronectin, which is abundant in the synovium. This trio of molecules, two on the activated endothelium and one on the lymphocytes, may be a sufficient mechanism to explain the homing of lymphocytes to synovium in rheumatoid arthritis. Within the synovium, the cytokines IL-4, TNFα, IL-1β, and IFNγ stimulate the adhesion of lymphocytes and monocytes to synovial fibroblasts.

There are other data supporting a distinct endothelial cell recognition system that controls lymphocyte traffic into inflamed synovium.[63] In an experimental model of proteoglycan-induced arthritis in mice, labeled lymphocytes from arthritic animals migrated primarily to synovial tissue of recipient mice, and their appearance there was associated with the onset of arthritis.[64]

In addition to VLA-4, there are other surface markers of lymphocytes that have significant enabling capabilities for migration in rheumatoid synovium. Those known are listed in Table 7–4. The presence of the CD29 and CD45RO phenotypes establishes lymphocytes as immature memory T cells previously activated by antigen. CD29$^+$ cells proliferate well when restimulated by homologous antigen, and the CD29 antigen itself may be important in endothelial cell binding.[64a] Using studies that identified the location in synovium of these lymphocytes, it has been observed that CD45RA$^+$ lymphocytes (nonactivated) were also present, but in perivascular locations; the inference is that, although both CD45RA$^+$ (nonactivated) and CD45RO$^+$ (activated) lymphocytes can enter the synovium, most of the resting cells become activated to CD45RO$^+$ phenotypes as they leave the

TABLE 7–4. Surface Antigen Phenotypes of Migrating CD4$^+$ Cells

LFA-1
CD58
VLA-2
VLA-4 (CD29)
VLA-5
CD44 (hyaluronate receptor)
Both naive (CD45RA$^+$) and early "memory" (CD45RO$^+$) markers

perivascular areas and become a part of the established synovitis.[65] Additional data suggest that, although activation increases the number of cells that migrate, the activated state is not essential for these cells to cross endothelial barriers.[66] As is apparent in Table 7–4, the adhesive molecule L-selectin, which probably is involved in the initial attachment of lymphocytes to endothelial cells, is not present on the migrating CD4+ cells. It may be stripped away or resorbed back into the cell.

CD8+ cells that transmigrate have a very similar surface phenotype, with the exception that fewer are memory T cells and many have less expression of β_1 integrins (VLAs).

T cells with a γ/δ receptor rather than α/β have a higher frequency of migration-competent cells than do CD4+ α/β T cells[67] and this may relate to their relative prominence within inflamed tissue, including rheumatoid synovium.[68] Nonactivated (naive) γ/δ T cells transmigrate more efficiently into synovium than do nonactivated cells with the α/β cell receptor.

Special Aspects of Adhesion Molecules in Rheumatoid Arthritis

The percentage of lymphocytes in perivascular infiltrates in synovium correlates positively with the "tallness" of the endothelial cells in adjacent capillaries and venules.[69] This has added support to the data showing that tall endothelium has a greater capacity to slow and bind circulating leukocytes than capillaries with flat endothelium. Indeed, there is increased expression of endothelial adhesion molecules (e.g., E-selectin, ICAM-1, VCAM-1) in the microvasculature of rheumatoid synovium but not in normal or osteoarthritic tissues.[43] Similarly, studies have demonstrated both an increased constitutive expression of E-selectin and ICAM-1 by synovial microvascular endothelial cells and a TNFα-inducible enhancement of E-selectin expression on these cells compared with similar endothelial cells from foreskins or umbilical veins.[70] In vitro, at least, synovial endothelial cells are more capable of binding leukocytes than similar cells from other sources.

E-selectin, the adhesion molecule found only on the surface of endothelial cells, exists in a soluble form as well. Soluble E-selectin is found in blood from normal individuals but is present in higher concentrations in blood of rheumatoid patients. There is a positive correlation between synovial fluid soluble E-selectin levels and both the degree of inflammation in the fluids (assayed by synovial

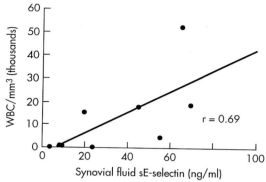

FIGURE 7–5. Positive correlation between synovial fluid soluble E-selectin (sE-selectin) and degree of inflammation as assayed by synovial fluid white blood cell (WBC) counts. (Modified from Koch, A. E., Turkiewicz, W., Harlow, L. A., et al.: Soluble E-selectin in arthritis. Clin. Immunol. Immunopathol. 69:29, 1993. Used by permission.)

fluid leukocyte counts[71]) and levels of soluble ICAM-1 (Fig. 7–5).

In the synovium, macrophage-like (type A) cells express high levels of ICAM-1, whereas the fibroblast-like (type B) synovial lining cells predominantly express VCAM-1.[72] In rheumatoid tissues, it has been shown that there is increased binding of synovial T lymphocytes from rheumatoid arthritis to E-selectin (ELAM-1) and VCAM-1.[73] Immunolocalization studies have demonstrated E-selectin in subsynovial blood vessels of rheumatoid synovium, in contrast to VCAM-1 and ICAM-1, which are found on synovial lining cells.[44] Just as in endothelium, VCAM-1 in synovial lining cells is significantly greater in rheumatoid tissue than in normal synovium.[58] It is possible that this differential expression, with higher densities of VCAM-1 in the lining layer rather than in the subsynovium, could determine cell distribution in rheumatoid tissues, as mentioned earlier. It is conceivable that exposure to activating substances in synovial fluid changes the phenotype of synovial fibroblasts sufficient to "transform" them into the characteristic intimal lining cells (Table 7–5).

Similar increases in concentrations of other adhesion molecules are found in the rheumatoid synovium, (Table 7–5) especially when compared with osteoarthritis. For example,

1. P-selectin is found on the surface of endothelium from rheumatoid synovium, but is only found deep within cells (and is less accessible) of osteoarthritis tissue.[11]

2. PECAM (CD31) is expressed within and on endothelial cells of both osteoarthritis and rheumatoid synovium, but is found more on lining cells and macrophages of the rheumatoid tissue.[74]

TABLE 7–5. Adhesive Molecules and Cytoattractants Found in Higher Density in Rheumatoid than Nonrheumatoid Joints

Microvasculature
  E-selectin
  ICAM-1
  VCAM-1
  P-selectin
  PECAM
Matrix
  Alternatively spliced fibronectin
Synovial Lining and Sublining Cells
  VCAM-1
  CD44
  ICAM-1
  VLA-4
Synovial Fluid
  IL-8
  Monocyte chemoattractant protein
  Soluble E-selectin

   3. Expression of CD44 in rheumatoid synovium is 10-fold greater than in synovium of patients with a noninflammatory synovitis, such as that resulting from joint trauma.[75]

   CD44 expression is markedly increased on synovial fluid T lymphocytes of rheumatoid patients relative to their peripheral blood T cells.[76] Because CD44 is a receptor for hyaluronan, and because hyaluronan is a major component of synovial fluid, this may implicate CD44 as a "homing" receptor for lymphocytes.

   ICAM-1, the adhesion molecule that is a ligand for the integrins LFA-1 and Mac-1, is prominently expressed by synovial fibroblasts[77] and more on rheumatoid synovial endothelial cells than on normal endothelium.[78] Cytokines reported to enhance expression of ICAM-1 on synoviocytes are IL-1β > TNFα > IFNγ >> platelet-derived growth factor > IL-6. GM-CSF and TGFβ had no effect.[77] The same cytokines that induce increased expression on these cells are the ones that augment shedding of ICAM-1 in vitro.[79] As noted earlier, soluble ICAM-1 is produced by mononuclear cells in rheumatoid synovial fluid in amounts greater than those produced by neutrophils or synovial tissue fibroblasts.[80]

   It is of interest that there are increased levels of circulating ICAM-1 in sera of patients with rheumatoid arthritis, and that these levels are significantly greater than those found in synovial fluid from rheumatoid patients or sera of osteoarthritic

patients.[81] The circulating ICAM-1 levels did not correlate with age, disease duration, duration of morning stiffness, global assessment of disease activity, C-reactive protein levels, IgM rheumatoid factor titers, or responses to nonsteroidal anti-inflammatory drug (NSAID) therapy.

   In the matrix of the inflamed synovium in rheumatoid arthritis, there are highly expressed adhesion proteins, just as there are on the circulating cells and endothelial cells. Stimulation of synovial cells with TNFα and IFNγ up-regulates expression of the VLA subgroup of the integrin family but has no effect upon the β_2 subgroup, which has been shown to be lymphocyte restricted.[47] These data are interesting in the context of experiments showing that fibronectin promotes the proliferation of naive and memory T cells by signaling through both the VLA-4 and VLA-5 integrin molecules.[82]

   T cells bind to synovial fibroblasts, and the avidity of the binding is affected by cytokines.[48] This interaction may contribute in vivo to the generation of inflammatory synovitis. In addition to enhancing synovitis, adhesion molecules may be involved in the invasive/destructive lesion of rheumatoid arthritis. VLA-4, VLA-5, and ICAM-1 have been identified on lymphocytes at the junction of the invasive pannus and cartilage.[83]

   The importance of having activation of synovial vessel endothelial cells in order for a true proliferative synovitis to develop was demonstrated in a study of clinically uninvolved joints in patients afflicted with rheumatoid arthritis in other joints.[84] A vascular proliferation index and high endothelial venule (HEV) index were calculated for use in histopathology from both involved and uninvolved joints. Neither vascular proliferation nor significant HEVs were seen in the uninvolved joints, adding support to the premise that, in the absence of new blood vessel formation and activated expression of adhesion molecules on synovial cells, the rheumatoid process has no scaffold on which to grow.

   As mentioned previously, once cells have bound to endothelium, there must be a strong cytoattractant in the extracellular space that entices cells to transmigrate into the synovium. In rheumatoid synovial fluid, IL-8 accounts for 25 to 60 per cent of neutrophil chemotactic bioactivity. Levels up to 15 μg/ml have been measured, whereas IL-8 has been undetectable in fluid from osteoarthritic joints.[85] MCP-1 is a major candidate for the chemoattractant that draws blood monocytes into rheumatoid synovium.[85] Up to 50 per cent of rheumatoid synovial macrophages express MCP-1 on their surfaces; it is likely that they are stimulated in a paracrine manner to produce this chemokine by IL-1 and TNFα. In response to stimulation by IL-1 and other inflammatory cytokines, articular chondrocytes express MCP-1; dexamethasone blunts the stimulation, whereas retinoic acid enhances it.[85]

Therapy Directed Against Adhesion Molecules: A Possibility for Rheumatoid Arthritis?

There are two strategies to be pursued for antiadhesion therapy, both of which have a rational basis for development. The first is a *direct interference* with adhesive interactions[86] using soluble receptors, surrogate ligands, or anti–adhesion molecule antibodies. Antibodies to ICAM-1 have ameliorated adjuvant arthritis.[87] In another system (experimental cardiac allografts), it was shown that antibodies against ICAM-1 and LFA-1, given together, permitted grafts to hold; given alone, neither antibody induced full tolerance.[88] Because of the multiple adhesion molecules involved in the transmigration of neutrophils, lymphocytes, and monocytes from synovial vasculature into the joints, the probabilities are that, to be truly effective, combined antibody therapy would be needed.

In patients with rheumatoid arthritis, trials of anti–ICAM-1 murine monoclonal antibodies have been done.[89] Of 13 patients given these antibodies, 9 achieved marked or moderate responses within 8 days, and 5 patients had efficacy that lasted for 2 months. This was a dose escalation study. The Westergren sedimentation rate did not change, but there were no infectious sequelae. A slight increase in circulating lymphocytes was noted in the patients, implying that lymphocytes were being denied egress from the circulation, although this was by no means proved.

The second strategy is *pharmacologic inhibition* of the synthesis or activity of adhesive molecules.[86] Possible approaches include

- Soluble carbohydrates that would inhibit L-selectin–mediated adhesive interactions.[90] Fucoidin—a fucose polymer—is a potent inhibitor of L-selectin binding to endothelial ligands.
- Exploitation of existing pharmacologic modulation of adhesion.[36] The problem with this second strategy, of course, is that these agents are being utilized fully at present. For example, although recent data have shown convincingly that dexamethasone inhibits TNFα-induced surface expression of ICAM-1, diminishes the accumulation of ICAM-1 mRNA in cultured human synovial cells, and inhibits adhesion of monocytes to TNFα-activated synovial cells, dexamethasone

is, and should be, used sparingly if at all in rheumatoid patients.[91] Similarly, NSAIDs, methotrexate, sulfasalazine, gold salts, and cyclosporine have each been demonstrated to inhibit, by varying mechanisms, leukocyte–endothelial cell adhesion.[92] This awareness may help us understand mechanisms of actions of these drugs, but will not alter the way in which we use them.

- Infusion of soluble adhesion molecules. They have been demonstrated in blood and synovial fluid,[79,81] and may well have a role in competing for cell or matrix-bound receptors.

SUMMARY

Once tiny new capillaries are formed within proliferating synovium, the endothelial cells are immediately exposed to cytokines that up-regulate expression of adhesive molecules. TNFα, IFNγ and IL-1β are the principal stimuli released by activated synovial cells, macrophages, and lymphocytes in the joint that induce the appearance of selectins and immunoglobulin superfamily adhesion molecules on the endothelium. The dominant adhesive interactions in established rheumatoid arthritis are probably VLA-4 to VCAM-1, LFA-1 to ICAM-1, and Hyaluronan to CD44. The sequence of leukocyte rolling in the vessels (primary adhesion) is followed by activation-dependent sticking of the cells to the endothelium. Chemoattractants such as chemokines (e.g., IL-8), activated complement components, and leukotriene B$_4$ lead to diapedesis/extravasation within the underlying synovial tissue. Because VLA-4, which binds so avidly to VCAM-1 on synovial lining cells, is not found on neutrophils, very few of this latter species stop in the synovium, but rather follow a chemoattractant gradient into the synovial fluid.

This process is highly redundant; more than one adhesive molecule can perform most functions on more than one cell. In addition, this process is an example of cyclic amplification in synovium; the migration of a few cells incites a slightly greater inflammatory response that draws more cells into a constantly proliferating vascular synovitis, and the cycle repeats itself again and again. It seems highly probable that specific inhibition of either angiogenesis or leukocyte homing to the synovium would be effective therapy for rheumatoid arthritis. Reviews of adhesion molecules in rheumatoid arthritis and other autoimmune diseases provide added detail on these processes.[56,93,94]

REFERENCES

1. Colville-Nash, P. R., and Scott, D. L.: Angiogenesis and rheumatoid arthritis: pathogenic and therapeutic implications. Ann. Rheum. Dis. 51:919, 1992.
2. Rooney, M., Condell, D., Quinlan, W., et al.: Analysis of the histologic variation in rheumatoid arthritis. Arthritis Rheum. 31:956, 1988.
3. Unemori, E. N., Bouhana, K. S., and Werb, Z.: Vectorial secretion of extracellular matrix proteins, matrix-degrading proteinases, and tissue inhibitor of metalloproteinases by endothelial cells. J. Biol. Chem. 265:445, 1990.
4. Folkman, J.: How is blood vessel growth regulated in normal and neoplastic tissue? Cancer Res. 46:467, 1986.
5. Vlodavsky, I., Folkman, J., Sullivan, R., et al.: Endothelial cell-derived basic fibroblast growth factor: synthesis and deposition into the subendothelial extracellular matrix. Proc. Natl. Acad. Sci. U.S.A. 84:2292, 1987.
6. Sano, H., Forough, R., Maier, J. A. M., et al.: Detection of high levels of heparin binding growth factor-1 (acidic fibroblast growth factor) in inflammatory arthritic joints. J. Cell Biol. 110:1417, 1990.
7. Moscatelli, D., and Rifkin, D. B.: Membrane and matrix localization of proteinases: a common theme in tumor cell invasion and angiogenesis. Biochim. Biophys. Acta 948:67, 1988.
8. Hull, M. A., Cullen, D. J. E., and Hawkey, C. J.: Basic fibroblast growth factor in gastric ulceration: mucosal levels and therapeutic potential. Gastroenterology 106: A97, 1994.
9. Koch, A. E., Polverini, P. J., and Leibovich, S. J.: Stimulation of neovascularization by human rheumatoid synovial tissue macrophages. Arthritis Rheum. 29:471, 1986.
10. Koch, A., Polverini, S., Kunkel, S., et al.: Interleukin-8 as a macrophage-derived mediator of angiogenesis. Science 258:1798, 1992.
11. Koch, A. E., Harlow, L. A., Haines, G. K., et al.: Vascular endothelial growth factor: a cytokine modulating endothelial function in rheumatoid arthritis. J. Immunol. 152: 4149, 1994.
12. Unemori, E. N., Ferrara, N., Bauer, E. A., et al.: Vascular endothelial growth factor induces interstitial collagenase expression in human endothelial cells. J. Cell. Physiol. 153:557, 1992.
13. Form, D. M., and Auerbach, R.: PGE_2 and angiogenesis. Proc. Soc. Exp. Biol. Med. 172:214, 1983.
14. Brown, R. A., Tomlinson, I. W., Hill, C. R., et al.: Relationship of angiogenesis factor in synovial fluid to various joint diseases. Ann. Rheum. Dis. 42:301, 1983.
15. McLaughlin, B., Cawston, T., and Weiss, J. B.: Activation of matrix metalloproteinase inhibitor by low molecular weight angiogenic factor. Biochim. Biophys. Acta 1073: 295, 1991.
16. Strieter, R. M., Kunkel, S. L., Elner, V. M., et al.: Interleukin-8: a corneal factor that induces neovascularization. Am. J. Pathol. 141:1279, 1992.
17. Takeuchi, M., Otsuka, T., Matsui, N., et al.: Aberrant production of gliostatin/platelet-derived endothelial cell growth factor in rheumatoid synovium. Arthritis Rheum. 37:662, 1994.
18. Dayer, J. M., and Arend, W. P.: Cytokines and growth factors. In Kelley, W. N., Harris, E. D., Jr., Ruddy, S., and Sledge, C. B. (eds.): Textbook of Rheumatology, 5th ed. Philadelphia, W. B. Saunders, (in press).
19. Roberts, A. B., Sporn, M. B., Assoian, R. K., et al.: Transforming growth factor-beta: rapid induction of fibrosis and angiogenesis in vivo and stimulation of collagen formation in vitro. Proc. Natl. Acad. Sci. U.S.A. 83:4167, 1986.
20. Norioka, K., Hara, M., Kitani, A., et al.: Inhibitory effects of human recombinant interleukin-1α and β on growth of human vascular endothelial cells. Biochem. Biophys. Res. Commun. 145:969, 1987.
21. Maione, T. E., Gray, G. S., Petro, J., et al.: Inhibition of angiogenesis by recombinant human platelet factor-4 and related peptides. Science 247:77, 1990.
22. Manicourt, D. -H., Triki, R., Fukada, K., et al.: Levels of circulating tumor necrosis factor α and interleukin-6 in patients with rheumatoid arthritis. Arthritis Rheum. 36: 490, 1993.

    Serum from 35 patients with rheumatoid arthritis and a group of age- and sex-matched control subjects was assayed for TNFα, IL-6, hyaluronic acid, (HA), and keratan sulfate. The serum level of HA correlated positively with the level of TNFα; the latter is a potent stimulator of HA biosynthesis by synovial fibroblasts. TNFα levels correlated well with concentrations of C-reactive protein, fibrinogen, and the erythrocyte sedimentation rate. TNFα and HA in serum correlated with joint scores (Lansbury index). Serum antigenic keratan sulfate did not correlate with serum TNFα, HA, or clinical activity. It is possible that serum levels of HA in rheumatoid arthritis may be markers for synovial proliferation.

23. Matsubara, T., and Ziff, M.: Inhibition of human endothelial cell proliferation by gold compounds. J. Clin. Invest. 79: 1440, 1987.
24. Matsubara, T., Saura, R., Hirohata, K., et al.: Inhibition of human endothelial proliferation in vitro and neovascularization in vivo by D-penicillamine. J. Clin. Invest. 83:158, 1989.
25. Folkman, J., Weisz, P. B., Joullié, M. M., et al.: Control of angiogenesis with synthetic heparin substitutes. Science 243:1490, 1989.
26. Buerin, C., Laterra, J., Masnyk, T., et al.: Selective endothelial growth inhibition by tetracyclines that inhibit collagenase. Biochem. Biophys. Res. Commun. 188:740, 1992.
27. Oliver, S. J., Banquerigo, M. L., and Brahn, E.: Suppression of collagen-induced arthritis using an angiogenesis inhibitor, AGM-1470, and a microtubule stabilizer, taxol. Cell. Immunol. 157:291, 1994.
28. Herron, G. S., Banda, M. J., Clark, E. J., et al.: Secretion of metalloproteinases by stimulated capillary endothelial cells. II. Expression of collagenase and stromelysin activities is regulated by endogenous inhibitors. J. Biol. Chem. 261:2814, 1986.
29. Haskard, D. O.: Cell adhesion molecules in rheumatoid arthritis. Curr. Opin. Rheumatol. 7:229, 1995.
30. Picker, L. J., and Butcher, E. C.: Physiological and molecular mechanisms of lymphocyte homing. Annu. Rev. Immunol. 10:561, 1992.

    This review expands in readable detail the interactions of lymphocytes and endothelial cells. Table 7–2 (see text) summarizes general knowledge about relevant molecules involved in this process.

31. Hemler, M. E., Elices, M. J., Parker, C., et al.: Structure of the integrin VLA-4 and its cell-cell and cell-matrix adhesion functions. Immunol. Rev. 114:45, 1990.
32. Ruoslahti, E., and Pierschbacher, M. D.: New perspectives in cell adhesion: RGD and integrins. Science 238:491, 1987.
33. Senior, R. M., Gresham, H. D., Griffin, G. L., et al.: Entactin stimulates neutrophil adhesion and chemotaxis through interactions between its Arg-Gly-Asp (RGD) domain and

the leukocyte response integrin. J. Clin. Invest. 90:2251, 1992.

34. Loeser, R. F.: Integrin-mediated attachment of articular chondrocytes to extracellular matrix proteins. Arthritis Rheum. 36:1103, 1993.

35. Davignon, D., Martz, E., Reynolds, T., et al.: Lymphocyte function-associated antigen 1 (LFA-1): a surface antigen distinct from Lyt-2,3 that participates in T lymphocyte-mediated killing. Proc. Natl. Acad. Sci. U.S.A. 78:4535, 1981.

36. Cronstein, B. N., and Weissmann, G.: The adhesion molecules of inflammation. Arthritis Rheum. 36:147, 1993.

    Mac-1 is a receptor for iC3b and mediates adhesion of leukocytes to endothelium; LFA-1 function includes cytotoxic T lymphocyte and natural killer cytotoxicity, antigen presentation and adhesion of lymphocytes to endothelium.

37. Fischer, A., Lisowska-Grospierre, B., Anderson, D. C., et al.: Leukocyte adhesion deficiency: molecular basis and functional consequences. Immunodefic. Rev. 1:39, 1988.

38. Chuluyan, H. E., and Issekutz, A. C.: VLA-4 integrin can mediate CD11/CD18-independent transendothelial migration of human monocytes. J. Clin. Invest. 92:2768, 1993.

39. Bevilacqua, M. P., and Nelson, R. M.: Selectins. J. Clin. Invest. 91:379, 1993.

40. Ley, K., Gaehtgens, P., Fennie, C., et al.: Lectin-like cell adhesion molecule 1 mediates leukocyte rolling in mesenteric venules *in vivo*. Blood 77:2553, 1991.

41. Grober, J. S., Bowen, B. L., Ebling, H., et al.: Monocyte-endothelial adhesion in chronic rheumatoid arthritis: *in situ* detection of selectin and integrin-dependent interactions. J. Clin. Invest. 91:2609, 1993.

42. Pober, J. S., Bevilacqua, M. P., Mendrick, D. L., et al.: Two distinct monokines, interleukin 1 and tumor necrosis factor, each independently induce biosynthesis and transient expression of the same antigen on the surface of cultured human vascular endothelial cells. J. Immunol. 136:1680, 1986.

43. Corkill, M. M., Kirkham, B. W., Haskard, D. O., et al.: Gold treatment of rheumatoid arthritis decreases synovial expression of the endothelial leukocyte adhesion receptor ELAM-1. J. Rheumatol. 18:1453, 1991.

44. Haynes, B. F., Telen, M. J., Hale, L. P., et al.: CD44: a molecule involved in leukocyte adherence and T-cell activation. Immunol. Today 10:423, 1989.

45. Vaporciyan, A. A., DeLisser, H. M., Yan, H.-C., et al.: Involvement of platelet-endothelial cell adhesion molecule-1 in neutrophil recruitment *in vivo*. Science 262:1580, 1993.

46. Koch, A. E., Burrows, J. C., Haines, G. K., et al.: Immunolocalization of endothelial and leukocyte adhesion molecules in human rheumatoid and osteoarthritic synovial tissues. Lab. Invest. 64:313, 1991.

47. Jalkanan, S., Jalkanan, M., Bargatze, R., et al.: Biochemical properties of glycoproteins involved in lymphocyte recognition of high endothelial venules in man. J. Immunol. 141:1615, 1988.

48. Cicuttini, F. M., Martin, M., and Boyd, A. W.: Cytokine induction of adhesion molecules on synovial type B cells. J. Rheumatol. 21:406, 1994.

49. Ziff, M.: Role of cellular adhesion in rheumatoid synovitis. *In* Smolen, K. and Maini, R. N. (eds.): Rheumatoid Arthritis. Berlin, Springer-Verlag, 1992, pp. 55–70.

50. Gerritsen, M. E., Kelley, K. A., Ligon, G., et al.: Regulation of the expression of intercellular adhesion molecule-1 in cultured human endothelial cells derived from rheumatoid synovium. Arthritis Rheum. 36:593, 1993.

51. Patel, K. D., Moore, K. L., Nollert, M. U., et al.: Neutrophils use both shared and distinct mechanisms to adhere to selectins under static and flow conditions. J. Clin. Invest. 96:1887, 1995.

52. Butcher, E. C.: Leukocyte-endothelial cell recognition: three (or more) steps to specificity and diversity. Cell 67:1033, 1991.

53. Oppenheimer-Marks, N., Davis, L. S., Bogue, D. T., et al.: Differential utilization of ICAM-1 and VCAM-1 during the adhesion and transendothelial migration of human T lymphocytes. J. Immunol. 147:2913, 1991.

54. Gimbrone, M. A., Jr., Oibin, M. S., Brock, A. F., et al.: Endothelial interleukin-8: a novel inhibitor of leukocyte-endothelial interactions. Science 246:1601, 1989.

55. Kishimoto, T. K., Jutila, M. A., Berg, E. L., et al.: Neutrophil Mac-1 and MEL-14 adhesion proteins inversely regulated by chemotactic factors. Science 245:1238, 1989.

56. Szekanecz, Z., Szegedi, G., and Koch, A. E.: Cellular adhesion molecules in rheumatoid arthritis: regulation by cytokines and possible clinical importance. J. Invest. Med. 44:124, 1996.

57. Hollingsworth, J. W., Siegel, E. R., and Creasey, W. A.: Granulocyte survival in synovial exudate of patients with rheumatoid arthritis and other inflammatory joint diseases. Yale J. Biol. Med. 39:289, 1967.

58. Morales-Ducret, J., Wayner, E., Elices, M. J., et al.: α_4/β_1 integrin (VLA-4) ligands in arthritis: vascular cell adhesion molecule-1 expression in synovium and on fibroblast-like synoviocytes. J. Immunol. 149:1424, 1992.

59. Laffon, A., Garcia-Vicuña, R., and Humbria, A.: Upregulated expression and function of VLA-4 fibronectin receptors on human activated T cells in rheumatoid arthritis. J. Clin. Invest. 88:546, 1991.

60. Lazarovits, A. I., and Karsh, J.: Differential expression in rheumatoid synovium and synovial fluid of $\alpha_4\beta_7$ integrin: a novel receptor for fibronectin and vascular cell adhesion molecule-1. J. Immunol. 151:6482, 1993.

61. Elices, M. J., Tsai, V., Strahl, D., et al.: Expression and functional significance of alternatively spliced CS1 fibronectin in rheumatoid arthritis microvasculature. J. Clin. Invest. 93:405, 1994.

62. Dinther-Janssen, A. C. H. M. E., Horst, G., Koopman, W. B., et al.: The VLA-4/VCAM-1 pathway is involved in lymphocyte adhesion to endothelium in rheumatoid arthritis. J. Immunol. 147:4207, 1991.

63. Jalkanen, S., Steere, A. C., Fox, R. I., et al.: A distinct endothelial cell recognition system that controls lymphocyte traffic into inflamed synovium. Science 233:556, 1986.

    In these experiments, binding of lymphocytes to rheumatoid synovial HEVs was not inhibited by a monoclonal antibody to lymphocyte receptors for lymph node HEV, and synovial HEVs failed to bind either lymph node HEV-specific or mucosal HEV-specific B lymphoblastoid cells. It seems possible either that small differences in adhesion molecules and their ligands on circulating CD4[+] memory cells, or else a completely different molecule yet to be defined, is involved in the synovial homing by lymphocytes.

64. Mikecz, K., and Glant, T. T.: Migration and homing of lymphocytes to lymphoid and synovial tissues in proteoglycan-induced murine arthritis. Arthritis Rheum. 37:1395, 1994.

64a. Martens, A. V., de Clerck, L. S., Moens, M. M., et al.: Lymphocyte activation status, expression of adhesion molecules and adhesion to human endothelium in rheumatoid arthritis—relationship to disease activity. Res. Immunol. 145:101, 1994.

A majority of lymphocytes in the synovial fluid of rheumatoid arthritis patients are known to be of the CD4/CD29 (memory helper cells)

65. Koch, A. E., Robinson, P. G., and Radosevich, J. A.: Distribution of CD45RA and CD45RO T-lymphocyte subsets in rheumatoid arthritis synovial tissue. J. Clin Immunol. 10:192, 1990.
66. Oppenheimer-Marks, N., and Lipsky, P. E.: Transendothelial migration of T cells in chronic inflammation. Immunologist 2(2):58, 1994.
67. Galea, P., Brezinschek, R., Lipskey, P. E., and Oppenheimer-Marks, N.: Phenotypic characterization of CD4 α/β TCR + and γ/δ TCR + cells with a transendothelial migratory capability. J. Immunol. 153:529, 1994.
68. Kjeldsen-Kragh, J., Quayle, A. J., Vinje, O., et al.: A high proportion of the V delta 1+ synovial fluid gamma delta T cells in JRA patients express the very early activation marker CD69, but carry the high molecular weight isoform of the lencocyte common antigen (CD45RA). Clin. Exp. Immunol. 91:202, 1993.
69. Iguchi, T., and Ziff, M.: Electron microscopic study of the distribution of T cell subsets in rheumatoid synovium. J. Exp. Med. 77:355, 1986.
70. To, S. S. T., Newman, P. M., Hyland, V. J., et al.: Regulation of adhesion molecule expression by human synovial microvascular endothelial cells in vitro. Arthritis Rheum. 39:467, 1996.
71. Koch, A. E., Turkiewicz, W., Harlow, L. A., et al.: Soluble E-selectin in arthritis. Clin. Immunol. Immunopathol. 69: 29, 1993.
72. Dinther-Janssen, A. C. H. M. E., Kraal, G., Soesbergen, R. M., et al.: Immunohistological and functional analysis of adhesion molecule expression in the rheumatoid synovial lining layer: implication for synovial lining cell destruction. J. Rheumatol. 21:1998, 1994.
73. Postigo, A. A., Garcia-Vicuña, R., Diaz-Gonzalez, F., et al.: Increased binding of synovial T lymphocytes from rheumatoid arthritis to endothelial-leukocyte adhesion molecule-1 (ELAM-1) and vascular cell adhesion molecule-1 (VCAM-1). J. Clin. Invest. 89:1445, 1992.
74. Johnson, B. A., Haines, G. K., Harlow, L. A., et al.: Adhesion molecule expression in human synovial tissue. Arthritis Rheum. 36:137, 1993.
75. Brooks, P. C., Clark, R. A. F., and Cheresh, D. A.: Requirement of vascular integrin $\alpha_v\beta_3$ for angiogenesis. Science 264:569, 1994.
76. Kelleher, D., Murphy, A., Hall, N., et al.: Expression of CD44 on rheumatoid synovial fluid lymphocytes. Ann. Rheum. Dis. 54:566, 1995.
77. Lindsley, H. B., Smith, D. D., Cohick, C. B., et al.: Proinflammatory cytokines enhance human synoviocyte expression of functional intercellular adhesion molecule-1 (ICAM-1). Clin. Immunol. Immunopathol. 68:311, 1993.
78. Szekanecz, Z., Haines, G. K., Lin, T. R., et al.: Differential distribution of intercellular adhesion molecules (ICAM-1, ICAM-2, and ICAM-3) and the MS-1 antigen in normal and diseased human synovia. Arthritis Rheum. 37:221, 1994.
79. Dooley, M. A., Cush, J. J., Lipsky, P. E., et al.: The effects of nonsteroidal anti-inflammatory drug therapy on serum levels of soluble IL-2R, CD4, and CD8 in early rheumatoid arthritis. J. Rheumatol. 20:1857, 1993.
80. Koch, A. E., Shah, M. R., Harlow, L. A., et al.: Soluble intercellular adhesion molecule-1 in arthritis. Clin. Immunopathol. 71:208, 1994.
81. Cush, J. J., Rothlein, R., Lindsley, H. B., et al.: Increased levels of circulating intercellular adhesion molecule 1 in the sera of patients with rheumatoid arthritis. Arthritis Rheum. 36:1098, 1993.
82. Springer, T. A., Dustin, M. L., Kishimoto, T. K., et al.: The lymphocyte function-associated LFA-1, CD2 and LFA-3 molecules: cell adhesion receptors of the immune system. Rev. Immunol. 5:223, 1987.
83. Ishiwawa, H., Hirata, S., Nishibayashi, Y., et al.: The role of adhesion molecules in synovial pannus formation in rheumatoid arthritis. Clin. Orthop. 300:297, 1994.
84. FitzGerald, O., Soden, M., and Yanni, G.: Morphometric analysis of blood vessels in synovial membranes obtained from clinically affected and unaffected knee joints of patients with rheumatoid arthritis. Ann. Rheum. Dis. 50: 792, 1991.
85. Strieter, R. M., Koch, A. E., Antony, V. B., et al.: The immunopathology of chemotactic cytokines: the role of interleukin-8 and monocyte chemoattractant protein-1. J. Lab. Clin. Med. 123:183, 1994.

Where does the IL-8 in synovial fluid of rheumatoid patients originate from? Synovial fibroblasts from rheumatoid patients tested in vitro did not constitutively produced IL-8 but were not induced to express more by TNF-α or IL-1. Immunolocalization studies of synovium suggest that the synovial macrophage generates most of the IL-8 in rheumatoid synovium. Monocyte chemoattractant protein is a member of a supergene family of chemokines characterized by having two cysteine amino acid residues linked together [C-C]. In contrast, IL-8 is a member of the C-X-C supergene chemokine family, wherein the first two cysteine residues are separated by a different amino acid.

86. Cronstein, B. N.: Adhesion molecules in inflammation: current research and new therapeutic targets. Clin. Immunonother. 1:323, 1994.
87. Jasin, H. E., Lightfoot, E., Davis, L. S., et al.: Amelioration of antigen-induced arthritis in rabbits treated with monoclonal antibodies to leukocyte adhesion molecules. Arthritis Rheum. 35:541, 1992.
88. Isobe, M., Yagita, H., Okumura, K., et al.: Specific acceptance of cardiac allograft after treatment with antibodies to ICAM-1 and LFA-1. Science 255:1125, 1992.
89. Kavanaugh, A. F., Nichols, L. A., and Lipsky, P. E.: Treatment of refractory rheumatoid arthritis with an anti-CD54 (intercellular adhesion molecule-1, ICAM-1) monoclonal antibody. Arthritis Rheum. 35:543, 1992.
90. Norgard-Summnicht, K. E., Varki, N. M., and Varki, A.: Calcium-dependent heparin-like ligands for L-selectin in nonlymphoid endothelial cells. Science 261:480, 1993.
91. Tessier, P., Audette, M., Cattaruzzi, P., et al.: Upregulation by tumor necrosis factor of intercellular adhesion molecule 1 expression and function in synovial fibroblasts and its inhibition by glucocorticoids. Arthritis Rheum. 11: 1528, 1993.
92. Pitzalis, C., Kingsley, G., and Panayi, G.: Adhesion molecules in rheumatoid arthritis: role in the pathogenesis and prospects for therapy. Ann. Rheum. Dis. 53:287, 1994.
93. McMurray, R. W.: Adhesion molecules in autoimmune disease. Semin. Arthritis Rheum. 25:215, 1996.
94. Folkman, J.: Clinical applications of research on angiogenesis. New Engl. J. Med. 333:1757, 1995.

8

Cytokines, Lymphokines, Growth Factors, and Chemokines

A striking characteristic of rheumatoid synovium is the heterogeneity of its cell population. Within the mature synovium there are lymphocytes that generate antibodies, macrophages that phagocytose and degrade products of red blood cells, endothelial cells actively proliferating to form new capillaries, and synovial cells that have proliferated and are producing proteases capable of destroying articular cartilage, bone, and tendons.

Although it seemed logical that these various cells should be "talking" with one another, it was not until about 20 years ago that the possible extent of paracrine communication—one cell type expressing and releasing soluble factors that could affect the phenotype of other cells in a local area—became rooted in fact rather than hypothesis.

As is often the case in the biologic sciences, the finding and characterization of one mediator leads to discovery of many more. The science of cytokines has been no exception, and now there are more than 30 different mediators acting in a paracrine or autocrine mode to alter phenotypic expression of cells. In studies of rheumatoid arthritis, different families of cytokines have been separated out according to diverse functions. For example, TNFα and IL-1β are increasingly considered the principal drivers of an inflammatory and proliferative response in the synovium, quite opposite from the reparative and phlogistic inhibitory effects of TGFβ. The relevance in pathogenesis of an imbalance between the Th1 and Th2 subsets of CD4$^+$ cells is becoming clear. IL-2 and IFNγ, lymphokines released by Th1 cells, enhance and propagate autoimmune responses, whereas IL-4 and IL-10, originating from Th2 cells, down-regulate cellular immune responses to antigens.

Indeed, there is much current interest in the concept and potential practice of "immune deviation." In this construct, it is believed that, if autoreactive Th2 cells could be induced in synovium of rheuma-

toid patients, the disease-associated Th1 response could be diminished (for a review of this concept, see ref. 1). Similarly, naturally occurring inhibitors have been isolated, the genes transcribing them cloned, and the protein expressed in recombinant systems. Now these inhibitors can be tried as therapy to oppose the inflammatory and proliferative effects of the "bad" cytokines.

For those interested in rheumatoid arthritis, two polypeptide biologic activities were most interesting as data on them emerged in the 1970s:

Criteria for Identification as a True Mediator of Tissue Damage in Autoimmune Diseases

Hollander[2] has outlined some reasonable standards for investigators and students to consider before labeling a particular cytokine as a principal participant in an autoimmune process such as rheumatoid arthritis:

1. Presence of the substance in diseased tissue
2. Evidence for damage to tissue induced by the mediator
3. Prevention of damage in vitro by inhibitors or antagonists of the mediator
4. Positive correlation of the mediator or its mRNA in diseased tissue with the extent of damage
5. Similar damage to tissue effected by recombinant mediators
6. Prevention of disease progression by treatment with inhibitors of the mediator(s)

The last criterion, obviously, is the hardest to achieve and a goal for both basic and clinical investigators in the field.

---

1. The substance released by activated T cells that enabled other T cells to proliferate and, so long as the substance was present, be "immortal." This was characterized subsequently and named **interleukin-2.**

2. The substance, initially designated as mononuclear cell factor, was found in culture medium of rheumatoid synovial tissue that induced other synovial fibroblasts to produce collagenase. This was characterized subsequently and named **interleukin-1**, and was found to have a multitude of different effects on biologic systems.

In the past 15 years, recombinant DNA technology linked with ingenious bioassays has enabled investigators to clone and synthesize multiple cytokines (often referred to as "lymphokines" when generated by lymphocytes) that have profound endocrine and paracrine effects on other cell types in the synovium. These investigations have given credibility to the hypothesis that, once the rheumatoid process has been initiated by an antigen-driven immune response, the complex network of cells and cytokines that collects around it is adequate to produce a cyclic automaticity sufficient to self-perpetuate chronic inflammation.

The task for clinical scientists interested in rheumatoid arthritis is now to determine which, if any, of the known cytokines triggers production of others and thus becomes of primary importance in initiating inflammation and amplifying immune responses in the synovial tissue. This challenge is compounded by the fact that many of these peptides

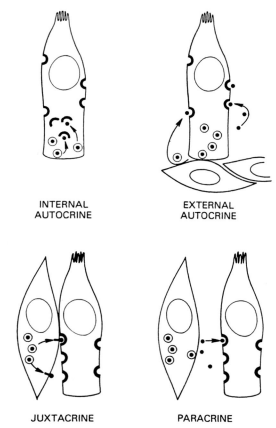

INTERNAL AUTOCRINE   EXTERNAL AUTOCRINE

JUXTACRINE   PARACRINE

FIGURE 8–1. Until 20 years ago, the endocrine mechanism was the principal pathway of information exchange known to investigators. Now there are more. In autocrine exchange, a cell produces a peptide that either acts internally or binds to a surface receptor of the same cell (internal and external autocrine, respectively). Paracrine stimulation is provided by a cytokine from one cell binding to another in the same vicinity. If cell-cell contact is essential, the pathway is a juxtacrine one. (From Sporn, M. B., and Roberts, A. B.: Autocrine secretion—10 years later. Ann. Intern. Med. 117:408, 1992. Used by permission.)

Autocrine and Paracrine Secretion

Awareness of the importance of these two mechanisms of phenotypic determination had to wait until techniques in cell biology had advanced sufficiently to isolate different cell types, sustain them in culture, and observe differences in biologic activity.

By *autocrine* action is meant the production or release by cell A of a regulatory peptide that has a major effect on the same cell type. An example is IL-2; released by activated CD4+ helper/inducer T cells, this lymphokine binds to the IL-2 receptor on the same cell or same cell type.

Paracrine secretion involves release of a regulatory peptide by one cell type that affects other cell types in the immediate environment. Variations in these mechanisms are shown in Figure 8–1.

---

and polypeptides have both up-regulatory and down-regulatory activity. As Sporn and Roberts point out, "Rather than doing what it is told in a rigid manner, a cell can take new information from its environment and, depending on the context of its past experience and its present stimuli, give an appropriate response."[3]

Predictably, the isolation and characterization of cytokines that have effects upon the phenotypic expression of cells have been followed by the discovery of additional molecules from blood or tissue that inhibit or modulate the biologic activities of cells. With proinflammatory actions of some cytokines, reparative actions of others, and inhibitors of both present in the tissues, the range of potential specific effects in rheumatoid synovium is enormous.

Modern immunohistochemical techniques have localized production of multiple cytokines and their inhibitors in rheumatoid synovial tissue, including IL-1α and -1β; interleukin-1 receptor antagonist (IL-1ra); IL-2, -3, -4, -5, -6, -8, -10, -13, -15, and other chemokines; GM-CSF and granulocyte colony-stimulating factor (G-CSF); TNFα and -β; IFNγ; and TGFβ.[4] Which are primary generators of the synovial inflammation? What are the additive, synergistic, or inhibitory effects of each one upon the others? Which are potentially reparative or healing cytokines?

One common denominator among many cytokines is emerging: The transcription factor nuclear factor κB (NF-κB) is responsible for activating genes for many of these. NF-κB has clearly been demonstrated within nuclei of rheumatoid synovial cells (Handel et al., Abstract 238). Another common denominator of cytokines is their interaction with specific cell surface receptors leading to activation of the JAK-STAT signaling pathway. There at least four tyrosine kinases known as JAKs, and a family of seven distinct latent cytosolic transcription factors known as STATs. JAK proteins link to intracellular domains of cytokine receptor subunits, are activated, and then phosphorylate tyrosines on STAT proteins. Activated STATs transocate to the cell nucleus, where they facilitate gene transcription of cytokine-inducible genes (R. D. Schreiber, Washington University School of Medicine, personal communication). This sequence has been best worked out through study of the IFNγ receptor/signal transduction mechanism.

INTERLEUKIN-1β AND TUMOR NECROSIS FACTOR α: POWERFUL DRIVING FORCES IN RHEUMATOID SYNOVITIS

This discussion of the relevance of cytokines focuses on a very few presented in detail because of their high degree of relevance to rheumatoid arthritis. IL-1 and TNFα are considered now to have true leadership roles in development of a sustained and destructive synovitis. Because it was isolated and studied earlier than TNFα, IL-1 is described first, although numerous studies suggest that TNFα is the more potent of the two and may induce expression of IL-1. Descriptions of other cytokines are provided later in a glossary section.

Interleukin-1

IL-1 is a small family of polypeptides—IL-1α, IL-1β, and IL-1ra—that are related structurally.[5] **IL-1α** is found principally within the cytosol of cells, although some may be found on cell membranes. Cells with dendritic morphology and bright staining for IL-1α, but not IL-1β, have been described circulating in blood from patients with rheumatoid arthritis.[6] **IL-1β,** in contrast, is released into the extracellular fluid, and measurable amounts find their way into the circulation in patients with infection, malignancy, or inflammation. Similar to many enzymes and other cytokines, IL-1β is synthesized in a "pro" form that must be enzymatically cleaved for full expression of activity; the ac-

FIGURE 8–2. Production and secretion of interleukin-1. A stimulant such as endotoxin activates a cell to transcribe the mRNA for IL-1α and IL-1β. Both forms are first synthesized as larger precursors. Most of the IL-1α remains within the cell or is expressed on the surface of the cell membrane. Extracellular proteases cleave the precursor into the mature form of IL-1α. The IL-1β precursor is cleaved by IL-1β–converting enzyme (ICE) to its mature form within the cell, after which it is secreted. However, some IL-1β precursor is found outside cells, where it is cleaved by other proteases. N, nucleus. (From Dinarello, C. A., and Wolff, S. M.: The role of interleukin-1 in disease. N. Engl. J. Med. 328:106, 1993. Used by permission of The New England Journal of Medicine. Copyright 1993, Massachusetts Medical Society.)

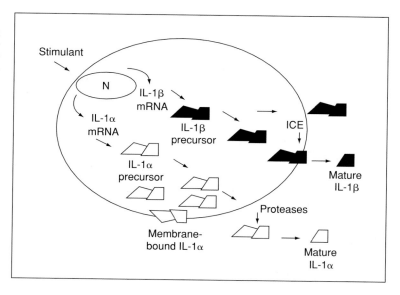

TABLE 8–1. Actions of IL-1 in Various Tissues

TISSUE	IL-1 ACTION
Central nervous system	Fever
	Somnolence
	Corticotropin and corticotropin-releasing hormone production
Liver	IL-6 and other acute phase protein synthesis
Capillaries and venules	Induction of proliferation of endothelial cells and expression of endothelial adhesive proteins
	Promotion of capillary leaking by inducing synthesis of nitrous oxide and platelet-activating factor
Bone	Stimulation of osteoblast/osteoclast activity
Fibroblasts, macrophages, and chondrocytes	Induction of proliferation
	Promotion of synthesis of metalloproteases, fibronectin, GAGs, plasminogen activator, and prostaglandins
	Induction of biosynthesis of other cytokines, including IL-6, GM-CSF, and G-CSF
	Decrease in production of type II collagen
Lymphocytes	Help in activation of both T and B cells
	Induction of IL-2 production by T cells
	Stimulation of cytokine receptor synthesis

tive form has a molecular weight of 17,500 Da (Fig. 8–2).

Monocyte-macrophages produce the greatest amounts of IL-1β, although endothelial cells and large granular lymphocytes can be induced to express it by a number of stimuli[7] including monocyte colony-stimulating Factor (M-CSF), TNFα, IFNγ, C5a, and endotoxin.

Both forms of IL-1 have a strong avidity for the two types of receptors on cells. Type I receptors are found on T cells, endothelial cells, keratinocytes, hepatocytes, and synovial fibroblasts.[8] Type II receptors are found on neutrophils and B cells but appear to have no recognized effector function. A high-affinity receptor for IL-1 has been demonstrated on cultured rheumatoid synovial cells.[9] Similar to IL-2, the receptor for IL-1 is a heterodimer. Both polypeptides contribute to ligand binding.[10] After binding with the receptor, the cells are activated and, depending on what type they are, undergo multiple phenotypic changes. The actions of IL-1 are listed in Table 8–1.[3,7,11,12]

Interleukin-1 and Experimental Synovitis

When injected into rabbit knee joints, IL-1 induces accumulation of neutrophils and mononuclear cells in the joint space and loss of proteoglycans from the articular cartilage[13] (Fig. 8–3). The degradative effect on proteoglycans is a direct effect of IL-1 on chondrocytes leading to diminished proteoglycan production as well as degradation, and not the result of release of enzymes from neu-

trophils. Subsequent studies[14] using recombinant IL-1β have revealed that, when high doses of cytotoxic drugs were administered to the rabbits, preventing neutrophil accumulation in the joints, there still was considerable proteoglycan and protease (stromelysin) released into the synovial fluid.

Interleukin-1 and Rheumatoid Arthritis

Studies linking IL-1 and rheumatoid arthritis are numerous. Many are linked with effects of TNFα, and the two cytokines are synergistic in many systems. The most important observations include the following:

1. Immunohistochemical studies reveal IL-1β in cells scattered among perivascular aggregates and in lining layer cells of rheumatoid synovium. The intensity of staining decreases after 12 weeks of intramuscular gold salt treatment.[15] Plasma IL-1β levels correlate weakly with progression of joint damage in rheumatoid arthritis.[16] A cautionary note for the relevance of measurements of IL-1β in tissues or fluids by immunoassays is the fact that, similar to the TNFα system, there are soluble forms of IL-1Rs that bind both IL-1β and IL-1ra with more avidity than either binds to each other.[17]

2. IL-1β stimulates production of IL-6 by rheumatoid synovial cells,[18] an effect inhibited by dexamethasone. IL-6, in turn, is a major inducer of the acute-phase response, plasminogen activator, and TIMP.[19] It also is involved in stimulation of immunoglobulin synthesis and T-cell activation. The stimulation of plasminogen activator biosynthesis

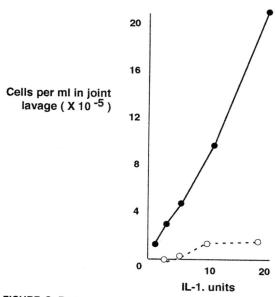

Cells per ml in joint lavage (X 10 $^{-5}$)

IL-1. units

FIGURE 8–3. Total leukocyte numbers in joint washes 24 hours after injection of highly purified human IL-1 into rabbit knee joints (●). Stock solutions of IL-1 (100 units/ml [1 unit of activity is defined as that amount of IL-1 required to double the proliferative response of mouse thymocytes stimulated with phytohemagglutinin alone at 1 μg/ml]) in 5% fetal calf serum were diluted with saline to give a constant injection volume of 0.5 ml. The contralateral joints received similar injections of diluted fetal calf serum alone (○). Each point is the mean ± 1 SEM of 4 to 10 estimations from separate animals. For all points, the total number of cells present in the IL-1–injected joints was significantly higher ($p<.01$) than in the vehicle-injected controls. The leukocytes present were predominantly (60 to 80 per cent) mononuclear. (From Pettipher, E. R., Higgs, G. A., and Henderson, B.: Interleukin-1 induces leukocyte infiltration and cartilage proteoglycan degeneration in the synovial joint. Proc. Natl. Acad. Sci. U.S.A. 83:8749, 1986. Used by permission.)

in human synovial cells by recombinant human IL-1β is inhibited by indomethacin.[20] One of the earliest defined effects of IL-1β (when it was still known as mononuclear cell factor) was the stimulation of synthesis of collagenase (metalloprotease I) and PGE$_2$; these effects also are inhibited by glucocorticoids.

3. A ''peri-articular bone destruction cascade'' around inflamed rheumatoid joints is set into motion by IL-1β and TNFα. These cytokines stimulate osteoblasts to secrete GM-CSF and IL-6, which, in turn, induce formation of osteoclasts from precursor cells.[21] 17β-Estradiol counteracts this sequence. The lack of this estrogen antagonism may be a major mechanism in the development of postmenopausal osteoporosis.

4. Anti–IL-1 antibody prevents degradation of living cartilage that normally is stimulated by rheumatoid synovial culture medium.[22] IL-1β sup-

presses proteoglycan synthesis in cartilage. In an unusual dissociation of effects of TNFα and IL-1β, TNFα does not exert this suppressive effect.[23]

Tumor Necrosis Factor α

TNFα (a 17,300-Da protein), similar to IL-1β, also exists in a secreted and a membrane-bound form. It is produced by activated T cells, mast cells, and macrophages after stimulation by endotoxin or other cytokines (e.g., GM-CSF, IFNγ).[7] Although first described as ''cachectin,'' which induced hypermetabolism, and as a tumor cytolytic factor, TNFα has effects on many biologic systems that are remarkably similar to, additive to, or synergistic with those of IL-1β. The TNFα receptor is found on activated T and B cells, fibroblasts, endothelial cells, NK cells, hepatocytes, osteoclasts, neutrophils, macrophages, and many tumor cells. The receptor has two polypeptide chains, one 55 and the other 75 kDa in size.

Recent work has defined the transcription factor responsible for regulation of biosynthesis of TNFα: It is a cAMP-responsive element binding protein (CEBPβ), a member of a family of transcription factors termed bZip proteins that bind DNA through a leucine ''zipper'' motif.[24] This transcription factor is probably responsible for regulating expression of other inflammatory cytokines and growth factors, raising the possibility of therapy through down-regulation of rheumatoid arthritis by development and use of inhibitors of CEBPβ activity.

The effects of TNFα on immune cells, macrophages, and fibroblasts are almost identical to those of IL-1β. In many systems, TNFα is synergistic with IL-1β.[25] For example, TNFα is synergistic with IL-1β in producing a synovitis when injected into rabbit joints.[26] Exceptions to this synergism are that IL-1β is a much more potent inducer of the metalloprotease stromelysin by cultured rheumatoid synovial cells, and is a more effective suppressor of proteoglycan biosynthesis by chondrocytes (see IL-1 discussion earlier) than is TNFα.[27]

Tumor Necrosis Factor α and Rheumatoid Arthritis

TNFα is a prime candidate for the principal driving cytokine in rheumatoid synovitis through its paracrine actions[28] (Fig. 8–4). The data that have given it this pivotal role include the following:

1. As an activator of the immune system, TNFα acutely enhances proliferation and IL-2 receptor expression by activated T cells, enhances proliferation and differentiation of B cells, and augments

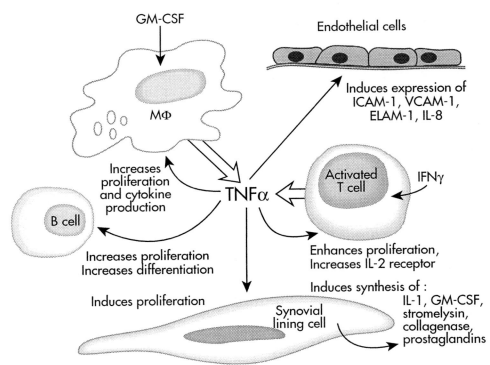

FIGURE 8–4. TNFα is a cytokine with multiple potentials for driving many engines of the inflammatory/proliferative processes in rheumatoid arthritis. It appears that both activated macrophages and T cells produce TNFα, which, in turn, can act back on these cells as well as on the synovial lining cells, endothelium, and B cells. All of the major activity of TNFα in model systems can be inferred to be proinflammatory. The fact that active TNFα enhances IL-1 production by cells is additional evidence for its primacy in generating and sustaining rheumatoid synovitis.

cytolytic activity of NK cells.[6] However, if activated T cells are exposed chronically to TNFα (as they must be in rheumatoid synovium), their capacity to respond to antigenic rechallenge becomes blunted and suboptimal.[29] This effect is reversed by anti-TNF. It is possible that antibodies against TNFα or soluble receptors of TNFα act in part by restoring immune responsiveness toward normal.

2. Synovial cells collected from synovial fluid of patients with inflammatory synovitis release amounts of TNFα sufficient to induce fibroblast proliferation.[30] TNFα induces expression of the potent metalloproteases, collagenase and stromelysin, and PGE$_2$ by synovial fibroblasts and fibrochondrocytes (from meniscal cartilages) in culture.[31]

3. With IL-1β, TNFα up-regulates expression of adhesion molecules (e.g., ICAM-1, endothelial leukocyte adhesion molecule 1 [ELAM-1]) on endothelium that enhance binding of neutrophils and leukocytes to vascular endothelium,[7] and of IL-8, a potent chemoattractant for inflammatory cells.[32] TNFα also up-regulates expression and function of ICAM-1 on synovial fibroblasts.[33] Because the adhesion of peripheral blood T lymphocytes within synovium is at least partially ICAM-1 dependent, this may help explain how and why lymphocytes accumulate in synovial tissue.

4. TNFα is found by immunostaining in the synovial membrane and in the cartilage-pannus junction,[31,34] and in both serum and synovial fluid from rheumatoid patients.[35] Serum TNFα levels correlate positively with joint scores on patient evaluations,[36] and with the erythrocyte sedimentation rate (ESR) and anemia.[37] Normal synovium does not express TNFα. Using specific immunoassays with monoclonal antibodies, soluble TNF receptors were found in synovial fluids of patients with rheumatoid arthritis (see later).[38]

5. Depletion of lean body mass in rheumatoid patients may be caused by TNFα. In one study, 16 of 24 patients with rheumatoid arthritis were cachectic by U.S. population norms, and the plasma TNFα levels correlated with weight loss as well as with demonstrable flares of disease.[39]

Perhaps most important in establishing a chain of importance of cytokines in rheumatoid arthritis are the observations that, in cultures of rheumatoid synovial membrane cells, biosynthesis and release of IL-1β, as well as GM-CSF, is dependent upon the presence of TNFα.[40] The inference is that TNFα may initiate the cytokine cascade in the synovium. IL-10 may be one of the only known down-regulators of TNFα production.[41]

The finding that anti–TNFα antibody ameliorated collagen-induced arthritis in mice,[42] plus the gene transfer experiments in which mice expressing the human TNF transgene develop arthritis from 4 weeks of age,[43] serve to support the primacy of TNFα in the pathogenesis of inflammatory synovitis.

INHIBITORS OF INTERLEUKIN-1β AND TUMOR NECROSIS FACTOR α: A POTENTIAL FOR THERAPY

As mentioned previously, naturally occurring inhibitors of a biologic activity cannot be identified until the agonist itself has been characterized. So it was that after IL-1 had been defined, discovery of a natural antagonist came not far behind. Since 1990, when IL-1ra was cloned, intense interest has been generated in the possibilities of using this or natural inhibitors of TNFα to control inflammatory conditions.

Interleukin-1 Receptor Antagonist

IL-1ra is structurally related to IL-1 and is produced by the same cells.[44,45] It exists in two forms that are different products of the same gene as a result of alternative splicing.[46,47] One form, secretory IL-1ra, is the predominant form in synovium and is effectively secreted by monocyte-macrophages. In its active form it is a nonglycosylated 17-kDa (153-amino-acid) molecule that has a 25 percent homology with IL-1β. The intracellular form is a product of fibroblasts (such as those in the synovial lining) and epithelial cells. Immunostaining and in situ hybridization located protein and mRNA for IL-1ra in the sublining of rheumatoid synovium, particularly in perivascular regions enriched for macrophages.[48] There was much less evidence for IL-1ra expression in osteoarthritic synovium.

Different stimuli have different effects on the relative expression by macrophages in culture of IL-1 and IL-1ra. For example, endotoxin generates equal amounts of the two, IgG induces expression only of IL-1ra, and IL-4 is of particular interest because it inhibits IL-1 production while enhancing IL-1ra expression.[49]

Because it is a competitive inhibitor of both IL-1α and IL-1β, a 10- to 100-fold greater concentration of IL-1ra than of IL-1 is needed to inhibit IL-1 activity. IL-1ra binds to cellular IL-1Rs but does not activate them. Given to normal human subjects, it produces no biologic responses, consistent with the belief that IL-1 does not play an important role in normal homeostasis.

Within rheumatoid synovial fibroblasts and macrophages, there is a large amount of IL-1ra, but it appears that very little is released from these cells. This factor, plus a probable defective production system for IL-1ra in rheumatoid synovium, generates a ratio of IL-1ra to IL-1 of less than 4, perhaps below the 10-fold excess of IL-1ra needed to inhibit IL-1 activity.[49,50] Rheumatoid patients have a significantly lower ratio of IL-1ra to IL-1β in plasma compared with osteoarthritic patients, and these differences are maintained through and after surgery in both types of patients.[51]

In contrast, and underscoring the compartmentalization between the joint space and the synovium, in rheumatoid synovial fluid there is more than enough IL-1ra to neutralize any IL-1 present. The reason for this is probably that the neutrophils in rheumatoid synovial fluid are contributing IL-1ra to the inflammatory ''soup'' there[52] (Fig. 8–5). When measured on the basis of cytokine production/content per cell, synovial fluid neutrophils produce less IL-1ra than do peripheral blood neutrophils. In contrast, synovial fluid neutrophils generate a much greater amount of other mediators (e.g., IL-8), than do peripheral blood neutrophils.[53]

It is apparent that, when delivered to sites of inflammation in sufficient quantity, IL-1ra can inhibit many actions attributable to IL-1. For example, IL-1ra inhibits IL-1–induced PGE$_2$ and collagenase production by cultured rheumatoid synovial cells,[54] reverses the depression of cartilage proteoglycaus induced by IL-2, and ameliorates the inflammatory effects of IL-1β on various forms of experimental arthritis, including type II collagen arthritis in mice.[55]

Interleukin-1β Blockade and Therapy

Although both gold salts and methotrexate are believed to have inhibitory effects upon IL-1 production, the clinical use of these therapies would not change based upon these findings alone. More specific therapeutic approaches[56] would be to (1) block production of IL-1, (2) prevent soluble IL-1 release from cells, (3) inhibit receptor binding, or

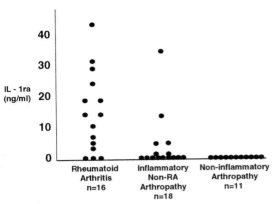

FIGURE 8–5. Relationship of synovial fluid (SF) IL-1ra concentration to the underlying rheumatologic disorder. SF samples were obtained from 15 patients with seropositive rheumatoid arthritis (RA) and 1 patient with seronegative RA. The mean SF IL-1ra concentration was 17.1 ng/ml for the 13 elevated values (SD = 12.6). Samples from patients with inflammatory non-RA arthropathy were from eight patients with acute gouty arthritis, four with reactive arthritis, two with ankylosing spondylitis, two with fungal arthritis, one with a Milwaukee shoulder syndrome, and one with an unclassified syndrome of recurrent monarticular aseptic pyarthrosis and pyoderma gangrenosum. The mean SF IL-1ra concentration in this group was 10.6 ng/ml for the six elevated values (SD = 13.4). Samples from patients with noninflammatory arthropathy were from 10 patients with osteoarthritis and 1 patient with a mechanical joint derangement. SF IL-1ra was undetectable in all samples in this category. (From Malyak, M., Swaney, R. F., and Arend, W. P.: Levels of synovial fluid interleukin-1 receptor antagonist in rheumatoid arthritis and other or thropathies: potential contribution from synovial fluid neutrophils. Arthritis Rheum. 36:781, 1993. Used by permission.)

(4) interfere with signal transduction after IL-1β binds to its specific receptors.

Prevention of IL-1 release from cells might be achieved if inhibition of its conversion from a larger inactive form to the secreted active form were possible; inhibitors of the converting enzyme are now being developed and tested. Similar to TNFα, there are soluble receptors for IL-1β within inflammatory fluids, and recombinant forms of these have been administered intra-articularly in active rheumatoid arthritis with beneficial results reported.[57]

A practical way to increase synthesis or activity of IL-1ra would obviate the challenge of delivering this useful molecule to patients. Use of enhancing cytokines (e.g., IL-4, IL-10) might result in harmful results from the multiple effects of these molecules on multiple different cells. The more specific, but complex, approach to gene therapy by transfer of IL-1ra transgene is being explored in experimental systems.

A disadvantage of using complex molecules such as IL-1ra in therapy is that it must be given by subcutaneous injection; this may be more than balanced by lack of toxicity other than injection site reactions. In a 6-month placebo-controlled, double-blind, randomized trial in Europe, doses of 50, 100, and 150 mg of recombinant IL-1ra were given by self-injection each day. All three doses produced a significant benefit (by ACR criteria) and there was a suggestive benefit on bone erosions, with slower progression in the treated group. Best of all, injection site reactions were the only significant toxicity.[58]

A Danish laboratory has studied autoantibodies directed against cytokines found in serum of patients and normal individuals. These are monospecific and have a high affinity for one particular cytokine.[59] Naturally occurring autoantibodies have been defined against IL-1α, IL-6, IL-10, IFNγ, and TNFα.[60] Interestingly, none against IL-1β has been described. The hypothesis has been raised that it is the presence of these anti-cytokine antibodies in pooled gamma globulin preparations that give therapeutic effects from intravenous IgG therapy in rheumatoid arthritis.

The Soluble Receptors of Tumor Necrosis Factor α

There are a number of reasons that soluble receptors for cytokines might be effective in therapy of rheumatoid arthritis. Soluble receptors

- Bind ligand with the same high affinity as surface-bound receptors (unlike IL-1ra)
- Are not immunogenic
- Perform well in vitro and in alleviating arthritis in some experimental models
- Have no side effects

A different approach from the relatively simple one of administering recombinant soluble TNF receptors (sTNFR) alone is the tactic of linking soluble receptors to the Fc portion of human Ig. Administration of such a dimeric soluble TNFα fusion protein (sTNFR-Fc) has been shown to decrease mortality in animals given endotoxin.[61] The possible ways that this beneficial effect could be made manifest are that sTNFR-Fc might

Inhibit soluble TNF in extravascular sites

Mask cell surface–expressed TNF

Dislodge TNF bound to surface receptors prior to complete signal transduction

In classical adjuvant arthritis, there is dose-dependent suppression of inflammation in joints injected with sTNFR-Fc and, most intriguing, in the contralateral joints as well. Consistent with the synergism observed between IL-1β and TNFα, adding a soluble IL-1R–Fc dimer to the sTNFR-Fc gives additive benefit in the experimental arthritis. Multicenter double blind trials[61a,61b] of TNFR-fusion protein given biweekly (subcutaneously), have proved useful in severe rheumatoid arthritis.

CYTOKINES RELEASED BY LYMPHOCYTES: THE LYMPHOKINES

Although it is apparent that T cells are proliferating in the rheumatoid process, and that B-cell production of rheumatoid factor and other antibodies is exuberant, it is both interesting and curious that these T-cell products are difficult to detect by assays for protein or mRNA in rheumatoid tissues.[62] Gene expression of IL-2, IL-2R, IL-6, IL-4, and IFNγ in T cells from fresh rheumatoid synovium and synovial fluid is low or absent compared with cells from control patients. The factors produced predominantly by macrophages and synovial fibroblasts, in contrast, are easy to measure; these include IL-1, IL-6, IL-8, TNFα, TGFβ, GM-CSF, M-CSF, and MCP-1.

Is it the relative lack of T cell factors that generates synovitis, or are there other reasons? These lower amounts of T cell factors are not common to all forms of inflammation. IFNγ, for instance, can be found in the tissues of patients with a number of inflammatory conditions. Other possible reasons for the relative decrease of lymphokines are

1. Synthesis of lymphokines is actually down-regulated by other cytokines (e.g., TGFβ, IL-10).
2. T-cell anergy exists; mRNA is present without protein production.
3. Lymphokines are produced in small quantities in a microenvironment, and immediately are sopped up by receptors that transduce signals and alter the phenotype of those particular effector cells.
4. T cells are not activated in the tissue.
5. T cells are maximally activated in the tissue; the CD45RB[dim] cells that are present in significant quantities in rheumatoid synovium give excellent B-cell help but produce few cytokines.
6. Other cytokines (e.g., IL-15) are additive or synergistic with small amounts of IL-2 to produce T-cell activation in synovium.

The relative intensity of forces pushing Th1 and Th2 cell development in rheumatoid synovitis may also affect cytokine secretion. For example, both IL-4 and IL-10 inhibit the ability of IL-12 to promote Th1 cell development. Although IL-4 is diffi-

cult to detect in rheumatoid tissues, IL-10 is present in abundant quantities in rheumatoid serum and synovial fluid, and it may contribute to the diminished production of IL-2 and IFNγ.[63]

IL-4, IL-10, and TGFβ appear to be the only known down-regulators of the inflammatory and proliferative cascade in rheumatoid synovium. IL-10, for example, can inhibit disease progression in collagen-induced arthritis in mice (Walmsley, et al., Abstract 767).

T-cell anergy is another possible explanation of lymphokine deficiency in rheumatoid tissues. It is likely that, after an initial specific antigen-driven T-cell response in synovium, T cells from multiple clones enter the joint. It may be that insufficient co-stimulatory molecules are present, and activation of these "bystander" T cells is incomplete. They do not express IL-2, IL-2R, or other lymphokines and are destined for apoptosis.

Studies have shown that many T cells are in an activated state. Chronic down-regulation is possible, but only after the immunoproliferative sequence has been set into motion. The most compelling evidence for a major T-cell role in rheumatoid arthritis is the abundant evidence for downstream activation of the full immune system.

Having admitted that a full and satisfactory explanation of why lymphokines are detected in unexpectedly low quantities in rheumatoid synovium cannot be provided, it nevertheless is important to focus on each lymphokine and review evidence for its involvement in the rheumatoid process.

Interleukin-2

As detailed in Chapter 5, CD4[+] T cells are composed of two functional subsets: Th1 and Th2. Th1 cells produce IL-2 and execute cell-mediated immune responses such as delayed hypersensitivity and activation of macrophages. Biosynthesis of both IL-2 and IFNγ is a result of stimulation by another cytokine, IL-12, that is produced by macrophages and B lymphocytes.[64]

IL-2 in its active form is a 133-amino-acid protein that exerts its effects on a specific receptor system found on T and B cells, NK cells, and lymphokine-activated killer (LAK) cells. The receptor (also known as Tac) has two subunits, α and β. Together they bind IL-2 with high affinity. A soluble IL-2R is released by activated T cells, and has been measured in synovial fluid in rheumatoid arthritis.[65] Joint inflammation is directly associated with soluble IL-2R levels in serum.[66]

T-cell activation fits into a "competence" and "progression" model: Stimulation of the TCR in the presence of co-stimulatory factors promotes entry into the G_1 phase of the cell cycle. Progression is dependent upon expression of both IL-2 and IL-2R. In addition to promoting T-cell growth, IL-2

- Augments B-cell growth and antibody production
- Induces IL-6 production by monocytes
- Modulates IL-2R expression

Interleukin-15

IL-15 has bioactivity similar to that of IL-2, and its actions are mediated through the IL-2R. IL-15 is a potent T-lymphocyte chemoattractant and has been implicated in T-lymphocyte migration and activation in rheumatoid arthritis. It has been demonstrated to be abundant in rheumatoid synovial lining cells (McInnes et al., Abstract 490) and in endothelial cells (Vita et al., Abstract 491). A portion of the chemotactic activity of rheumatoid synovial fluids has been attributed to the presence of IL-15. In a murine model, injection of recombinant IL-15 was found to induce a local tissue inflammatory infiltrate consisting predominantly of T lymphocytes.[67] In this same study, it was shown that the presence of IL-15 at immunologically active levels in rheumatoid joints provides another mechanism—driven by macrophages, not IL-2 from lymphocytes—for activation of T cells.

Interferon γ

This "immune interferon" is produced primarily by CD4[+] and CD8[+] lymphocytes after mitogen or antigen stimulation, or in response to IL-2 or IL-12. It induces MHC class I and II expression on synovial macrophages[68] and generally sensitizes these cells for cytotoxicity. An effect not directly related to the immune system is the ability of IFNγ to inhibit collagen synthesis.[69]

The impaired capacity for rheumatoid peripheral blood lymphocytes to synthesize IFNγ in response to IL-2 appears to be a distinct cellular effect not directly related to suppressive effects of prostaglandins or other well-characterized mechanisms.[70]

Interleukin-4 and Interleukin-10

IL-4 is produced principally by CD4[+] T cells, specifically the Th2 subset. It has numerous activities:[62]

- IL-4 is required for production of IgE and is responsible for B-cell switching to this heavy chain isotype.
- IL-4 inhibits macrophage activation, blocking

most of the activating influences of IFNγ. Thus, activation of Th2 cells is often associated with a suppression of macrophage-mediated immune reactions.

- IL-4 enhances growth and differentiation of Th2 cells.
- IL-4 stimulates expression of endothelial cell adhesion molecules.
- IL-4 induces MCP-1 (see later) secretion by endothelial cells.
- IL-4 inhibits bone resorption. The mechanism is related to a reduction of IL-6 production and decrease in the numbers of osteoclasts present.[71]
- Recombinant IL-4 produced a rapid down-modulation of TNFα receptor on rheumatoid synovial fibroblasts, indicating that the potentials of IL-4 are not confined to inhibiting monokine production but also include the ability to interfere with their action on the major effector cells of the synovium in rheumatoid arthritis.[72]

IL-10 is an anti-inflammatory cytokine secreted by activated T cells, monocytes, and B cells. It is constitutively produced by synovial fluid mononuclear cells from rheumatoid patients, and has been found in most rheumatoid synovial fluids. Interesting experiments have shown that, although *endogenous* IL-10 produced by synovial fluid mononuclear cells inhibits the production of HLA-DR, IL-1, TNFα, and GM-CSF,[73] the levels of these cytokines can be further down-regulated by *exogenous* IL-10.[74] In these same studies, neutralization of endogenously produced IL-10 by anti–IL-10 mononuclear antibodies resulted in increased production of the inflammatory cytokines and HLA-DR expression. The only exception to consistent anti-inflammatory and proliferative activities of IL-10 is the observation that IL-10 down-regulates collagen type I expression by fibroblasts while enhancing production of collagenase and stromelysin.[75]

When added to T-cell culture systems, IL-10 inhibits production of IL-2,[76] and it significantly inhibited proliferation of synovial fluid mononuclear cells, even in the presence of IL-2.[74] In B-cell systems, IL-10 stimulates proliferation and production of immunoglobulin by purified cells, perhaps by induction of synthesis of Bcl-2, the molecule that saves germinal center B cells from apoptosis.[77] Because prolonged B-cell survival in *bcl-2* transgenic mice favors autoantibody production,[78] it remains to be tested whether IL-10 is involved in sustained rheumatoid factor production. The IL-10 levels in serum and synovial fluid from rheumatoid patients correlated significantly with serum rheumatoid factor and amounts of IgM rheumatoid factor production by B cells from these patients.[63] Direct evidence for the power of IL-10 in suppressing inflammation in arthritis is the finding that IL-10 reverses the cartilage degradation induced by antigen-stimulated activated mononuclear cells of rheumatoid arthritis patients. IL-4 has an additive effect on this process. In addition, IL-10 has a direct stimulatory effect on cartilage proteoglycan synthesis, quite opposite from the inhibitory influence of IL-1.[79]

Taken together with the fact that IL-10 can produce immune deviation away from Th1 modes toward Th2, and the observation that exogenous IL-10 added to in vitro systems gives additive suppression of inflammatory mediators and mechanisms for antigen presentation, this molecule deserves serious trials as a therapy for active rheumatoid arthritis.

Interleukin-13

IL-13 is a product of activated T cells that shares "anti-inflammatory" qualities with IL-4 and IL-10 but acts primarily on B cells and monocytes. It has been found to inhibit rheumatoid synovial fibroblast proliferation stimulated by IL-1, but it augmented IL-1 stimulation of IL-6 production in these cells. IL-4, IL-10, and IL-13 suppress production of IL-1, TNFα, and IL-8; IL-13 and IL-4 enhance production of IL-1ra. Although IL-13 down-regulates macrophage and fibroblast activity similar to IL-4, it is weaker than IL-4 or IL-10 as a modulator of Th1-mediated immune responses (Morita et al., Abstract 1197).

TRANSFORMING GROWTH FACTOR β: A MAJOR "REPARACTIVE" CYTOKINE

In rheumatoid arthritis, the polypeptide TGFβ can be considered a prototype of "counter-regulatory molecules." In some pathologic states, such as atherosclerosis, in which TGFβ appears to stimulate matrix formation that can close off lumens of coronary arteries, or possibly in scleroderma, in which excessive collagen deposition is a prominent feature, the "dark side" of what may be an excess of TGFβ may be dominant.[80] In synovial inflammation, however, there is a potential role for TGFβ in repair, inhibition of cartilage and bone destruction, and down-regulation of the immune response.

Structurally, TGFβ is a homodimer of 25 kDa (112 amino acids). It is a member of the "chemokine" gene family that shares nine cysteine residues. It is expressed by most cell types and is released in a latent form (391 amino acids).[81–83] (Ref. 81 to 83 are excellent reviews of the biologic, pathologic, and potential therapeutic activities of TGFβ.) There are striking differences between the latent and active forms, the principal one being the biologic half-lives of the two. Latent TGFβ has a much longer half-life than the active form, so much so that the latent form may be thought of as having an endocrine mechanism for action, whereas the active form exerts its effect in the immediate environment in autocrine/paracrine fashion.

In the extracellular space after release from cells, TGFβ is associated with a 135-kDa modulator protein that is important for "docking" of the cytokine to cells. Once cleaved to an active form, TGFβ is available to bind to its receptors on virtually all cells in the synovial environment; however, it also can be engulfed by α_2-macroglobulin, bind to extracellular matrix proteoglycans such as betaglycan, or reassociate with the latency protein from which it was recently separated (Fig. 8–6).

Some of the major activities of TGFβ are as follows:[62]

- Inhibition of T-cell activation and activated T-cell proliferation, in part by down-regulating expression of the IL-2R
- Down-regulation of B-cell proliferation and differentiation
- Inhibition of collagen breakdown by
  –inhibiting biosynthesis of collagenase
  –enhancing production of TIMP
- Acceleration of bone and soft tissue repair by enhancement of collagen and GAG production
- Protection of articular cartilage from the effects of IL-1 that induce breakdown of proteoglycan[84] and repression of its synthesis
- Stimulation of hyaluronan synthesis in human synovial lining cells[85]
- Counteraction of effects of TNFα by inhibition of its secretion from macrophages
- "Deactivation" of macrophages, with a decrease in HLA-DR on their surfaces, and interruption of oxygen free radical formation
- Blockade of neutrophil binding to endothelium
- Increase of microvascular blood flow into wounds and other sites for active repair by enhancing release of angiogenic factors from macrophages

In normal human T lymphocytes, dexamethasone causes an increase in TGFβ production. This enhancement is augmented by cycloheximide, a compound that inhibits protein synthesis from

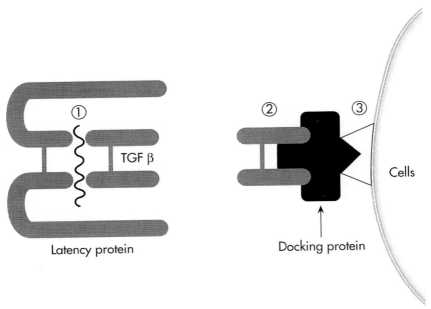

FIGURE 8–6. The biology of TGFβ is complex. The large latent form of this cytokine has a long circulating half-life. When the active segment of the molecule is separated from its associated latency protein (1), it then must combine with a docking protein (2) in order for it to bind to its receptor on cells (3). Although active TGFβ is susceptible to entrapment by α_2-macroglobulin, it also can return to the protection of its latency protein, presumably to await subsequent reactivation.[81–83]

mRNA, suggesting that glucocorticoids may inhibit synthesis of a protein(s) that decreases TGFβ gene transcription or translation.[86]

Transforming Growth Factor β and Rheumatoid Arthritis

In studies specific for rheumatoid arthritis, TGFβ has been demonstrated by immunostaining at the cartilage-pannus junction and within the synovium[87] in both type A and type B cells. Monocyte-macrophages isolated from rheumatoid synovium and nurtured in culture generated sufficient TGFβ to block the activity of considerable amounts of IL-1 on synovial cells.[88] TGFβ counteracted IL-1–induced suppression of articular cartilage proteoglycan synthesis in animals but—in a singular example of a phlogistic effect of this compound—was synergistic with IL-1 in attracting inflammatory cells into the joint into which the cytokines were injected.[66] The counteraction by TGFβ of IL-1 effects on cartilage may be accomplished by reduction of IL-1R expression on chondrocytes.[89]

Using streptococcal cell wall–induced experimental arthritis, it was observed that systemic administration of TGFβ significantly suppressed both the acute and chronic phases of inflammation of

disease in joints[90] (Fig. 8–7). Inflammatory cell infiltration, pannus formation, joint erosion, and leukocytosis all were diminished, and no toxicity was observed. Similar benefit was noted for collagen-induced arthritis in mice, where it was noted that

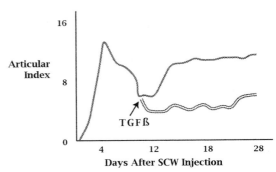

FIGURE 8–7. The effect of TGF-β1 treatment on the chronic phase of the arthritis. Lewis rats were injected on day 0 with streptococcal cell wall (SCW) and their articular index was determined daily thereafter. On day 10, half of the animals (double lines) were begun on a daily dosing regimen of 5 μg TGF-β1/animal (intraperitoneally). This regimen suppressed the chronic phase of arthritis, as indicated by the lower articular index values for these animals. (Modified from Brandes, M. E., Allen, J. B., Ogawa, Y., et al.: Transforming growth factor β1 suppresses acute and chronic arthritis in experimental animals. J. Clin. Invest. 87:1108, 1991. Used by copyright permission of The American Society for Clinical Investigation, 1991.)

"TGFβ has powerful anti-inflammatory effects, mimicking in some respects the beneficial effects of immunosuppressive drugs in these experimental models of autoimmune disease, but without discernible adverse effects."[91]

If subcutaneous injection each day is accepted to patients with active, progressive arthritis in a trade-off for having no side effects, TGFβ could be an important molecule to use in clinical trials.

GLOSSARY OF CYTOKINES, GROWTH FACTORS, AND CHEMOKINES

The initial sections of this chapter focused on four different types of cytokines:

IL-1β and TNFα, which enhance both the immune and proliferative lesions of rheumatoid arthritis

IL-2 and IFNγ, which enhance lymphocyte proliferation

IL-4 and IL-10, which deviate the immune system from a Th1 to a Th2 setting

TGFβ, which diminishes many of the inflammatory, immune, and proliferative effects of the inflammatory cytokines.

There are many more activities associated with specific proteins in rheumatoid synovitis, however. It is appropriate to mention many of these, albeit briefly. In future years, as understanding of the rheumatoid process grows and changes, some of these may be assigned more, or less, important roles in the mechanisms of pathogenesis of this disease. Table 8–2, from a review by Lipsky et al.,[7] summarizes details of many of them. IL-4 and IL-10 were discussed previously.

Cytokines

Interleukin-6 and Interleukin-11

IL-6 is a 26-kDa polypeptide produced by monocytes, T lymphocytes, and fibroblasts. It facilitates activation of T cells and differentiation of B cells, and is the primary inducer of acute-phase protein synthesis in hepatocytes.[92] IL-6 can be considered in the second tier of cytokines; it probably is driven by IL-1β, and augments effects of IL-1β and TNFα. It does appear to be a reasonable index of rheumatoid activity, correlating in blood with the ESR or C-reactive protein level,[93] with local IgM production in synovial fluid,[94] and with the general examination of patients (joint scores and duration

of morning stiffness).[95] Consistent with their putative role in suppressing inflammatory (Th1-mediated) activities, both IL-4 and IL-10 suppress production of IL-6 by rheumatoid synovium and by monocyte-macrophages from rheumatoid synovial tissue.[96]

Similar to IL-6, another cytokine, IL-11, acts synergistically with IL-3 or IL-4 to stimulate colony-forming units for granulocytes and macrophages and megakaryocytes in the bone marrow. IL-11, independently of other cytokines, induces functional osteoclast formation.[97] In estrogen-deficient states, increased amounts of cytokines from stromal cells and peripheral blood mononuclear cells and osteoblasts lead to osteoclast formation and excess bone resorption.

Granulocyte/Macrophage Colony-Stimulating Factor

GM-CSF has been exploited for its role in inducing proliferation and differentiation of bone marrow cells. Macrophages constitutively produce it in synovium, and synovial fibroblasts are induced to express it by IL-1. Once produced by these cells, GM-CSF may have a major role in stimulating the induction of HLA class II antigens on APCs in early synovitis.[98]

Growth Factors

Platelet-Derived Growth Factor

In addition to platelets, macrophages and endothelial cells produce this very potent mitogen for fibroblasts and smooth muscle cells. In rheumatoid arthritis, it is the ability of platelet-derived growth factor (PDGF) to stimulate proliferation of synovial fibroblasts (type B cells) and to induce metalloprotease production and PGE_2, which helps establish and perpetuate the increase in cell mass associated with rheumatoid synovitis.[11] TNFα may induce expression of PDGF by synovial type A cells, the macrophage-like lining cells.

Fibroblast Growth Factor

Fibroblast growth factor (FGF) is a family of polypeptides that has both acidic (aFGF) and basic (bFGF) forms. Within inflammatory and proliferative tissue such as rheumatoid synovium, their angiogenic capacities are probably their most important qualities.[99] Synovial lining cells and vascular endothelial cells have been shown to produce bFGF in rheumatoid patients.[100]

TABLE 8–2. Cytokines Potentially Involved in Rheumatoid Inflammation

CYTOKINE	ABBREV.	OTHER NAMES	M_r OF NATURAL PROTEIN ($\times 10^3$)	AMINO ACIDS OF MATURE PROTEIN	CHROMOSOME	MAJOR SOURCE	PROBABLE SOURCE WITHIN SYNOVIUM
Interleukin-1α	IL-1α	Lymphocyte-activating factor (LAF)	17.5	159	2	Monocyte-macrophage, fibroblast, keratinocyte, endothelial cell, many others	Monocyte-macrophage, fibroblast, endothelial cell,
Interleukin-1β	IL-1β	B cell–activating factor (BAF) Leukocyte endogenous mediator (LEM) Endogenous pyrogen (EP) Hemopoietin I Catabolin Mononuclear cell factor (MCF) Osteoclast-activating factor (OAF) Activating factor (ETAF) Epidermal cell–derived thymocyte	17.5	153	2		
Interleukin-2	IL-2	T-cell growth factor (TCGF)	15–17	133	4	T cell	T cell
Interleukin-4	IL-4	B-cell–stimulatory factor 1 (BSF-1) B-cell differentiation factor-γ (BCDF-γ) T-cell growth factor 2 (TCGF-2) Mast cell growth factor 2 (MCGF-2)	20	129	5	T cell, mast cell	Not detected
Interleukin-5	IL-5	B-cell growth factor II (BCGF-II) T-cell replacing factor (TRF) Killer helper factor (KHF) Eosinophil differentiation factor (EDF) Eosinophil colony-stimulating factor (Eo-CSF) IgA-enhancing factor (IgA-EF)	50–60	113	5	T cell	Not demonstrated
Interleukin-6	IL-6	Interferon β2 (IFNβ2) B-cell–stimulatory factor 2 (BSF-2)	26	184	7	Monocyte-macrophage, fibroblast, T cell, smooth muscle cell, endothelial cell	T cell, macrophage, fibroblast

Name	Abbreviation	Other names				Source	
		Hepatocyte stimulatory factor II (HSF-II); Hybridoma plasmacytoma growth factor (HPGF, IL-HP1); Myeloma cell growth factor (MCGF); 26-kDa protein					
Interleukin-8	IL-8	Mononuclear cell–derived neutrophil chemotactic factor; Macrophage inflammatory protein 2 (MIP-2)	6–8	72	4	Macrophage	Not demonstrated
Tumor necrosis factor α	TNFα	Cachectin	17	157	6	Monocyte-macrophage, fibroblast, T cell, smooth muscle cell	Monocyte-macrophage, T cell
Lymphotoxin	LT	Tumor necrosis factor β (TNFβ)	25	171	6	T and B cell	Not detected
Interferon α	IFNα		16–27	166	9	Macrophage	Not detected
Interferon β	IFNβ		20	166	9	Fibroblast	Not detected
Interferon γ	IFNγ	Macrophage-activating factor (MAF)	20–25	146	12	T and NK cells	T cell
Interleukin-3	IL-3	Multipotential colony-stimulating factor (Multi-CSF); Hematopoietic cell growth factor (HCGF); P-cell growth factor (PSP); Mast cell growth factor (MCGF); Erythroid colony-stimulating factor (ECSF); Megakaryocyte colony-stimulating factor (Meg-CSF); Eosinophil colony-stimulating factor (Eo-CSF); Burst-promoting activity (BPA)	20–26	133	5	T cell	Not detected
Granulocyte colony–G-CSF stimulating factor	G-CSF	Colony-stimulating factor β (CSFβ); Pluripoietin	19.6	177	17	Monocyte-macrophage, fibroblast, endothelial cell	Not detected

Table continued on following page

TABLE 8-2. *Continued*

CYTOKINE	ABBREV.	OTHER NAMES	M_r OF NATURAL PROTEIN ($\times 10^3$)	AMINO ACIDS OF MATURE PROTEIN	CHROMOSOME	MAJOR SOURCE	PROBABLE SOURCE WITHIN SYNOVIUM
Granulocyte/macrophage colony-stimulating factor	GM-CSF	Colony-stimulating factor α Pluripoietin Colony stimulating factor 2 Neutrophil migration inhibitory factor from T cells (NIF-T)	22	127	5	T cell, fibroblast, endothelial cell	T cell, fibroblast, endothelial cell
Macrophage colony-stimulating factor	M-CSF	Colony-stimulating factor (CSF-1) Urinary colony-stimulating factor	70–90	224	5	Fibroblast, monocyte, endothelial cell	Synoviocyte
Epidermal growth factor	EGF	Urogastrone	6	53	4	Macrophage	Synoviocyte
Fibroblast growth factor, acidic	aFGF	Heparin-binding growth factor Tumor angiogenesis factor	14–18	149	5	Platelet, macrophage, endothelial cells	Platelet, macrophage, endothelial cell
Fibroblast growth factor, basic	bFGF	Eye growth factor Retina growth factor Cartilage growth factor Endothelial cell growth factor	16	146			
Insulin-like growth factor I	IGF	Somatomedin C	7	70	12	Macrophage	Macrophage
Platelet-derived growth factor 1	PDGF-1		14–18	104	7	Platelet, endothelial cell, monocyte-macrophage	Endothelial cell, platelet, macrophage
Platelet-derived growth factor 2	PDGF-2		16	109	22		
Transforming growth factor α	TGFα		5–8	50	2	Macrophage	Not detected
Transforming growth factor β	TGFβ		25	2×112	19	Platelet, T cell, endothelial cell, fibroblast, monocyte-macrophage, mast cell	Fibroblast, mononuclear cell

Modified from Lipsky, P. E., Davis, L. S., Cush, J. J., et al.: The role of cytokines in the pathogenesis of rheumatoid arthritis. Semin. Arthritis Rheum. 11:123, 1989. Used by permission.

Vascular Endothelial Growth Factor

Vascular endothelial growth factor (VEGF) is a polypeptide that appears to affect only endothelial cells, and acts as a mitogen and endothelial cell chemoattractant. It is produced by synovial macrophages and, as with the other factors discussed here, has been identified in synovial tissues or fluid.[101]

Leukemia Inhibitory Factor

Leukemia inhibitory factor (LIF) can be considered as a catabolic factor that was first found to induce differentiation of murine leukemia cells. In connective tissue, LIF stimulates bone resorption by stimulating maturation and activity of osteoclasts through an effect on osteoblasts, which have receptors for this cytokine. It also stimulates synovial production of metalloproteases. Rheumatoid synovial fluids contain LIF, and it is produced by both synovial cells and chondrocytes in response to a variety of other cytokines, including IL-1β and TNFα.[102]

Osteopontin

Osteopontin (Eta-1) is an extracellular phosphoprotein secreted by activated T cells as well as by osteoblasts and macrophages. It has chemoattractant activity and has a potential role in cell adhesion. Data have shown that osteopontin is, in addition to hyaluronan, a ligand for CD44.[103] It is a reasonable hypothesis that, depending which ligand binds CD44, a different effect is generated; osteopontin (but not hyaluronan) can induce CD44-dependent chemotaxis, whereas hyaluronan (but not osteopontin) induces CD44-dependent aggregation of cells within connective tissue. These data enhance the potential importance in rheumatoid arthritis of CD44. It may mediate translocation of activated lymphocytes and monocytes out of the bloodstream into the synovium and then fix these cells in that area, preventing their migration into the synovial fluid.

Chemokines

This interesting family of small polypeptides has more than 15 members in two subfamilies. In the C-X-C subfamily, two conserved cystine residues are separated by an unrelated amino acid, whereas the C-C subfamily has no intervening amino acid between cysteine residues. Virtually all of the known chemokines have chemoattractant (chemotactic) activity. They attract leukocytes by binding to 7-transmembrane receptors expressed on the leukocyte surface. Injection of chemokines (e.g., IL-8 and MCP-1) attracts the appropriate cell types to the site, and antibodies that neutralize the same molecules reduce the inflammation in tissues. As with many of these cytokines, additional effects that overlap with actions of other biologic substances have been found for the chemokines. For example, chemokines may contribute to cell adhesion and regulation of angiogenesis as well as attracting cells to inflammatory sites.

Interleukin-8 and Epithelial Neutrophil-Activating Peptide-78

IL-8 is a potent chemoattractant for, and activator of, neutrophils that become adherent to the addressins on tall endothelial venules in rheumatoid synovial capillaries. More IL-8 activity is found in rheumatoid synovial fluid than in fluids from patients with osteoarthritis.[104] It is produced by synovial tissue macrophages, fibroblasts, and chondrocytes in response to IL-1β or TNFα,[105] which are synergistic in their enhancing effects upon IL-8 synthesis. IL-8 accounts for more than 40 per cent of the chemoattractant activity in rheumatoid synovial fluid,[104] and it is a powerful magnet for lymphocytes and endothelial cells.[106] In addition to acting as a chemoattractant, IL-8 (in nanomolar concentrations) inhibits neutrophil adhesion to endothelial cells, enabling the neutrophils to slip through the endothelium of synovial capillaries into the extravascular space. There is enhanced production of IL-8 by rheumatoid mononuclear cells after stimulation. Inhibition of IL-8 activity is mediated by IFNγ and by glucocorticoids.[107]

ENA-78 is homologous to IL-8, is produced by synovial fibroblasts, and has molar concentrations in rheumatoid synovial fluid 15 times that of IL-8 while accounting (similar to IL-8) for about 40 per cent of the chemotactic activity for neutrophils in these fluids.[108]

Connective Tissue–Activating Peptide III

Connective tissue–activating peptide III (CTAP-III) is a growth factor chemokine from α-granules of platelets that is powerful and abundant, and has properties that link it with TGFβ as a reparative cytokine.[109] It stimulates synthesis of DNA, hyaluronan, sulfated GAGs, and other matrix components, and is produced by synovial fibroblasts.

Monocyte Chemoattractant Protein 1 and Macrophage Inflammatory Protein 1α

MCP-1 is a member of the C-C chemokine family. It is produced by rheumatoid synovial fibroblasts in response to IL-1β or TNFα.[110] Injection of MCP-1 into animal joints causes a marked influx of macrophages into the synovium.[111] This chemokine is believed to work with IL-8 to overcome circulating leukocyte adhesion to endothelium, leading to transmigration into the extravascular space. Although first described as an endogenous pyrogen, MIP-1α may have an important role as a chemotactic cytokine for macrophages within rheumatoid synovium,[112] accounting for more than 35 per cent of the chemoattractant force for monocytes in rheumatoid synovial fluid. It joins other chemokines in being induced by IL-1β or TNFα in synovial fibroblasts and macrophages.

REFERENCES

1. Röcken, M., Racke, M., and Shevach, E. M.: IL-4 -induced immune deviation as antigen-specific therapy for inflammatory autoimmune disease. Immunol. Today 17: 225, 1996.
2. Hollander, A. P.: Criteria for identifying mediators of tissue damage in human autoimmune diseases. Autoimmunity 9:171, 1991.
3. Sporn, M. B., and Roberts, A. B.: Autocrine secretion—10 years later. Ann. Intern. Med. 117:408, 1992.
4. Ulfgren, A.-K., Lindblad, S., and Klareskog, L.: Detection of cytokine producing cells in the synovial membrane from patients with rheumatoid arthritis. Ann. Rheum. Dis. 54:654, 1995.
5. Dinarello, C. A., and Wolff, S. M.: The role of interleukin-1 in disease. N. Engl. J. Med. 328:106, 1993.
6. Barkley, D. E. H., Feldmann, M., and Maini, R. N.: Cells with dendritic morphology and bright interleukin-1α staining circulate in the blood of patients with rheumatoid arthritis. Clin. Exp. Immunol. 80:25, 1990.
7. Lipsky, P. E., Davis, L. S., Cush, J. J., et al.: The role of cytokines in the pathogenesis of rheumatoid arthritis. Semin. Arthritis Rheum. 11:123, 1989.
8. Dower, D. L. U. S. K.: The interleukin-1 receptor. Immunol. Today 8:46, 1987.
9. Chin, J., Rupp, E., Cameron, P. M., et al.: Identification of a high-affinity receptor for interleukin 1α and interleukin 1β on cultured human rheumatoid synovial cells. J. Clin. Invest. 82:420, 1988.
10. Kroggel, R., Martin, M., Pingoud, V., et al.: Two-chain structure of the interleukin 1 receptor. FEBS Lett. 229: 59, 1988.
11. Koch, A. E., Kunkel, S. L., and Strieter, R. M.: Cytokines in rheumatoid arthritis. J. Invest. Med. 43:28, 1995.
12. Leizer, T., Cebon, J., Layton, J. E., et al.: Cytokine regulation of colony-stimulating factor production in cultured human synovial fibroblasts: I. Induction of GM-CSF and G-CSF production by interleukin-1 and tumor necrosis factor. Blood 76:1989, 1990.
13. Pettipher, E. R., Higgs, G. A., and Henderson, B.: Interleukin 1 induces leukocyte infiltration and cartilage proteoglycan degradation in the synovial joint. Proc. Natl. Acad. Sci. U.S.A. 83:8749, 1986.
14. Mc Donnell, J., Hoerrner, L. A., Lark, M. W., et al.: Recombinant human interleukin-1β-induced increase in levels of proteoglycans, stromelysin, and leukocytes in rabbit synovial fluid. Arthritis Rheum. 35:799, 1992.
15. Kirkham, B.: Interleukin-1, immune activation pathways,

16. North, J., Situnayake, R. D., and Tikly, M.: Interleukin 1β, hand and foot bone mineral content and the development of joint erosions in rheumatoid arthritis. Ann. Rheum. Dis. 53:543, 1994.
17. Arend, W. P., Malyak, M., Smith, M. F. Jr., et al.: Binding of IL-1α, IL-1β and IL-1ra by soluble IL-1 receptors and levels of soluble IL-1 receptors in synovial fluids. J. Immunol. 53:4766, 1994.
18. Rosenbaum, J. T., Cugnini, R., Tara, D. C., et al.: Production and modulation of interleukin 6 synthesis by synoviocytes derived from patients with arthritic disease. Ann. Rheum. Dis. 51:198, 1992.
19. Ito, A., Itoh, Y., Sasaguri, Y., et al.: Effects of interleukin-6 on the metabolism of connective tissue components in rheumatoid synovial fibroblasts. Arthritis Rheum. 35: 1197, 1992.
20. Leizer, T., Clarris, B. J., Ash, P. E., et al.: Interleukin-1β and interleukin-1α stimulate the plasminogen activator activity and prostaglandin E$_2$ levels of human synovial cells. Arthritis Rheum. 30:562, 1987.
21. Horowitz, M. C.: Cytokines and estrogen in bone: antiosteoporotic effects. Science 260:626, 1993.
22. Yodlowski, M. L., Hubbard, J. R., Kispert, J., et al.: Antibody to interleukin 1 inhibits the cartilage degradative and thymocyte proliferative actions of rheumatoid synovial culture medium. J. Rheumatol. 17:1600, 1990.
23. van de Loo, F. A. J., Joosten, L. A. B., van Lent, P. L. E. M., et al.: Role of interleukin-1, TNFα, and interleukin-6 in cartilage proteoglycan metabolism and destruction. Arthritis Rheum. 38:164, 1995.
24. Pope, R. M., Leutz, A., and Ness, S. A.: C/EBPβ regulation of the tumor necrosis factor α gene. J. Clin. Invest. 94: 1449, 1994.
25. Le, J., and Vilcek, J.: Tumor necrosis factor and interleukin 1: cytokines with multiple overlapping biological activities. Lab. Invest. 56:234, 1987.
26. Henderson, B., and Pettipher, E. R.: Arthritogenic actions of recombinant IL-1 and tumour necrosis factor α in the rabbit: evidence for synergistic interactions between cytokines in vivo. Clin. Exp. Immunol. 75:306, 1989.
27. Firestein, G. S., and Paine, M. M.: Stromelysin and tissue inhibitor of metalloproteinases gene expression in rheumatoid arthritis synovium. Am. J. Pathol. 140:1309, 1992.
28. Brennan, F. M., Maini, R. N., and Feldmann, M.: TNFα—a pivotal role in rheumatoid arthritis? Br. J. Rheumatol. 31:293, 1992.
29. Cope, A. P., Londei, M., Chu, N. R., et al.: Chronic exposure to tumor necrosis factor (TNF) in vitro impairs the activation of T cells through the T cell receptor/CD3 complex; reversal in vivo by anti-TNF antibodies in patients with rheumatoid arthritis. J. Clin. Invest. 94:749, 1994.
30. Thornton, S. C., Por, S. B., Penny, R., et al.: Identification of the major fibroblast growth factors released spontaneously in inflammatory arthritis as platelet derived growth factor and tumour necrosis factor-alpha. Clin. Exp. Immunol. 86:79, 1991.
31. Jasser, M. Z., Mitchell, P. G., and Cheung, H. S.: Induction of stromelysin-1 and collagenase synthesis in fibrochondrocytes by tumor necrosis factor-α. Matrix Biol. 14: 241, 1994.
32. Strieter, R. M., Kunkel, S. L., Showell, H. J., et al.: Endothelial cell gene expression of a neutrophil chemotactic factor by TNFα, lipopolysaccharide, and IL-1β. Science 243:1467, 1989.

33. Tessier, P., Audette, M., Cattaruzzi, P., et al.: U-regulation by tumor necrosis factor α of intercellular adhesion molecule 1 expression and function in synovial fibroblasts and its inhibition by glucocorticoids. Arthritis Rheum. 36:1528, 1993.

34. Feldmann, M., Brennan, F. M., Williams, R. O., et al.: Evaluation of the role of cytokines in autoimmune disease: the importance of TNFα in rheumatoid arthritis. Prog. Growth Factor Res. 4:247, 1992.

35. Saxne, T., Palladino, M. A. Jr., Heinegard, D., et al.: Detection of tumor necrosis factor α but not tumor necrosis factor β in rheumatoid arthritis synovial fluid and serum. Arthritis Rheum. 31:1041, 1988.

36. Manicourt, D.-H., Triki, R., Fukuda, K., et al.: Levels of circulating tumor necrosis factor α and interleukin-6 in patients with rheumatoid arthritis. Arthritis Rheum. 36:490, 1993.

37. Tetta, C., Camussi, G., Modena, V., et al.: Tumor necrosis factor in serum and synovial fluid of patients with active and severe rheumatoid arthritis. Ann. Rheum. Dis. 49:665, 1990.

38. Roux- Lombard, P., Punzi, L., Hasler, F., et al.: Soluble tumor necrosis factor receptors in human inflammatory synovial fluids. Arthritis Rheum. 36:485, 1993.

39. Roubenoff, R., Roubenoff, R. A., Ward, L. M., et al.: Rheumatoid cachexia: depletion of lean body mass in rheumatoid arthritis. Possible association with tumor necrosis factor. J. Rheumatol. 19:1505, 1992.

40. Brennan, F. M., Chantry, D., Jackson, A., et al.: Inhibitory effect of TNFa antibodies on synovial cell interleukin 1 production in rheumatoid arthritis. Lancet 2:244, 1989.

41. Kalscher, P.D., Chu, C.-Q., Brennan, F.M., et al.: Immunoregulatory role of IL-10 in rheumatoid arthritis. J. Exp. Med. 179:1517, 1994.

42. Williams, R. O., Feldmann, M., and Maini, R. N.: Anti-TNF ameliorates joint disease in murine collagen-induced arthritis. Proc. Nat. Acad. Sci. U.S.A. 89:9784, 1992.

43. Keffer, J., Probert, L., Cazlaris, H., et al.: Transgenic mice expressing human tumour necrosis factor—a predictive genetic model of arthritis. EMBO J. 13:4025, 1991.

44. Arend, W. P.: Interleukin 1 receptor antagonist: a new member of the interleukin 1 family. J. Clin. Invest. 88:1445, 1991.

45. Arend, W. P.: Interleukin-1 receptor antagonist. Adv. Immunol. 54:167, 1993.

46. Malyak, M., Smith, M. F. Jr., Abel, A. A., et al.: Peripheral blood neutrophil production of interleukin-1 receptor antagonist and interleukin-1β. J. Clin. Immunol. 14:20, 1994.

47. Haskill, S., Martin, G., Van Le, L., et al.: cDNA cloning of an intracellular form of the human interleukin 1 receptor antagonist associated with epithelium. Proc. Nat. Acad. Sci. U.S.A. 88:3681, 1991.

48. Firestein, G. S., Berger, A. E., Tracey, D. E., et al.: IL-1 receptor antagonist protein production and gene expression in rheumatoid arthritis and osteoarthritis synovium. J. Immunol. 149:1054, 1992.

49. Jenkins, J. K., and Arend, W. P.: Interleukin 1 receptor antagonist production in human monocytes is induced by IL-1α, IL-3, IL-4 and GM-CSF. Cytokine 5:407, 1993.

50. Firestein, G. S., Boyle, D. L., Yu, C., et al.: Synovial interleukin-1 receptor antagonist and interleukin-1 balance in rheumatoid arthritis. Arthritis Rheum. 37:644, 1994.

51. Chikanza, I. C., Roux-Lombard, P., Dayer, J.-M., et al.: Dysregulation of the *in vivo* production of interleukin-1

receptor antagonist in patients with rheumatoid arthritis. Arthritis Rheum. 38:642, 1995.

52. Malyak, M., Swaney, R. E., and Arend, W. P.: Levels of synovial fluid interleukin-1 receptor antagonist in rheumatoid arthritis and other arthropathies: potential contribution from synovial fluid neutrophils. Arthritis Rheum. 36:781, 1993.

53. Beaulieu, A. D., and McColl, S. R.: Differential expression of two major cytokines produced by neutrophils, interleukin-8 and the interleukin-1 receptor antagonist, in neutrophils isolated from the synovial fluid and peripheral blood of patients with rheumatoid arthritis. Arthritis Rheum. 37:855, 1994.

54. Seckinger, P., Kaufmann, M.-T., and Dayer, J.-M.: An interleukin-1 inhibitor affects both cell-associated interleukin-1-induced T cell proliferation and PGE$_2$/collagenase production by human dermal fibroblasts and synovial cells. Immunobiology 180:316, 1990.

55. Wooley, P. H., Whalen, J. D., Chapman, D. L., et al.: The effect of an interleukin-1 receptor antagonist protein on type II collagen-induced arthritis and antigen-induced arthritis in mice. Arthritis Rheum. 36:1305, 1993.

56. Arend, W. P., and Dayer, J.-M.: Inhibition of the production and effects of IL-1 and TNFα in rheumatoid arthritis. Arthritis Rheum. 38:151, 1995.

57. Dreylow, B., Capezio, J., Lovis, R., et al.: Phase I study of recombinant human interleukin-1 receptor (RHU IL-1R) administered intra-articularly in active rheumatoid arthritis. Arthritis Rheum. 34:S45, 1993.

58. Bresnihan, B. and collaborators. Treatment with recombinant human interleukin-1 receptor antagonist (rh IL-1ra) in rheumatoid arthritis: results of a randomized double-blind placebo controlled multi center trial. Arthritis Rheum. 39:S73, 1996.

59. Bendtzen, K., Svenson, M., Jønsson, V., et al.: Autoantibodies to cytokines—friends or foes? Immunol. Today 11:167, 1990.

60. Bendtzen, K., Hansen, M. B., Diamant, M., et al.: Naturally-occurring autoantibodies to IL-1α, IL-6, IL-10 and IFNα. J. Interferon Res. 14:157, 1994.

61. Mohler, K. M., Torrance, D. S., Smith, C. A., et al.: Soluble tumor necrosis factor receptors are effective therapeutic agents in lethal endotoxemia and function simultaneously as both TNF carriers and TNF antagonists. J. Immunol. 151:1548, 1993.

61a. Baumgartner, S., Moreland, L. W., Schiff, M. H., et al.: Double-blind, placebo controlled trial of TNF receptor (p80) fusion protein (TNFR:Fc) in active rheumatoid arthritis. Arthritis Rheum. 39:S74, 1996.

61b. Hasler, F., van de Putte, L., Bandin, M., et al.: Chronic TNF neutralization (up to 1 year) by Lenercept (TNFRSS-IgG, Ro45-2081) in patients with rheumatoid arthritis: results of an open-label extension of a double-blind single dose phase 1 study. Arthritis Rheum. 39:S243, 1996.

62. Firestein, G. S.: Pathogenesis of rheumatoid arthritis. *In* Kelley, W. N., Harris, E. D. Jr., Ruddy, S., and Sledge, C. B. (eds.): Textbook of Rheumatology, 5th ed. Philadelphia, W. B. Saunders, 1996, in press.

63. Cush, J. J., Splawski, J. B., Thomas, R., et al.: Elevated interleukin-10 levels in patients with rheumatoid arthritis. Arthritis Rheum. 38:96, 1995.

64. Scott, P.: IL-12: initiation cytokine for cell-mediated immunity. Science 260:496, 1993.

65. Wood, N., Symons, J., and Duff, G.: Serum interleukin-2 receptor in rheumatoid arthritis: a prognostic indicator of disease activity? J. Autoimmun. 1:353, 1988.

66. Harrington, L., Affleck, G., Urrows, S., et al.: Temporal

covariation of soluble interleukin-2 receptor levels, daily stress, and disease activity in rheumatoid arthritis. Arthritis Rheum. 36:199, 1993.

67. McInnes, I. B., Al-Mughales, J., Field, M., et al.: The role of interleukin-15 in T-cell migration and activation in rheumatoid arthritis. Nature Med. 2:175, 1996.

68. Pober, J. S., Gimbrone, M. A., Cotran, R. S., et al.: Ia expression by vascular endothelium is inducible by activated T cells and by human interferon. J. Exp. Med. 157:1339, 1983.

69. Granstein, R. D., Murphy, G. F., Margolis, R. J., et al.: Gamma-interferon inhibits collagen synthesis *in vivo* in the mouse. J. Clin. Invest. 79:1254, 1987.

70. Hasler, F., and Dayer, J.-M.: Diminished IL-2-induced gamma-interferon production by unstimulated peripheral-blood lymphocytes in rheumatoid arthritis. Br. J. Rheumatol. 27:15, 1988.

71. Miossec, P., Chaomarat, P., Dechanet, J., et al.: Interleukin 4 inhibits bone resorption through an effect on osteoclasts and proinflammatory cytokines in an *ex vivo* model of bone resorption in rheumatoid arthritis. Arthritis Rheum. 12:1715, 1994.

72. Taylor, D. J.: Interleukin-4 induces down-modulation and shedding of the p55 tumor necrosis factor receptor and inhibits TNFα's effect on rheumatoid synovial fibroblasts. Rheumatol. Int. 14:21, 1994.

73. de Waal Malefyt, R., Haanen, J., Spits, H., et al.: Interleukin 10 (IL-10) and viral IL-10 strongly reduce antigen-specific human T cell proliferation by diminishing the antigen-presenting capacity of monocytes via downregulation of class II major histocompatibility complex expression. J. Exp. Med. 174:915, 1991.

74. Isomäki, P., Luukkainen, R., Saario, R., et al.: Interleukin-10 functions as an antiinflammatory cytokine in rheumatoid synovium. Arthritis Rheum. 39:386, 1996.

75. Reitamo, S., Remitz, A., Tamai, K., et al.: Interleukin-10 modulates type I collagen and matrix metalloprotease gene expression in cultured human skin fibroblasts. J. Clin. Invest. 94:2489, 1994.

76. de Waal Malefyt, R., Yssel, H., and de Vries, J. E.: Direct effects of IL-10 on subsets of human CD4 + T cell clones and resting T cells. J. Immunol. 150:4754, 1993.

77. Levy, Y., and Brouet, J.-C.: Interleukin-10 prevents spontaneous death of germinal center B cells by induction of the *bcl-2* protein. J. Clin. Invest. 93:424, 1994.

78. Strasser, A., Whittingham, S., Vaux, D. L., et al.: Enforced BCL2 expression in B-lymphoid cells prolongs antibody responses and elicits autoimmune disease. Proc. Nat. Acad. Sci. U.S.A. 88:8661, 1991.

79. van Roon, J. A. G., van Roy, J. L. A. M., Gmelig-Meyling, F. H. J., et al.: Prevention and reversal of cartilage degradation in rheumatoid arthritis by interleukin-10 and interleukin-4. Arthritis Rheum. 39:829, 1996.

80. Border, W. A., and Ruoslahti, E.: Transforming growth factor-β in disease: the dark side of tissue repair. J. Clin. Invest. 90:1, 1992.

81. Roberts, A. B., and Sporn, M. B.: Physiological actions and clinical applications of transforming growth factor-β (TGF-β). Growth Factors 8:1, 1993.

82. Border, W. A., and Noble, N. A.: Transforming growth factor β in tissue fibrosis. N. Engl. J. Med. 331:1286, 1994.

83. Panayi, G. S.: Cytokines and anticytokines. Clin. Exp. Rheumatol. 8(Suppl. 5):65, 1990.

84. van Beuningen, H. M., van der Kraan, P. M., Arntz, O. J., et al.: Protection from interleukin-1 induced destruction of articular cartilage by transforming growth factor

beta: studies in anatomically intact cartilage *in vitro* and *in vivo*. Ann. Rheum. Dis. 52:185, 1993.

85. Haubeck, H.-D., Kock, R., Fischer, D.-C., et al.: Transforming growth factor beta 1, a major stimulator of hyaluronan synthesis in human synovial lining cells. Arthritis Rheum. 38:669, 1995.

86. Ayanlar Batuman, O., Ferrero, A. P., Diaz, A., et al.: Regulation of transforming growth factor-β1 gene expression by glucocorticoids in normal human T lymphocytes. J. Clin. Invest. 88:1574, 1991.

87. Chu, C. Q., Field, M., Abney, E., et al.: Transforming growth factor-β1 in rheumatoid synovial membrane and cartilage/pannus junction. Clin. Exp. Immunol. 86:380, 1991.

88. Wahl, S. M., Allen, J. B., Wong, H. L., et al.: Antagonistic and agonistic effects of transforming growth factor-β and IL-1 in rheumatoid synovium. I. Immunol. 145: 2514, 1990.

89. Redini, F., Mauviel, A., and Pronost, S.: Transforming growth factor B exerts opposite effects from interleukin-1b on cultured rabbit articular chondrocytes through reduction of interleukin-receptor expression. Arthritis Rheum. 36:44, 1993.

90. Brandes, M. E., Allen, J. B., Ogawa, Y., et al.: Transforming growth factor β1 suppresses acute and chronic arthritis in experimental animals. J. Clin. Invest. 87:1108, 1991.

In these experiments on rats susceptible to streptococcal cell wall arthritis, TGFβ initiated 1 day before an arthritogenic dose of antigen virtually eliminated joint swelling. More significantly, however, TGFβ suppressed evolution of arthritis even when it was given after the acute phase of disease.

91. Kuruvilla, A. P., Shah, R., Hochwald, G. M., et al.: Protective effect of transforming growth factor β1 on experimental autoimmune disease in mice. Proc. Natl. Acad. Sci. U.S.A. 88:2918, 1991.

92. Le, J., and Vilcrek, J.: Interleukin 6: a multifunctional cytokine regulating immune reactions and the acute phase protein response. Lab. Invest. 61:588, 1989.

93. Wendling, D., Racadot, E., and Wijdenes, J.: Treatment of severe rheumatoid arthritis by anti-interleukin-6 monoclonal antibody. J. Rheumatol. 20:259, 1993.

94. Helle, M., Boeije, L., de Groot, E., et al.: Sensitive ELISA for interleukin-6. Detection of IL-6 in biological fluids: synovial fluids and sera. J. Immunol. Methods 138:47, 1991.

95. Madhok, R., Crilly, A., Murphy, E., et al.: Gold therapy lowers serum interleukin 6 levels in rheumatoid arthritis. J. Rheumatol. 20:630, 1993.

96. Chaomarat, P., Banchereau, J., and Moissec, P.: Differential effects of interleukins 10 and 4 on the production of interleukin-6 by blood and synovium monocytes in rheumatoid arthritis. Arthritis Rheum. 38:1046, 1995.

97. Girasole, G., Passeri, G., Jilka, R. L., et al.: Interleukin-11: a new cytokine critical for osteoclast development. J. Clin. Invest. 93:1516, 1994.

98. Alvaro-Garcia, J. M., Zvaifler, N. J., and Firestein, G. S.: Granulocyte/macrophage colony-stimulating factor-mediated induction of class II MHC antigen on human monocytes: a possible role in rheumatoid arthritis. J. Exp. Med. 170:865, 1989.

99. Klagsbrun, M., and D' Amore, P. A.: Regulators of angiogenesis. Ann. Rev. Physiol. 53:217, 1991.

100. van Beuningen, H. M., van der Kraan, P. M., Arntz, O. J., et al.: *In vivo* protection against interleukin-1-induced articular cartilage damage by transforming growth fac-

tor beta 1: age related differences. Ann. Rheum. Dis. 53:593, 1994.

101. Koch, A. E., Harlow, L. A., Haines, G. K., et al.: Vascular endothelial growth factor: a cytokine modulating endothelial function in rheumatoid arthritis. J. Immunol. 152: 4149, 1994.

102. Lotz, M., Moats, T., and Villiger, C.: Leukemia inhibitory factor is expressed in cartilage and synovium and can contribute to the pathogenesis of arthritis. J. Clin. Invest. 90:88, 1992.

103. Weber, G. F., Ashkar, S., Glimcher, M. J., and Cantor, H.: Receptor-ligand interaction between CD44 and osteopontin (Eta-1). Science 271:509, 1996.

104. Koch, A. E., Kunkel, S. L., Burrows, J. C., et al.: Synovial tissue macrophage as a source of the chemotactic cytokine IL-8. J. Immunol. 147:2187, 1991.

105. Rathanaswami, P., Hachicha, M., Wong, W. L., et al.: Synergistic effect of interleukin-1β and tumor necrosis factor α on interleukin-8 gene expression in synovial fibroblasts. Arthritis Rheum. 36:1295, 1993.

106. Koch, A. E., Polverini, P. J., Kunkel, S. L., et al.: Interleukin-8 as a macrophage-derived mediator of angiogenesis. Science 258:1798, 1992.

107. Seitz, M., Dewald, B., Gerber, N., et al.: Enhanced production of neutrophil-activating peptide-1/interleukin-8 in rheumatoid arthritis. J. Clin. Invest. 87:463, 1991.

108. Koch, A. E., Kunkel, S. L., Harlow, L. A., et al.: Epithelial neutrophil activating peptide-78: a novel chemotactic cytokine for neutrophils in arthritis. J. Clin. Invest. 94: 1012, 1994.

109. Castor, C. W., Andrews, P. C., Swartz, R. D., et al.: The origin, variety, distribution, and biologic fat of CTAP-III isoforms: characteristics in patients with rheumatic, renal, and arterial disease. Arthritis Rheum. 36:1142, 1993.

110. Villiger, P. M., Terkeltaub, R., and Lotz, M.: Production of monocyte chemoattractant protein-1 by inflamed synovial tissue and cultured synoviocytes. J. Immunol. 149:722, 1992.

111. Akahoshi, T., Wada, C., Endo, H., et al.: Expression of monocyte chemotactic and activating factor in rheumatoid arthritis. Arthritis Rheum. 36:762, 1993.

112. Koch, A. E., Kunkel, S. L., Harlow, L. A., et al.: Macrophage inflammatory protein-1a: a novel chemotactic cytokine for macrophages in rheumatoid arthritis. J. Clin. Invest. 93:921, 1994.

9

Rheumatoid Synovium: Complex, and More Than the Sum of Its Parts

Being in the operating room during a synovectomy of a boggy knee joint of a rheumatoid patient is the best way to appreciate this tissue. One is struck first by its convoluted layers and fronds (Fig. 9–1). The color is café au lait with a tinge of orange, streaked occasionally with bright red dilated venules. Occasionally, particularly at the tips of fronds, white and atrophic patches are indications of infarction and subsequent fibrin deposition where trauma and hemorrhage have occurred. The texture is soft and pliable. Unlike a tumor, it cuts easily as would a raw salmon fillet. One feels no grittiness as when tumors are cut, and it is not friable.

Grossly, there is a clear demarcation at various depths between the soft tan tissue and the tough white collagenous subsynovial tissue and capsule. If the surgery is performed before major damage is done, there is a notable localization of erosions at the periphery of the cartilage, where synovium inserts just at the junction of cartilage and bone (Fig. 9–2). Vascular tissue with elements of gray and white amid the tan adheres to and can be seen to invade this area.

In more advanced disease, luxurious tan synovium still is present in recesses of the joint, but in areas where cartilage is being destroyed on the articular surface, the invading pannus is rarely thicker than 1 mm on the surface, while probing extensions of it dig deeper in.

In end-stage disease, the proliferative rich fronds have often become thin and white. Subchondral bone—sometimes marrow—can be seen where the cartilage has been completely destroyed.

The histology of the tan, velvety fronds varies from one area to another, but there are commonalities in almost every section. These include:

1. A definite lining layer of cuboid/columnar cells rich in cytoplasm that is 2 to 10 cell layers thick. Considering that there is no formal basement membrane between these mesenchymal lining cells and underlying mesenchymal stromal cells and lymphocytes, this "layer" is remarkably demarcated from the underlying tissue.

2. A network of capillaries and venules, often dilated, and lined by tall endothelium. These vessels enrich the sublining layers.

3. Foci of lymphocytes of variable density are found around most of the small blood vessels. Some foci are diffuse and not in a pseudofollicular formation. In other areas the volume and organization of lymphocytes may resemble, microscopically, a typical lymphoid follicle. Plasma cells appear as well.

4. Plump macrophages are found diffusely throughout the sublining layers. Frequently, these cells have phagocytosed particulate material or hemosiderin.

5. Neutrophils are rarely seen in these synovial fronds.

It is important to recognize that this classical appearance of the rheumatoid synovial fronds is different from the histology of the invasive front, where cartilage and bone is being destroyed. Here, lymphocytes are rare. Cells that are not polarized but have stellate extensions of cytoplasm penetrate cartilage, with several-cubic-micron areas of virtually no matrix surrounding each cell where collagen and proteoglycans have been degraded. Capillaries do not accompany the cells leading the invasive pannus. The network of blood vessels usually begins 10 to 50 μ from the invasive edge. The implications of this histopathology are discussed in Chapter 11.

This tissue, the proliferative and heterogeneous mass described, has the capacity to erode bone and destroy cartilage and tendons much like a localized malignancy. This was first demonstrated 25 years ago by culturing rheumatoid synovium on sterile, inverted, mouse gut segments in a highly enriched culture medium[1] (see Fig. 2 in the Introduction).

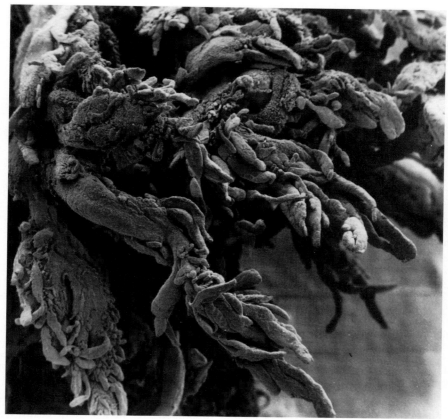

FIGURE 9–1. Low-power scanning electron micrograph of proliferative villi in moderately advanced rheumatoid synovium. The fine irregularity of the surface, barely visible, is the synovial lining cell layer. ($\times 160$) (Courtesy of Gilbert Faure, Vandoeuvre, France.)

The rheumatoid tissue invaded and destroyed gut mucosa and collagenous serosa as rapidly as did specimens from very invasive human cancers.

The analogies between rheumatoid synovial tissue and cancer do not end with these observations. It was found that dissociated rheumatoid synovial cells survived and coalesced into organized, vascularized nodules when implanted into nude mice.[2] More recently, two studies dealing with proto-oncogenes within rheumatoid synovial cells suggest that they have the phenotype of transformed cells. It was demonstrated that c-*fos* and c-*jun* products have a role in activating translation of mRNA for metalloproteases generated by rheumatoid synovial cells in culture,[3] and both Ras and Myc proteins have been localized by immunofluorescence studies in proliferating synovial lining cells and in those cells attached to cartilage and bone at the sites of joint destruction in rheumatoid patients.[4] These oncoproteins have been linked to altered cell proliferation and/or differentiation.[5]

There are different ways of approaching the rela-

tionship of histopathology to pathogenic function in rheumatoid synovium, ranging from focus on the gross characteristics of the tissue to the biology of individual cells. However, it is important to keep in mind that the principal distinguishing characteristic of rheumatoid synovium is the heterogeneity of its cellular composition. We know now that there are multiple communications among the macrophages, synovial fibroblasts, lymphocytes, mast cells, and endothelial cells in this tissue through the pathways made by cytokines.

Separating out one species of cell from the others takes it from the network of cross-talk essential for its activity in vivo. A classical example of this occurred in the late 1960s and early 1970s. It was known that, in organ culture, bits of rheumatoid synovial tissue released collagenase into the culture medium. However, when fibroblasts growing out from the synovium were subcultured, no collagenase was present in medium of the passaged cells. It was only when the cells of fresh rheumatoid synovium were dissociated and plated en masse that

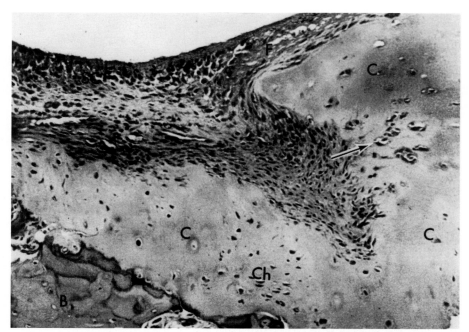

FIGURE 9–2. Photomicrograph showing the initial process of cartilage (C) destruction in rheumatoid arthritis. The mesenchymal cells proliferate and penetrate the lateral borders of articular cartilage near the chondral-bone (B) interface. Chondrocytes (Ch) are activated as well and tend to proliferate within lacunae as well as to release proteases into the surrounding matrix. The arrow indicates the direction of the synovial invasion into the cartilage. (Courtesy of Kingsley Mills.)

collagenase could be found in these primary cultures. We know now that the synovial fibroblasts needed cytokines (e.g., IL-1) produced by macrophages to express measurable amounts of this degradative enzyme.

With the caveat accepted that it is impossible to understand the whole of rheumatoid synovium well simply by study of its individual parts (i.e., cell types), let us consider it from several different perspectives.

GROSS PATTERNS OF SYNOVIAL INVOLVEMENT IN RHEUMATOID ARTHRITIS AND THEIR RELATIONSHIP TO JOINT DESTRUCTION

Double-contrast arthrography has been used to classify patterns of synovial proliferation in rheumatoid knee joints.[6,7] These patterns in turn revealed different patterns of synovial distribution within affected joints, and these have been correlated with the extent of destruction.

Panarticular disease: All surfaces of the joint space show proliferative tissue, including the suprapatellar pouch. Joint destruction is rapid and severe in these patients.

Suprapatellar pouch—isolated disease: If synovitis is confined to the suprapatellar pouch, cartilage destruction is rare.

Posterior pouch/recess—isolated disease: Same as suprapatellar pouch disease: cartilage erosion is rare.

Destroyed joints: In joints in which the cartilage is completely destroyed, there is little evidence of proliferative synovitis in any compartment of the joint.

These observations match those reported by orthopedic surgeons in rheumatoid patients followed after total joint replacement: If all residual cartilage is removed, that joint does not participate in flares of synovitis affecting other joints, even when ample amounts of synovium have been left in situ at surgery.

CORRELATION OF ARTHROSCOPY AND RADIOGRAPHS

Use of arthroscopy has enabled rheumatologists and orthopedic surgeons to directly examine the synovium and to correlate the appearance of the tissue and cartilage destruction in the knee[8] with radiographic changes. It has been possible to stage the progression of disease in this manner.

Stage I. Visible evidence of pathology is seen in the synovium; although villous fronds are apparent, there is no invasion of meniscal or articular cartilage.

Stage II. Proliferative synovium encroaches on cartilage surfaces, and erosions of meniscal and articular cartilage at the periphery are apparent. No narrowing of the joint space or erosions are apparent on radiographic examination. Because conventional radiographs cannot detect the early synovial invasion of cartilage, physicians often underestimate the progression of disease at this stage.

Stage III. Full-thickness craters lined with proliferative synovial tissue are found. Free-floating debris and meniscal tears and erosions are prominent. Radiographic appearance of the apparent joint space is normal in 75 percent of patients at this stage.

Stage IV. Only when articular cartilage is irreversibly damaged and many meniscal cartilages almost completely dissolved are radiographic changes significant.

Lessons from these broad morphologic studies are that radiographic changes lag much behind the formation of a progressively invasive synovitis, and that the worst prognosis is for those with pan-articular disease (Fig. 9–3).

HISTOPATHOLOGIC ANALYSIS OF DEFINITE RHEUMATOID SYNOVIUM

Synovial sampling using closed-needle biopsy has provided tissue from early disease in rheumatoid arthritis. Certain correlations have been made between histopathology found in samples from untreated patients and current status and later outcome:

1. Endothelial cell "tallness," an index of activated cells expressing numerous adhesion molecules, is greater in patients with active disease who have not yet received second-line therapy.[9]

2. In patients presenting with relatively mild disease, there is a correlation of synovial lining cell thickness with outcome at 1 year measured by a composite index of disease activity.[10] At 3 years a correlation between activity and both the initial synovial lining layer thickness and T-cell infiltration exists.

In a 1-year uncontrolled, prospective study of 12 active rheumatoid patients, synovial biopsies at time 0 were correlated with radiographic progression 1 year later; there was a positive correlation between the number of infiltrating synovial tissue macrophages and radiologic deterioration.[11] It is likely that cytokines produced by these macrophages are the driving force upon the synovial lining cells to produce metalloproteases that can destroy the joints. In another prospective study, both

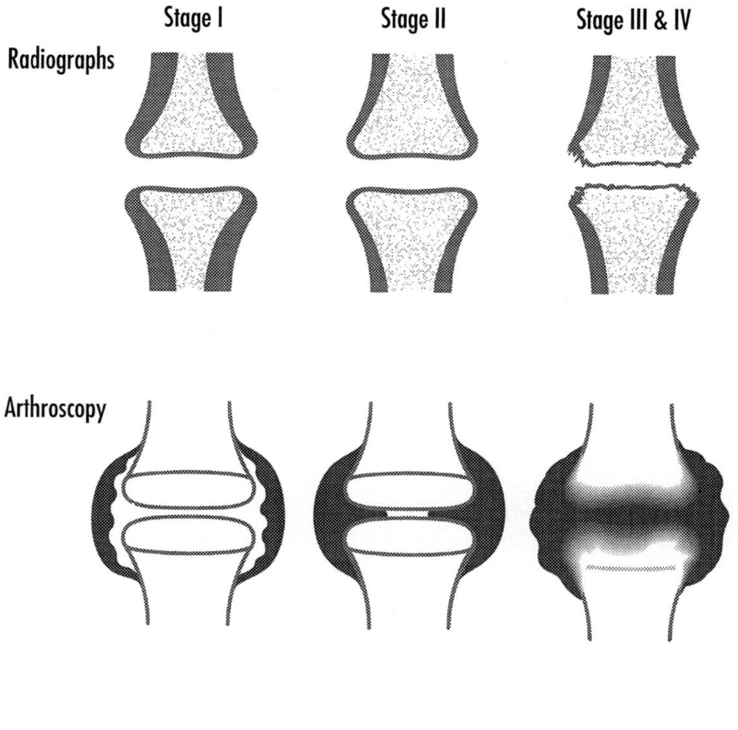

FIGURE 9–3. Radiographic changes of joint space narrowing and erosions appear at a time significantly *after* proliferative synovium begins encroachment upon cartilage and depletion of proteoglycans occurs. (From Harris, E. D. Jr.: A collagenolytic system produced by primary cultures of rheumatoid nodule tissue. J. Clin. Invest. 51:2973, 1972. Used by copyright permission of The Rockefeller University Press, 1972.)

the synovial lining cell layer depth and the $CD14^+$ macrophage infiltrate in the sublining layers correlated with the radiologic progression of the disease.[12]

Although there are, as expected, wide variations among samples taken from different patients using criteria such as synovial hyperplasia, fibrosis, proliferation of blood vessels, lymphocyte infiltrate, and presence or absence of focal infiltrates, no such variation exists in multiple biopsies of the same joint.[13] This validates use of sequential biopsies of the same individual for staging disease in the synovium.

3. An assumption that cell density within rheumatoid synovium is greater than that in noninflammatory synovitis has been made by most investigators, but has been proved by morphometric comparisons only recently[14] (Fig. 9–4).

4. Ultrastructural analysis of the synovial lining layers in established rheumatoid arthritis shows a marked increase in the numbers of type B synovial fibroblast-like cells that have a cellular organelle system directed at synthesis, as opposed to phagocytosis.

These data support the belief that it is the heterogeneity of cell types—activated endothelium, proliferating T cells, macrophages, synovial lining cells—and the communications among them amplifying inflammation that lead to destroyed joints in rheumatoid arthritis.

Sequence of Development of Rheumatoid Synovitis—From Microns to Centimeters Thick

Surface Morphology

Viewed with a dissecting microscope or scanning electron microscope, the synovial surface early in development is rippled but has few folds and no villous fronds. As the synovitis matures, the surface area appears to increase almost exponentially, compared with a simple volume measurement. This happens by formation of redundant and overlapping villi, a process probably dictated by a need for efficient arborization of blood supply. The ripples evolve into folds, and the folds into flaps of redundant tissue, and the flaps eventually develop into villous fronds. Within each villous structure there are microvilli. Individual cells can be visualized by scanning electron microscopy, and many of these have cellular processes extending out into the synovial fluid (Fig. 9–5).

Histology of Early Synovitis—Mononuclear Cells and Synoviocytes

Synovial samples from early synovitis are difficult to find. The best examples come from needle biopsies of knee joints after just a few weeks of symptoms.[15] The principal point gained from these

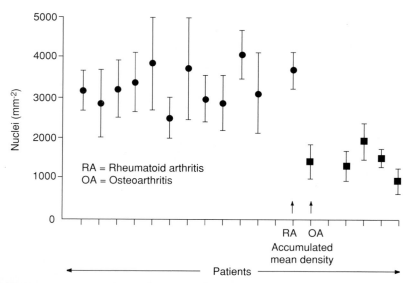

FIGURE 9–4. Mean nuclear density ($\times 10^3$ nuclei/mm^2) and 95 per cent confidence interval (vertical bars) of accumulated and individual representative samples taken from the upper synovial region of osteoarthritic and rheumatoid arthritic synovium. (From Kennedy, T. D., Plater-Zyberk, C., Partridge, T. A., et al.: Morphometric comparison of synovium from patients with osteoarthritis and rheumatoid arthritis. J. Clin. Pathol. 41:847, 1988. Used by permission. Copyright 1988 by the BMJ Publishing Group.)

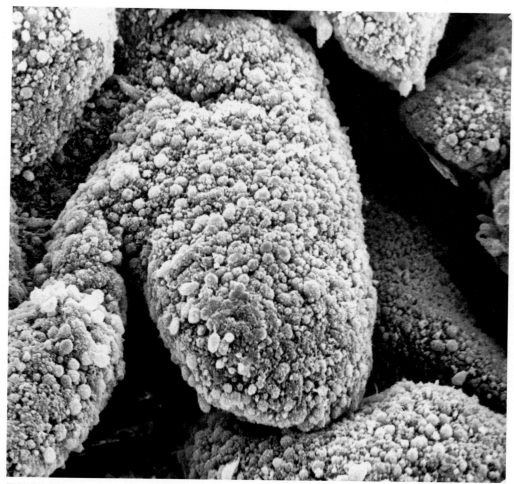

FIGURE 9–5. The well-formed ''mitten-like'' synovial villi are evident in this scanning electron microscopic view of rheumatoid synovium. There is marked variation in the size of synovial cells, seen projecting as confluent papules from the surface. (×300) (Courtesy of Gilbert Faure, Vandoeuvre, France.)

analyses is that a proliferation of macrophages and synovial lining cells dominates early rheumatoid synovitis. As determined by expression of mRNA for metalloproteases, these cells are activated. It is later that aggregates of lymphocytes appear.

Beginning shortly after rheumatoid arthritis begins, almost antedating symptoms, edema and a proliferation of synoviocytes is observed. Scattered lymphocytes are found, but they are not congregated in follicles. Neutrophils are rarely seen as they quickly traverse the area between synovial vasculature and their destination, the joint fluid.[10] Subintimal mononuclear cells are more numerous than lymphocytes.[16] New blood vessels proliferate along with this nonspecific synovitis.[17] The endothelial cells become full, deep, and tall, consistent with their activated state.

After these changes appear, synovial lining cells proliferate even more, as do cells in the sublining areas. Mingled among them are macrophages that have been attracted from the bone marrow. Of all factors tested that can stimulate synoviocyte proliferation, including aFGF, bFGF, TGFβ, IL-1α, TNFα, PDGF, and IFNγ, it was PDGF—released by activated macrophages—that was clearly the most potent stimulant of long-term growth of human synoviocytes.[18] The lining cells are morphologically very distinct from sublining cells of the same apparent mesenchymal lineage, yet there is no basement membrane separating them. This feature is reflected in their function (Fig. 9–6).

As the volume of cells increases in the synovium, the matrix structural proteins (e.g., collagen) of the subsynovial layers and joint capsule begin to accumulate. Mast cells, multinucleate giant cells, and hemosiderin-laden macrophages accumulate along

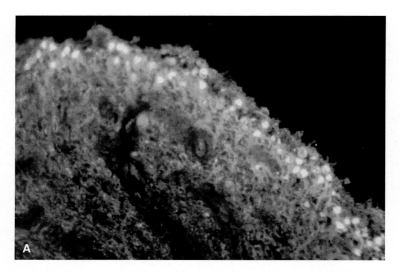

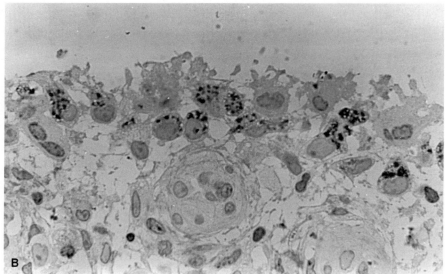

FIGURE 9–6. *A,* This section of a rheumatoid synovial villus identifies cells by immunohistochemistry that are synthesizing matrix metalloprotease 3 (stromelysin). If the sample had been stained for collagenase, hyaluronan, type VI collagen, or inflammatory cytokines, the same pattern would appear. The *reasons why* it is the cells fronting on the synovial fluid, and not sublining cells, that produce so much of these proteases, cytokines, and matrix components is not known. (Immunohistochemical photomicrograph courtesy of Yasunori Okada.) *B,* A 1-μm epon-embedded section of rheumatoid synovium stained with toluidine blue and with antibody to stromelysin. The same localization to the synovial lining cells is seen as is evident in *A.*

with the foci of lymphocytes, proliferating synovial lining cells, and new blood vessels. The mature active synovitis is a heterogeneous mixture of mesenchymal and marrow-derived cells. One cell type—epithelium—is missing.

Before discussion of the pathology at the invasive front where synovial tissue is actively degrading bone and cartilage, it is relevant to focus on the individual cell types in the fully developed synovium and the proteins that they express.

CELLS AND MATRIX OF THE NORMAL AND RHEUMATOID SYNOVIUM: THE LINING LAYER, SUBLINING CELLS, IMMUNOCYTES, AND SPECIAL CELLS

The **normal synovial lining**, a few cells in depth, is a mixture of cell types: type A cells (macrophage-like), which have prominent vacuoles, vesicles, and filopodia but only a poorly developed endoplasmic reticulum; and type B cells (fibroblast-like), which have a well-developed rough endoplasmic reticulum and few vesicles and vacuoles or cell processes, and which appear to be involved in synthesis of gene products for secretion from the cell (see Fig. 1–14 in Chapter 1).

Studies using a genetic "tracer"—leukocyte common antigen (LCA), expressed by all cells derived from the hematopoietic stem cell—confirm the impression inferred from histomorphology that only 10 per cent of the lining cells are derived from the marrow, and the remaining 90 per cent are specialized fibroblasts derived from the mesenchyme.[19]

The number of cells within **rheumatoid synovium** is enormously increased over normal, and immunocytes are a significant component of the increased cellularity. However, whether cells other than immunocytes and easily recognizable mast cells and endothelial cells are macrophages that have transmigrated from extrasynovial sites, or whether they are resident mesenchymal cells (synovial fibroblasts) that have multiplied within the tissue, is still contested.

An equation represents cellularity in rheumatoid synovium:

Number of cells in synovium

$$= \left(\begin{array}{c} \text{Resident cell} \\ \text{proliferation} \end{array} + \begin{array}{c} \text{Transmigrating} \\ \text{cells} \end{array} \right)$$

$$- \left(\begin{array}{c} \text{Cell death by apoptosis} \\ \text{or killing} \end{array} + \begin{array}{c} \text{Transmigration} \\ \text{out of the joint} \end{array} \right)$$

On the *minus* side of the equation, cells in synovium die from loss of blood supply, infarction, trauma, cell-mediated cytotoxicity, complement-mediated death, and apoptosis. Utilizing agarose gel electrophoresis of DNA to identify patterns characteristic for apoptosis, there were significant numbers of apoptotic cells in the synovial lining.[20] Those programmed for cell death were primarily macrophages and fibroblasts. T cells in lymphoid aggregates in sublining areas express large amounts of *bcl-2* and are spared from apoptosis (see Chapter 6). Macrophage and fibroblast production of Fas, the possible receptor that could induce apoptosis when linked with Fas ligand, was demonstrated. There is no evidence that significant numbers of cells leave the joint by the way they came in to survive in the circulation.

The *plus* side of the equation, however, is of special interest, because it could give leads to ways physicians could interfere with development of this invasive tissue. Those who hold to the tenet that

macrophages from extrasynovial sources make up most of the population of other-than-immunocytes point to the following pieces of evidence[21]:

1. During routine histologic examination of rheumatoid synovium, mitoses are rarely observed; when tritiated thymidine is used to label dividing cells, only 4 per cent of cells take up this isotope.[22] In studies using a monoclonal antibody that is reported to recognize dividing cells, the number of labeled cells is less than 1:2,000.

2. In studies using monoclonal antibodies that recognize mononuclear phagocytes derived from marrow, most cells in the synovial lining other than lymphocytes bind these antibodies.[23,24] Many cells in the rheumatoid synovium appear to express "activation" antigens common to macrophages.[25] LCA is found on many more rheumatoid synovial lining cells than in normal synovium.[19] The question is whether this is proof that these cells are macrophages, or whether highly activated fibroblasts could express the same surface antigens. In another example of the fact that there is questionable specificity of cell markers, the "macrophage-specific" surface molecule, CD68, has been shown to be expressed as well by synovial fibroblasts in rheumatoid arthritis.[26]

3. Using a variety of culture conditions and passage numbers, monoclonal antibodies, and immunocytochemistry, one laboratory has demonstrated that synovial lining cells coexpress fibroblast (prolyl hydroxylase) and macrophage markers (CD68) (El-Gabalawy et al., Abstract 24), supporting the concept that the distinction between synovial A and B cells may reflect different differentiation states of the same cell line.

In contrast, many other data support the concept that the synovial cells that are not immunocytes resemble much more the phenotype of activated synovial fibroblasts than of immigrant macrophages:

1. Using the same data that emphasize the low mitotic rate of cells in the synovium, it was demonstrated that there are four- to fivefold more cells that take up tritiated thymidine in rheumatoid arthritis than in "normal" synovium.[22] This has been recently confirmed.[27] Recombinant human cytokines (e.g., IL-1β, TNFα) stimulate RNA synthesis of human synovial fibroblast-like cells.[28] It has been shown that neutrophils are rarely seen moving through thick synovium to the joint space during one instant in time represented by a biopsy, yet up to 1 billion neutrophils may enter a 30-ml synovial effusion containing 25,000 cells/mm^3 each day.[29] Similarly, if apoptosis and cell killing are even fractionally less in rheumatoid synovium than is cell

proliferation—as expressed in the equation presented earlier—cell volume within the soft tissue of the joint will increase steadily.

2. Early-passage synoviocytes from rheumatoid joints grow in vitro under anchorage-independent conditions (i.e., they form colonies in soft agar).[30] This is a characteristic of transformed cells that correlates closely with potential for in vivo tumorigenicity. These cells have a fibroblast, not macrophage, phenotype. It is a reasonable hypothesis that these synovial cells, "transformed" by intense cytokine stimulation, could express multiple different cell membrane markers, even those usually expressed on macrophages.

Using rheumatoid synovial cells dissociated from matrix and assayed for phenotypic expression of cell surface markers, three classes of cells have been recognized[31]:

Type I: macrophage-like cells with DR antigens, Fc receptors, monocyte lineage differentiation antigens, and a capability for phagocytosis

Type II: nonphagocytic cells that have DR antigens but lack Fc receptors and expresses neither monocyte nor fibroblast antigens

Type III: fibroblast-like cells without phagocytic activity, DR antigens, or monocyte markers

These different types have been cloned successfully[32]; types I and II grow slowly, and type III cells have a 1- to 2-day doubling time typical of fibroblasts. When incubated with PGE_2, type III cells take on a phenotype of a stellate appearance with long, thin cell processes, not unlike that observed as synovial cells invade cartilage.[33] Cells with the stellate phenotype also produce significant quantities of IL-1.[32]

In cultures of enzymatically dissociated rheumatoid tissue, these stellate cells are always found. As shown in Figure 9–7, they have contracted cytoplasm around the nucleus, radial cytoplasmic extensions with knobby inclusions, and terminal adherent pseudopodia. In Chapter 11, the association of these unusual cells with matrix metalloproteases is demonstrated. They represent activated cells, are found in psoriatic arthritis and aggressive juvenile arthritis, and are present in numbers roughly proportional to the degree of inflammoproliferative activity of the synovium.

The data suggest that the nonimmune cells of the synovial lining are a mixture of highly activated macrophages that have transmigrated from the marrow, and proliferating resident fibroblast-like cells that have a slow but steady doubling rate and become—when activa- **ted—the aggressive metalloprotease-producing cell of invasive synovitis.**

A Special Phenotype: Superficial Synovial Lining Cells

The name "superficial synovial lining (or intimal) cells" refers specifically to those cells separating synovial fluid from subsynovial lining cells. On the usual hematoxylin and eosin stains of tissue, they are plump and tall, with a faint blue tinge and many thin cell processes (Fig. 9–8). Although, as mentioned earlier, they are mesenchymal in origin and derived from the same cells as those in the sublining areas, they appear to have a highly differentiated function (see the box on page 136).

These lining cells, unlike underlying fibroblasts in the synovial tissue, have a high content of uridine diphosphoglucose dehydrogenase (UDPGD).[36] This enzyme synthesizes uridine diphosphate (UDP)-glucuronate, which is co-polymerized with UDP-N-acetylglucosamine to form hyaluronan. When using antibodies against prolyl hydroxylase, an enzyme specific for collagen synthesis, many of these cells are double-labeled. Although many sublining fibroblasts have abundant prolyl hydroxylase, very few expressed UDPGD. Intimal cells produce chondroitin 4- and 6-sulfate, essential GAGs for aggrecan.[37] Thus, although the synovial phenotype in this disease is a destructive one, these lining cells can express matrix and structural elements as well (Fig. 9–9).

A marker for lysosomes, anti-CD68, labels macrophage-like cells in the intimal layer that did not stain for cells producing enzymes involved in connective tissue biosynthesis, supporting the concept that the intimal lining, as well as mixtures of cells from the entire synovial villi, have a mixture of both activated fibroblasts and macrophages.[36] About 60 per cent of the lining cells, but very few stromal cells in the sublining layers, stain positively for metalloproteases, the enzymes that degrade proteoglycans and collagen.[38] Thus these lining cells synthesize and release both matrix components and the enzymes that degrade them. Because the proteases are produced as latent proforms, this is possible without immediate danger to newly synthesized collagen or proteoglycans (see Fig. 9–6).

The extensive cytoplasmic extensions of synovial lining cells with the "stellate" phenotype has been emphasized. In addition, scanning electron micrograph images suggest that cytoplasmic bridges may link synovial lining cells that are otherwise independent of each other (Fig. 9–10).

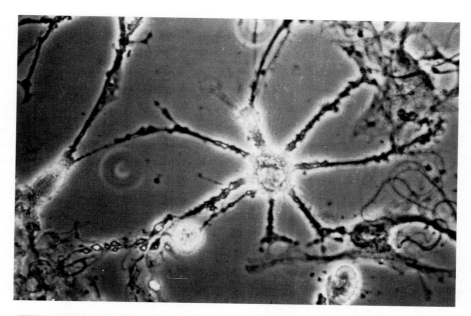

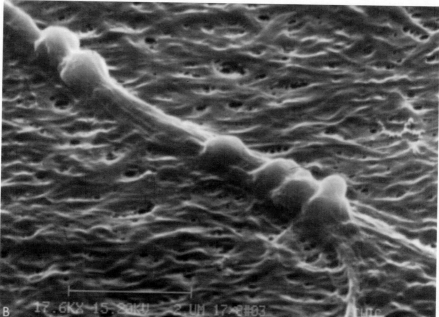

FIGURE 9–7. Various views of stellate cells from rheumatoid synovium. These cells are derived from fragments of rheumatoid synovium dissociated by brief exposure to bacterial collagenase and trypsin, and plated on either plastic (*A*) and incubated in serum-enriched culture medium. Up to 40 per cent of adherent cells from active rheumatoid synovitis have this stellate appearance. Photomicrograph *A* is taken in phase contrast. *B*, Scanning electron microscopic view. In addition to the knobbly expanded areas in this high-power ($\times 17,600$) view, thin filaments running under the plasma membrane are visible, as is the flat terminal portion (at right) of the long cell process adherent to the collagen gel. (*B* from Harris, E. D. Jr.: Etiology and pathogenesis of rheumatoid arthritis. *In* Kelley, W. N., Harris, E. D. Jr., Ruddy, S., and Sledge, C. B. [eds.]: Textbook of Rheumatology, 4th ed., Vol. 1. Philadelphia, W. B. Saunders, 1993, pp. 833–873. Used by permission.)

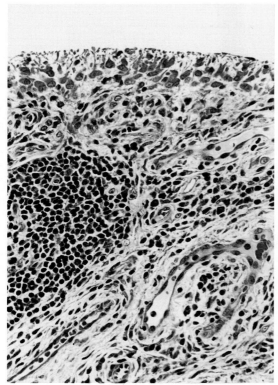

FIGURE 9–8. Light photomicrograph of rheumatoid synovial tissue showing hyperplastic synovial lining cells and lymphocyte aggregations in the sublining cell layer. (Hematoxylin and eosin stain; ×165) (Courtesy of Dr. Yasunori Okada.)

Activation of the Synovial Lining Cell

As is mentioned often in this book, there are many suggestions that the synovial lining cells are transformed, much as are cancer cells, yet are distinguished from malignancy in their inability to metastasize while expressing a powerful capability to invade connective tissue locally. Data to support the concept that these cells have a ''transformed phenotype'' include finding protein or mRNA of proto-oncogenes c-*fos, jun-B, ras,* and c-*myc* in synovial cells.[4,39] These genes are induced by many stimuli but must be regarded as indicators of cellular activation. The majority of the activated cells appear to be of fibroblast, not macrophage, lineage.[40] Although not malignant, the lingering unanswered question is: Are these activated synovial cells autonomous in their capability of producing excessive proteases and cytokines, thereby having an unregulated capacity to degrade cartilage, tendons, and bone (Fig. 9–11)?

In an interesting study that confirmed the role of c-*fos* and c-*jun* as constituitive signal transducers

---

Transcription Factor Activation in the Rheumatoid Synovial Lining Cell

The cascade of events that leads to expression by synovial lining cells of cytokines and proteases begins by activation of transcription factors such as NF-κB and activator protein 1 (AP-1). NF-κB enhances gene expression of M-CSF, G-CSF, GM-CSF, VCAM-1, E-selectin, TNFα, IL-1β, IL-6, IL-8, IL-2, MCP-1, and nitric oxide synthase. Fos and Jun are the subunits of AP-1, which has a major role in inducing biosynthesis of the metalloproteases that destroy cartilage, tendons, and bone in this disease.

In nonstimulated cells, NF-κB is inactive and in the cytosol of cells. When activated, it translocates to cell nuclei and binds to DNA. Consistent with data on the phenotype of synovial lining cells, NF-κB was found in nuclei of subsynovial endothelial cells and in CD14+ (macrophage-like) lining cells, whereas Jun/Fos was seen in CD14− type B fibroblasts.[34,35]

Prostaglandins
Cytokines (IL-6, IL-1)
Types I, III, IV, V, VI collagens
Metalloproteases
Chondroitin 4 and 6 sulfate
Hyaluronan

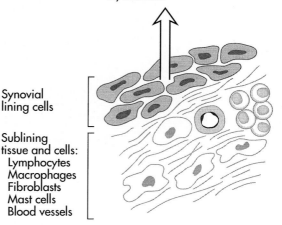

Synovial lining cells

Sublining tissue and cells:
Lymphocytes
Macrophages
Fibroblasts
Mast cells
Blood vessels

FIGURE 9–9. Sketch illustrating the quantitative and qualitative differences between synovial lining cells and the subsynovium. The lining cells are phenotypically characterized as activated cells producing many products for export. Cytokines and other molecules enter the joint space as well as remaining in the synovium.

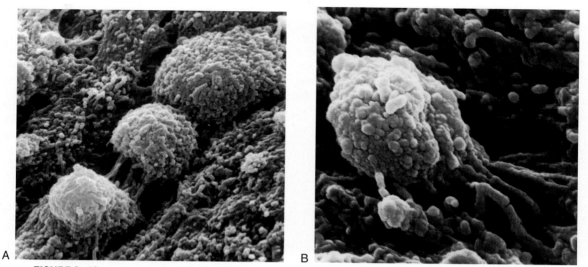

FIGURE 9–10. Scanning electron micrographs of the synovial lining surface illustrating cytoplasmic extensions that may contact other cells and possibly allow sharing of information/activation stimuli among these cells. (*A*, ×4800; *B*, ×12,000) (Courtesy of Gilbert Faure, Vandoeuvre, France.)

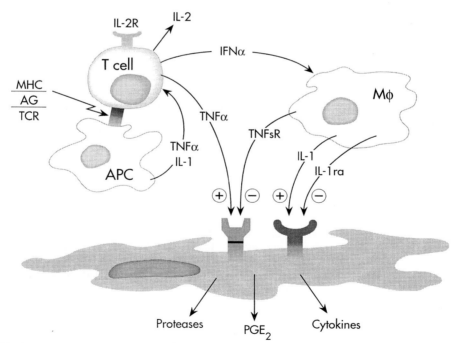

FIGURE 9–11. The balance between stimulation and down-regulation of synovial lining cells. Only two activators of synovial cells are sketched in here: TNFα and IL-1. Both are prime candidates for activation of the synovial lining cells to produce proteases (metalloproteases [e.g., collagenases, stromelysin]), protease inhibitors (TIMP), prostaglandins and leukotrienes, and other cytokines. Both TNFα and IL-1 have endogenous inhibitors (IL-1ra and soluble TNFR [TNFR]) that have been characterized. It is possible that, with time and more investigation, specific endogenous inhibitors of other cytokines will be identified as well. This schema implies appropriately that both activated T cells and macrophages (Mπ) drive the proliferation and activation of the synovial cells. Many of the synovial lining cells (probably type B) become dendritic cells following activation.

in rheumatoid synovial tissues, it was demonstrated that there was a 30-fold decrease (compared with control specimens) of the potential metastasis suppressor gene *nm23-H1* in 90 per cent of rheumatoid synovial tissues[41] and a activation of the *ets-2* nuclear oncogene in one third of rheumatoid tissues. Expression of these gene products may lead to the "locally malignant" phenotype of aggressive rheumatoid arthritis.

Monocyte-Macrophages: Cells of Central Importance in Driving Proliferation in Rheumatoid Synovitis

Why are monocytes attracted to joints early in rheumatoid arthritis, and how are they activated? It is likely that monocytes are recruited in response to chemotactic agents produced at the foci of inflammation in response to various cytokines upon resident cells. One monocyte-macrophage chemoattractant present in rheumatoid synovitis is **monocyte chemotactic and activating factor** (MCAF) a peptide of 76 amino acids.[42] IL-1 and TNFα are among the cytokines that induce synthesis and release of MCAF from type B synovial fibroblasts and synovial lining cells. High levels of MCAF have been measured in synovial fluid of rheumatoid patients. Another cytokine, **MIP-1α**, not only is a chemoattractant for macrophages but is produced by them, as well as by synovial lining cells of rheumatoid synovium.[43] It has structural homologies with MCAF; both are members of the chemokine gene superfamily (see Chapter 8). MIP-1α has been found to do more than attract macrophages; it is an endogenous pyrogen with a different mechanism of action from IL-1, it regulates stem cell proliferation, and it is chemotactic for T lymphocytes. Acting on the cell that produces it, MIP-1α stimulates macrophage production of IL-1α, TNFα, and IL-6. TGFB, PDGF, and GM-CSF also have the capacity to attract macrophages into the joint.

It is probable that many monocytes become activated by exposure to substances such as GM-CSF, IFNγ, IL-1, TNFα, and neuropeptides substance P and substance K[44] almost as soon as, if not before, they enter the synovium. MCAF, induced to form by IL-1, is a potent activator as well. A qualitative difference between the response of resting monocytes (CD14$^-$) from bone marrow of rheumatoid and osteoarthritis patients has been demonstrated.[45] Spontaneous generation of CD14$^+$ from CD14$^-$ cells and HLA-DR was seen in samples from rheumatoid patients, but not from controls. The stimulus

for this transition is not known, but appears to be a factor(s) other than GM-CSF.

Once activated, macrophages synthesize and release a phenomenally broad spectrum of cytokines (e.g., IL-1, IL-6, IL-8, TGFβ, TNFα), growth factors (colony stimulating factors G-CSF and GM-CSF), and enzymes (collagenase, stromelysin, elastase, gelatinase). They generate prostaglandins and activate generation of oxygen-derived free radicals. Their presence almost guarantees enhancement and perpetuation of the proliferative synovitis in rheumatoid arthritis.[46]

Phenotype of the Immunocytes in the Subintimal Layers of Rheumatoid Synovitis

Immunocytes, which are not present in the lining layers and are found clustered principally around small vessels in the subintima, are a driving force of the immune response that takes place in synovium. As reviewed in Chapter 5, their most striking aspect is their activated state. One careful set of data using flow cytometry summarizes their phenotypes.[47] Compared with lymphocytes from peripheral blood of both normal persons and rheumatoid patients, synovial tissue lymphocytes from rheumatoid patients have the same percentages ($\pm$47 per cent) of CD3$^+$ and CD4$^+$ cells, but fewer CD8$^+$ cells (22 per cent compared with 30 to 35 per cent in peripheral blood).

Applying immunohistology and a cell-specific, nonradioactive in situ hybridization technique for IL-2 mRNA in synovial specimens from inflammatory arthritis, transcripts of mRNA—but no expressed IL-2 protein—are found in rheumatoid synovium. In contrast, IL-2 is produced by spondyloarthritic and psoriatic synovium,[48] suggesting that there may be a difference in central immunoregulatory activity in patients with different types of inflammatory synovitis. One difference may be that the lymphocytes in rheumatoid tissue are terminally differentiated CD45RB^{dim} cells that produce little IL-2 or IFNγ. Also, although cells from peripheral blood and synovium of rheumatoid patients have a higher expression of HLA-DR, relatively few cells from control patients or rheumatoid blood or synovium express IL-2 receptors[47] or as much mRNA for IL-3 as do cells from noninflammatory synovitis.[49]

In contrast, there is a large increase in the expression of the adhesion antigens LFA-1 and very late antigen 1 (VLA-1) on synovial tissue lymphocytes from rheumatoid patients, compared with peripheral blood lymphocytes or cells from control patients. These adhesion molecules have a central role in lymphocyte function, helping to mediate cytotoxicity and antigen recognition by T cells, as well as helping them fix in tissues after transmigration from vessels to the synovium.[47] Separate studies have indicated that activated T cells from inflammatory synovitis bind to fibroblast-like synovial cells in culture.[50]

Cytotoxic lymphocytes are found in rheumatoid synovium as well. Using in situ hybridization techniques on synovial tissue, significant messenger RNA for both granzyme A and perforin are found. In rheumatoid arthritis, but not osteoarthritis, synovium mRNA for both of these molecules is detected in 10 to 50 per cent of lymphocytes, most of which are expressing a mature memory phenotype.[51] Both granzyme A and perforin are expressed by activated cytotoxic T lymphocytes and NK cells. Because these cells have a major antiviral function, these data support the hypothesis that there may be active retroviruses in synovium of rheumatoid patients.

As with T cells, there are in rheumatoid synovial tissues a higher percentage of differentiated B cells and plasma cells.[52] compared with peripheral blood of the same patients, consistent with the supposition that these tissues are significant sources of autoantibodies.

Phenotype of the Subintimal Cells of Rheumatoid Synovial Villi

There are many suggestions (some mentioned earlier and others discussed in Chapter 11) that the lining (intimal) cells of rheumatoid synovium "behave" neither as macrophages nor as fibroblasts, but as an activated hybrid of each. The greatest numbers of nonimmunocytes in a typical synovial villous structure are those that are distributed through the subintimal layers in proximity to lymphocytes and small blood vessels, eventually becoming continuous with the joint capsule.

The cells resembling activated fibroblasts that can be dissociated from the matrix and grown in culture have a modulated pattern of gene activation that can persist through many passages of cells.[49] Compared with cells isolated from osteoarthritic synovial tissue, the rheumatoid fibroblastoid cells express significantly higher mRNA of the following proteins and cytokines[38,49]:

- Stromelysin, the most critical of destructive metalloproteases in rheumatoid tissue
- Vimentin, the cytoskeletal fibrillar protein that

may be responsible for the stellate or dendritic morphology in these cells
- TIMP, the specific inhibitor of collagenase, stromelysin, and gelatinase
- IL-6
- IL-1
- Collagen types I, III, IV, V, and VI
- Hyaluronan
- Fibronectin
- Laminin
- Chondroitin 4-/6-sulfate, heparin sulfate, and keratan sulfate

It is interesting that, in these same studies, mRNA for the proto-oncogene c-*myc* was only weakly expressed in cell cultures from inflammatory synovitis.[49] Because c-*myc* may have a dual function of promoting apoptosis as well as driving cell proliferation,[53] its absence in these cells may enhance their proliferation in the synovium.

mRNA transcripts for both PDGF and HBGF are found to be elevated in rheumatoid synovium.[54] After cells bind either of these growth factors to their respective receptors, cellular activation occurs and proto-oncogenes such as *fos* and *myc* are expressed. Both factors impart to the synovial cells a transformed phenotype.

Other studies, using radioimmunoprecipitation and other sensitive methods that measure amounts of expressed gene products rather than mRNA levels, support these data and indicate expression of additional proteins and cytokines by rheumatoid synovial fibroblasts. There is a positive correlation between IL-1 production by organ cultures of synovium obtained at arthroscopy and erosive changes on roentgenograms.[55] βFGB, TGFβ, and GM-CSF are also produced by synovial fibroblasts from inflamed synovial tissues.[56] In a demonstration of the complexity of cytokine interaction in synovial tissues, IL-1β—although unable to stimulate synoviocyte DNA synthesis by itself—does synergize with PDGF in stimulating DNA synthesis if prostaglandin production is inhibited.[57]

Large amounts of HLA-DR are expressed on rheumatoid monocytes, but low amount of HLA-DQ.[58] Because HLA-DQ may be involved in activation of sT cells, a defect in its production could help tip the balance toward inflammation and an excessive immune response in the tissue.

The activated fibroblasts and macrophages in sublining areas of rheumatoid synovium also generate substantial numbers of cytokines (refer also to Chapter 8). IL-6 is elevated in synovial fluid and serum from rheumatoid patients as well as from patients with nonrheumatoid inflammatory synovitis.[59] IL-6, which promotes T- and B-lymphocyte growth and differentiation and acute-phase protein synthesis, is also produced by synoviocytes in culture, a phenomenon enhanced by TNFα and IL-1.[60] Rheumatoid synovial tissue in culture generates monocyte growth factors (e.g., GM-CSF) that can induce DR expression on cells.[61] The same tissue samples produce a mast cell growth factor, an interesting finding in light of the excessive numbers of those cells in rheumatoid synovium (see later). Macrophages isolated from rheumatoid synovial tissue constitutively express IL-8, the cytokine that is responsible for about half of the neutrophil chemotactic activity in rheumatoid synovial fluid.[62] Synovial fibroblasts produce very little IL-8.

Stimulated peripheral blood monocytes induce human synovial fibroblasts to produce and release plasminogen activator that has cross-reactivity with the urokinase-type enzyme. Plasminogen activator is an important mediator of processes of cell migration, tissue remodeling, and inflammation; it is likely that this expression by synovial fibroblasts is intrinsically important for progression of rheumatoid disease.[63,64]

TGFβ is produced by rheumatoid synovial cells,[65] and it is reasonable to assume that this reparative growth factor is in part responsible for the large amounts of proteoglycans and hyaluronan generated by cultures of synovial cells.[66] To focus again on the complexity of cytokine networks in synovial tissue, TGFβ1 and -β2 inhibit both anchorage-dependent and -independent synovial fibroblast growth stimulated by PDGF that is produced in significant amounts, and in parallel quantities with HBGF (precursor of aFGF), by explants of rheumatoid synovium.[67]

Although these cells in culture have the appearance of fibroblasts, not macrophages, they also have a striking capability for phagocytosis (see Fig. 9–12).

Extracellular Matrix of the Synovium: An Active Participant in the Architecture of Inflamed Synovium

It has been emphasized often in this book that there is no basement membrane in synovium. This deserves clarification. The intact basement membrane is a complex of four molecules: type IV collagen, entactin, laminin, and heparin sulfate proteoglycans. Entactin is the ''glue'' that laces these components into a formed membrane in most tissues, and it is absent in rheumatoid synovium (N. Zvaifler, personal communication). Thus, although

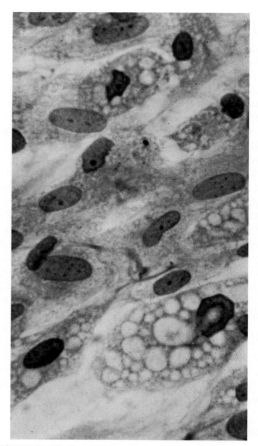

FIGURE 9–12. Synovial fibroblasts in cell culture were passage subcultured three times. Stellate cells were not visible after the first passage. The cells had the appearance in culture of fibroblasts. Sterile latex particles were added to the cultures on the fourth day of the third subculture. Coverslips were stained (hematoxylin and eosin) on the fifth day. Approximately 30 per cent of cells demonstrated significant phagocytic capability, as shown by the white spherical intracellular particles in the cells.

type IV collagen and laminin and proteoglycans are present,[68] there is no structure for a full membrane. It is likely, however, that the three molecules that are present give an anchor to the intimal cells and affect their phenotypic expression.

The distribution of collagen types in the superficial synovial lining layer is different from that in the subsynovium as well. Type VI collagen, appearing as filamentous structures with 100-nm periodicity, is not degraded by the matrix metalloproteases secreted by synovial lining cells and appears to serve as an anchoring structure for these specialized intimal cells; it is not present below the lining layer.[69] That type VI collagen chains do have cell attachment properties has been carefully demonstrated,[70] and it is probable that these molecules serve as a surrogate basement membrane for the lining cells. The fibronectin present in rheumatoid synovium has complex effects on both synovial cell proliferation and attachment.[71]

One of the most important of matrix molecules, hyaluronan, appears to have many more functions than serving to link aggrecans together in a super-molecule and serving as a soft tissue lubricant. A pericellular layer of hyaluronan surrounds synovial fibroblasts. It may protect the cells from attack by infectious agents or immune cells, and prevent dysfunctional cell-cell contact.[72] One of the isoforms of CD44, a lymphocyte homing receptor, binds hyaluronan.[73] Finally, hyaluronan has been implicated in functions of mitosis, angiogenesis, cell migration, and phagocytosis, but the extent of its role in these and other synovial processes has not yet been clarified.[74]

Adhesive Molecules on Synovial Cells

Although, as detailed earlier, there are ample quantities of matrix molecules that can attract, bind, and support growth of cells in the synovium, the intimal and subintimal cells are also involved in binding cells that immigrate into the synovium through the activated endothelium in rheumatoid tissue. For example, VCAM-1, CD44, and β_1 integrin have been demonstrated on cell membranes of the lining cells.[75–77] ICAM-1 is up-regulated on synovial lining cells in rheumatoid arthritis.[78] The combined effects of these molecules and the cell-binding domains of the matrix macromolecules are largely responsible for the characteristic distribution of immigrant cells within synovial fronds.

Unusual Cells in the Rheumatoid Synovium

Multinucleate giant cells and mast cells are found scattered through the subintimal regions of rheumatoid synovium. Although neither comprises more than a fraction of 1 per cent of the total cells, they are found in much higher numbers in rheumatoid compared with normal tissue (Fig. 9–13).

The **multinucleate cells** are probably derived from both fibroblasts and macrophages, and a lymphokine has been identified that generates formation of multinucleate giant cells from human monocyte precursors.[79] Using cytochemical and immunohistochemical techniques, the cells of origin of giant cells in the intimal layers of rheumatoid synovium were inferred to be either true synoviocytes (fibroblasts) or macrophages. Those with macrophage lineage have tartrate-resistant acid phospha-

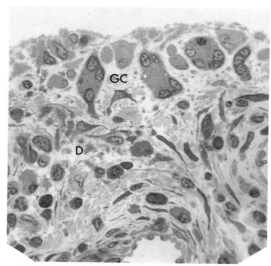

FIGURE 9–13. Thin section of rheumatoid synovium prepared for transmission electron microscopy. In addition to the high density of multinucleate cells (GC), several other features of rheumatoid synovitis are apparent:

- Endothelial cells bulge into the small vessel lumen at the bottom of the photograph.
- The lymphocytes and plasma cells (few in number) are the darkly staining cells in the perivascular areas.
- Relatively few nuclei of synovial lining cells are seen, but the surface is interlaced by cell processes from these cells.
- ''D'' marks amorphous debris.

(Prepared by Donald DiBona, Ph.D., Massachusetts General Hospital.)

tase activity and probably serve as chondroclasts, cells that are involved in active cartilage degradation (see Chapter 11).[80] Other studies in vitro have demonstrated that multinucleate cells can be formed in cultures of synovial fibroblasts by adding small quantities of membrane-lysing agents for a short time.[81] These cells then generate very large quantities of collagenase, much more than control cells, for many weeks (Fig. 9–14).

Mast cells appear to have a role in activation of the destructive processes at the pannus-cartilage junction in rheumatoid arthritis and are discussed in more detail in Chapter 11. They are present throughout the synovial lesions.[82] In a histomorphometric study, 49 mast cells/20 high power fields were found in rheumatoid synovium, compared with only 4 in samples from patients undergoing meniscectomy. Measurable histamine is found in rheumatoid synovial fluids.[83] There is a strong positive correlation between the number of mast cells per cubic millimeter of synovial tissue and the degree of lymphocyte infiltration.[84] The pathogenic function of these mast cells is related both to the preformed granule-associated components that they

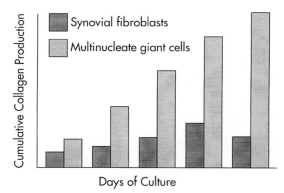

FIGURE 9–14. Multinucleate giant cells formed in cultures of synovial fibroblasts by short exposure to polyethylene glycol have a sustained and active capability of producing matrix metalloprotease 1 (interstitial collagenase).[81] Because giant cells are found in histopathology of numerous destructive lesions, it is reasonable to assume that, in situ, these cells contribute significantly to matrix degradation. It is untested, yet assumed, that these cells also produce significant quantities of stromelysin as well (see Chapter 11).

release and to newly synthesized mediators induced by many different ligands. A grand potpourri of molecules is secreted by these cells[85] (see Table 9–1). A schematic illustration of the potential consequences of mast cell activation in rheumatoid synovium is shown in Fig. 9–15.[86]

As an activator cell, the mast cell has a multifaceted capability. For example, in the region of the invasive pannus, the mast cell, TNFα, and other components of the granule and cytoplasmic secretion can activate fibroblasts to assume the stellate, invasive phenotype. The activated stellate cells generate prometalloproteases. Prostromelysin is activated by mast cell tryptase and by plasmin generated from mast cell plasminogen activator. The active stromelysin, along with plasmin, can then activate procollagenase. Mast cell heparin, cytokines, and growth factors also can activate macrophages.

Recent data have shown that fibroblasts and endothelial cells produce a cytokine named stem cell factor that enables mast cell precursors to migrate,

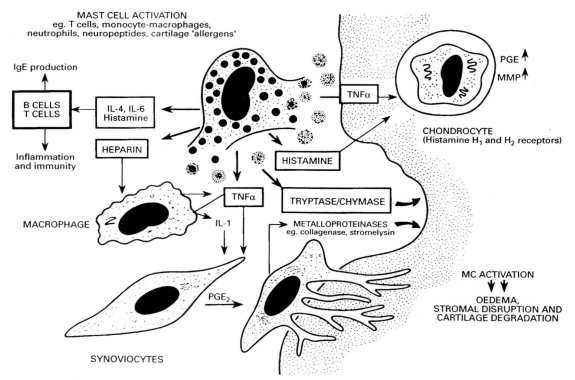

FIGURE 9–15. Schematic illustration of potential cellular interactions that may result from mast cell activation at the rheumatoid lesion. Mast cell (MC) stimulation of synoviocytes results in both morphologic transformation and enhanced metalloprotease and prostanoid production.[110] Moreover, the MC proteases tryptase and chymase activate precursor forms of the metalloproteases.[111] MC stimulation of chondrocytes via histamine and TNFα promotes prostanoid (PGE) and metalloprotease (MMP) production.[110] MC stimulation of monocyte-macrophages mediated via heparin promotes IL-1 production.[110] MC stimulation of lymphocytes via histamine and IL-4 modulates antibody production and the inflammatory cycle.[112–114] (From Woolley, D. E.: Mast cells in the rheumatoid lesion—ringleaders or innocent bystanders? Ann. Rheum. Dis. 54:533, 1995. Used by permission.)

TABLE 9–1. Molecules Secreted by Mast Cells

Preformed granule-associated mast cell products
  Heparin
  Chondroitin sulfate
  Chymase and tryptase
  Plasminogen activator
  Elastase, carboxypeptidase A, peroxidase, and superoxide dismutase
Preformed rapidly eluted mast cell products
  Histamine
  Serotonin
  Chemoattractants for circulating neutrophils and lymphocytes
  Exoglycosidases
Genes transcribed by activated mast cells
  Cytokines (TNFα, IL-1, IL-6, GM-CSF, TGFβ)
  Prostaglandins
  Leukotrienes
  Adenosine, superoxide, platelet-activating factor

survive, and proliferate and induces secretion of numerous mediators from mature mast cells.[87]

Iron—a Product of Erythrocyte Breakdown—and Its Role in Rheumatoid Synovitis[88]

Virtually every specimen of synovium from rheumatoid arthritis has evidence for extraerythrocytic iron (Fig. 9–16). Special stains reveal large quantities of it, and iron can be found on regular hematoxylin and eosin stains as brown inclusions within phagocytic cells. The iron is present in the ferric rather than ferrous form in most rheumatoid tissue,[89] and the extent of a patient's anemia correlates with histologic estimates of iron stores.[90] These deposits can amount to a large iron store, yet rheumatoid patients usually have an anemia characterized by a decrease in serum iron and iron-binding capacity. Transferrin saturation is diminished, but there is a marked increase in serum ferritin. All these indices point to an inability of the rheumatoid patient to reutilize iron stores within the reticuloendothelial system. This may be related to an in-

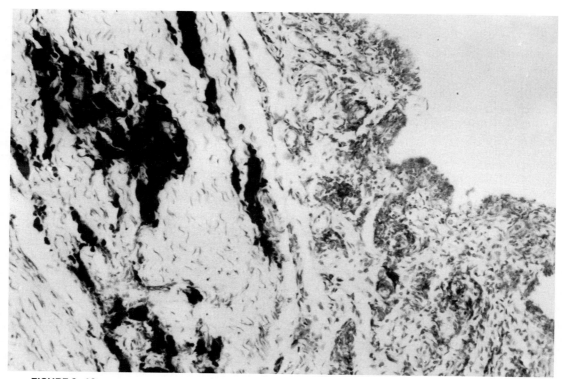

FIGURE 9–16. Section of rheumatoid synovium prepared with Prussian blue stain showing large collections of iron, the product of many microhemorrhages, found deep in the subsynovial tissue. (×315) (Courtesy of K. Muirden, M. D.) (From Harris, E. D. Jr.: Etiology and pathogenesis of rheumatoid arthritis. *In* Kelley, W. N., Harris, E. D. Jr., Ruddy, S., and Sledge, C. B. [eds.]: Textbooks of Rheumatology, 4th ed., Vol. 1. Philadelphia, W. B. Saunders, 1993, pp. 833–873. Used by permission.)

creased synthesis of the iron storage protein apoferritin, which behaves as an acute-phase reactant; this apoferritin provides a storage depot for incoming iron delivered through lactoferrin or from dead erythrocytes. This diversion produces hypoferremia[91] and, matched with the increased ferritin synthesis, results in inaccessible iron stores.

In addition to contributing to anemia, these sequestered iron stores may have an active role in the inflammatory process in rheumatoid synovium:

- In both particulate and soluble forms, iron induces biosynthesis of collagenase by synovial cells in vitro.[92] As an in vivo corollary, the destructive and proliferative synovitis that develops in hemophiliacs after multiple recurrent hemarthroses may well be driven by the proliferative stimulus of fragmented red blood cells and their hemoglobin breakdown products.[93] Amid the immunologic activity in rheumatoid synovium, the same stimulatory effect of extravasated erythrocytes may be a major factor in rheumatoid synovial proliferation.
- Iron catalyzes oxidative radical reactions, leading to the formation of toxic hydroxyl ($\cdot$OH) radicals and subsequent lipid peroxidation, both of which have the potential to disrupt cellular organelle membranes.[94]
- There is a significant correlation between synovial fluid ferritin concentration, synovial immune complexes, and other indices of inflammatory activity in rheumatoid patients.[95] It is possible that this association is related to a direct toxic effect of excess iron within synovial macrophages, rendering them unable to clear immune complexes.
- In a group of seven patients given infusions of iron dextran to improve their anemia, five had distinct flares of their rheumatoid synovitis within 24 hours after the therapy.[95] This phenomenon corresponded with a saturation of serum iron-binding capacity in another group of patients given intravenous iron.[96]
- Iron in both ionic and particulate forms may have effects upon lymphocytes that up-regulate their responses in a deleterious manner for patients.[88]

The presence of ferritin and hemosiderin iron in the synovium of rheumatoid patients implies a poor prognosis. The synovial hemorrhages could be a marker for a more aggressive and proliferative synovitis; conversely, the excess iron itself may be driving proliferative responses and cellular toxicity within the already inflamed villi.

RHEUMATOID NODULES

Although these characteristic nodules are, on occasion, seen in histologic sections of synovium, they are most commonly found in the subcutaneous tissue overlying bony prominences. They have a more simple organization than does the synovium: A central area of necrosis is rimmed by palisades of radially arranged macrophages, lymphocytes, and activated fibroblasts surrounded by relatively vascular connective tissue containing many lymphocytes.

There are interesting similarities between rheumatoid nodules and rheumatoid synovium:

1. When placed in organ culture, fragments of the palisading arcades generate large quantities of collagenase, implying that these cells are driven by cytokines in the same way that the synovial lining cells are. These observations led to a hypothesis that the central necrosis of these nodules is related to proteolytic degradation of the collagenous scaffold that normally holds cells in the palisading layers in place.[97]

2. A similar percentage of cells in the palisading arcades show positive staining with antibodies for LCA, HLA-DR, and macrophage markers as do nonlymphoid cells in the synovium.[98]

3. T lymphocytes are found among the palisading macrophages and fibroblasts. Only a minority express IL-2Rs.[99] This indicates that they either are resting cells or, more likely, are terminally differentiated, similar to the CD45RB^{dim} cells of rheumatoid synovium that express little IL-2 but provide strong help to B-cell differentiation and immunoglobulin synthesis.

4. Multinucleate giant cells are occasionally visible among the palisading cells.[99]

5. Plasma cells, although comprising less than 5 percent of the palisading cells, in rheumatoid nodules produce IgG in greater quantities than IgM or IgA.[98]

Although not yet proved, a reasonable hypothesis is that, as a result of microtrauma in a sensitized mesenchymal cell population in extra-articular locations in active rheumatoid disease, a cytokine network becomes active in the subcutaneous tissue in the same way that it is active within synovium. New blood vessels develop, monocytes and lymphocytes are recruited from the circulation to join activated mesenchymal cells, and extracellular matrix immunoglobulins, metalloproteases, and cytokines become dominant products of the cells as the rheumatoid nodule grows. Necrosis begins, and extends, by a combination of microvascular ischemia and stromelysin/collagenase activity on the matrix surrounding the palisading layers. The nodules enlarge as matrix synthesis dominates loss of tis-

sue, and regress as central necrosis dominates over matrix synthesis.

CYTOKINE ANTAGONISM: POSSIBLE EFFECTS IN RHEUMATOID SYNOVITIS

Natural inhibitors of cytokines have been isolated and characterized (e.g., IL-1ra and soluble TNFα receptors), and it is probable that these have a role in modulation of the inflammatory capabilities of IL-1 and TNFα (see Chapter 8). Similarly, it is increasingly appreciated that the actions of one cytokine within tissues can either amplify or diminish those of another. Synergism between cytokines is exemplified by the combined effects of IL-1 and TNFα, but what about antagonism of one cytokine by another? Examples are given here of the impact each may have in the rheumatoid synovium.

Interleukin-10 and Interleukin-4 versus Interleukin-1

IL-10 is produced by the Th2 subset of CD4+ T-helper cells, and helps suppress the production of inflammatory cytokines generated by the Th1 group of T cells. IL-10 is also produced by monocytes and T cells in both rheumatoid and osteoarthritic synovium.[100] In addition to inhibiting IL-1 and TNFα synthesis by monocytes,[101] IL-10 generated by Th2 cells induces IL-1ra protein and mRNA expression in these cells.[102] IL-4 also inhibits IL-1 production by human monocytes.[103] This combined effect of IL-4 and IL-10 may be sufficient to alter the IL-1β:IL-1ra ratio sufficiently to diminish the effective inflammatory enhancement of IL-1.

Interleukin-1 and Platelet-Derived Growth Factor

These two cytokines are generally considered to have similar effects within synovium, each enhancing synovial cell proliferation and destructive enzyme production. The interactions of both added to the same system are complicated, however[57]:

- IL-1 inhibits PDGF-stimulated synoviocyte proliferation, possibly by enhancing PGE$_2$ production by IL-1–driven synoviocytes. Exogenous PGE$_2$ inhibits PDGF-induced synovial cell proliferation.
- PDGF antagonizes IL-1–stimulated mRNA collagenase transcription.

Transforming Growth Factor β and Interleukin-1β/Tumor Necrosis Factor α

From the list of TGFβ actions delineated in Chapter 8, it is easy to surmise that these cytokines are antagonistic. TGFβ not only suppresses the growth factor/IL-1/TNFα–stimulated production of collagenase by synovial cells, but also induces expression of the tissue inhibitor of collagenase and TIMP.[104] In vivo models of arthritis in mice show that intra-articular TGFβ counteracts IL-1–induced suppression of articular cartilage proteoglycan synthesis.[105] An associated observation that this effect was manifested primarily in young mice underscores the fact that young matrix tissues have a greater sensitivity to cytokines. Because it has been demonstrated that the IL-1ra:IL-1 ratios in rheumatoid tissues are, at most, around 4—below the 10-fold excess of IL-1ra needed to inhibit IL-1 bioactivity[106]—the counteractive effects of reparative cytokines such as TGFβ may be essential for regulation of the destructive capabilities of IL-1.

Other Cytokine Antagonisms

In a study of a broad array of cytokines potentially involved in rheumatoid arthritis, the following interactions were observed[107]:

- TNFα inhibited IFNγ–mediated HLA-DR expression by rheumatoid synovial cells.
- IFNγ inhibited TNFα–induced synovial cell proliferation and collagenase production, but not these same functions initiated by IL-1. This and the previous antagonisms mentioned between TNFα and IFNγ could be an effective homeostatic control mechanism that is defective in rheumatoid arthritis because the terminally differentiated memory T cells from rheumatoid arthritis patients have a specific defect in IFNγ biosynthesis.[108]
- An ex vivo model of bone resorption using human tissue has facilitated biochemical and histomorphometric parameters of bone resorption, the regulation of the production of IL-6, and the collagen cross-link pyridinoline (a marker for bone resorption). IL-4 induced a 70 percent reduction of IL-6 production by bone cultures, a decrease in pyridinoline, and a 35 percent increase in the mean total bone area after 7 days of IL-4 treatment.[109] Possibly, IL-4 should be developed as a treatment for postmenopausal osteoporosis.

These are only a few of the known antagonisms between cytokines, and no doubt many have not been delineated yet. The key for investigators is to exploit and amplify the reparative and immunosuppressive effects of cytokines in order to break into the cycle of inflammation of rheumatoid arthritis and lead the joint toward normal cellularity.

REFERENCES

1. Harris, E. D., Jr., Evanson, J. M., DiBona, D. R., et al.: Collagenase and rheumatoid arthritis. Arthritis Rheum. 13:83, 1970.
2. Brinckerhoff, C. E., and Harris, E. D., Jr.: Survival of human rheumatoid synovium implanted into nude mice. Am. J. Pathol. 103:411, 1981.
3. Conca, W., Kaplan, P. B., and Krane, S. M.: Increases in levels of procollagenase messenger RNA in cultured fibroblasts induced by human recombinant interleukin 1 beta or serum follow c-jun expression and are dependent on new protein synthesis. J. Clin. Invest. 83:1753, 1989.
4. Trabandt, A., Aicher, W. K., Gay, R. E., et al.: Expression of the collagenolytic and Fas-induced cysteine proteinase cathepsin L and proliferation-associated oncogenes in synovial cells of MRL/1 mice and patients with rheumatoid arthritis. Matrix 10:349, 1990.
5. Sibbitt, W., Jr.: Oncogenes, normal cell growth, and connective tissue disease. Ann. Rev. Med. 39:123, 1988.
6. Fujikawa, K.: Arthrographic study of the rheumatoid knee. Part 1. Synovial proliferation. Ann. Rheum. Dis. 40: 332, 1981.
7. Fujikawa, K., Tanaka, Y., Matsubayashi, T., et al.: Arthrographic study of the rheumatoid knee. Part 2. Articular cartilage and menisci. Ann. Rheum. Dis. 40:344, 1981.
8. Salisbury, M. D., and Nottage, W. M.: A new evaluation of gross pathologic changes and concepts of rheumatoid articular cartilage degeneration. Clin. Orthop. Rel. Res. 199:243, 1985.
9. Yanni, G., Whelan, A., Feighery, C., et al.: Morphometric analysis of synovial membrane blood vessels in rheumatoid arthritis: associations with the immunohistologic features, synovial fluid cytokine levels and the clinical course. J. Rheumatol. 20:634, 1993.
10. Soden, M., Rooney, M., Whelan, A., et al.: Immunohistological analysis of the synovial membrane: search for predictors of the clinical course in rheumatoid arthritis. Ann. Rheum. Dis. 50:673, 1991.
11. Yanni, G., Whelan, A., Feighery, C., et al.: Synovial tissue macrophages and joint erosion in rheumatoid arthritis. Ann. Rheum. Dis. 53:39, 1994.
12. Mulherin, D., Fitzgerald, O., and Bresnihan, B.: Synovial tissue macrophage populations and articular damage in rheumatoid arthritis. Arthritis Rheum. 39:115, 1996.
13. Rooney, M., Condell, D., Quinlan, W., et al.: Analysis of the histologic variation of synovitis in rheumatoid arthritis. Arthritis Rheum. 31:956, 1988.
14. Kennedy, T. D., Plater-Zyberk, C., Partridge, T. A., et al.: Morphometric comparison of synovium from patients with osteoarthritis and rheumatoid arthritis. J. Clin. Pathol. 41:847, 1988.
15. Zvaifler, N. J., Boyle, D., and Firestein, G. S.: Early synovitis—synoviocytes and mononuclear cells. Semin. Arthritis Rheum. 23(suppl. 2):11, 1994.
16. Soden, M., Rooney, M., Cullen, A., et al.: Immunohistologic features in the synovium obtained from clinically uninvolved knee joints of patients with rheumatoid arthritis. Br. J. Rheumatol. 28:287, 1989.
17. Kulka, P. J.: Microcirculation impairment as a factor in inflammatory tissue damage. Ann. N.Y. Acad. Sci. 116: 1018, 1964.
18. Remmers, E. F., Lafyatis, R., Kumkumian, G. K., et al.: Cytokines and growth regulation of synoviocytes from patients with rheumatoid arthritis and rats with streptococcal cell wall arthritis. Growth Factors 2:179, 1990.
19. Athannasou, N. A., and Quinn, J. M.: Immunocytochemical analysis of human synovial lining cells: phenotypic relation to other marrow-derived cells. Ann. Rheum. Dis. 50:311, 1991.
20. Firestein, G. S., Yeo, M., and Zvaifler, N. J.: Apoptosis in rheumatoid arthritis synovium. J. Clin. Immunol. 96: 1631, 1995.
21. Henderson, B., Revell, P. A., and Edwards, J. C. W.: Synovial lining cell hyperplasia in rheumatoid arthritis: dogma and fact. Ann. Rheum. Dis. 47:348, 1988.
22. Mohr, W., and Beneke, G.: Proliferation of synovial lining cells and fibroblasts. Ann. Rheum. Dis. 34:219, 1975.
23. Hogg, N., Palmer, D. G., and Revell, P. A.: Mononuclear phagocytes of normal and rheumatoid synovial membrane identified by monoclonal antibodies. Immunology 56:673, 1985.
24. Palmer, D. G., Selvendran, Y., Allen, C., et al.: Features of synovial membrane identified with monoclonal antibodies. Clin. Exp. Immunol. 59:529, 1985.
25. Koch, A. E., Burrows, J. C., Skoutelis, A., et al.: Monoclonal antibodies detect monocyte/macrophage activation and differentiation antigens and identify functionally distinct subpopulations of human rheumatoid synovial tissue macrophages. Am. J. Pathol. 138:165, 1991.
26. Mulder, A. H. L., Westra, J., Barendsen, B. C., et al.: Expression of CD68 by synovial fibroblasts in rheumatoid arthritis [abstract]. Ann. Rheum. Dis. 54:525, 1995. (not in Medline)
27. Nykanen, P. J.: Cell proliferation in rheumatoid arthritis synovial membrane and synovial fluid. Thesis, University of Helsinki, 1992.
28. Butler, D. M., Piccoli, D. S., Hart, P. H., et al.: Stimulation of human synovial fibroblast DNA synthesis by recombinant human cytokines. J. Rheumatol. 15:1463, 1988.
29. Hollingsworth, J. W., Siegel, E. R., and Creasey, W. A.: Granulocyte survival in synovial exudate of patients with rheumatoid arthritis and other inflammatory joint diseases. Yale J. Biol. Med. 39:289, 1967.
30. Lafyatis, R., Remmers, E. F., Roberts, A. B., et al.: Anchorage-independent growth of synoviocytes from arthritic and normal joints: stimulation by exogenous platelet-derived growth factor and inhibition by transforming growth factor-beta and retinoids. J. Clin. Invest. 83:1267, 1989.
31. Burmester, G. R., Dimitriu-Bona, A., Waters, S. J., et al.: Identification of three major synovial lining cell populations by monoclonal antibodies directed to Ia antigens and antigens associated with monocytes/macrophages and fibroblasts. Scand. J. Immunol. 17:69, 1983.
32. Goto, M., Sasano, M., Yamanaka, H., et al.: Spontaneous production of an interleukin 1-like factor by cloned rheumatoid synovial cells in long-term culture. J. Clin. Invest. 80:786, 1987.
33. Baker, D. G., Dayer, J.-M., Roelke, M., et al.: Rheumatoid synovial cell morphologic changes induced by a mononuclear cell factor in culture. Arthritis Rheum. 26:8, 1983.
34. Handel, M. L., McMorrow, L. B., and Gravallese, E. M.: Nuclear factor-κB in rheumatoid synovium: Localization of p50 and p56. Arthritis Rheum. 38:1762, 1995.

35. Marok, R., Winyard, P. G., Coumbe, A., et al.: Activation of the transcription factor nuclear factor-κB in human inflamed synovial tissue. Arthritis Rheum. 39:583, 1996.

36. Wilkinson, L. S., Pitsillides, A. A., Worral, J. G., et al.: Light microscope characterization of the fibroblast-like synovial intimal cell (synoviocyte). Arthritis Rheum. 35: 1179, 1992.

37. Revell, P. A., Al-Saffar, N., Fish, S., et al.: Extracellular matrix of the synovial intimal cell layer. Ann. Rheum. Dis. 54:404, 1995.

38. Okada, Y., Takeuchi, N., Tomita, K., et al.: Immunolocalisation of matrix metalloproteinase 3 (stromelysin) in rheumatoid synovioblasts (B cells): correlation with rheumatoid arthritis. Ann. Rheum. Dis. 48:645, 1989.

39. Kinne, R. W., Palombo-Kinne, E., and Emmrich, F.: Activation of synovial fibroblasts in rheumatoid arthritis. Ann. Rheum. Dis. 54:501, 1995.

40. Kinne, R. W., Boehn, S., Iftner, T., et al.: Expression of jun-B and c-fos proto-oncogenes by activated fibroblast-like cells in synovial tissue of rheumatoid arthritis and osteoarthritis patients. Arthritis Rheum. 36:S264, 1993.

41. Dooley, S., Herlitzka, I., Hanselmann, R., et al.: Constitutive expression of c-fos and c-jun, overexpression of ets-2, and reduced expression of metastasis suppressor gene nm23-H1 in rheumatoid arthritis. Ann. Rheum. Dis. 55:298, 1996.

42. Akahoshi, T., Wada, C., Endo, H., et al.: Expression of monocyte chemotactic and activating factor in rheumatoid arthritis. Arthritis Rheum. 36:762, 1993.

43. Koch, A. E., Kunkel, S. L., Harlow, L. A., et al.: Macrophage inflammatory protein-1α. J. Clin. Invest. 93:921, 1994.

44. Lotz, M., Vaughan, J. H., and Carson, D. A.: Effect of neuropeptides on production of inflammatory cytokines by human monocytes. Science 241:1218, 1988.

45. Hirohata, S., Yanagida, T., Itoh, K., et al.: Accelerated generation of CD14+ monocyte-lineage cells from the bone marrow of rheumatoid arthritis patients. Arthritis Rheum. 39:836, 1996.

46. Thomas, R., and Lipsky, P. E.: Monocytes and macrophages. In Kelley, W. N., Harris, E. D. Jr., Ruddy, S., and Sledge, C. B. (eds.): Textbook of Rheumatology, 4th ed., Vol. 1. Philadelphia, W. B. Saunders, 1993, pp. 286–303.

47. Cush, J. J., and Lipsky, P. E.: Phenotypic analysis of synovial tissue and peripheral blood lymphocytes isolated from patients with rheumatoid arthritis. Arthritis Rheum. 31:1230, 1988.

48. Howell, W. M., Warren, C. J., Cook, N. J., et al.: Detection of IL-2 at mRNA and protein levels in synovial infiltrates from inflammatory arthropathies using biotinylated oligonucleotide probes in situ. Clin. Exp. Immunol. 86:393, 1991.

49. Ritchlin, C., Dwyer, E., Bucala, R., et al.: Sustained and distinctive patterns of gene activation in synovial fibroblasts and whole synovial tissue obtained from inflammatory synovitis. Scand. J. Immunol. 40:292, 1994.

50. Haynes, B. F., Grover, B. J., Whichard, L. P., et al.: Synovial microenvironment–T cell interactions: human T cells bind to fibroblast-like synovial cells in in vitro. Arthritis Rheum. 31:947, 1988.

51. Muller-Ladner, U., Kriegsmann, J., Tschopp, J., et al.: Demonstration of Granzyme A and perforin messenger RNA in the synovium of patients with rheumatoid arthritis. Arthritis Rheum. 38:477, 1995.

52. Nakao, H., Eguchi, K., Kawakami, A., et al.: Phenotypic characterization of lymphocytes infiltrating synovial tissue from patients with rheumatoid arthritis: analysis of lymphocytes isolated from minced synovial tissue by dual immunofluorescent staining. J. Rheumatol. 17:142, 1990.

53. Evan, G. I., Wyllie, A. H., Gilbert, C. S., et al.: Induction of apoptosis in fibroblasts by c-myc protein. Cell 69: 119, 1992.

54. Remmers, E. F., Sano, H., and Wilder, R. L.: Platelet-derived growth factors and heparin-binding (fibroblast) growth factors in the synovial tissue pathology of rheumatoid arthritis. Semin. Arthritis Rheum. 21:191, 1991.

55. Miyasaka, N., Sato, K., Goto, M., et al.: Augmented interleukin-1 production and HLA-DR expression in the synovium of rheumatoid arthritis patients: possible involvement in joint destruction. Arthritis Rheum. 31:480, 1988.

56. Bucala, R., Ritchlin, C., Winchester, R., et al.: Constitutive production of inflammatory and mitogenic cytokines by rheumatoid synovial fibroblasts. J. Exp. Med. 173:569, 1991.

57. Kumkumian, G. K., Lafyatis, R., Remmers, E. F., et al.: Platelet-derived growth factor and interleukin-1 interactions in rheumatoid arthritis: regulation of synoviocyte proliferation, prostaglandin (PGE$_2$) production, and collagenase transcription. J. Immunol. 143:833, 1989.

58. Bergroth, V., Zvaifler, N. J., and Firestein, G. S.: Cytokines in chronic inflammatory arthritis. III. Rheumatoid arthritis monocytes are not usually sensitive to γ-interferon, but have defective γ-interferon–mediated HLA-DQ and HLA-DR induction. Arthritis Rheum. 32:1074, 1989.

59. Houssiau F. A., Devogelaer, J.-P, Van Damme, J., et al.: Interleukin-6 in synovial fluid and serum of patients with rheumatoid arthritis and other inflammatory arthritides. Arthritis Rheum. 31:784, 1988.

60. Guerne, P.-A., Zuraw, B. L., Vaughan, J. H., et al.: Synovium as a source of interleukin 6 in vitro: contribution to local and systemic manifestations of arthritis. J. Clin. Invest. 83:585, 1989.

61. Firestein, G. S., Xu, W.-D., Townsend, K., et al.: Cytokines in chronic inflammatory arthritis. I. Failure to detect T cell lymphokines (interleukin 2 and interleukin 3) and presence of macrophage colony-stimulating factor (CSF-1) and a novel mast cell growth factor in rheumatoid synovitis. J. Exp. Med. 168:1573, 1988.

62. Koch, A. E., Kunkel, S. L., Burrows, J. C., et al.: Synovial tissue macrophage as a source of the chemotactic cytokine IL-8. J. Immunol. 147:2187, 1991.

63. Hamilton, J. A., and Slywka, J.: Stimulation of human synovial fibroblast plasminogen activator production by mononuclear cell supernatants. J. Immunol. 126:851, 1981.

64. Hamilton, J. A., Bootes, A., Phillips, P. E., et al.: Human synovial fibroblast plasminogen activator. Arthritis Rheum. 24:1296, 1981.

65. Goddard, D. H., Grossman, S. L., Williams, W. V., et al.: Regulation of synovial cell growth: coexpression of transforming growth factor β and basic fibroblast growth factor by cultured synovial cells. Arthritis Rheum. 35:1296, 1992.

66. Bassols, A., and Massague, J.: Transforming growth factor-beta regulates the expression and structure of extracellular matrix chondroitin/dermatan sulfate proteoglycans. J. Biol. Chem. 262:3039, 1988.

67. Remmers, E. F., Sano, H., Lafyatis, R., et al.: Production of platelet derived growth factor B chain (PDGF-B/c-sis) mRNA and immunoreactive PDGF B-like polypeptide by rheumatoid synovium: coexpression with hepa-

rin binding acidic fibroblast growth factor-1. J. Rheumatol. 18:7, 1991.

68. Pollock, L. E., Lalor, P., and Revell, P. A.: Type IV collagen and laminin in the synovial intimal layer: an immunohistochemical study. Rheumatol. Int. 9:277, 1990.

69. Okada, Y., Naka, K., Minamoto, T., et al.: Localization of type VI collagen in the lining cell layer of normal and rheumatoid synovium. Lab. Invest. 63:647, 1990.

70. Aumailley, M., Mann, K., von der Mark, H., et al.: Cell attachment properties of collagen type VI and Arg-Gly-Asp dependent binding to its α 2 (VI) and α 3 (VI) chains. Exp. Cell. Res. 181:463, 1989.

71. Carsons, S. E., and Wolf, J.: Interaction between synoviocytes and extracellular matrix *in vitro*. Ann. Rheum. Dis. 54:413, 1995.

72. Clarris, B. J., and Fraser, J. R. E.: On the pericellular zone of some mammalian cells *in vitro*. Exp. Cell. Res. 49:181, 1968.

73. Lesley, J., Hyman, R., and Kincade, P. W.: CD44 and its interaction with extracellular matrix. Adv. Immunol. 54:271, 1993.

74. Laurent, T. C., Laurent, U. B. G., and Fraser, J. R. E.: Functions of hyaluronan. Ann. Rheum. Dis. 54:429, 1995.

75. Henderson, K. F., Pitsillides, A. A., Edwards, J. C. W., et al.: Reduced expression of CD44 in rheumatoid synovial cells. Br. J. Rheumatol. 32:25, 1993.

76. Wilkinson, L. S., Edwards, J. C. W., Poston, R., et al.: Cell populations expressing VCAM-1 in normal and diseased synovium. Lab. Invest. 68:82, 1993.

77. Al-Saffar, N., Hah, J. T. L., Kadoya, Y., et al.: Neovascularisation and the induction of cell adhesion molecules in response to degradation products from orthopaedic implants. Ann. Rheum. Dis. 54:201, 1995.

78. Szekanecz, Z., Haines, G. K., Lin, T. R., et al.: Differential distribution of intercellular adhesion molecules (ICAM-1, ICAM-2, and ICAM-3) and the MS-1 antigen in normal and diseased human synovium: the possible pathogenetic and clinical significance in rheumatoid arthritis. Arthritis Rheum. 37:221, 1994.

79. Postlethwaite, A. E., Jackson, B. K., Beachey, E. H., et al.: Formation of multinucleated giant cells from human monocyte precursors. J. Exp. Med. 155:168, 1982.

80. Wilkinson, L. S., Pitsillides, A. A., and Edwards, J. C. W.: Giant cells in arthritic synovium. Ann. Rheum. Dis. 52:182, 1993.

81. Brinckerhoff, C. E., and Harris, E. D. Jr.: Collagenase production by cultures containing multinucleated cells derived from synovial fibroblasts. Arthritis Rheum. 21:745, 1978.

82. Crisp, A. J., Chapman, C. M., Kirkham, S. E., et al.: Articular mastocytosis in rheumatoid arthritis. Arthritis Rheum. 27:845, 1984.

83. Malone, D. G., Irani, A.-M., Schwartz, L. B., et al.: Mast cell numbers and histamine levels in synovial fluids from patients with diverse arthritides. Arthritis Rheum. 29:956, 1986.

84. Malone, D. G., Wilder, R. L., Saavedra-Delgado, A. M., et al.: Mast cell numbers in rheumatoid synovial tissues. Arthritis Rheum. 30:130, 1987.

85. Woolley, D. E.: Mast cells and histopathology of the rheumatoid lesion. *In* Balint, G., et al. (eds.): Rheumatology: State of the Art. New York, Elsevier, 1992, pp. 112–114.

86. Woolley, D. E.: Mast cells in the rheumatoid lesion—ringleaders or innocent bystanders? Ann. Rheum. Dis. 54:533, 1995.

87. Valent, P.: The riddle of the mast cell: Kit(CD117)-ligand as the missing link. Immunol. Today 15:111, 1994.

88. Dabbagh, A. J., Trenam, C. W., Morris, C. J., et al.: Iron in joint inflammation. Ann. Rheum. Dis. 52:67, 1993.

89. Giordano, N., Vaccai, D., Cintorino, M., et al.: Histopathological study of iron deposit distribution in the rheumatoid synovium. Clin. Exp. Rheumatol. 9:463, 1991.

90. Muirden, K. D.: The anaemia of RA: the significance of iron deposits in the synovial membrane. Aust. Ann. Med. 2:97, 1970.

91. Konijn, A. M., and Hershko, C.: Ferritin synthesis in inflammation: pathogenesis of impaired iron release. Br. J. Haematol. 37:7, 1977.

92. Okazaki, I., Brinckerhoff, C. E., Sinclaire, J. F., et al.: Iron increases collagenase production by rabbit synovial fibroblasts. J. Lab. Clin. Med. 97:396, 1981.

93. Mainardi, C. L., Levine, P. H., Werb, Z., et al.: Proliferative synovitis in hemophilia. Arthritis Rheum. 21:137, 1978.

94. Blake, D. R., Gallagher, P. J., Potter, A. R., et al.: The effect of synovial iron on the progression of rheumatoid disease. Arthritis Rheum. 27:495, 1984.

95. Blake, D. R., and Bacon, P. A.: Synovial fluid ferritin in rheumatoid arthritis: an index or cause of inflammation? Br. Med. J. 282:189, 1981.

96. Reddy, P. A., and Lewis, M.: Adverse effect of intravenous iron-dextran in rheumatoid arthritis. Arthritis Rheum. 12:454, 1969.

97. Harris, E. D. Jr.: A collagenolytic system produced by primary cultures of rheumatoid nodule tissue. J. Clin. Invest. 51:2973, 1972.

98. Athanasou, N. A., Quinn, J., Woods, C. G., et al.: Immunohistology of rheumatoid nodules and rheumatoid synovium. Ann. Rheum. Dis. 47:398, 1988.

99. DeKeyser, F., Verbruggen, G., Veys, E. M., et al.: T-cell receptor Vβ usage in rheumatoid nodules: marked oligoclonality among IL-2 expanded lymphocytes. Clin. Immunol. Immunopathol. 68:29, 1993.

100. Katsikis, P. D., Chu, C.-Q., Brennan, F. M., et al.: Immunoregulatory role of interleukin 10 in rheumatoid arthritis. J. Exp. Med. 179:1517, 1994.

101. Ralph, P., Nakoinz, I., Sampson-Hohannes, A., et al.: IL-10, T lymphocyte inhibitor of human blood cell production of IL-1 and tumor necrosis factor. J. Immunol. 148:808, 1992.

102. Jenkins, J. K., Malyak, M., and Arend, W. P.: The effects of interleukin-10 on interleukin-1 receptor antagonist and interleukin-1β production in human monocytes and neutrophils. Lymphokine Cytokine Res. 13:47, 1994.

103. Donnelly, R. P., Fenton, M. J., Kaufman, J. D., et al.: IL-1 expression in human monocytes is transcriptionally and posttranscriptionally regulated by IL-4. J. Immunol. 146:3431, 1991.

104. Edwards, D. R., Murphy, G., Reynolds, J. J., et al.: Transforming growth factor beta modulates the expression of collagenase and metalloproteinase inhibitor. EMBO J. 6:1899, 1987.

105. van Beuningen, H. M., van der Kraan, P. M., Arntz, O. J., et al.: *In vivo* protection against interleukin-1-induced articular cartilage damage by transforming growth factor β1: age-related differences. Ann. Rheum. Dis. 53:593, 1994.

106. Firestein, G. S., Boyle, D. L., Yu, C., et al.: Synovial interleukin-1 receptor antagonist and interleukin-1 balance in rheumatoid arthritis. Arthritis Rheum. 37:644, 1994.

107. Alvaro-Gracia, J. M., Zvaifler, N. J., and Firestein, G. S.: Cytokines in chronic inflammatory arthritis. V. Mutual

antagonism between interferon-gamma and tumor necrosis factor-alpha on HLA-DR expression, proliferation, collagenase production, and granulocyte macrophage colony-stimulating factor production by rheumatoid arthritis synoviocytes. J. Clin. Invest. 86: 1790, 1990.

108. Hasler, F., Bluestein, H. G., Zvaifler, N. J., et al.: Analysis of the defects responsible for the impaired regulation of Epstein-Barr virus-induced B cell proliferation by rheumatoid arthritis lymphocytes. I. Diminished gamma interferon production in response to autologous stimulation. J. Exp. Med. 157:173, 1983.

109. Miossec, P., Chomarat, P., Dechanet, J., et al.: Interleukin-4 inhibits bone resorption through an effect on osteoclasts and proinflammatory cytokines in an *ex vivo* model of bone resorption in rheumatoid arthritis. Arthritis Rheum. 37:1715, 1994.

110. Woolley, D. E., Bartholomew, J. S., Taylor, D. J., and Evanson, J. S.: Mast cells and rheumatoid arthritis. *In* Galli, S. J., Austen, F. K. (eds.): Mast Cell and Basophil Differentiation and Function in Health and Disease. New York, Raven Press, 1989, pp. 183–193.

111. Lees, M., Taylor, D. J., and Woolley, D. E.: Mast cell proteinases activate precursor forms of collagenase and stromelysin, but not gelatinases A and B. Eur. J. Biochem. 223:171, 1994.

112. White, M., and Kaliner, M. A.: Histamine. *In* Gallin, J. I., Goldstein, I. M., and Snyderman, R. (eds.): Inflammation: Basic Principles and Clinical Correlates. New York, Raven Press, 1988, pp. 169–193.

113. Romagnani, S.: Regulation and deregulation of human IgE synthesis. Immunol. Today 11:316, 1990.

114. Schwartz, L. B.: Mast cells: function and contents. Curr. Opin. Immunol. 6:91, 1994.

10
Cartilage and the Mechanisms for Its Destruction

Protection of the anatomic and functional integrity of articular cartilage is the principal underlying goal of physicians treating rheumatoid arthritis. The logic of this is based upon two facts:

1. Each of the many inflammatory and proliferative cycles set in motion during rheumatoid synovial inflammation converge in collaborative collusion upon articular cartilage; together, they amass a potent capability for destruction.

2. Articular cartilage is a terminally differentiated tissue, and cannot be regenerated effectively. Once it is lost, the joint is destroyed.

Articular cartilage has some special qualities that explain why it is so vulnerable, why rheumatoid synovitis moves centripetally to destroy cartilage, and, perhaps, why rheumatoid arthritis affects joints in the first place. First, the function of articular cartilage depends not only upon normal metabolism of its cells (chondrocytes) but also upon the integrity of its complex matrix structure. Second, articular cartilage, in the normal adult, has no blood supply. This affects its normal mechanisms for nutrition and homeostasis, and also may lead to sequestration of potential autoantigens, giving it "immunologic privilege."

The first of these two qualities, the complexity of its matrix structure, is a function primarily of the collagens and proteoglycans within the joint. The proteoglycans, with their negatively charged side chains of GAGs, confer upon cartilage the ability to rebound from a deforming load. Very early in joint inflammation of any etiology, including that resulting from relatively minor trauma, proteoglycans are depleted from cartilage. This does not result in any difference in gross appearance of the cartilage; it still retains its glistening surface and volume. The difference, however, is that water replaces the GAGs and changes the texture and stiffness of the cartilage (normally not unlike that of a peeled and sliced almond); it becomes flimsy and deformable and cannot rebound from compression as does normal cartilage[1,2] (Fig. 10–1).

The loss of cartilage collagens can be equated with loss of physical volume. Collagen loss is much slower than is GAG loss. If, after GAG loss, inflammation stops (e.g., during healing of an acute injury), GAG is replaced by chondrocyte biosynthesis, and a normal tissue is the result. In contrast, loss of collagens means permanent loss of cartilage.

When considering cartilage and the effects upon it of inflammation, it is important to remember that, in its natural, unharmed state, it has special properties that are crucial for its normal function. When the normal structure is altered or deformed, cartilage becomes vulnerable. For instance, intact cartilage is protected from binding of anti–type II collagen antibodies by a proteinaceous material synthesized by resident chondrocytes and bound noncovalently to the underlying intercellular matrix. When this material is degraded, antibody binding may take place.[3]

The enzyme primarily responsible for degradation of proteoglycans in cartilage, as well as for primary activation of collagenase, is stromelysin. Treatment of cartilage explants with 3 days' exposure to 20-nM stromelysin leads to significant loss of proteoglycans, cleavage of type IX collagen that leads to tissue swelling, and loss of compressive stiffness—that crucial functional property of cartilage that enables it to quickly rebound from a deforming load.[4]

COLLAGENS AND GLYCOSAMINOGLYCANS OF CARTILAGE

As mentioned in brief in the section on **collagen** in Chapter 1, there are at least six genetic types of

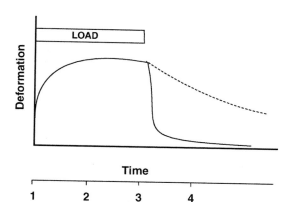

FIGURE 10–1. Graphic presentation of data from cartilage compression experiments[1] in which the rate of return to normal volume of cartilage after a deforming load was applied was measured. The solid line, after load was removed, represents the response of normal cartilage. The dotted line represents the response of cartilage depleted of proteoglycans. The slow response of proteoglycan-depleted cartilage interferes with normal mechanisms for nutrient exchange in this tissue. (Modified from Harris, E. D. Jr., Parker, H. G., Radin, E. L., et al.: Effects of proteolytic enzymes on structural and mechanical properties of cartilage. Arthritis Rheum. 15:497, 1972. Used by permission.)

collagen in cartilage, five of which (type XII is not shown) are portrayed schematically in Fig. 10–2 as they are aggregated in fibril form.[5] Four (types II, IX, X, and XI) are cartilage specific, not found in significant amounts in other tissues. Another, type VI, is more ubiquitous and may play a role in fixing synovial lining cells in place.

Type II collagen is the major fibrous collagen of cartilage, representing 80 to 90 per cent of the collagen in this tissue. It is closely linked (Fig. 10–2) with **type XI collagen,** with which it has striking sequence homology. The globular domains of type XI and the increased glycosylation of type II collagen compared with types I and III may have a role in determination of fibril diameter. The major function of type II collagen is providing the tensile strength and toughness of cartilage.

The *fibril-associated collagens* with *interrupted triple helices* (FACIT collagens) are **types IX and XII collagens.** They contribute to forming the stable meshwork with GAG in the cartilage. Type IX, for example, appears to be woven into the fibril structure with type II collagen, and also to bind strongly to GAG. As shown in Figure 10–2, the globular, amino-terminal domains project out from the fibril surface into the perifibrillar matrix. There is a site on type IX collagen molecules for specific binding of either a chondroitin sulfate or a dermatan sulfate GAG molecule. Type XII collagen is homologous to type IX and has similar structure and functions.

Type X collagen molecules form a hexagonal lattice structure that appears to be involved not in stable adult cartilage, but in the mineralization of hypertrophic cartilage and the endochondral ossification process in fracture repair.[6]

Type VI collagen has a short triple-helical domain flanked on both ends by larger globular domains. It forms beaded microfilaments and is believed to play an important role in bridging between cells and the extracellular matrix.[4] The helical portion contains numerous sequences that can support binding to cells. It also develops specific noncovalent interactions with hyaluronan.[5] It is found laced throughout the intimal lining layer of synovial cells in rheumatoid arthritis.

Surrounding the network of collagen fibrils and microfibrils in cartilage is a mesh of **hyaluronan** of high molecular weight; a large proteoglycan, **aggrecan,** binds to hyaluronan through stabilization by **link protein**[7] (see Chapter 1). Attachment regions for keratan sulfate and chondroitin sulfate polysaccharide side chains are found on the protein core of aggrecan. These proteoglycans constitute up to 10 per cent of the wet weight of cartilage, and the GAGs can absorb up to 50 times their weight in water, all of which is constrained by the network of collagens.

FORCES OF DESTRUCTION AGAINST CARTILAGE IN INFLAMMATORY ARTHRITIS

Acute joint inflammation, such as that found in the early stages of rheumatoid arthritis, can be reproduced in animals by inducing adjuvant (antigen-induced) arthritis or by injections of interleukin-1 (Fig. 10–3). In adjuvant arthritis, there is a 40 per cent loss of proteoglycan from cartilage in 1 week after the arthritis is induced; this levels off to about 50 per cent loss after 3 weeks as synthesis increases to match degradation.[8] The point of emphasis is that the damage occurs very early to proteoglycans, and the degraded GAG can be measured within the joint fluid. Neutrophil-depleted animals still had significant GAG in the joint fluid and depletion of this matrix from cartilage. The interpretation must be that inflammation induces cytokine formation by synovial cells, and that these (probably IL-1 and TNFα) induce production of enzymes (probably stromelysin) by synovial cells and chondrocytes, initiating degradation of the proteoglycan molecules. The clipped, small-molecular-weight GAGs diffuse into synovial fluid. In antigen- (ovalbumin-) induced arthritis, the synovium and not the chon-

Collagen
type

Supramolecular
structure

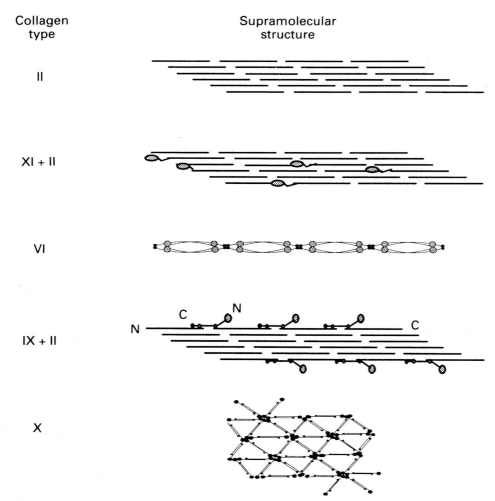

FIGURE 10–2. Diagrammatic representation of the supramolecular assemblies adopted by the cartilage collagens. Unless otherwise indicated, the molecules are oriented with their amino termini to the left. *Type II* collagen is organized into fibrils illustrated as an array of individual triple helices with a quarter-stagger of 67 nm. *Type XI* collagen forms heterotypic fibrils with type II collagen (see text), but is distinguished from type II collagen by retaining the amino-terminal NC domains as illustrated. *Type VI* collagen forms beaded microfibrils by antiparallel association of monomers into dimers, lateral association of dimers into tetramers, and end-on association of tetramers. *Type IX* collagen does not form multimeric aggregates on its own, but associates, via cross-links, with the surface of type II collagen fibrils in an antiparallel fashion (see text). The globular NC4 domain and the triple-helical COL2 domain project out from the fibril surface. *Type X* collagen molecules are thought to associate laterally and via their carboxyl-terminal NC domains to form a regular hexagonal lattice. (From Thomas, J. T., Ayad, S., and Grant, M. E.: Cartilage collagens: strategies for the study of their organisation and expression in the extracellular matrix. Ann. Rheum. Dis. 53:488, 1994. Used by permission.)

drocytes produce metalloproteases; in contrast, in a polycation- (poly-D-lysine–) induced arthritis, both the synovial lining and articular cartilage synthesize neutral metalloproteases.[9]

The same sequence must occur in rheumatoid arthritis. Cartilage from the disease taken early in the course shows normal gross appearance of the tissue but a marked depletion of proteoglycans on histologic examination[10] (Fig. 10–4).

If IL-1 is injected into rabbit knee joints, there is immediate and extensive loss of proteoglycan. If no further insults are directed at the joint, GAG synthetic rates double and the GAG is replaced to normal amounts within 3 or 4 weeks with no permanent damage to the collagen network.[11] The implications for rheumatoid arthritis are clear: If effective therapy could inhibit the immunoinflammatory reaction in the joint

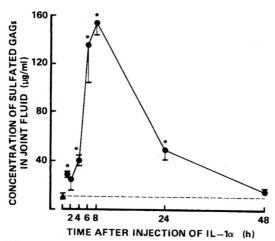

FIGURE 10-3. Levels of sulfated GAGs in fluid from joints of normal rabbits at various time points after intra-articular injection of 25 ng of IL-1α. Values are the mean and SEM of data from 3 to 10 animals. Closed triangle with bars and dashed line represents the mean $\pm$ SEM value in control, contralateral joints. *, $p<.01$ versus control. (From Pettipher, E. R., Henderson, B., Hardingham, T., et al.: Cartilage proteoglycan depletion in acute and chronic antigen-induced arthritis. Arthritis Rheum. 32:601, 1989. Used by permission.)

within the window of time before the collagen network of the cartilage is damaged, joint destruction could be avoided.

Modulation of Chondrocyte Gene Expression: A Basis for Self-Destruction of Cartilage

Human chondrocytes can be immortalized by specific transfection techniques.[12] These cells look like chondrocytes and express mRNAs that encode cartilage-specific collagens (II, IX, and XI) and proteoglycans for long periods of time. When added to these cells, IL-1β decreases the levels of type II collagen mRNA, increases the mRNAs for collagenase and stromelysin, and retards the rate of new GAG synthesis.

In cultures of fresh human chondrocytes, a definite autocrine effect of IL-1 has been noted: IL-1β induces more IL-1β production by the same cells, as well as G-CSF and GM-CSF. IL-1β is also a potent inducer of metalloproteases. IL-6 and IL-8 are produced constitutively by fresh chondrocytes in culture, and not induced by IL-1.[13]

Both tissue- and urokinase-type plasminogen activator biosynthesis are induced by IL-1 in human chondrocyte cell layers.[14] The importance of plasminogen activator in the schema of matrix destruction is as follows: Collagenase and stromelysin that are produced by chondrocytes (and synovial cells)

are in a proenzyme form. In plasma-free cultures, the proteases remain inactive unless plasminogen is added.[15] The inference must be that, as in rheumatoid synovial cell systems,[16] plasminogen activator produces plasmin from plasminogen, and the plasmin activates the stromelysin and aids stromelysin in activation of collagenase. Evidence gathered from other studies measuring IL-1–induced cartilage proteoglycan degradation suggests that cathepsin B (a lysosomal protease with a spectrum of activity near neutral pH) is also expressed by IL-1–activated chondrocytes and is capable of proteoglycan degradation.[17]

Unlike many other systems in which IL-1 and TNFα are additive, and occasionally synergistic, in

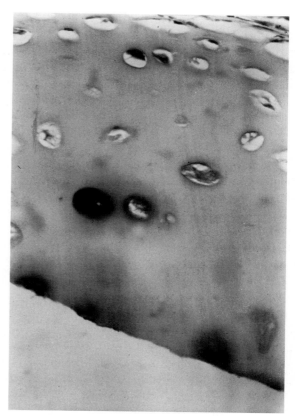

FIGURE 10-4. Human articular cartilage from active rheumatoid arthritis removed at joint arthroplasty and stained for metachromasia. The only dark metachromatic stain surrounds a few chondrocytes, which, presumably, are actively making proteoglycan only to have it broken down by proteases derived from synovial fluid, chondrocytes, or synovial tissue. The form of this depleted cartilage is normal; however, its functional capacity to rebound from a deforming load is seriously impaired. (From Harris, E. D. Jr.: Etiology and pathogenesis of rheumatoid arthritis. *In* Kelley, W. N., Harris, E. D. Jr., Ruddy, S., and Sledge, C. B. [eds.]: Textbook of Rheumatology, 4th ed., Vol. 1. Philadelphia, W. B. Saunders, 1993, pp. 833–873. Used by permission.)

the induction of inflammatory responses, these two cytokines have different effects on cartilage. For example, intra-articular IL-1 suppresses chondrocyte proteoglycan biosynthesis effectively, whereas high doses of TNFα only marginally inhibit this function.[18] Injection of antibodies against IL-1, but not anti-TNFα or anti–IL-6, prevents suppression of proteoglycan biosynthesis. In isolation, IL-6 is 1,000 times less potent than IL-1 as an inhibitor of chondrocyte proteoglycan production,[19] but there is evidence that IL-1 requires IL-6 in order to inhibit proteoglycan biosynthesis in cartilage.[20]

Protection against the Effects of Interleukin-1 on Cartilage

If IL-1 has such a major role in initiating the destructive effects upon cartilage, studies of natural or exogenous substances that inhibit IL-1 effects upon cartilage may give useful leads for therapy. One of the most promising natural substances is TGFβ. Pretreatment of cartilage explants with TGFβ prevented both IL-1–induced breakdown of collagen and IL-1–induced decrease in synthesis of collagen and GAG.[21] Good evidence has been presented that at least part of the mechanism is down-regulation of the high-affinity IL-1R on chondrocytes. In addition, TGFβ decreases metalloprotease expression by inducing a protein that binds to a specific TGFβ inhibitor element in the metalloprotease gene, resulting in a decrease in transcription.[22,23]

In organ cultures, high-molecular-weight hyaluronan prevents release of proteoglycans from cartilage matrix in the presence of IL-1 or TNFα, although it is not known whether this is an effect of inhibiting proteases, increasing synthesis, or retarding diffusion of proteoglycan fragments from the matrix.[24] These data are provocative in light of the use of high-molecular-weight hyaluronan in Europe for treatment of osteoarthritis.

An unusual protein that may have chondroprotective capabilities is produced by synovial cells, mononuclear cells, and chondrocytes during inflammatory states[25,26] and is found in high titers in synovial fluids of most arthritis patients[25]; it is named TNF-stimulated gene 6 [(TSG-6)]. This polypeptide is a member of the family of hyaluronan-binding proteins that include cartilage link protein, aggrecan, and the adhesion protein CD44.[27] Its synthesis is induced in chondrocytes by IL-1β, TNFα, PDGF, and TGFβ; this represents a rare example of TNFα, IL-1β, and TGFβ each influencing a gene expression in the same manner. Of potential importance to rheumatoid arthritis are the data showing that TSG-6 forms a stable complex

with a circulating protein inter-α-inhibitor (IαI). This binding potentiates the inhibitory effect of IαI on the activity of plasmin.[28] TSG-6 may serve as a marker for chondrocyte activation as well as being an endogenous suppressor of cartilage degradation in rheumatoid arthritis.

Glucocorticoids remain the standard against which to measure the potential of pharmacologic effects of inflammatory cytokines on cartilage. Induction of proteases from chondrocytes in culture by IL-1 is moderately well inhibited by prednisone in low doses.[29] In vivo, using experimental models of osteoarthritis, intra-articular methylprednisolone reduced pathologic lesions as well as chondrocyte stromelysin synthesis.[30] The cellular mechanism of this effect of glucocorticoids on metalloproteases is at the transcriptional level.[31] In the collagenase gene, glucocorticoids exert their action through an interaction of the glucocorticoid receptor with the activator AP-1 (Fos/Jun), leading to down-regulation of IL-1β transcription.[32]

Another antirheumatic drug, Tenidap (CP-66,248),[33] appears to suppress IL-1–induced stromelysin and collagenase production by reducing the number of IL-1 receptors,[34] not unlike a part of the actions of TGFβ. Similar effects were produced by indomethacin and naproxen, but only at concentrations well above their therapeutic ones. Glucocorticoids had no effect on IL-1R expression.

A recent European trial has examined effects on clinical measures and bone erosions of daily subcutaneous injections of IL-1ra over a 6-month period. Clinical outcome measures were reported to improve, there were no significant side effects, and a measureable slowing of progression of bone erosions (and, by extrapolation, cartilage destruction) was found. These provocative data demand confirmation, and could lead to a new adjunct in therapy of the destructive component of rheumatoid arthritis (see Chapter 8).

Influence of Inflammatory Cells in Synovial Fluid on the Destruction of Cartilage

Adding to the proteases generated by activated chondrocytes are the trapped millions of neutrophils in rheumatoid synovial fluid that have direct access to the cartilage. Once synovial inflammation begins, there are several events that facilitate this access to the macromolecules in cartilage:

- Normally, molecules such as fibromodulin and decorin, which are part of the group of glycoproteins found in cartilage matrix near the surface, prevent neutrophil adhesion or binding to collagen of anti–type II collagen antibodies. Cartilage from rheumatoid patients, more than that from those with osteoarthritis, lacks the protective surface coat[35] that prevents cells as well as immunoglobulins from binding to collagen. Neutrophil elastase, and perhaps other proteases from the neutrophil granules, disrupts the surface of articular cartilage by degrading these protective proteins.[36]

- Attachment of cells and degradation of both proteoglycans and collagens is facilitated by immunoglobulins adherent to the cartilage surface and by the synergistic action of neutrophil serine and metalloproteases released during activation of neutrophils by the surface-associated immunoglobulin.[37] Cartilage from rheumatoid patients has much more immunoglobulin bound within the surface layers than does cartilage from osteoarthritis.[38] Anti-type II collagen antibodies bind to the epitopes exposed by protease action. It also is possible that as yet poorly characterized epitopes on proteoglycans in cartilage (e.g., gp 39) exposed by proteases may act as autoantigens that draw in immunoglobulins and attract synovial cells to become invasive.[39]
- Evidence has been presented that superficial GAG loss from cartilage by neutrophils is not caused by toxic oxygen species, but rather by neutrophil proteases[40] (Fig. 10–5).
- Direct damage to cartilage by cell-free rheumatoid synovial fluid has been demonstrated, and occurs at a rate roughly proportional to the activity of disease in a given patient.[41] Normal fluids contain sufficient protease inhibitors (e.g., α_2-macroglobulin) to bind and neutralize active proteases, but 25 years ago it was demonstrated that, when synovial fluid counts of neutrophils exceeded 50,000/mm³ in synovial fluids, the protease inhibitors were saturated, allowing free metalloproteases to break down cartilage without normal restraint.[42]
- Lymphocytes within rheumatoid synovial fluid may be another cause of cartilage loss. More lysis of chondrocytes was produced by cells from rheumatoid synovial fluid than from fluids from osteoarthritis, or rheumatoid synovial tissues or blood.[43] The chondrocytolytic activity was isolated to cells that did not form rosettes with erythrocytes or express the CD3 antigen; this classifies them as NK cells. In addition, cells from rheumatoid synovium that expressed a high density of T-cell markers become endowed with chondrocytolytic activity after being incubated with recombinant IL-2. In vivo, however, there is no access for lymphocytes to chondrocytes until they are exposed, and probably dead.

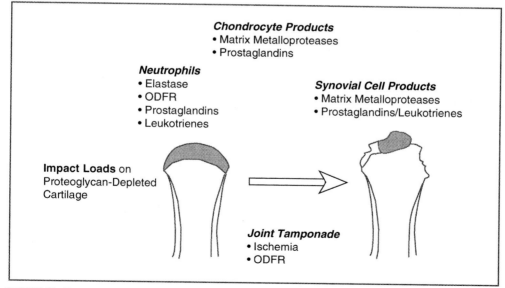

FIGURE 10–5. The diarthrodial joint is destroyed by multiple forces in rheumatoid arthritis. Proteases released by synovial cells, chondrocytes, and neutrophils are dominant, but the abnormal physiology induced by proteoglycan depletion from cartilage and ischemia from ''joint tamponade'' (see Chapter 13) contribute as well. Many processes induce formation of oxygen-derived free radicals (ODFR) (see Chapter 14). Not mentioned here are the effects of osteoclastic destruction of the underlying subchondral bone, which undermine cartilage (see Chapter 11).

Hypothesis: A Sequence That Results in Destruction of Articular Cartilage

The first assumption is that a self-sustaining synovitis begins within multiple joints. As noted previously, this involves an immune response within an immunogenetically susceptible host. It could be initiated by a retrovirus, or by an immune response against a superantigen that has epitopes mimicking host proteins, or by another cause.

Once inflammation in the synovium begins, and neutrophils follow a chemoattractant gradient to the joint fluid, cartilage degradation can occur. Neutrophils activated within the synovial fluid release proteases, particularly elastase, that degrade the glycoproteins forming a protective coat over the cartilage surface. At the same time, the neutrophil enzymes degrade proteoglycan molecules within the type II collagen matrix; the loss of these proteoglycans alters the physical properties of the cartilage. No longer can it resist the forces of a compressive load and spring back to its original size. The collagen network adsorbs water, and the cartilage swells.

Cytokines, particularly IL-1, diffuse from the activated fibroblasts and macrophages in the synovial lining into the accessible cartilage matrix, activating chondrocytes to produce collagenase and stromelysin, initiating a process of destruction from within. Immunoglobulin, particularly anti–type II collagen that has formed in response to exposed epitopes usually not seen by the adult immune system, precipitates in the cartilage surface layers. Synovial cells and macrophages find attachment sites on collagen in the exposed matrix, and begin moving as a localized malignancy into the cartilage, destroying it bit by bit.

REFERENCES

1. Harris, E. D. Jr., Parker, H. G., Radin, E. L., et al.: Effects of proteolytic enzymes on structural and mechanical properties of cartilage. Arthritis Rheum. 15:497, 1972.
2. Kempson, G. E., Muir, H., Swanson, S. A. V., et al.: Correlations between stiffness and the chemical constituents of cartilage of the human femoral head. Biochim. Biophys. Acta 215:70, 1970.
3. Jasin, H. E., Noyori, K., Takagi, T., et al.: Characteristics of anti-type II collagen antibody binding to articular cartilage. Arthritis Rheum. 36:651, 1993.
4. Bonassar, L. J., Frank, E. H., and Murray, J. C.: Changes in cartilage composition and physical properties due to stromelysin degradation. Arthritis Rheum. 38:173, 1995.
5. Thomas, J. T., Ayad, S., and Grant, M. E.: Cartilage colla-
gens: strategies for the study of their organisation and expression in the extracellular matrix. Ann. Rheum. Dis. 53:488, 1994.
6. Grant, W. T., Wang, G.-J., and Balian, G.: Type X collagen synthesis during endochondral ossification in fracture repair. J. Biol. Chem. 263:9844, 1987.
7. Rizkalla, G., Reiner, A., Bogoch, E., et al.: Studies of the articular cartilage proteoglycan aggrecan in health and osteoarthritis. J. Clin. Invest. 90:2268, 1992.
8. Pettipher, E. R., Henderson, B., Hardingham, T., et al.: Cartilage proteoglycan depletion in acute and chronic antigen-induced arthritis. Arthritis Rheum. 32:601, 1989.
9. Henderson, B., Pettipher, E. R., and Murphy, G.: Metalloproteinases and cartilage proteoglycan depletion in chronic arthritis: comparison of antigen-induced and polycation-induced arthritis. Arthritis Rheum. 33:241, 1990.
10. Hamerman, D.: Cartilage changes in the rheumatoid joint. Clin. Orthop. 64:91, 1969.
11. Page Thomas, D. P., King, B., Stephens, T., et al.: In vivo studies of cartilage regeneration after damage induced by catabolin/interleukin-1. Ann. Rheum. Dis. 50:75, 1991.
12. Goldring, M. B., Birkhead, J. R., Suen, L.-F., et al.: Interleukin-1β-modulated gene expression in immortalized human chondrocytes. J. Clin. Invest. 94:2307, 1994.
13. Seid, J. M., Rahman, S., Graveley, R., et al.: The effect of interleukin-1 on cytokine gene expression on cultured human articular chondrocytes analyzed by messenger RNA phenotyping. Arthritis Rheum. 36:35, 1993.
14. Campbell, I. K., Piccoli, D. S., Butler, D. M., et al.: Recombinant human interleukin-1 stimulates human articular cartilage to undergo resorption and human chondrocytes to produce both tissue- and urokinase-type plasminogen activator. Biochim. Biophys. Acta 967:183, 1988.
15. Cruwys, S. C., Davies, D. E., and Pettipher, E. R.: Cooperation between interleukin-1 and the fibrinolytic system in the degradation of collagen by articular chondrocytes. Br. J. Pharmacol. 100:631, 1990.
16. Werb, Z., Mainardi, C. L., Vater, C. A., et al.: Endogenous activation of latent collagenase by rheumatoid synovial cells: evidence for a role of plasminogen activator. N. Engl. J. Med. 296:1017, 1977.
17. Buttle, D. J., Handley, C. J., Ilic, M. Z., et al.: Inhibition of cartilage proteoglycan release by a specific inactivator of cathepsin B and an inhibitor of matrix metalloproteinases. Arthritis Rheum. 36:1709, 1993.
18. van de Loo, F. A. J., Joosten, L. A. B., van Lent, P. L. E. M., et al.: Role of interleukin-1, tumor necrosis factor alpha, and interleukin-6 in cartilage proteoglycan metabolism and destruction. Arthritis Rheum. 38:164, 1995.
19. Nietfeld, J. J., Wilbrink, B., Helle, M., et al.: Interleukin-1-induced interleukin-6 is required for the inhibition of proteoglycan synthesis by interleukin-1 in human articular cartilage. Arthritis Rheum. 33:1695, 1990.
20. Nietfeld, J. J., Duits, A. J., Tilanus, M. G. J., et al.: Antisense oligonucleotides, a novel tool for the control of cytokine effects on human cartilage: focus on interleukins 1 and 6 and proteoglycan synthesis. Arthritis Rheum. 37:1357, 1994.

    In this study, a modified antisense oligonucleotide was used to block IL-6 production by chondrocytes in cartilage explants. An 18-mer was chosen to optimize specificity, and the phosphate backbone was modified into phosphorothioates to give a longer half-life and better cell penetration.

21. Redini, F., Mauview, A., Pronost, S., et al.: Transforming growth factor beta exerts opposite effects from interleukin-1β on cultured rabbit articular chondrocytes through

reduction of interleukin-1 receptor expression. Arthritis Rheum. 36:44, 1993.

22. Werb, Z., and Alexander, C. M.: Proteinases and matrix degradation. *In* Kelley, W. N., Harris, E. D. Jr., Ruddy, S., and Sledge, C. B. (eds.): Textbook of Rheumatology, 4th ed., Vol. 1. Philadelphia, W. B. Saunders, 1993, pp. 248–268.

23. Kerr, L. D., Miller, D. B., and Matrisian, L. M.: TGF-β1 inhibition of transin/stromelysin gene expression is mediated through a *fos* binding sequence. Cell 61:267, 1990.

24. Shimazu, A., Jikko, A., Iwamoto, M., et al.: Effects of hyaluronic acid on the release of proteoglycan from the cell matrix in rabbit chondrocyte cultures in the presence and absence of cytokines. Arthritis Rheum. 36:247, 1993.

25. Wisniewski, H.-G., Maier, R., Lotz, M., et al.: TSG-6 a TNF-, IL-1, and LPS-inducible secreted glycoprotein associated with arthritis. J. Immunol. 151:6593, 1993.

26. Maier, R., Wisniewski, H.-G., Vilcek, J., and Lotz, M.: TSG-6 expression in human articular chondrocytes. Arthritis Rheum. 39:552, 1996.

27. Lee, T. H., Wisniewski, H.-G., and Vilcek, J.: A novel secretory tumor necrosis factor-inducible protein (TSG-6) is a member of the family of hyaluronate binding proteins, closely related to the adhesion receptor CD44. J. Cell Biol. 116:545, 1992.

28. Wisniewski, H.-G., Burgess, W. H., Oppenheim, J. D., and Vilcek, J.: TSG-6, an arthritis-associated hyaluronan binding protein, forms a stable complex with the serum protein inter-α-inhibitor. Biochemistry 33:7432, 1994.

29. Lane, N. E., Williams, R. J. III, Schurman, D. J., et al.: Inhibition of interleukin 1 induced chondrocyte protease activity by a corticosteroid and a nonsteroidal antiinflammatory drug. J. Rheumatol. 19:135, 1992.

30. Pelletier, J.-P., Mineau, F., Raynauld, J.-P., et al.: Intraarticular injections with methylprednisolone acetate reduce osteoarthritic lesions in parallel with chondrocyte stromelysin synthesis in experimental osteoarthritis. Arthritis Rheum. 37:414, 1994.

31. Frisch, S. M., and Ruley, H. E.: Transcription from the stromelysin promoter is induced by interleukin-1 and repressed by dexamethasone. J. Biol. Chem. 262:16300, 1987.

    This paper identifies nucleotide sequences that confer inducibility of stromelysin by IL-1 and repression by glucocorticoids.

32. Jonat, C., Rahmsdorf, H. J., Park, K. K., et al.: Antitumor promotion and anti-inflammation: down-modulation of AP-1 (Fos/Jun) activity by glucocorticoid hormone. Cell 62:1189, 1990.

33. Moilanen, E., Alanko, J., Asmawi, M. Z., et al.: CP-66,248, a new anti-inflammatory agent, is a new potent inhibitor of leukotriene B4 and prostanoid synthesis in human polymorphonuclear leukocytes *in vitro*. Eicosanoids 1:35, 1988.

34. Pelletier, J.-P., McCollum, R., Dibattista, J., et al.: Regulation of human normal and osteoarthritic chondrocyte interleukin-1 receptor by antirheumatic drugs. Arthritis Rheum. 36:1517, 1993.

35. Noyori, K., Koshino, T., Takagi, T., et al.: Binding characteristics of anti-type II collagen antibody to the surface of diseased human cartilage as a probe for tissue damage. J. Rheumatol. 21:293, 1994.

36. Jasin, H. E., and Taurog, J. D.: Mechanisms of disruption of the articular cartilage surface in inflammation: neutrophil elastase increases availability of collagen type II epitopes for binding with antibody on the surface of articular cartilage. J. Clin. Invest. 87:1531, 1991.

37. Chatham, W. W., Swaim, R., Frohsin, H. Jr., et al.: Degradation of human articular cartilage by neutrophils in synovial fluid. Arthritis Rheum. 36:51, 1993.

38. Jasin, H. E.: Autoantibody specificities of immune complexes sequestered in articular cartilage of patients with rheumatoid arthritis and osteoarthritis. Arthritis Rheum. 28:241, 1985.

39. Goodacre, J. A., and Pearson, J. P.: Human cartilage proteoglycans as T cell autoantigens. Ann. Rheum. Dis. 51:1094, 1992.

40. Moore, A. R., Iwamura, H., Larbre, J. P., et al.: Cartilage degradation by polymorphonuclear leukocytes: in vitro assessment of the pathogenic mechanisms. Ann. Rheum. Dis. 52:27, 1992.

41. Larbre, J.-P., Moore, A. R., Da Silva, J. A. P., et al.: Direct degradation of articular cartilage by rheumatoid synovial fluid: contribution of proteolytic enzymes. J. Rheumatol. 21:1796, 1994.

    More than half of rheumatoid synovial fluids induced significant GAG loss from cartilage, as did 3 of 15 osteoarthritic synovial fluids. Serine protease inhibitors, as well as a specific elastase inhibitor, blocked this element of cartilage destruction.

42. Harris, E. D. Jr., DiBona, D. R., and Krane, S. M.: Collagenases in human synovial fluid. J. Clin. Invest. 48:2104, 1969.

43. Yamaga, K. M., Bolen, H., Kimura, L., et al.: Enhanced chondrocyte destruction by lymphokine-activated killer cells. Arthritis Rheum. 36:500, 1993.

11

The Pannus-Cartilage Junction: Focus of the Destructive Process

The many steps in the pathophysiology of rheumatoid arthritis that have been described thus far combine to provide a mechanism for the destruction of cartilage (see Chapter 10) and the subchondral bone. In analyzing this process of joint destruction, there are three major questions for which answers are needed to make the process comprehensible:

1. Does the histopathology of the invasive process give clues about the cellular mechanisms of joint destruction?

2. What are the elements attracting the proliferative synovium toward and into the cartilage and bone?

3. What are the principal enzymes involved in the destruction of joints?

The first two questions are discussed in this chapter; the enzymes that are involved in joint destruction are the subject of Chapter 12.

HISTOPATHOLOGY OF JOINT DESTRUCTION AND INFERENCES GAINED FROM IT

The histologic appearance of the zone in which cartilage is being destroyed varies both within a single joint and among different joints. An example of *interjoint* variations is found in studies of the cartilage-pannus junction from multiple sections of many joints.[1] In small, non-weight-bearing joints, such as the metacarpophalangeal joints, invasive stellate cells are observed in close contact with cartilage collagen in a matrix largely depleted of proteoglycans (Fig. 11–1). In contrast, in weight-bearing joints such as the knee, a transitional zone of fibroblast-like cells with a matrix rich in both collagen and keratan sulfate separates the cartilage from the more cellular pannus.[1] In those areas where a

well-defined, invasive cartilage-pannus junction is found, the underlying cartilage is depleted of chondrocytes and in poor condition, whereas chondrocytes underlying the transitional fibroblastic zone are abundant and functioning well, judging by the abundant proteoglycans that they are synthesizing. Understanding the reasons for these differences in appearance of the cartilage-pannus junction at different sites may provide significant help in sorting out the mechanisms of joint destruction.

A good argument can be made that there are three elements that determine the histopathology of the cartilage-pannus junction, and therefore the manner in which joints are destroyed:

- The **rate** at which the destructive process moves
- The degree of **protective response** mounted by cartilage and bone
- An intrinsic **cycling** or **pulsing** of the process so that, in one area of the joint, rapid destruction may be followed by a quiescent phase of relatively little enzymatic destruction and increased matrix formation (a reparative process).

That there are differences in *rate* of joint destruction is the element best defended. In one joint, for example, there may be pockets of neutrophils forming true abscesses in small foci, generating necrotic holes in cartilage in front of the encroaching pannus.[2] This is a rare finding in rheumatoid arthritis because neutrophils are not a common finding in the synovium or pannus. However, when present, tissue destruction at the base of these abscesses is rapid. Also rare, but equally indicative of rapid destruction of cartilage, is the finding by electron microscopy of infiltrating pannus cells containing intact fragments of cartilage collagen within phagolysosomes[3] (Fig. 11–2). Direct contact with the cartilage collagen was made by invasive cells that were sufficiently aggressive to engulf entire

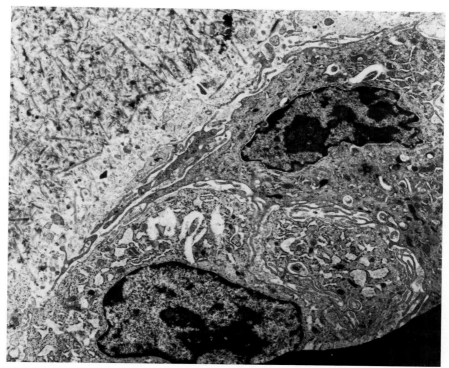

FIGURE 11–1. Low-power electron micrograph illustrating the synovial cell–cartilage junction from a metacarpophalangeal joint replaced at surgery in a 52-year-old woman. The articular cartilage is on the left. Linear, dark-staining collagen fibers are visible. On the right are two invading cells with different morphology. The upper right cell has more cell processes and vacuoles; it resembles a macrophage. The lower cell has a highly developed endoplasmic reticulum and resembles a fibroblast. The light-staining area, no more than 5 to 10 μm wide, represents the area of cartilage destruction by enzymes secreted from the invasive pannus. There is no transitional zone of fibroblast-like cells. (Courtesy of D. R. DiBona, Ph.D., Massachusetts General Hospital.)

components of fibrils and begin a process of intra-lysosomal degradation of them.

The most common mechanism of cartilage degradation takes place at a moderate, well-regulated pace. On histopathology, one observes pannus cells close to the cartilage margin. A narrow zone (no more than 5 to 10 μm wide) (Fig. 11–3) containing amorphous debris exists between pannus cell processes and the collagen fibers, and amorphous material representing proteoglycans and their breakdown products. The amorphous zone represents an area where cartilage destruction is taking place[4] at a steady rate, but not as fast as destruction characterized by microabscesses or cartilage collagen fragments found in phagolysosomes. These areas of penetration by stellate cells are trailed by collections of immunocytes, fibroblasts, and macrophages. Capillaries follow as well, but rarely penetrate closer than 100 μm from the pannus-cartilage junction; nevertheless, they are the supply line of nutrients and oxygen for these active invasive cells.

This form of invasion—cellular fingers composed of activated synovial lining cells (Fig. 11–4)—is probably the one operating at the beginning of cartilage destruction at the periphery near the cartilage-bone junction[5] that commences within months after the rheumatoid synovial inflammation becomes sustained. In areas such as these, many of the chondrocytes adjacent to the invasive front and in deeper zones of cartilage as well have much larger than normal lacunae surrounding them (Fig. 11–5), suggesting that they have responded to cytokine diffusion from the synovitis in a way to activate their expression of metalloproteases. It is in areas such as these, stripped of protective proteoglycans and near capillaries, that antibodies can interact with antigens. These immune complexes are then deposited in superficial layers of cartilage. The development of specific antibodies that react with degraded type II collagen peptides has enabled immunoelectron microscopic localization of these cleaved fragments in cartilage from rheumatoid joints. It has been confirmed that morphologically recognizable damage to type II collagen fibrils accompanies antibody binding.[6]

Slower rates of cartilage loss probably occur in

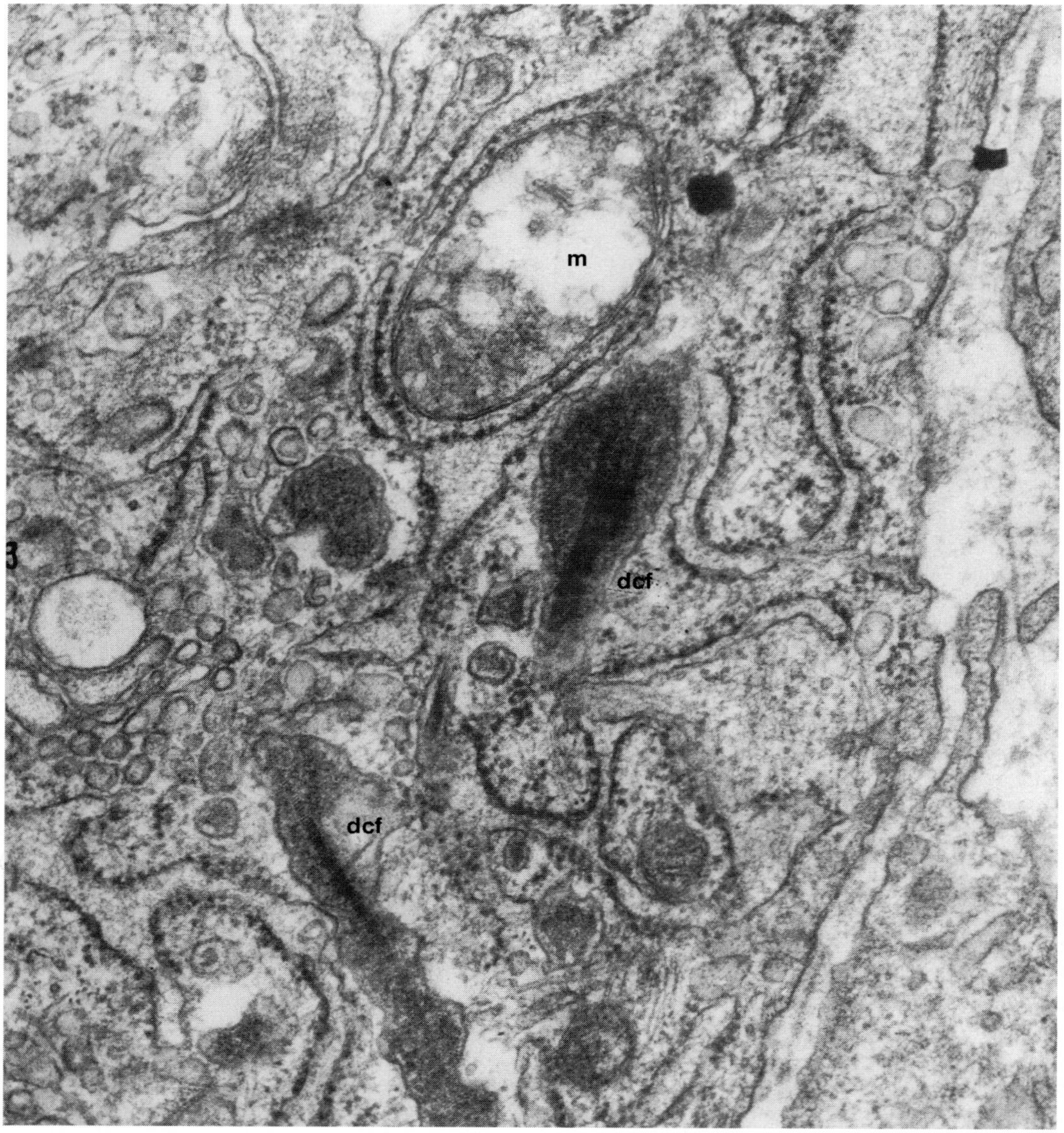

FIGURE 11–2. *A*, High-power transmission electron micrograph showing detail from a cell closely abutting (without any "clear zone" as in Fig. 11–1) articular cartilage at a focus of fast erosion in rheumatoid arthritis. Within lysosomes are collagen fibrils (dcf) being degraded. In this case an aggressive pannus has phagocytosed particulate collagen rather than "waiting" as enzymes released into the extracellular space degrade the cartilage. At the right (top to bottom) is the gap between the cell on the left and another cell. g, Golgi apparatus; m, mitochondrion. (Courtesy of Audrey Glauert, Ph.D., Strangeways Laboratory, Cambridge, England.) *Illustration continued on opposite page*

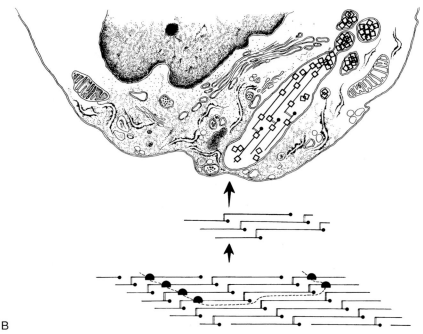

B

FIGURE 11–2. *Continued B*, Illustration of the probable sequence leading to active phagocytosis of collagen fragments by invasive synovial tissue. Molecules are either cleaved at cross-linked regions (vertical lines in schematized fiber) or cleaved by collagenase (at the dark half-circles) to make aggressive phagocytosis possible.

areas mentioned earlier, characterized by a layer of transitional fibroblasts between cartilage and more cellular pannus,[1] or in areas of relatively avascular pannus adjacent to invasive tongues of pannocytes (Fig. 11–5). It can be inferred that there is only minimal activity of free and active proteases in these areas, and that "reparative" cytokines, such as TGFβ, are dominant, inducing synthesis of more matrix proteins. It is in these areas that the reparative attempts by chondrocytes are apparent. Because the fibroblast-like cells in this transitional zone have been shown to be capable of producing keratan sulfate, it is believed that they are derived from articular cartilage rather than from the adjacent synovial membrane.[7] Chondrocytes in cartilage below this transitional fibroblastic zone are metabolically active, stimulated to produce matrix proteoglycans and collagen in response to cytokines from the synovium. This is a protective response. In considering why this transitional fibroblastic zone is more commonly found in larger joints, such as the knees and hips, it has been argued that weight bearing itself may induce chondrocytes to generate more matrix collagen and proteoglycans than are produced by chondrocytes in finger joints.[1] A more vigorous reparative response could retard the finger-like penetration of synovial invasion. This could explain why erosions are more commonly seen earlier in non-weight-bearing than in weight-bearing joints.

It is virtually impossible to have access to tissue from the same area of a pannus-cartilage junction in the same joint at different time periods. Therefore, the possibility that there is an ebb and flow of invasiveness at the same place at the interface between synovium and cartilage cannot be tested. A best guess is that it does happen, that periods of a rapid rate of destruction at one site by aggressive phagocytosis of collagen type II fibers and maximal production by stellate cells of metalloproteases could be followed by a quiet period when more reparative mechanisms dominate, a transitional fibroblastic zone is produced, and matrix synthesis—but ineffective repair—exceeds release of destructive enzymes.

Subchondral Mechanisms of Bone and Cartilage Destruction

Joint destruction also occurs from the subchondral areas of joints. One apparent mechanism is large multinucleate cells that have been called "**chondroclasts**." They are directly involved in degradation of articular cartilage.[8] Special stains show abundant acid phosphatase, and electron micrographs reveal ruffled borders at the interface

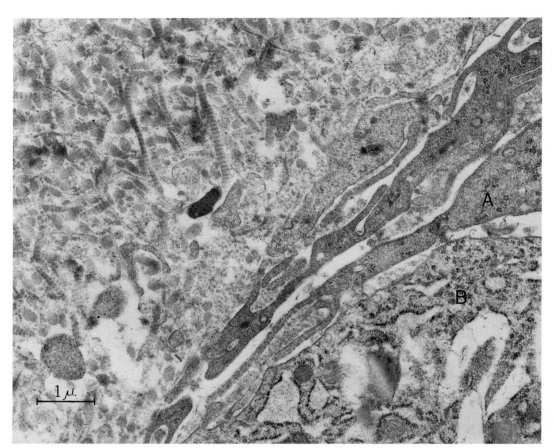

FIGURE 11–3. Higher power view of the pannus-cartilage junction from a proximal interphalangeal joint of a 45-year-old man with rheumatoid arthritis. The 760-Å periodicity of cartilage collagen is visible. There are portions of two "pannocytes" on the right, one (A) with darker cytoplasm and multiple cell processes, the other (B) with a well-developed endoplasmic reticulum. There is a distinct amorphous zone between the cells and collagen fibrils where it can be inferred that proteases released into the extracellular space have degraded both collagen and GAGs. (Courtesy of D. R. DiBona, Ph.D., Massachusetts General Hospital.)

with cartilage, just as ruffled borders at the bone-osteoclast interface are found.

Although metalloproteases are necessary and sufficient to destroy cartilage and other soft connective tissues, additional mechanisms are necessary to break down bone. Mineral (i.e., calcium hydroxyapatite) must be dissolved before collagen and matrix glycoproteins can be degraded. The very specialized **osteoclast** does both jobs. Osteoclasts are derived from a primitive cell in the monocyte lineage. They are formed through a combination of effects of a cytokine (M-CSF), differentiation factors generated by stromal cells in response to PGE_2, parathyroid hormone, and inflammatory cytokines such as IL-6 and IL-11. Bradykinin elaborated by neutrophils may stimulate osteoclastic bone degradation by enhancing endogenous prosta-

glandin formation in the local areas adjacent to bone.[9] Essential for dissolving mineral is having a tight junction between the bone and the leading edge (the ruffled border) of the osteoclast. This is accomplished by adherence of the $\alpha V \beta 3$ integrin on the cell to osteopontin on the bone surface. The osteoclast pumps protons into the extracellular pocket, decreasing pH. The mineral dissolves, and then matrix metalloproteases (MMPs) 1, 3, and 9, and acid proteases such as cathepsin B and L, degrade the matrix glycoproteins and collagen. Studies using in situ hybridization and an antisense probe have revealed MMP-9 in high density within osteoclasts at the border between bone and invasive synovial tissue osteoclasts.[10] MMP-9 cleaves cross-link–containing amino-terminal telopeptides of collagen chains, denatured colla-

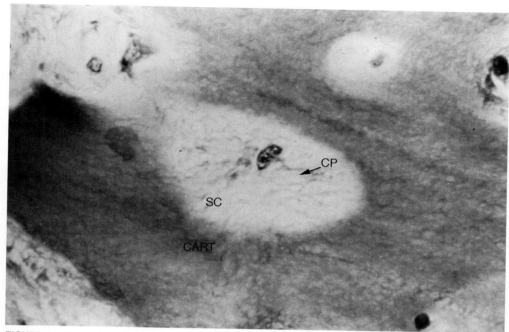

FIGURE 11–4. Specimen from a proximal interphalangeal joint in a 34-year-old man with active rheumatoid arthritis. This single invasive cell (SC) has penetrated the cartilage matrix (CART) from the invasive pannus off the left upper part of the photomicrograph. The clear area is a large area representing matrix degraded to soluble ''soup'' by stromelysin, collagenase, cathepsin B, and possibly other proteases. (Courtesy of Forst Brown, M.D., Dartmouth-Hitchcock Medical Center.)

FIGURE 11–5. Several important features of invasive rheumatoid arthritis are visible in this photomicrograph from a metacarpophalangeal joint. This section includes the surface of the pannus (P) and extends down through the subchondral plate into the bone marrow.

- A portion of subchondral bone has been totally resorbed (B).
- The cellular pannus that has peninsulas of invasion is very vascular (V), whereas a less cellular, less invasive component (PC) has very few blood vessels.
- Chondrocytes and invasive fingers of pannocytes look very similar, but the larger-than-normal lacunae around the chondrocytes imply that they have been activated sufficiently to produce proteases that have degraded pericellular matrix.
- Although the apparent joint space could look normal radiographically, this cartilage is completely nonfunctional.

(Courtesy of Drs. Forst Brown and Charles Faulkner, Dartmouth-Hitchcock Medical Center.)

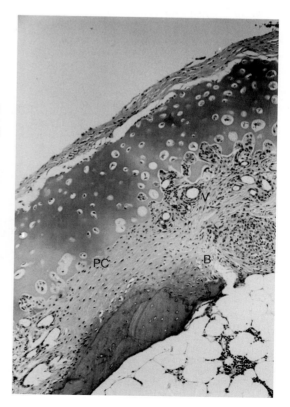

gen (all types), and native collagen types III, IV, and V.

In rheumatoid arthritis, synovial inflammation and proliferation are responsible for the osteoclastic erosion of bone in the same way that they cause the invasion of cartilage. Macrophages isolated from rheumatoid synovium are capable of producing extensive "roughening" of bone.[11] Although not the same as resorptive pit formation by osteoclasts or chondroclasts found in this tissue, this process independently resorbs bone (Fig. 11-6). Indeed, the cellular and enzymatic machinery for bone degradation may be more efficient than that for cartilage, because it is not unusual for a "lip" of articular cartilage to form as underlying subchondral bone is degraded faster than the overlying cartilage. One

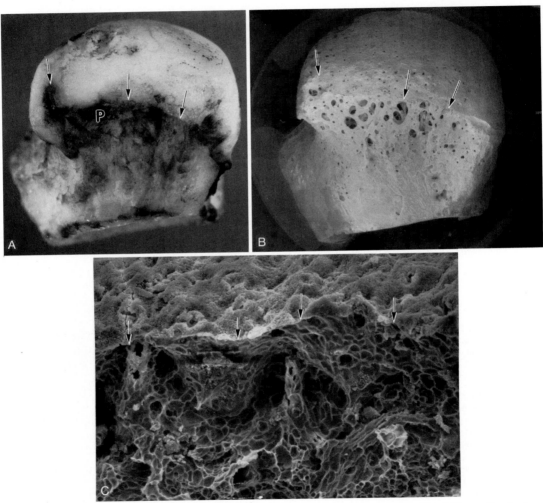

FIGURE 11-6. *A*, Gross view of the volar (palmar) surface of a left third finger metacarpal head. The eroding front (arrows) of the pannus (P) stained with India ink is shown. (×8) *B*, Gross view of the volar surface of the same left third finger metacarpal head after chemical maceration. The eroding front adjacent to the pannus is delineated (arrows). Various-sized holes, which differ from penetrations through the subchondral plate, are seen in the bony surface originally covered by the pannus. (×8) *C*, The eroding front (arrows) at the junction of pannus with the layer of calcified cartilage and subchondral bone is obvious in the macerated sample viewed with the scanning electron microscope at a higher magnification. The calcified cartilage and subchondral bone originally covered by the pannus show confluent lacunae typical of the pattern of osteoclastic resorption. (×270) (Courtesy of J. C. C. Leisen, M.D., and Howard Duncan, M.D., Henry Ford Hospital.) (From Harris, E. D. Jr.: Etiology and pathogenesis of rheumatoid arthritis. *In* Kelley, W. N., Harris, E. D. Jr., Ruddy, S., and Sledge, C. B. [eds.]: Textbook of Rheumatology, 4th ed., Vol. 1. Philadelphia, W. B. Saunders, 1993, pp. 833–873. Used by permission.)

factor retarding cartilage degradation may be the endogenous protease inhibitors synthesized in this tissue.[12,13]

FORCES ATTRACTING RHEUMATOID SYNOVIUM INTO CARTILAGE

Were it not for the centripetal polarization of the invasion of joints, rheumatoid synovium would spread as a tumor in all directions, perhaps even degrading the joint capsule and eroding into the fascia. Of course, that does not happen; the destructive synovitis moves toward the center of each joint. In contrast, in the sublining layers of rheumatoid synovium and joint capsule there is a proliferative (reparative) response. Much new collagen and matrix glycoproteins are laid down in a relatively acellular pattern. Fibroblasts there produce matrix, not active metalloproteases. Although it is not documented in a quantitative manner, we can assume that, while at the pannus-cartilage junction, the synovial cells are stimulated to produce proteases by cytokines such as IL-1 and TNFα,[14,15] leading to an excess of active proteases over tissue- and fluid-phase inhibitors of proteases. The reverse must be true in the deep synovium and capsule. Here one can hypothesize that TGFβ and other "reparative" cytokines induce new matrix biosynthesis, and that tissue inhibitor of metalloproteases (TIMP) is generated in quantities sufficient to cancel out active proteases.

What attracts the synovium to cartilage and bone? For cartilage, the standing hypothesis is that immune complexes or chondrocyte membrane components act as cytoattractants for the pannus. A high proportion of patients with rheumatoid arthritis have immunoglobulins and complement in the superficial layers of articular cartilage[16] (see Chapter 10). These deposits extend deep into the cartilage, and extraction studies have suggested that IgG is bound to cartilage by antigen-antibody bonds.[17] IgG deposits are virtually absent in areas of cartilage directly under invasive synovial cells; the inference is that synovial macrophages have ingested them.[18] It is a logical hypothesis that these immune deposits activate macrophages near the synovial lining layer, and that the gradient of cytokines generated by these macrophages impels the synovial lining and dendritic cells toward and into the cartilage (Fig. 11–7).

There are additional candidate stimuli for generating this polarization of the pannus. One is related to the striking T-cell reactivity toward chondrocyte

The Invasion of Cartilage by Rheumatoid Synovium

From data now available, the following sequence is a reasonable hypothesis as to why rheumatoid synovium begins and continues invasion of cartilage (this extends the hypothesis in the box on page 156):

1. As the synovium consolidates into fronds with activated lining cells and subsynovial lymphocyte foci, several actions affect the articular cartilage:
   a. Elastase and other proteases from neutrophils in the joint fluid degrade the proteoglycans in the superficial layers of cartilage.
   b. Depletion of proteoglycans enables immune complexes (both preformed and those of IgG/type II cartilage collagen) to precipitate in the superficial layers of collagen.
   c. Loss of cartilage proteoglycans exposes previously "hidden" chondrocytes; synovial lymphocytes proliferate in response to chondrocyte membranes.
2. Macrophages are drawn to the immune complexes, and lymphocytes to the chondrocytes. It is possible that they "drag" the pannocytes (the specialized mesenchymal cells on the synovial lining surface) over the partially damaged cartilage, where they bind to fibronectin and collagen via their expressed adhesion molecules.
3. Metalloproteases released by the stellate pannocytes begin the sequence of collagen loss and pannus spread. As the process continues micron by micron, synovial macrophages phagocytose cartilage-bound immune complexes, renewing activation.
4. Chondrocytes activated by cytokines (e.g., TNFα and IL-1) from the synovium express metalloproteases that cause loss of matrix and collagen around them. This exposure makes their immunogenic cell membrane proteins more accessible to APCs, leading to subsequent activation of T-cell clones.
5. Depending on the *intensity* of the forces driving the proliferative lesion, the *rate* of destruction of cartilage will vary, leading to differences (see earlier) in the histopathologic appearance of the pannus-cartilage junction.

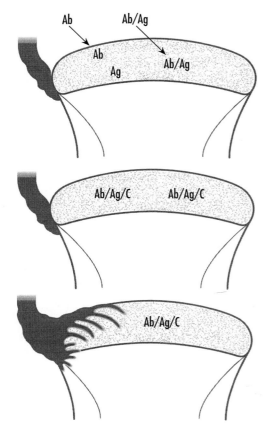

FIGURE 11–7. Is the deposition of antigen (Ag), antibody (Ab), and complement (C) within superficial layers of articular cartilage an attractant for the invasive synovial pannus in rheumatoid arthritis? Another possible attractant is an autoimmune response against some chondrocyte membrane component.

cell membranes. This reactivity, found both in peripheral blood T cells and in synovial T cells in rheumatoid arthritis, far exceeds responses of the same cells to contact with cell membranes from fibroblasts or epithelial cells.[19] These studies were initiated by the finding of serum autoantibodies against chondrocyte cell surface proteins in patients with osteoarthritis or rheumatoid arthritis.[20] Other studies have suggested that, after proteases from inflammation deplete surface proteoglycans and glycoproteins from cartilage, fibronectin in these superficial regions of cartilage enables binding of pannocytes to the altered cartilage.[21]

REFERENCES

1. Allard, S. A., Muirden, K. D., and Maini, R. N.: Correlation of histopathological features of pannus with patterns of damage in different joints in rheumatoid arthritis. Ann. Rheum. Dis. 50:278, 1991.
2. Mohr, W., and Wessinhage, D.: The relationship between polymorphonuclear granulocytes and cartilage destruction in rheumatoid arthritis. J. Rheumatol. 37:81, 1978.
3. Harris, E. D. Jr., Glauert, A. M., and Murley, A. H. G.: Intracellular collagen fibers at the pannus-cartilage junction in rheumatoid arthritis. Arthritis Rheum. 20:657, 1977.
4. Harris, E. D. Jr., DiBona, D. R., and Krane, S. M.: A mechanism for cartilage destruction in rheumatoid arthritis. Trans. Assoc. Am. Physicians 83:267, 1970.
5. Kingsley-Mills, W. M.: Pathology of the knee joint in rheumatoid arthritis. J Bone Joint Surg. 52:746, 1970.
6. Dodge, G. R., Pidoux, I., and Poole, A. R.: The degradation of type II collagen in rheumatoid arthritis: an immuno-electron microscopic study. Matrix 11:330, 1991.
7. Muirden, K. D., Allard, S. A., Rogers, K., et al.: Immuno-electron microscopy of chondrocyte-derived cells in the rheumatoid cartilage-pannus junction. Rheumatol. Int. 8:231, 1988.
8. Bromley, M., and Woolley, D. E.: Chondroclasts and osteoclasts at subchondral sites of erosion in the rheumatoid joint. Arthritis Rheum. 27:968, 1984.
9. Lerner, U. H., Jones, I. L., and Gustafson, G. T.: Bradykinin, a new potential mediator of inflammation-induced bone resorption. Arthritis Rheum. 30:530, 1987.
10. Okada, Y., Naka, K., Kawamura, K., et al.: Localization of matrix metalloproteinase 9 (92-kilodalton gelatinase/type IV collagenase = gelatinase B) in osteoclasts: implications for bone resorption. Lab. Invest. 72:311, 1995.
11. Chang, J. S., Quinn, J. M., Demaziere, A., et al.: Bone resorption by cells isolated from rheumatoid synovium. Ann. Rheum. Dis. 51:1223, 1992.
12. Kuettner, K. E., Harper, E. J., and Eisenstein, R.: Protease inhibitors in cartilage. Arthritis Rheum. 20:5124, 1977.
13. Fassbender, H. G., Seibel, M., and Herbert, T.: Pathways of destruction in metacarpal and metatarsal joints of patients with rheumatoid joints. Scand. J. Rheumatol. 21:10, 1992.

   In this study, 219 metatarsal and 69 metacarpal heads obtained during surgery on rheumatoid patients were evaluated histologically. In 15 per cent, invasion by proliferative synovium of only the articular cartilage was found; in 49 per cent, invasion exclusively of the cortical subchondral bone was observed; and in 36 per cent, a "forceps-like" invasion of both cartilage and bone, sometimes producing a "lip" of cartilage, was seen.

14. Deleuran, B. W., Chu, C.-Q., Field, M., et al.: Localization of tumor necrosis factor receptors in the synovial tissue and cartilage-pannus junction in patients with rheumatoid arthritis: implications for local actions of tumor necrosis factor α. Arthritis Rheum. 35:1170, 1992.

   The two TNFα receptor components—p55 and p75 TNFR—were searched for in rheumatoid synovial membranes using monoclonal antibodies and immunofluorescent staining techniques. The receptor(s) were detectable in 90 per cent of the cells in the lining layer, particularly in pannus cells invading cartilage, in close proximity to cells expressing the ligand, TNFα. In osteoarthritic and normal synovial samples, the expression of TNFR was at a much lower intensity.

15. Deleuran, B. W., Chu, C. Q., Field, M., et al.: Localization of interleukin-1α, type 1 interleukin-1 receptor and interleukin-1 receptor antagonist in the synovial membrane and cartilage/pannus junction in rheumatoid arthritis. Br. J. Rheumatol. 31:801, 1992.

   Using monoclonal antibodies and immunofluorescence, it was observed that, although 90 per cent of the cells at the pannus-cartilage junction expressed IL-1 and IL-1R, the antagonist (inhibitor) of the IL-1R (IL-1ra) was present in less than 10 per cent of the cells. IL-1ra was much more abundant in sublining cells of the synovium.

16. Cooke, T. D., Hurd, E. R., Jasin, H. E., et al.: Identification of immunoglobulins and complement in rheumatoid articular collagenous tissues. Arthritis Rheum. 18:541, 1975.

17. Mannik, M., and Person, R. E.: Immunoglobulin G and serum albumin isolated from the articular cartilage of patients with rheumatoid arthritis or osteoarthritis contain covalent heteropolymers with proteoglycans. Rheumatol. Int. 13:121, 1993.

18. Shiozawa, S., Jasin, H. E., and Ziff, M.: Absence of immunoglobulins in rheumatoid cartilage-pannus junction. Arthritis Rheum. 33:768, 1980.

19. Alsalameh, S., Mollenhauer, J., Hain, N., et al.: Cellular immune response toward human articular chondrocytes: T cell reactivities against chondrocyte and fibroblast membranes in destructive joint diseases. Arthritis Rheum. 33:1477, 1990.

20. Mollenhauer, J., von der Mark, K., Burmester, G. R., et al.: Serum autoantibodies against chondrocyte cell surface proteins in osteoarthritis and rheumatoid arthritis. J. Rheumatol. 15:1811, 1988.

21. Shiozawa, S., Yoshihara, R., Kuroki, Y., et al.: Pathogenic importance of fibronectin in the superficial region of articular cartilage as a local factor for the induction of pannus extension on rheumatoid articular cartilage. Ann. Rheum. Dis. 51:869, 1992.

12

Enzymes Responsible for Joint Destruction

In the early 1960s, there was a basic understanding of the nature of the proteins forming the cartilage, bone, and tendons in and around joints. Collagen was recognized as the principal structural protein of these tissues, but there was no known enzymatic mechanism for destruction of cartilage, despite the ample evidence from rheumatoid histopathology that it was happening, sometimes at a rapid rate.

Drawing on techniques developed to demonstrate a true collagenase in amphibian tissues,[1] collagenase activity was found in explants of rheumatoid synovium placed in culture upon a substratum of native collagen.[2] The rheumatoid collagenase, as well as similar enzymes identified later from many other mammalian tissues from healthy and diseased animals or humans, had a unique mechanism of action. At neutral pH, it cleaved native collagen at one locus on the molecule, approximately three quarters from the amino-terminal end (see Figs. 1–8, 1–9, and 1–10 in Chapter 1). After being cleaved at physiologic temperatures, the two fragments of the native collagen denatured from their triple-helical structure to gelatin, and could be further degraded by many different proteases in tissues or within lysosomes. The rate-limiting step of collagen breakdown is the initial cut through the triple-helical collagen molecule.

In subsequent years, active collagenase was identified in culture medium from explants of synovitis of many different etiologies. Active collagenase was found in rheumatoid synovial fluid, although it was not known whether its source was synovium or neutrophils that contained a similar collagenase in specific granules.

Active collagenase could not be demonstrated in extracts of rheumatoid synovium, however, generating the concern that finding such enzymes in culture medium from explants of tissue was little more than an artifact of tissue culture. This problem was solved in the 1970s by the demonstration that collagenase was released into the extracellular space as a latent enzyme. The latent enzyme was shown to be a proenzyme that could be activated in tissues by specific and nonspecific mechanisms. The conformational integrity of this zinc-containing protease, interstitial collagenase, was dependent upon the presence of calcium ions. It has been labeled MMP-1. (For a review of factors involved in the regulation of mammalian collagenases, see ref. 3.)

The MMP family is now at least 13 in number. The important ones for considering damage to tissue in rheumatoid arthritis are

MMP-1—interstitial collagenase

MMP-2—gelatinase/type IV collagenase

MMP-3—stromelysin 1

MMP-8—neutrophil collagenase

MMP-9—gelatinase/type V collagenase

MMP-13—interstitial collagenase with capability to degrade cross-link region; active against type II collagen more than is MMP-1 (H. Welgus, personal communication)

Stromelysin may be the most important of these enzymes because it is needed in active form for full activation of collagenase, and because it can degrade proteoglycan core protein, types IV and IX collagens, denatured types I and II collagens, fibronectin, and other matrix components. A new epitope created only by cleavage of aggrecan by stromelysin (VDIPEN[4]) can be found very early by immunochemical techniques deep in cartilage of mice immunized to develop collagen-induced arthritis. The neoepitope appears before any histologic damage or clinical symptoms are present, establishing that activity of stromelysin in breaking down proteoglycans must be one of the earliest events in what is to become a destructive inflammatory arthritis.[4]

Stromelysin is more abundant and is found more consistently in different samples from different rheumatoid synovium than is either **gelatinase** or **collagenase**.[5,6] Stromelysin and collagenase are both found in more abundant quantities in the synovial lining layers than in underlying subsynovial mesenchymal tissue, underscoring the phenotyping differences between these lining cells of rheumatoid synovium and other connective tissue cells in the same tissue (see Chapter 10).

A direct correlation between amounts of stromelysin mRNA and collagenase mRNA has been found in rheumatoid lining cells.[7] The cells responsible for secretion of stromelysin in the synovial lining have the phenotype of synovial fibroblasts (type B cells) rather than synovial macrophages.[8] In a comprehensive study of synovial fluid and synovial tissue biopsies using ELISA assays and immunohistochemical stains, the following correlations were made[9]:

- Collagenase (MMP-1) levels in synovial fluid correlated positively with the degree of synovial inflammation.
- Collagenase levels in synovial fluid increased with increasing numbers of cells staining positively for collagenase in synovial lining cells.
- The ratios of collagenase to TIMP correlated with collagenase activity in the fluids.
- Synovial fluid collagenase concentrations did not correlate with C-reactive protein levels in serum, supporting observations that there often is a dichotomy between the inflammatory and proliferative components of rheumatoid arthritis.

In immunohistologic sections of the pannus-cartilage junction, both collagenase and stromelysin are present in much greater quantity there than in tissue only 20 to 50 μm on either side of this junction.[10,11] It is presumed that localized higher concentrations of metalloprotease inducers are present at the narrow interface zone between invasive tissue and cartilage. Using a double-antibody ELISA assay for prostromelysin (MMP-3), it has been shown that serum levels of this proenzyme are increased up to ninefold in the inflammatory arthritides, but not in sera from patients with noninflammatory arthritis or from patients with heightened acute-phase reactants as a result of multiple organ failure.[12]

Studies of procollagenase and prostromelysin mRNA in adult articular cartilage samples give results that are consistent with what one sees in histologic sections early in rheumatoid arthritis. mRNA for stromelysin is abundant and rapidly induced by IL-1, whereas neither collagenase mRNA nor TIMP mRNA is found in significant quantities.[13] The inference is that, in response to IL-1 from inflamed synovium, stromelysin is produced by chondrocytes. The activated enzyme degrades proteoglycans in the matrix, harming the functional capabilities of the cartilage and perhaps facilitating degradation of the collagen at the cartilage-pannus interface by collagenase.

As in many systems, the balance between an agonist and its inhibitors is of great importance in determining which direction a pathway will go. For the metalloproteases, the ratio of TIMP to active enzymes is believed to be important. Although immunostaining cannot be absolutely quantitated, interesting data have come from studies of expression of stromelysin and TIMP mRNAs in various areas of rheumatoid synovium[14]:

- Both stromelysin and TIMP are expressed in synovial lining cells, similar to collagenase.
- In subsynovial tissues, many TIMP-positive/stromelysin-negative cells are seen.
- In synoviocyte cultures, unstimulated cells do not express the stromelysin gene, whereas TIMP is constitutively expressed.

The interpretation is that, in normal and subsynovial tissues, the balance is in favor of minimal remodeling; in areas near the cartilage-pannus junction and wherever stimulators of induction are present, stromelysin—the key enzyme in connective tissue remodeling—is abundant.

INDUCTION OF BIOSYNTHESIS OF TISSUE METALLOPROTEASES

The metalloproteases are expressed only weakly, if at all, in resting tissues. However, synovial cells and explants in culture respond to many different inductive stimuli by generating mRNA for collagenase and stromelysin. After being exposed to an inductive stimulus, synovial fibroblasts transcribe collagenase mRNA within 6 hours,[15] and, within 45 minutes after protein synthesis of collagenase is initiated, the proenzyme is secreted.[16] Major inductive stimuli that are likely to be present in rheumatoid joints include[17,18]:

- Cytokines (e.g., IL-1, TNFα, PDGF)
- Particulate material that is phagocytosed
- Cell-cell interactions
- Formation of multinucleate giant cells
- Serum amyloid A–like protein and β_2-microglobulin–like protein[19] produced by synovial fibroblasts in an autocrine induction model
- Iron (soluble and particulate)
- Bacterial toxins
- IL-10[20]
- Direct contact between T lymphocytes and monocytes[21]

Not all inductive stimuli turn on expression of each enzyme in the same cells. For example, although PDGF was able to stimulate rheumatoid synovial fibroblasts to secrete collagenase (MMP-1), it did not induce expression of MMP-9, the 92-kDa gelatinase/type V collagenase.[22] In addition, stimuli that enhance collagenase biosynthesis may down-regulate collagen synthesis; IL-10 is one of these. Consistent with the analogy between rheumatoid synovium and a localized malignancy are the data showing that, when rheumatoid cells are induced by peptides such as PDGF, the proto-oncogenes c-*fos* and c-*jun* are activated. The proteins (Jun/Fos) that they express bind as transactivating factors to the AP-1 binding site on DNA upstream from the coding regions.[23] Although the AP-1 sequence is both important and essential, it is not the only contributor to promotion of induction.[24]

Not all inductive stimuli exert transcriptional effects on the collagen gene. IL-10, for example, induces collagenase by post-transcriptional mechanisms,[25] and IL-1β induces collagenase gene expression by both transcriptional and post-translocational mechanisms. Relaxin, the peptide hormone found in serum during pregnancy that may have a role in loosening pelvic ligaments to create a larger birth canal, can cause significant collagen turnover both by stimulating collagenase expression and by down-modulating collagen synthesis and secretion.[26]

The induction of procollagenase synthesis in monocytes by direct contact with T cells or fragments of previously activated T-cell membranes is intriguing.[21] In contrast to the release of soluble mediators that act in an autocrine or paracrine fashion, direct cell-cell contact is a potent vehicle only for paracrine activation (see Chapter 9). Characterizing the membrane component(s) that mediate MMP induction in monocytes will give useful information about stimulatory signal transduction.

ACTIVATION OF PROMETALLOPROTEASES TO THEIR ACTIVE FORMS

Once it was realized that collagenase was released from cells as a latent enzyme, it was rapidly determined that protease treatment by trypsin or other proteases converted the inactive species to active ones at a lower molecular weight. The mechanisms for activation were confusing, however, when it became apparent that organomercurial agents could activate latent collagenase, and that activation of procollagenase was poorly accomplished by any of these agents unless stromelysin in active form was present. The mechanism of activation has been sorted out and can be explained as follows[27] (Fig. 12–1):

- Latency of procollagenase is maintained by a cysteine-Zn^{2+} bond that links the unpaired propeptide cysteine residues to the active site.

- Enzymes such as mast cell tryptase can activate prostromelysin to stromelysin, but have no effect upon procollagenase unless prostromelysin is present.[28]

- Stromelysin (MMP-3) is capable of activating procollagenase directly; this reaction is slow. It involves removal of residues 1 to 80 from procollagenase.

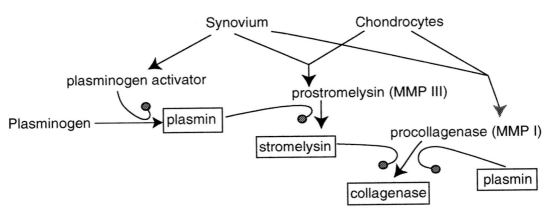

FIGURE 12–1. Activation of metalloproteases in the rheumatoid joint. Both synovial lining cells and chondrocytes produce zymogens of these enzymes, and the synovial cells express plasminogen activator. The combined effects of plasmin and stromelysin are sufficient to activate procollagenase. Between them, collagenase and stromelysin can degrade (at variable rates) almost all proteins in joints.

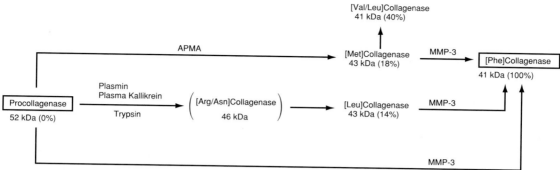

FIGURE 12–2. Activation pathways of procollagenase. Various forms of collagenase generated during in vitro activation are shown. Procollagenase is activated by MMP-3 directly, but this process is slow. Proteinases and aminophenyl mercuric acetate (APMA) partially activate procollagenase by removing portions of the propeptide region. Full activation is achieved by MMP-3 resulting in complete removal of 80 amino acid residues from the amino terminus. In the case of protease treatment, 46,000-M_r intermediates are first formed, which are then processed to M_r 43,000. The action of MMP-3 on partially activated collagenase is rapid. Amino acid residues in brackets indicate the amino terminus of each collagenase species. [Leu]Collagenase of M_r 43,000 was identified only with plasma kallikrein or plasmin-treated procollagenase. In the absence of MMP-3, APMA-treated collagenase of M_r 43,000 is converted to a 41,000-M_r species by autolysis at the Phe[81]-Val[82] and the Val[82]-Leu[83] bonds. Collagenolytic activity of each species is shown in parentheses. (From Suzuki, K., Enghild, J. J., Morodomi, T., et al.: Mechanisms of activation of tissue procollagenase by matrix metalloproteinase 3 (stromelysin). Biochemistry 29:10261, 1990. Used by permission. Copyright 1990, American Chemical Society.)

- Organomercurial compounds (e.g., aminophenyl mercuric acetate) induce an intramolecular self-cleavage at a different site.
- Proteolytic cleavage of procollagenase by proteases such as plasmin or plasma kallikrein open the conformation of the molecule, enabling stromelysin (MMP-3) to rapidly activate collagenase (Fig. 12–2). The combined action of plasmin and

MMP-3 results in sequential cleavage of the pro-enzyme,[27] producing the active form.

In rheumatoid synovium, the activation of metalloproteases is likely to occur as follows (Fig. 12–3). Plasmin is produced by the action of synovial plasminogen activator on plasminogen that is abundant in synovial fluid.[29] Plasmin activates prostromelysin and cleaves a piece of procollagenase so that

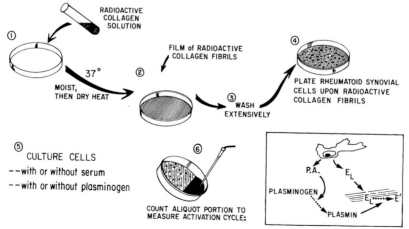

FIGURE 12–3. This in vitro system is a probable model for how procollagenase is activated through a cascade from plasminogen activator. If rheumatoid synovial cells are plated on beds of radiolabeled collagen and plasminogen is added, the collagen is degraded. Sufficient controls support the hypothesis that plasminogen activator generated by the synovial cells is sufficient to activate plasmin, which, through its combined effect with stromelysin (and activation of prostromelysin), activates procollagenase. (From Werb, Z., Mainardi, C. L., Vater, C. A., et al.: Endogenous activation of collagenase secreted by rheumatoid synovial cells: evidence for the role of plasminogen activator. N. Engl. J. Med. 296:1017, 1977. Copyright 1977, Massachusetts Medical Society. All rights reserved. Used by permission.)

active stromelysin can complete catalytic cleavage of procollagenase to the active form. Mast cell tryptase is an efficient activator of prostromelysin, and thus indirectly can activate procollagenase[28] as well. The complexity of this process is an indication of how tightly collagenolysis is regulated. The same complexity gives added opportunity for biologic regulation of synovial collagenase. For example, if IFNγ is added to cultures of rheumatoid synovial fibroblasts in the presence of IL-1β, procollagenase protein secretion is augmented as expected by IL-1β, but active collagenase yields are very small. This is because IFNγ significantly inhibits prostromelysin production by these cells,[30] and procollagenase is poorly activated in the absence of stromelysin.

OTHER PROTEASES INVOLVED IN CONNECTIVE TISSUE DEGRADATION

Although the involvement of metalloproteases in a very attractive story because of the inductive and activating sequences as well as the remarkable substrate specificities of these enzymes, they are not the only proteases involved in cartilage destruction. Three other classes of proteases, classified by their catalytic mechanisms, are potentially involved in joint destruction.

Aspartic Proteases

This group of enzymes, often referred to as *acid hydrolases*, are involved in intracellular destruction of protein in lysosomes. They depend upon an aspartic acid residue in the catalytic mechanism. *Cathepsin D* is found in lysosomes of phagocytic cells. During states of active tissue destruction, it is excreted from the cells, and, in micropockets of inflammation where lactic acid and carbon dioxide production is sufficient to lower extracellular pH, it could be active. At pH 5, its optimum, it degrades cartilage proteoglycans.[18]

Cysteine Proteases

Cysteine proteases are similar to papain, and depend upon cysteine and histidine residues for activity. *Cathepsin B* and *cathepsin L* are the best known in this family. Cathepsin B cleaves the nonhelical cross-link regions of interstitial collagens, and may cleave proteoglycans, fibronectin, and elastin. Along with stromelysin, it could be involved in decreasing the compressive stiffness of cartilage,

making it susceptible to mechanical and other enzymatic degradation. An enhanced transcription of cathepsin B mRNA has been demonstrated in rheumatoid synovial cells compared with that in normal fibroblasts of tumor cells. Immunolocalization shows it restricted to synovial cells attached to cartilage and bone at sites of joint erosion.[31]

Interest in cathepsin L has been spawned by the information that it is the major induced protein in *ras*-transformed cells in culture. It also has been found by immunolocalization in synovial cells at the cartilage-pannus junction,[32] along with *ras* oncogene transcripts. The presence and potential activity of these oncoproteins gives support to the concept that synovial cells transformed by retroviruses are the driving force of rheumatoid arthritis.

Serine Proteases

Serine proteases are the largest class of mammalian proteases. Active at neutral pH, their importance is underscored by the fact that inhibitors of serine proteases represent 10 per cent of all plasma proteins.[18] Most of the coagulation cascade proteins, those initiating fibrinolysis, and the complement cascade are serine proteases. Specific serine proteases found in inflammatory joint tissues and fluids include thrombin, plasminogen activator, plasmin, kallikrein, and neutrophil elastase. In synovial fluid, for example, *plasminogen* has a high affinity for fibrin that forms as a result of many microhemorrhages on the synovial surface; this provides a ready mechanism for lysis when plasminogen activator (bound to the surface of macrophages and fibroblasts by specific receptors) contacts the plasminogen.

Kallikrein, in addition to acting on high-molecular-weight kininogen to produce bradykinin, can activate prostromelysin, setting into motion the cascade that ends in formation of active collagenase.[33]

Neutrophil elastase is found in the azurophil granules of both neutrophils and monocytes. It is uniquely capable of degrading elastin, and degrades link protein and other components of proteoglycans in synovial tissue and cartilage. Elastase also may be involved in collagen degradation by degrading the aminoterminal nonhelical peptides in collagen that contain cross-links. Because the extent of cross-linking of collagen is inversely related to the rapidity with which collagenase can degrade it, elastolytic removal of cross-linking regions of the molecule may hasten the collagenolytic process. Through its capability to degrade laminin and collagen type IV, elastase is one of the most potent destroyers of basement membranes.

Mast cell chymase and *tryptase* have broad reactivity against noncollagenous matrix proteins, and can activate prostromelysin.

INHIBITORS OF PROTEASE ACTIVITY

The major inhibitor of collagenases and other proteases in plasma and synovial fluids is α_2-macroglobulin (α_2M). α_2M is a large protein 725,000 kDa) and inhibits almost all proteases from all four catalytic classes of proteins. Its activity depends upon the protease attacking a "bait" region within α_2M. This cleavage triggers a conformational change that entraps the enzyme within folds of α_2M but does not block its active site, while preventing its contact with large protein substrates. MMP-1 (collagenase) binds to α_2M very rapidly. α_2M serves as a far better substrate than any other protein for collagenase, including collagen.[34] Although it is an effective scavenger of proteases in synovial fluid, its capacity is limited, and, in a severe synovial inflammation such as that associated with sepsis, it may become saturated, resulting in free and active proteases within the joint fluid and no measurable inhibitory activity.[35]

The large size of α_2M may restrict its activity to the fluid phase as a scavenger of proteases that have diffused from tissues. Fibroblasts within cartilage, synovium, and tendons produce a lower molecular weight (28,000) metalloprotease inhibitor known as tissue inhibitor of metalloproteases (TIMP). TIMP was first purified from human tendons.[36] It is synthesized and secreted by chondrocytes, synovial fibroblasts, and endothelial cells. TIMP has at least two molecular forms (TIMP-1 and TIMP-2), both of which bind active metalloproteases to form 1:1 noncovalent complexes that inactivate the enzymes. The ratio of TIMP to MMP synthesis by cells in various tissues probably has an important role in determining the rate of connective tissue degradation in that tissue, and is a function of the stimulus to biosynthesis. For example, TNFα induces collagenase and stromelysin synthesis but not TIMP, while IL-6 enhances TIMP but not metalloprotease expression. TGFβ increases TIMP expression while repressing metalloprotease expression.[18] Chondrocytes produce large amounts of TIMP, an important factor in the relative resistance to degradation of this crucial tissue. Studies of mRNA expression for TIMP in rheumatoid synovial cells have found a relative decrease of TIMP compared with proteinase levels.[13]

Inhibitors of Metalloprotease Biosynthesis

The stromelysin/collagenase/gelatinase metalloproteases not only are induced by numerous compounds but can be down-regulated as well. Whereas TNFα and IL-1β increase MMP biosynthesis, TGFβ, glucocorticoid hormones, and retinoid compounds suppress it.[37] The mechanisms are transcriptional as well as post-transcriptional.[38]

Tetracyclines are potent inhibitors of metalloproteases and, in combination with NSAIDs, can produce substantial normalization of radiographic joint damage in animal models of arthritis[39]; this has been a rationale for using tetracyclines as therapy in rheumatoid arthritis (see Chapter 34).

Inhibitors of Metalloproteases in the Treatment of Rheumatoid Arthritis

The approaches to inhibiting matrix destruction by metalloproteases include interference with biosynthesis, activation, or activity of the enzymes.[25] The challenge lies in delivery of inhibitors to the pannus-cartilage junction, where destruction of cartilage takes place in a zone only a few microns in width. In addition, there is a problem with specificity; chelators of zinc and calcium rapidly and completely inactivate metalloproteases in vitro but cannot be used in vivo (other than on the cornea in treatment of abrasions or burns) for fear of inhibiting multiple essential cellular processes.

Inhibitors of biosynthesis of MMP include the naturally occurring compounds such as TGFβ and all-*trans*-retinoic acid, and synthetic derivatives of retinoic acid and glucocorticoids.[25] For the most part, these substances act by interfering with transcription of mRNA for metalloproteases by interfering with elements within the promoter regions of DNA for these proenzymes. For example, the glucocorticoid receptor–hormone complex interacts with the *fos-jun* element in the MMP promoter region in such a way that transcription regresses.[40] The problem with glucocorticoids is not their *sensitivity* as potential inhibitors; they are active at micromolar concentrations. The problem is *specificity;* the multiple other actions of these hormones when given chronically lead to toxicity that supersedes beneficial effects.

Interference with adenine-uridine (AU)–rich regions of mRNA may effectively inhibit protein synthesis in a post-translational manner, and because certain inducers of MMP (e.g., IL-1) appear to exert their effects post-translationally, it may be reasonable to attempt blocking these RNA-binding regions.

Inhibitors of activity that have potential for therapeutic use include the tetracyclines (mentioned earlier). Although the results of trials are somewhat inconclusive (see Chapter 34), these compounds have a low toxicity and therefore even a modicum of efficacy may give a favorable cost-benefit analysis. Different derivatives of the tetracycline molecule may give better results.

Much effort in pharmaceutical laboratories is being invested in creation of synthetic peptides that will specifically inhibit MMP. The challenges are to produce compounds that can be given by mouth, resist degradation in the gut, not be immunogenic, and find their way to inflamed joints.[41] One such compound, a hydroxamate developed as a chelator of zinc that mimics the substrate for MMP, has shown promise in diminishing cartilage degradation in animal models of arthritis.[42]

A pair of heptanoic acid methyl esters of low molecular weight that have thiol moieties capable of binding essential zinc residues in metalloproteases have been shown to decrease degradation of both proteoglycans and collagen in a novel animal model.[43] At this time, however, there are no MMP inhibitors available that are effective given by mouth.

REFERENCES

1. Gross, J., and Lapiere, C. M.: Collagenolytic activity in amphibian tissues: a tissue culture assay. Proc. Natl. Acad. Sci. U.S.A. 48:1014, 1962.
2. Evanston, J. M., Jeffrey, J. J., and Krane, S. M.: Studies on collagenase from rheumatoid synovium in tissue culture. J. Clin. Invest. 47:2639, 1968.
3. Harris, E. D. Jr., Welgus, H. G., and Krane, S. M.: Regulation of the mammalian collagenases. Collagen Rel. Res. 4:493, 1984.
4. Singer, I. I., Kawka, D. W., Bayne, E. K., et al.: VDIPEN, a metalloproteinase-generated neoepitope, is induced and immunolocalized in articular cartilage during inflammatory arthritis. J. Clin. Invest. 95:2178, 1995.
5. Hembry, R. M., Bagga, M. R., Reynolds, J. J., et al.: Immunolocalisation studies on six matrix metalloproteinases and their inhibitors, TIMP-1 and TIMP-2, in synovia from patients with osteo- and rheumatoid arthritis. Ann. Rheum. Dis. 54:25, 1995.
6. Walakovits, L. A., Moore, V. L., Bhardwaj, N., et al.: Detection of stromelysin and collagenase in synovial fluid from patients with rheumatoid arthritis and posttraumatic knee injury. Arthritis Rheum. 35:35, 1992.
7. Gravallese, E. M., Darling, J. M., Ladd, A. L., et al.: *In situ* hybridization studies of stromelysin and collagenase messenger RNA expression in rheumatoid synovium. Arthritis Rheum. 34:1076, 1991.
8. Okada, Y., Takeuchi, N., Tomita, K., et al.: Immunolocalisation of matrix metalloproteinase 3 (stromelysin) in rheumatoid synovioblasts (B cells): correlation with rheumatoid arthritis. Ann. Rheum. Dis. 48:645, 1989.
9. Maeda, S., Sawai, T., Uzuki, M., et al.: Determination of interstitial collagenase (MMP-1) in patients with rheumatoid arthritis. Ann. Rheum. Dis. 54:970, 1995.
10. Woolley, D. E., Crossley, M. J., and Evanson, J. M.: Collagenase at sites of cartilage erosion in the rheumatoid joint. Arthritis Rheum. 20:1231, 1977.
11. Hasty, K. A., Reife, R. A., Kang, A. H., et al.: The role of stromelysin in the cartilage destruction that accompanies inflammatory arthritis. Arthritis Rheum. 33:388, 1990.
12. Taylor, D. J., Cheung, N. P., and Dawes, P. T.: Increased serum proMMP-3 in inflammatory arthritides: a potential indicator of synovial inflammatory monokine activity. Ann. Rheum. Dis. 53:768, 1994.
13. Nguyen, Q., Mort, J. S., and Roughley, P. J.: Preferential mRNA expression of prostromelysin relative to procollagenase and *in situ* localization in human articular cartilage. J. Clin. Invest. 89:1189, 1992.
14. Firestein, G. S., and Paine, M. M.: Stromelysin and tissue inhibitor of metalloproteinases gene expression in rheumatoid arthritis synovium. Am. J. Pathol. 140:1309, 1992.
15. Brinckerhoff, C. E., and Auble, D. T.: Regulation of collagenase gene expression in synovial fibroblasts. Ann. N. Y. Acad. Sci. 580:355, 1990.
16. Nagase, H., Brinckerhoff, C. E., Vater, C. A., et al.: Biosynthesis and secretion of procollagenase by rabbit synovial fibroblasts. Biochem. J. 214:281, 1983.
17. Harris, E. D. Jr., and Krane, S. M.: Effects of colchicine on collagenase in cultures of rheumatoid synovium. Arthritis Rheum. 14:669, 1971.
18. Werb, Z., and Alexander, C. M.: Proteinases and matrix degradation. *In* Kelley, W. N., Harris, E. D. Jr., Ruddy, S., and Sledge, C. B., (eds.): Textbook of Rheumatology, 4th ed., Vol. 1. Philadelphia, W. B. Saunders, 1993, pp. 248–268.
19. Brinckerhoff, C. E., Mitchell, T. I., Karmilowicz, M. J., et al.: Autocrine induction of collagenase by serum amyloid A-like and β_2-microglobulin-like proteins. Science 243: 655, 1989.
20. Reitamo, S., Remitz, A., Tamai, K., et al.: Interleukin-10 modulates type I collagen and matrix metalloprotease gene expression in cultured human skin fibroblasts. J. Clin. Invest. 94:2489, 1994.
21. Lacraz, S., Isler, P., Vey, E., et al.: Direct contact between T lymphocytes and monocytes is a major pathway for induction of metalloproteinase expression. J. Biol. Chem. 269:22027, 1994.
22. Unemori, E. N., Hibbs, M. S., and Amento, E. P.: Constitutive expression of a 92-kD gelatinase (type V collagenase) by rheumatoid synovial fibroblasts and its induction in normal human fibroblasts by inflammatory cytokines. J. Clin. Invest. 88:1656, 1991.
23. Conca, W., Kaplan, P. B., and Krane, S. M.: Increases in levels of procollagenase messenger RNA in cultured fibroblasts induced by human recombinant interleukin-1β or serum follow *c-jun* expression and are dependent on new protein synthesis. J. Clin. Invest. 83:1753, 1989.
24. Sirum, C. K., and Brinckerhoff, C. E.: Interleukin-1 or phorbol induction of the stromelysin promoter requires an element that cooperates with AP-1. Nucleic Acids Res. 19:335, 1991.
25. Vincenti, M. P., Clark, I. M., and Brinckerhoff, C. E.: Using inhibitors of metalloproteinases to treat arthritis: easier said than done? Arthritis Rheum. 37:1115, 1994.
26. Unemori, E. N., and Amento, E. P.: Relaxin modulates synthesis and secretion of procollagenase and collagen by human dermal fibroblasts. J. Biol. Chem. 265:10681, 1990.
27. Suzuki, K., Enghild, J. J., Morodomi, T., et al.: Mechanisms of activation of tissue procollagenase by matrix metalloproteinase 3 (stromelysin). Biochemistry 29:10261, 1990.

28. Gruber, B. L., Marchese, M. J., Suzuki, K., et al.: Synovial procollagenase activation by human mast cell tryptase dependence upon matrix metalloproteinase 3 activation. J. Clin. Invest. 84:1657, 1989.

29. Werb, Z., Mainardi, C. L., Vater, C. A., et al.: Endogenous activation of collagenase secreted by rheumatoid synovial cells: evidence for the role of plasminogen activator. N. Engl. J. Med. 296:1017, 1977.

30. Unemori, E. N., Bair, M. J., Bauer, E. A., et al.: Stromelysin expression regulates collagenase activation in human fibroblasts: dissociable control of two metalloproteinases by interferon-γ. J. Biol. Chem. 266:23477, 1991.

31. Trabandt, A., Gay, R. E., Fassbender, H.-G., et al.: Cathepsin B in synovial cells at the site of joint destruction in rheumatoid arthritis. Arthritis Rheum. 34:1444, 1991.

32. Trabandt, A., Aicher, W. K., Gay, R. E., et al.: Expression of the collagenolytic and Ras-induced cystine proteinase cathepsin L and proliferation-associated oncogenes in synovial cells of MRL/1 mice and patients with rheumatoid arthritis. Matrix 10:349, 1990.

33. Nagase, H., Cawston, T. E., Desilva, M., et al.: Identification of plasma kallikrein as an activator of latent collagenase in rheumatoid synovial fluid. Biochim. Biophys. Acta 702:133, 1982.

34. Enghild, J. J., Salvesen, G., Brew, K., et al.: Interaction of human rheumatoid synovial collagenase (matrix metalloproteinase 1) and stromelysin (matrix metalloproteinase 3) with human α_2-macroglobulin and chicken ovostatin: binding kinetics and identification of matrix metalloproteinase cleavage sites. J. Biol. Chem. 264:8779, 1989.

35. Cawston, T. E., Weaver, L., Coughlan, R. J., et al.: Synovial fluids from infected joints contain active metalloproteinases and no inhibitory activity. Br. J. Rheumatol. 28:386, 1989.

36. Vater, C. A., Mainardi, C. L., and Harris, E. D. Jr.: An inhibitor of mammalian collagenases from cultures *in vitro* of human tendon. J. Biol. Chem. 254:3045, 1979.

37. Woessner, J. J.: Matrix metalloproteinases and their inhibitors in connective tissue remodeling. FASEB J. 5:2145, 1991.

38. Delany, A. M., and Brinckerhoff, C. E.: Post-transcriptional regulation of collagenase and stromelysin gene expression by epidermal growth factor and dexamethasone in cultured human fibroblasts. J. Cell. Biochem. 50:400, 1992.

39. Greenwald, R. A., Moak, S. A., Ramamurthy, N. S., et al.: Tetracyclines suppress matrix metalloproteinase activity in adjuvant arthritis and in combination with flurbiprofen, ameliorate bone damage. J. Rheumatol. 19:927, 1992.

40. Schule, R., Rangarajan, P., Kliewer, S., et al.: Functional antagonism between oncoprotein c-Jun and the glucocorticoid receptor. Cell 62:1217, 1990.

41. Henderson, B., and Davies, D. E.: The design of inhibitors of cartilage breakdown. *In* Russel, R. G. G., and Dieppe, P. A. (eds.): Osteoarthritis: Current Research and Perspectives for Pharmacological Intervention. London, IBC Technical Services, 1991, pp. 372–398.

42. DiMartino, M. J., Wolff, C. E., High, W., et al.: Antiinflammatory and chondroprotective activities of a potent metalloproteinase inhibitor. J. Cell. Biochem. Suppl. 19E:179, 1991.

43. Karran, E. H., Young, T. J., Markwell, R. E., et al.: *In vivo* model of cartilage degradation—effects of a matrix metalloproteinase inhibitor. Ann. Rheum. Dis. 54:662, 1995.

SECTION V

ABNORMAL PHYSIOLOGY OF THE JOINT AND SYNOVIAL FLUID IN RHEUMATOID ARTHRITIS

For rheumatologists in clinics and hospitals, synovial fluid is the window of access for an approximation of what is going on in the synovium. The degree of inflammation in synovial fluid, monitored by counts of neutrophils, provides indirect measure of the degree of cellular activation. The number of neutrophils, for example, is a better index of the proliferative index in synovium than are the symptoms of pain and signs of swelling of joints. In contrast, the amount of synovial fluid within a rheumatoid joint has little relationship to neutrophil count or to synovial inflammation, but the increase in intra-articular pressure that high volumes of fluid in a joint can generate affects, in a major way, the oxygenation of synovial tissue and cartilage. The next two chapters provide a guide to how synovial physiology is altered in this disease, and how findings in the synovial fluid can be exploited to provide a sense of what is happening in synovium.

13

Intra-articular Pressure, Blood Flow, and pH in the Rheumatoid Joint

It is easier to access blood from rheumatoid patients than it is to obtain synovial fluid or synovial cells. Even more difficult, however, is to study the physiology of the intact joint, or to appreciate how the relative imbalances between blood flow, cellular metabolism, and pressures developed within rheumatoid joints influence the state of cartilage and synovium. Nevertheless, these factors are important contributions to the pathology of rheumatoid arthritis and the disability that can result from it.

NORMAL PHYSIOLOGY OF THE SYNOVIUM

Within the normal diarthrodial joint cavity there is a small amount of synovial fluid. This fluid coats either synovial lining, cartilage, or small "bare" areas of bone where a gap of bone exists between where the synovium/joint capsule inserts and articular cartilage begins. Because synovial tissue is mesenchymal in origin, there is no well-defined basement membrane separating the lining cells of the synovium from sublining cells. Thus, the organization of the "synovial membrane" is informal. There are no tight junctions among the specialized fibroblasts that line the joint cavity.[1,2]

Ultrastructural studies have shown that the synovial capillaries in humans have many fenestrations, suggesting a high permeability to water on the side facing the joint cavity (for review see ref. 3). These may be essential for facilitating diffusion of oxygen and nutrients in a complicated journey from the circulation, into the synovium, through the synovial layer into the synovial fluid, and finally into cartilage itself to nourish the relatively isolated chondrocytes.

The unusual feature of diarthrodial joints, of course, is that they are often moving. There is suffi-cient redundancy in the synovium to prevent it from being stretched even in extreme ranges of motion. To facilitate this movement, synovium needs lubrication to move upon itself. It is **hyaluronan,** the very large nonsulfated polysaccharide, that provides efficient lubrication among these folds of synovial tissue,[4] whereas it is the specialized glycoprotein **lubricin,** produced by synovial cells, that lubricates the cartilage-cartilage interfaces.

In the position providing maximum volume of the normal joint space (e.g., slight flexion of the knee), pressure is subatmospheric.[5] In contrast, intra-articular pressure was positive in all 24 rheumatoid joints examined (8 metacarpophalangeal joints, 4 ankles, 8 wrists, 4 elbows), and was subatmospheric in 15 normal joints.[6] Exercise increased pressure in the rheumatoid joints but not the controls.

Although difficult to prove, it seems logical that in normal subjects this negative pressure, alternating with increased pressure during flexion, has a role in the flux of metabolites and nutrients to the synovium as well as to the cartilage. Chondrocytes must receive all their nutrients from synovial capillaries, and their metabolites must diffuse back to the same capillaries for removal, recycling, and discharge.

ARTICULAR ISCHEMIA: AN ACCOMPANIMENT OF ACTIVE SYNOVITIS

The early pathology in rheumatoid arthritis is marked by new blood vessel formation, proliferation of synovial cells, and influx of mononuclear cells and neutrophils from the circulation into the lining and synovial fluid. The inflammation breaks down barriers to diffusion of solutes and water; the result is synovial effusions. In active disease, intra-

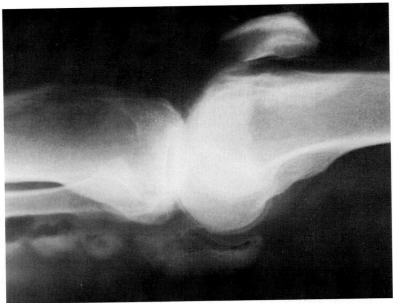

FIGURE 13–1. This is an arthrogram in a patient who developed a popliteal (Baker's) cyst. On a Saturday morning he was carrying a heavy box up a flight of stairs when he had an "explosive" pain in his proximal calf behind and below his knee. By Monday morning he was unable to walk and had pitting edema of the lower leg and foot and marked tenderness on palpation of the calf. His Baker's cyst had disappeared.

The air-dye arthrogram (shown here) revealed the convoluted appearance of rupture or pseudorupture of the popliteal cyst into the gastrocnemius-soleus muscle bundles. He was treated effectively with rest, ice, and an injection into the anterior knee of 60 mg triamcinolone hexacetonide.

articular pressure may build to levels sufficient to rupture the joint capsule (e.g., a ruptured Baker's cyst) (Fig. 13–1). It is not surprising that a direct result of this increased pressure resulting from increased volume of synovial fluids is impairment of the influx of oxygen and nutrients into the joint, as well as the efflux of carbon dioxide, lactate, and other metabolites from chondrocytes and synovium back out of the joints. Hypoxic reperfusion-mediated joint injury is very likely a reality.

As inflammation increases, the synovial physiology becomes ischemic; there is a low pO_2, increased pCO_2, low pH, high lactate, and low glucose[7,8] (Fig. 13–2). Almost 30 percent of 55 patients studied with rheumatoid arthritis had measurements of synovial fluid pO_2 that were less than 15 mm Hg. Several factors accelerate ischemia of the rheumatoid joint. One is motion itself, resulting in an increase in neutrophils drawn into the joint. The other is that, when effusions are more than minimal, any flexion of an involved joint increases intra-articular pressures to levels that exceed intra-capillary pressure.[9] The practical importance of these findings is borne out by the data showing that resting synovial fluid pH is inversely related to radiologic evidence for cartilage and bone de-

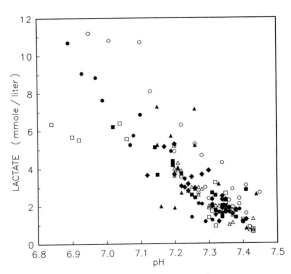

FIGURE 13–2. Correlation between synovial fluid lactate concentration and pH ($r = -.83$, $p < .001$). The data in this figure were taken from seven separate studies. (From Simkin, P. A., and Bassett, J. E.: Lactate in synovial effusions. J. Rheumatol. 19:1017, 1992. Used by permission.)

struction in rheumatoid arthritis.[10] In this study there appeared to be relatively little contribution from neutrophils in the fluid to the acidosis.

How much the low pH and lactate directly damage tissue, and how much they are no more than an accurate reflection of the intensity of the inflammatory/destructive process is not known, but the best bet would be that hypoxia within synovium, and therefore within cartilage, is additive if not synergistic with the destructive potential of metalloproteases.

Another potential factor in contributing to synovial hypoxia and acidosis is the excessive oxygen consumption of rheumatoid synovial tissue, estimated at 20-fold normal.[11] This is in part related to the increased numbers of glycolytically active cells and to the fact that rheumatoid synovial cells have enzymatic machinery that favors the less efficient anaerobic glycolysis.[12]

EXERCISE AND ITS EFFECTS ON BLOOD FLOW OF THE JOINT

It has long been appreciated that, in prescribing a program of physical exercise for rheumatoid patients, the goal must be to establish a careful balance between sufficient muscle exertion to keep or increase muscle tone and strength, and too much stress on involved joints. It is a reasonable hypothesis that during exercise there is sufficient ''tamponade'' of blood flow within a boggy, fluid-filled joint to produce endothelial damage. Indeed, it has been shown that a marker for hypoxic reperfusion endothelial cell injury—plasma von Willebrand factor level—is significantly increased after exercise in rheumatoid patients compared with controls[13] (Fig. 13–3).

It is probable, although not directly demonstrated as yet, that tissue hypoxia results in release of platelet-activating factor, endothelin, nitric oxide (also called endothelial relaxing factor), superoxide radicals, and lipoxygenase metabolites.[14] It also is probable that the driving force for new capillary formation may be as much a response to hypoxia as to growth factors.[15]

IMPLICATIONS FOR TREATMENT FROM STUDIES OF PHYSIOLOGY OF INFLAMED JOINTS

Perhaps the most important lesson for therapy is not to let synovial effusions, especially in an acces-

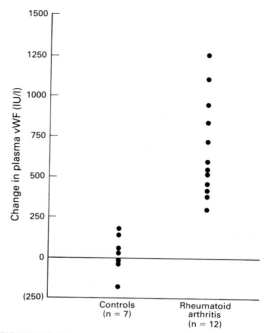

FIGURE 13–3. Exercise-induced change in plasma von Willebrand factor (vWF) levels in controls and patients with rheumatoid arthritis. (From Farrell, A. J., Williams, R. B., Stevens, C. R., et al.: Exercise induced release of von Willebrand factor: evidence for hypoxic reperfusion microvascular injury in rheumatoid arthritis. Ann. Rheum. Dis. 51:1117, 1992. Used by permission.)

sible joint such as the knee, become too tense and full. The danger of rupture is exceeded by the pressure-induced microvascular tamponade that the effusion generates. Too much exercise will increase the quantity of neutrophils in the joint and also contribute to hypoxia and acidosis in a rheumatoid joint, whereas too little exercise impairs achieving much-needed muscle tone and strength.

REFERENCES

1. Simkin, P. A.: Physiology of normal and abnormal synovium. Semin. Arthritis Rheum. 21:179, 1991.
2. Henderson, B., and Edwards, J. C. W.: The Synovial Lining in Health and Disease. London, Chapman and Hall, 1987.
3. Levick, J. R., and McDonald, J. N.: Fluid movement across synovium in healthy joints: role of synovial fluid macromolecules. Ann. Rheum. Dis. 54:417, 1995.
4. Swann, D. A., Radin, E. L., Nazimiec, M., et al.: Role of hyaluronic acid in joint lubrication. Ann. Rheum. Dis. 33:318, 1974.
5. Levick, J. R.: Joint pressure-volume studies: their importance, design and interpretation. J. Rheumatol. 10:353, 1983.
6. Gaffney, K., Williams, R. B., Jolliffe, V. A., et al.: Intra-articular pressure changes in rheumatoid and normal peripheral joints. Ann. Rheum. Dis. 54:670, 1995.
7. Simkin, P. A., and Bassett, J. E.: Lactate in synovial effusions. J. Rheumatol. 19:1017, 1992.

The correlation between synovial fluid lactate concentration and pH is remarkably linear, even when multiple studies are analyzed ($r = -.83$). The data in Figure 13–2 (see text) are entirely consistent with synovial hypoxia. Insufficient oxygen in tissues results in anaerobic glycolysis that generates lactic acid as an end product. Thus, synovial lactate concentrations reflect the balance (or lack of it) between net synovial production and microvascular clearance of lactate.

8. Falchuk, K. H., Goetzl, E. J., and Kulka, J. P.: Respiratory gases of synovial fluids. Am. J. Med. 49:223, 1970.

   This study, one of the first to correlate joint pathology and physiology, showed that joints with the lowest pO_2 (as low as 9 mm Hg) also had the highest levels of pCO_2 and lactate. These same joints showed pathologic changes of microvascular obliteration.

9. James, M. J., Cleland, L. G., Rofe, A. M., et al.: Intraarticular pressure and the relationship between synovial perfusion and metabolic demand. J. Rheumatol. 17:521, 1990.
10. Geborek, P., Saxne, T., Petterson, H., et al.: Synovial fluid acidosis correlates with radiological joint destruction in rheumatoid arthritis knee joints. J. Rheumatol. 16:468, 1989.
11. Dingle, J. T. M., and Page-Thomas, D. P.: *In vitro* studies in human synovial membrane: a metabolic comparison of normal and rheumatoid disease. Br. J. Exp. Pathol. 37:318, 1956.
12. Henderson, B., Bitensky, L., and Chayen, I.: Glycolytic activity in human synovial lining cells in rheumatoid arthritis. Ann. Rheum. Dis. 38:63, 1979.
13. Farrell, A. J., Williams, R. B., Stevens, C. R., et al.: Exercise induced release of von Willebrand factor: evidence for hypoxic reperfusion microvascular injury in rheumatoid arthritis. Ann. Rheum. Dis. 51:1117, 1992.
14. Stevens, C. R., Williams, R. B., Farrell, A. J., et al.: Hypoxia and inflammatory synovitis: observations and speculation. Ann. Rheum. Dis. 50:124, 1991.
15. West, D. C., Hampson, I. N., Arnold, F., et al.: Hyaluronan and angiogenesis. *In* Evered, D., and Whelan, J. (eds.): The Biology of Hyaluronan. Chichester, England, Wiley, 1985, pp. 187–207.

14

Synovial Fluid: A Sink for Neutrophils and Inflammatory Mediators

Synovial fluid is the most valuable material available for diagnostic testing in rheumatoid arthritis. Ample evidence exists that the joint fluid reflects more accurately than does blood the pathophysiology as well as the stage and activity of disease. In this chapter, the analysis of fluid from rheumatoid joints will be linked with the pathophysiology of the disease process.

SYNOVIAL FLUID ANALYSIS

It is not within the planned scope of this book to describe the techniques of aspiration of joints. These approaches are described well in the textbooks.[1] Considering the large number of arthrocenteses performed by primary care physicians, rheumatologists, and orthopedic surgeons, the incidence of complications from the procedure is very low. The most serious is that of introducing bacterial infection, and yet the frequency of this outcome is probably less than $1:50,000$ aspirations, when performed carefully. The ACR guidelines[2] for performing office synovial fluid examinations are reproduced in Table 14–1.

Routine and Useful Studies on Synovial Fluid

For *diagnosis*, synovial fluid examination can provide much information and be useful in ruling out other entities[3] that are listed in Tables 14–2 and 14–3. The following components of synovial fluid analysis are important for differential diagnosis.

General Appearance

A rough estimate of the number of cells can be arrived at by simple examination of the fluid. One can read large letters through the clear fluid from noninflammatory synovitis. In contrast, septic ar-

thritis or severe rheumatoid arthritis may yield fluid that is white or yellow and opaque. Rice bodies, which are hyalinized fibrin nodules containing macrophages within their fibrillar networks, are much more common in rheumatoid effusions than in those from other diagnoses[4] (Table 14–4). Blood in the fluid that is dark or does not clear during aspiration suggests trauma. Fat in bloody fluid is almost always associated with fracture through the subchondral plate into the bone marrow. Other causes of hemarthroses are listed in Table 14–5.

White Blood Cell Count

The white blood cell (WBC) count is the most helpful test but the least specific. The number of cells gives an important index of the strength of the inflammation within the joint at the time of aspiration. Cell counts can range from more than 100,000 cells/mm^3, found in sepsis, gout, Reiter's syndrome, and severe rheumatoid arthritis, to less than 200 cells/mm^3 with mild trauma or osteoarthritis[3] (Tables 14–2 and 14–3). The number of WBCs per cubic millimeter has relevance for joint destruction when the counts are high. Active proteases capable of degrading cartilage matrix and collagen are usually not measurable in synovial fluid because they are inhibited by α_2M and other protease inhibitors. However, collagenase and other proteases can be detected in synovial fluid when the neutrophil count exceeds 50,000/mm^3. At these levels, available inhibitors become saturated.

Neutrophils can have a turnover rate of more than 1 billion cells/day in an inflamed knee joint. Their numbers in fluid can be influenced markedly by large doses of glucocorticoids, but by few other compounds. Intravenous injection of 1000 mg of methylprednisolone produces a marked temporary improvement in joint symptoms in patients; this is associated with a highly significant inhibition of neutrophil ingress into inflamed knee joints that oc-

TABLE 14–1. American College of Rheumatology Office Synovial Fluid Examination Guidelines

I. Occupational Safety and Health Administration guidelines should be followed according to the universal precaution standards for exposure for bloodborne pathogens as published in the Federal Register on December 6, 1991.

II. EQUIPMENT AND MAINTENANCE MINIMA FOR PERFORMING SYNOVIANALYSIS
   A. Required list.
   1. A microscope of laboratory grade with a condenser.
   2. An ordinary white light source should be used without colored filters.
   3. $10\times$ eye piece, low power, high power, and oil immersion objectives.
   4. Polarizer and analyzer must be obtained commercially; ''home-made'' options are not acceptable.
   5. First-order red plate compensator; this must be a commercial product.
   6. The microscope must be cleaned annually.
   7. Appropriate maintenance after each use (cleaning of objectives and covering the microscope).
   8. Glass slides and coverslips.
   B. Recommended features.
   1. A binocular microscope.
   2. Phase light condenser.
   3. All components built into the microscope.
   4. The microscope is dedicated for joint fluid examination only.
   5. The annual cleaning of the microscope is done professionally.

III. REAGENT MINIMA FOR PERFORMING SYNOVIANALYSIS
   A. The Neubauer hemocytometer is preferred over automated counting systems to avoid artifact.
   B. Reagent grade 0.3% saline solution, stored in a closed container.
   C. Wright stain to be performed in accordance with any standard reference manual for joint fluid.

IV. REFERENCE STANDARDS MINIMA ON SITE
   A. A microscopic slide of a gouty tophus.
   B. Color photographs of the following, with the orienting (length slow) line of the compensator clearly marked. Examples of these may be found in reference texts, . . .
   1. Monosodium urate monohydrate crystals in yellow and blue positions, both intracellularly and extracellularly.
   2. Monoclinic and triclinic calcium pyrophosphate dihydrate crystals in the yellow and blue positions, both intracellularly and extracellularly.
   3. Corticosteroid crystals for intra-articular use, at least four common types.
   4. Cholesterol crystals.

V. JOINT FLUID EXAMINATION
   A. All specimens should be examined within two hours of aspiration to ensure the accuracy of the evaluation.
   B. Specimen should be placed in green top (*sodium* heparin) tubes, except for small volume specimen.
   C. Small specimens, less than 0.3 mL, should not be placed in a green top (*sodium* heparin) tube. These specimens should be placed in a red top (non-anticoagulated) tube and taken to the laboratory immediately. Minute specimens, i.e., a few drops only, should not be transported to the laboratory in the needle and syringe. Slides should be made at the bedside, covered with a coverslip and sealed with nail polish. This slide should then be transported to the laboratory according to current OSHA guidelines and promptly examined.
   D. Wet preparations should be examined immediately.
   E. Slides should be dust free or cleaned with lint-free wipes and glass coverslips should be used. Slides and coverslips should be used only once. . . .
   G. In appropriate instances, Gram stain and culture will be indicated to clarify the differential diagnosis.

VI. THE FOLLOWING TESTS ARE OF NO CLINICAL VALUE
   A. Mucin clot (viscosity provides equivalent information).
   B. Chemistries (e.g., protein, glucose, enzymes, electrolytes, pH).
   C. Immunologic studies (e.g., LE cell prep, immunoglobulins, complements, ANA, rheumatoid factor).

VII. PERSONNEL REQUIREMENTS
   The rheumatologist or other physician with comparable training in synovial fluid evaluation serves as the consultant or director of the laboratory for these tests. The ''testing personnel'' as defined by Clinical Laboratory Improvement Amendments (CLIA) 1988 are trained by the consultant to perform the gross examination, the wet prep for crystals, and the total white cell count. The differential white blood cell (WBC) count must be performed by a qualified technician using a Wright stain according to a standard reference for joint fluid staining. The consultant or director will conduct ongoing review of the proficiency of the testing personnel and technicians as defined by current CLIA regulations.

Table continued on opposite page

TABLE 14–1. *Continued*

VIII. **CURRENT PROCEDURAL TERMINOLOGY (CPT) CODING 1994**
    A. **Gross examination (CPT85810).**
        1. Viscosity.
        2. Color.
        3. Clarity.
    B. **Cell count.**
        1. Total white cell count (CPT89050).
        2. Total white cell count plus differential (CPT89051).
    C. **Polarizing light microscopy for crystal identification (CPT89060).**

IX. **ACCREDITATION AND MONITORING**
    Accreditation for synovial fluid evaluation by a laboratory should be granted in accordance with standards established by the American College of Rheumatology. Proficiency testing should be done on a regular periodic basis, at least annually. Recertification should occur every 2 years.

From Gatter, R. A., Andrews, R. P., Cooley, D. A., et al.: American College of Rheumatology guidelines for performing office synovial fluid examinations. J. Clin. Rheumatol. 1:194, 1995. Used by permission. Copyright 1995 by Williams & Wilkins.

curs within 90 minutes after injection and can continue for up to 2 weeks. No effect on egress was seen.[5]

The differential WBC count in synovial fluid is rarely of help in differential diagnosis, principally because, as the total number of cells increases, the number of neutrophils as a percentage of the total increases as well. In noninflammatory effusions the neutrophil–mononuclear cell ratio may be as low as $1:1$, but once the cell number exceeds $5,000/mm^3$, neutrophils will comprise more than 70 per cent of the total, and when counts exceed $50,000/mm^3$, a $10:1$ neutrophil excess over other cell types can be expected. There are exceptions to this guideline, of course. Occasionally, early rheumatoid effusions may have a predominance of mononuclear cells, as

TABLE 14–2. Relatively Noninflammatory Joint Effusions (Leukocyte Count <2,000/mm³)

Osteoarthritis	Aseptic necrosis
Traumatic arthritis	Ehlers-Danlos syndrome
Acromegaly	Sickle cell disease
Gaucher's disease	Amyloidosis
Hemochromatosis	Hypertrophic pulmonary
Hyperparathyroidism	osteoarthropathy
Ochronosis	Pancreatitis
Paget's disease	Osteochondritis dissecans
Mechanical	Charcot's joints
derangement	Wilson's disease
Erythema nodosum	Epiphyseal dysplasias
Villonodular synovitis,	Glucocorticoid withdrawal
tumors	

From Schumacher, H. R. Jr.: Synovial fluid analysis and synovial biopsy. *In* Kelley, W. N., Harris, E. D. Jr., Ruddy, S., and Sledge, C. B. (eds.): Textbook of Rheumatology, 4th ed., Vol. 1. Philadelphia, W. B. Saunders, 1993, pp. 562–578. Used by permission.

will fluids from the arthritis of early systemic lupus erythematosus. A Wright's stain preparation of fluid prepared on a slide by a cytocentrifuge is the best way to see detailed morphology of the cells. Synovial lining cells are large and round. Those with homogeneous blue cytoplasm are more often fibroblast-like type B cells; those with vacuoles and granules are usually macrophage-like type A cells. Large granular lymphocytes are similar to the large vacuolated lymphocytes associated with viral infections, and may be cytotoxic T cells or NK cells (Fig. 14–1).[6] Macrophages are usually more dense than synovial cells; they have granules, refractile organelles, and material within phagolysosomes.

Crystals and Debris in Wet Mount Preparations

By light and polarized light microscopy, much can be learned from a thorough search of a well-prepared wet mount.[3] It is important to look first at noncellular material by regular light microscopy. Fragments of cartilage, metal fragments in patients who have had replacement arthroplasty, fibrin, and lipids should be acknowledged, if present. Microscopic rice bodies are common in rheumatoid patients.[4] Inclusions in cells may be immune complexes. Compensated polarized light microscopy aids enormously in definition of the nine or more species of crystals that can be seen inside or outside cells in multiple different forms of arthritis. Parenthetically, it should be noted that gout and rheumatoid arthritis are rarely present in the same patient, perhaps because—for unknown reasons—hyperuricemia exerts anti-inflammatory actions.

Other Tests of Synovial Fluid

The "mucin clot" test is of historical interest; it gives no useful information that a WBC count and

TABLE 14–3. Inflammatory Joint Effusions (Leukocyte Count >2,000/mm³)

Rheumatoid arthritis
Psoriatic arthritis
Reiter's syndrome
Ulcerative colitis
Regional enteritis
Post–ileal bypass arthritis
Ankylosing spondylitis
Juvenile rheumatoid arthritis
Rheumatic fever
Collagen-vascular disease
    Systemic lupus erythematosus
    Scleroderma
    Polymyositis
    Polychondritis
    Polyarteritis
Polymyalgia rheumatica
Giant cell arteritis
Sjögren's syndrome
Wegener's granulomatosis
Goodpasture's syndrome
Henoch-Schönlein purpura
Familial Mediterranean fever
Whipple's disease
Behçet's syndrome
Erythema nodosum
Sarcoidosis
Multicentric reticulohistiocytosis
Erythema multiforme (Stevens-Johnson)
Post-*Salmonella*, post-*Shigella*, post-*Yersinia* arthritis
Infectious arthritis
    Parasitic
    Viral (hepatitis, mumps, rubella, human immunodeficiency
        virus, others)
    Fungal
    Mycoplasmal
    Bacterial (staphylococcal or gonococcal infection, tuberculo-
        sis, others)
    Spirochetal (Lyme disease, syphilis)
Carcinoid
Subacute bacterial endocarditis
Crystal-induced arthritis
    Gout
    Pseudogout
    Post–intra-articular steroid injection
    Apatite arthritis
    Oxalosis
Hyperlipoproteinemias
Serum sickness
Hypogammaglobulinemia
Leukemia
Hypersensitivity angiitis
Palindromic rheumatism

From Schumacher, H. R. Jr.: Synovial fluid analysis and synovial biopsy. *In* Kelley, W. N., Harris, E. D. Jr., Ruddy, S., and Sledge, C. B. (eds.): Textbook of Rheumatology, 4th ed., Vol. 1. Philadelphia, W. B. Saunders, 1993, pp. 562–578. Used by permission.

TABLE 14–4. Relationship between Diagnosis and Presence/Absence of Microscopic Rice Bodies in Synovial Fluid

	RICE BODIES		
	PRESENT (%)	ABSENT (%)	TOTAL SAMPLES
Rheumatoid arthritis	45 (34.9)*	84 (65.1)	129
Microcrystalline arthritis	3 (4)	72 (96)*	75
Osteoarthritis	1 (3.1)†	31 (96.9)**	32
Infectious arthritis	2 (15.4)	11 (84.6)	13
Seronegative spondyloarthropathies	2 (5.1)	37 (94.9)**	39
Juvenile chronic arthritis	0 (0)	10 (100)	10
Miscellany	0 (0)	8 (100)	8
Total samples	53 (17.3)	253 (82.7)	306

From Gálvez, J., Sola, J., Ortuño, G., et al.: Microscopic rice bodies in rheumatoid synovial fluid sediments. J. Rheumatol. 19:1851, 1992. Used by permission.

† The critical revision of the preparations demonstrated that they corresponded to synovium fragments coated with fibrin.
* $p<.001$.
** $p<.05$.

smear examination does not provide. The reason that inflammatory fluids do not form a firm, ropy clot when acidified (i.e., a "positive" mucin clot test) is that enzymatic destruction of hyaluronan has reduced this abundant component of synovial fluid to small fragments that disperse as a fine precipitate in these samples. Similarly, it is of historical interest that glucose levels in rheumatoid joint

TABLE 14–5. Hemarthroses

Trauma with or without fractures
Pigmented villonodular synovitis
Tumors
Hemangioma
Charcot's joint or other severe joint destruction
Hemophilia or other bleeding disorders
Von Willebrand's disease
Anticoagulant therapy
Myeloproliferative disease with thrombocytosis
Thrombocytopenia
Scurvy
Ruptured aneurysm
Arteriovenous fistula
Idiopathic
Intense inflammatory disease

From Schumacher, H. R. Jr.: Synovial fluid analysis and synovial biopsy. *In* Kelley, W. N., Harris, E. D. Jr., Ruddy, S., and Sledge, C. B. (eds.): Textbook of Rheumatology, 4th ed., Vol. 1. Philadelphia, W. B. Saunders, 1993, pp. 562–578. Used by permission.

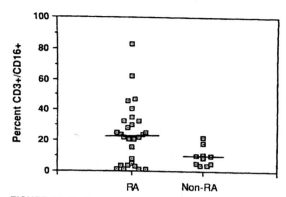

FIGURE 14–1. Scatter plot of the percentage of CD3[+]/CD16[+] cells obtained from the synovial fluid of rheumatoid arthritis (RA) ($n = 30$) and non-RA ($n = 10$) patients. (From Bray, R. A., Pope, R. M., and Landay, A. L.: Identification of a population of large granular lymphocytes obtained from the rheumatoid joint coexpressing the CD3 and CD16 antigens. Clin. Immunol. Immunopathol. 58:409, 1991. Used by permission.)

effusions are often low, related to problems in diffusion of glucose from blood vessels into the joint space, but there is no correlation between activity of disease and joint fluid glucose. As mentioned in Chapter 13, accurate pH measurements and lactate concentration in synovial fluids correlate with radiographic damage and can be useful to assess the current activity of synovitis. Cultures should be done routinely, and with special care when one joint in an established rheumatoid arthritis patient has an acute flare of disease. Complement, lactate dehydrogenase, and protein assays are not helpful in diagnosis or staging. Results of assays for immune complexes have not correlated with clinical findings or joint fluid WBC counts.

Assays of Joint Fluid with Relevance for Pathophysiology but Not for Diagnosis

The lack of enthusiasm expressed here for doing analyses other than culture, WBC count and differential, and wet mount crystal examination for clinical purposes should not discourage investigators from analyses of multiple aspects of cellular expression in synovial fluid. The synovial fluid is a mirror of disease in the synovium. For example, the local production of GM-CSF was demonstrated in synovial fluid and believed to be the first description of this cytokine at a site of disease activity.[7] This cytokine is a principal activator of macrophages. Other cytokines are elevated as well. Fifty per cent of rheumatoid patients in one series had measurable levels of TNFα,[8] the cytokine that may induce expression of IL-1, IL-6, and other proinflamma-

tory factors. In rheumatoid patients, soluble IL-2R levels in synovial fluid were significantly higher than in sera from the same patients.[9]

One interesting molecule that has multiple biologic activities and is present in rheumatoid synovial fluids is **platelet-activating factor** (PAF, PAF-acether). This small compound, 1-*O*-alkyl-2-acetyl-sn-glycero-3-phosphocholine, has been implicated as a phospholipid mediator in many different inflammatory diseases. Activation of phospholipase A_2 leads to release of both the precursors of PAF and arachidonic acid. PAF is

- a potent platelet-aggregating agent
- a neutrophil-activating factor and chemoattractant
- a stimulant of leukotriene and prostaglandin release from numerous cell types

Lipo-PAF is PAF bound to lipoprotein as a storage form. In blood and synovial fluid samples, lipo-PAF is present in much higher concentrations in specimens from rheumatoid arthritis than from other rheumatologic processes.[10] Lipo-PAF is probably the most important form of PAF in active rheumatoid arthritis.

Components or breakdown products of matrix macromolecules within synovial fluid are reminders of the marked remodeling of extracellular connective tissue that goes on in synovium and cartilage. Careful studies have shown that the fragments of **aggrecan** that are in synovial effusions from all types of inflammatory diseases as well as trauma have a similar structure. They are large, and evidence is good that they are generated by limited proteolysis of the core cartilage aggrecan protein. It is interesting that the ''aggrecanase'' has not yet been defined; the cleavage site appears not to be the same as those produced by many of the well-characterized metalloprotenases, the cathepsins, or leukocyte elastase.[11] If identified, the aggrecanase would be an appropriate therapeutic target in rheumatoid arthritis.

Hyaluronan is degraded after synthesis by synovial lining cells to smaller fragments in rheumatoid synovial fluid. The mechanism for fragmentation may be enzymatic, or nonenzymatic involving action of toxic oxygen radicals. It is speculated that the small fragments of this nonsulfated polysaccharide may interfere with normal hyaluronan-cell–matrix glycoprotein interactions in cartilage, thereby accelerating cartilage damage.[12] This is an intriguing hypothesis, and is bolstered by the reported beneficial effects of injections of high-molecular-weight hyaluronan into joints in osteoarthritis.[13]

Concentrations of antigens related to fibrinolysis (e.g., **plasminogen activator, plasminogen activator inhibitor, and plasminogen activator receptor**) have been reported to be elevated in synovial fluids of rheumatoid patients compared with those found in control fluids or fluid from osteoarthritis. There was no direct correlation of these levels with clinically assessed inflammation of the joints from which fluid was aspirated, nor were there changes in the ratio of plasminogen activator to its inhibitor.[14]

Type VI collagen microfibrils that bind to hyaluronan and are produced by synovial cells can be found by immunostaining in synovial fluid.[15] Type VI collagen may serve as anchoring matrix for synovial lining cells.

NEUTROPHILS IN RHEUMATOID ARTHRITIS

As emphasized in Chapters 7 and 9, neutrophils are an important cell in synovial fluid in rheumatoid arthritis, but rarely are they found in rheumatoid synovium. The most direct evidence to explain this is that chemoattractants for neutrophils are abundant in the fluid phase, and that these cells do not express the necessary surface adhesion molecules that would enable them to remain on matrix or cells in the synovium after their arrival through HEVs. The other sites for finding neutrophils in rheumatoid arthritis are in vasculitis, wherein vessel walls in rheumatoid vasculitis show infiltration with neutrophils, and in rheumatoid lung disease.[16]

Neutrophil Physiology

After maturing within the bone marrow for several weeks while acquiring granules, neutrophils are released into the circulation.[17] There are three types of granules in these cells:

Primary (azurophil) granules: contain myeloperoxidase, lysozyme, acid hydrolases, and elastase. Elastase is a powerful protease; in addition to elastin, it degrades aggrecan and types III and IV collagen.

Secondary (specific) granules: contain lysozyme, vitamin B_{12}–binding protein, and collagenase (capable of degrading types I, II, and III collagen).

"C" particles: contain gelatinase (capable of degrading types IV and V collagen as well as denatured fragments of all collagens).

Neutrophils degranulate after engulfing a particle too large for complete consumption or after being activated on a matrix surface. This type of "overt degranulation" can be diffusely harmful to the local environment and has been called "regurgitation during feeding."[18] In addition to degranulation, neutrophils produce both prostaglandins and leukotrienes. One of the latter, leukotriene B_4, is a strong chemoattractant for neutrophils.[19]

Activated Neutrophils in Rheumatoid Arthritis

Activation of neutrophils occurs after specific ligands bind to neutrophil receptors. These ligands include both soluble and insoluble aggregates of IgG or immune complexes, the Fc portion of immunoglobulin, leukotriene (LT) B_4, PAF, IL-8, and the C5a component of complement. Phagocytosis of particulate material, including cell membranes and fibrin, is also sufficient to activate these cells, setting into motion the release of tissue-damaging granule proteases and reactive oxygen species.[20]

Specific plasma membrane receptors on neutrophils are expressed, and others are down-regulated when these cells are activated within the joint space. **Complement receptors** (CR1 and CR3) are upregulated in neutrophils from rheumatoid synovial fluids.[21] The **FcRIII** receptor for immunoglobulins is shed from the cell surface, while expression of **FcRI**—which requires active biosynthesis—is increased.[22] Contrary to previous reports, recent evidence suggests that signaling responses of Fc receptors (**FcγRII and FcγRIII**) are identical to those in neutrophils from rheumatoid and control patients.[23] The measures used were intracellular free calcium concentrations, which rise as one of the first measurable changes after neutrophil activation. When the FyγRII or FCγRIII were blocked or removed from neutrophil surfaces, activation by soluble immune complexes did not occur, whereas blockade by insoluble aggregates of IgG was inhibited less. The inference is that the II and III Fc receptors are essential for neutrophil activation by soluble immune complexes.[24] IFNγ may be necessary for induction of synthesis of the FcRI immunoglobulin receptor.[25] **FcRII** expression remains constant on synovial fluid neutrophils. Higher numbers of activation-associated antigens (e.g., CD64 [FcγRI], CD67, CD24, and M5) were found on synovial fluid neutrophils compared to autologous peripheral blood neutrophils.[26]

Thus, it is likely that as neutrophils respond to chemotactic substances in the joint and transmigrate through the endothelium and synovial lining to the joint space, they are activated by cytokines and immune complexes, contributing significantly to synovial inflammation.[17,27] Many of them are actively synthesizing proteins such as gelatinase, fibronectin,[28] and the prototype of inflammatory cytokines, IL-1.[28a]

Another important accompaniment of neutrophil activation is mobilization of membrane phospholipids to arachidonic acid and subsequent oxidation to prostaglandins and leukotrienes. There is enhanced phospholipase activity in rheumatoid patients, and rheumatoid synovial fluid contains substantially more phospholipase A_2–activating protein compared with other inflammatory arthropathies.[29] The stable prostaglandins can produce vasodilation and increase vascular permeability within the synovium. LTB_4 may be the most relevant of arachidonic acid metabolites for pharmacologic attempts at inhibition. It is chemotactic for neutrophils, eosinophils, and macrophages; it promotes neutrophil aggregation; and it enhances neutrophil adherence to endothelial cells and NK cell cytotoxic activity.[30] Prostaglandins and leukotrienes are discussed in more detail in Chapter 17.

The active role in rheumatoid inflammation played by prostaglandins and leukotrienes is underscored by the beneficial effects of diet therapy that is rich in fish oil ω-3 fatty acids, which inhibit formation of cyclo-oxygenase products and LTB_4.[31] It is generally agreed that the principal mechanism of the anti-inflammatory actions of NSAIDs may be that of inhibiting early intracellular events that govern activation of neutrophils.[32]

Although, as stressed earlier, neutrophils rarely accumulate in the synovium, it is of interest that, at the invasive edge between synovium and cartilage, there are found occasional pockets of neutrophils[33] (see Chapter 11). These observations are consistent with the hypothesis that there is something within cartilage that serves to attract invasive cells in rheumatoid arthritis. Whether the putative ''something'' is aggregates of immune complexes, a matrix component, or an unusual surface glycoprotein on chondrocytes is not known. It has been noted that, in vitro, neutrophils attach to cartilage fragments from rheumatoid patients and invade the matrix to engulf immune complexes trapped in the tissue.[34] It is possible that activated neutrophils release both latent proteases and oxygen-derived free radicals (ODFRs); the latter could activate the former, and cartilage would be destroyed, bit by bit. By morphometric analyses, it has been estimated that no more than 10 per cent of the pannus-cartilage junction is surfaced by neutrophils, but no one knows the relative rate of tissue destruction by fibroblasts/macrophages compared with that of neutrophils.

OXYGEN-DERIVED FREE RADICALS

A free radical is defined as any atom, group of atoms, or molecule with an unpaired electron occupying an outer orbit (see ref. 35 for a good review oriented to rheumatology). Biologically, the following free radicals derived from oxygen may have relevance to pathology in connective tissue and rheumatoid arthritis:

- superoxide anion (O_2^-; O_2 plus one electron)
- singlet oxygen ($O_2^{\cdot}$, oxygen with reverse electron spin)
- hydroxyl radical ($^{\cdot}OH$; the most reactive oxy radical)
- hydrogen peroxide (H_2O_2, the 2-electron reduction product of O_2)

Although enzymes such as xanthine oxidase generate superoxide as part of their catalytic effects, the greatest sources of ODFRs are activated phagocytes and tissue damaged by ischemia-reperfusion.

The particularly aggressive hydroxyl ion can be generated by a reaction of hydrogen peroxide with ferrous iron:

$$Fe^{2+} + H_2O_2 \rightarrow Fe^{3+} + OH^- + {}^{\cdot}OH$$

Additional reactive species—N-chloroamines and hypochlorous acid (i.e., bleach)—are formed by action upon hydrogen peroxide of myeloperoxidase and halide ions.[36] Although N-chloroamines have a much lower oxidizing potential than does hypochlorous acid, these species have relatively long half-lives and the possibility of causing damage at distant sites.

Phagocytic cells (neutrophils, monocyte-macrophages) produce superoxide and hydrogen peroxide as part of a ''respiratory burst'' when they ingest particulate matter or are otherwise activated by C5a, aggregated IgG, or another stimulus. The superoxide generation that leads the process is driven by a cell membrane–associated reduced nicotinamide adenine dinucleotide phosphate (NADPH) oxidase.[20] There are data to suggest that cytokines such as GM-CSF in synovial fluid are sufficient to ''prime'' the neutrophils so that subsequent exposure to soluble immunoglobulin aggregates completely activates the cells, resulting in granule release and activation of the NADPH oxidase on the plasma membrane.[37]

Ischemia-reperfusion is the sequence that occurs in many tissues when blood supply is cut off briefly and then restored. This happens in rheumatoid synovium when the intra-articular pressures increase as joint fluid accumulates[38] (see Chapter 13).

The sequence is initiated by ischemia that precipitates activation of xanthine oxidase; when oxygen re-enters the tissue (e.g., reperfusion), xanthine oxidase acts on xanthine or hypoxanthine and superoxide is formed.

Role of Oxygen-Derived Free Radicals in Rheumatoid Arthritis

The unanswered question is: Are ODFRs involved in tissue damage in rheumatoid arthritis? Positive evidence to support a pathogenic role for ODFRs is primarily circumstantial because the half-life of most of free radical species is measured in milliseconds. The exception to this is the stable end product of the hydrogen peroxide–myeloperoxidase reaction: **hypochlorous acid**. Synovial fluid from rheumatoid patients can activate this system.[39]

Some additional circumstantial evidence to link up ODFRs to pathogenesis of the destructive components of rheumatoid arthritis has accumulated from a number of laboratories. For example, iron levels in rheumatoid synovial fluid samples correlate roughly with joint clinical counts and C-reactive protein levels[40] and are sufficient to catalyze the **superoxide–hydroxyl ion** conversion. Other data link damage to structural molecules in joints to ODFRs. Thus, as shown in Table 14–6, ODFRs can damage the macromolecules in connective tissue, all of the cells in synovium and cartilage, enzymes and protease inhibitors (particularly α_1-protease inhibitor), and immunoglobulins. **Hyaluronan** is depolymerized by superoxide-generating systems.[41] **Neutrophil collagenase** is activated from its latent pro-form by hypochlorous acid (HOCL/OCL$^-$)[42] This oxidant also has the capacity to degrade protease inhibitors, such as α_1-antitrypsin,[36,43] as well as directly damaging collagen, making it more susceptible to collagenases. As a balance to this, one of the reactive and stable end products of oxygen metabolism, N-chlorotaurine, actually inhibits collagenase activity in millimolar concentrations; thus this metabolite may help minimize damage brought about by hypochlorous acid and other chloramines. **Hydrogen peroxide**, a very diffusible compound, can inhibit cartilage proteoglycan synthesis[44] and can be generally toxic to chondrocytes.

Inflamed rheumatoid synovium, in vitro, produces more reactive oxygen species when subjected to an ischemia-reperfusion cycle than do noninflamed tissues. The method used to demonstrate this was electron spin resonance spectroscopy plus

TABLE 14–6. Substrates of Rheumatic Disease Relevance Reported To Be Susceptible to Action of ODFRs

SUBSTRATE	REPORTED EFFECT
Structural Macromolecules	
Hyaluronic acid	Depolymerization, chemical changes to saccharide components
Collagen	Impaired gelation, low-grade solubilization, proteolytic susceptibility, stimulated synthesis
Proteoglycans	Degradation, impaired synthesis
Cells and Tissues	
Endothelial cells	Membrane damage/leakage
Neutrophils	"Suicide"
Chondrocytes	Impaired growth, decreased PG synthesis
Fibroblasts	Impaired/stimulated growth
Lymphocytes	Decreased blast transformation, altered subsets
Miscellaneous Targets	
Immunoglobulins	Aggregation, changes in fluorescence, altered amino acids
Collagenase	Activation
α_1-Antiprotease	Inactivation
Serum -SH groups	Decrease
Uric acid crystal	Dissolution
Arachidonic acid and/or serum albumin–lipid complex	Generation of chemotactic products

From Greenwald, R. A.: Oxygen radicals, inflammation, and arthritis: pathophysiological considerations and implications for treatment. Semin. Arthritis Rheum. 20:219, 1991. Used by permission.

a compound that traps reactive oxygen species. Because xanthine oxidase inhibitors (e.g., oxypurinol) diminish production of oxidizing species, it has been inferred that this oxidase in endothelial cells is principally responsible for generating these reactive species.[45] It appears that, compared with circulating neutrophils from controls, most of the circulating and synovial fluid neutrophils in patients with rheumatoid arthritis are in a state of "readiness" to generate superoxide radicals upon activation by inflammatory stimuli; substances such as PAF can prime these cells.[46]

Regulation of Oxygen-Derived Free Radicals

It is likely that the only path to determine the role of the products of oxygen metabolism in pathogenesis is to utilize specific inhibitors of oxygen radical formation and activity in experimental situations and, eventually, in patients.

Superoxide Dismutase

Superoxide dismutase is an intracellular protein found primarily in erythrocytes. It is induced by high oxygen tensions and acts as an effective scavenger of free radicals. The antioxidant capability of ceruloplasmin is useful as an adjunct free-radical scavenger.[47]

Drugs

There has not been a drug utilized that acts specifically as a scavenger of ODFRs or as an inhibitor of their formation. Glucocorticoids, for example, have a net effect of diminishing the capabilities of cellular production of oxygen radicals, but there is no suggestion that this effect is other than one related to generalized suppression of leukocyte function. Gold, similarly, has been identified as diminishing oxygen production by macrophages.[35]

Orgotein

Orgotein, a protein isolated from liver, was found to be superoxide dismutase after it had been touted as an anti-inflammatory agent. The fact that it cannot be given by mouth has inhibited its pharmacologic use. In the future, purified and possibly recombinant versions of superoxide dismutase, altered chemically or in ''packaging,'' might be available for oral therapy and serve to minimize free radical damage in rheumatoid joints.

REFERENCES

1. Owen, D. S. Jr.: Aspiration and injection of joints and soft tissues. In Kelley, W. N., Harris, E. D. Jr., Ruddy, S., and Sledge, C. B., (eds.): Textbook of Rheumatology, 4th ed., Vol. 1, Philadelphia, W. B. Saunders, 1993, pp. 545–561.
2. Gatter, R. A., Andrews, R. P., Cooley, D. A., et al.: American College of Rheumatology guidelines for performing office synovial fluid examinations. J. Clin. Rheumatol. 1:194, 1995.
3. Schumacher, H. R. Jr.: Synovial fluid analysis and synovial biopsy. In Kelley, W. N., Harris, E. D. Jr., Ruddy, S., and Sledge, C. B., (eds.): Textbook of Rheumatology, 4th ed. Vol. 1. Philadelphia, W. B. Saunders, 1993, pp. 562–578.
4. Gálvez, J., Sola, J., Ortuño, G., et al.: Microscopic rice bodies in rheumatoid synovial fluid sediments. J. Rheumatol. 19:1851, 1992.
5. Youssef, P. P., Cormack, J., Evill, C. A., et al.: Neutrophil trafficking into inflamed joints in patients with rheumatoid arthritis, and the effects of methylprednisolone. Arthritis Rheum. 39:216, 1996.
6. Bray, R. A., Pope, R. M., and Landay, A. L.: Identification

of a population of large granular lymphocytes obtained from the rheumatoid joint coexpressing the CD3 and CD16 antigens. Clin. Immunol. Immunopathol. 58:409, 1991.

In this study of synovial fluid mononuclear cells, there was an increased percentage of large granular lymphocytes (LGL) within the population of mononuclear cells obtained from rheumatoid patients compared to those without rheumatoid arthritis (Table 14–7). The LGLs expressed an unusual phenotype, that has been associated with efficiency in mediating antibody-dependent cytotoxicity without significant NK function. Several reports have noted the association of an expanded population of LGL and polyarthritis, and approximately 25 per cent of patients with this lymphoproliferative disorder may also have rheumatoid arthritis.

7. Xu, W. D., Firestein, G. S., Taetle, R., et al.: Cytokines in chronic inflammatory arthritis. II. Granulocyte-macrophage colony-stimulating factor in rheumatoid synovial effusions. J. Clin. Invest. 83:876, 1989.
8. Saxne, T., Palladino, M. A., Heinegård, D., et al.: Detection of tumor necrosis factor α but not tumor necrosis factor β in rheumatoid arthritis synovial fluid and serum. Arthritis Rheum. 31:1041, 1988.
9. Keystone, E. C., Snow, K. M., Bombardier, C., et al.: Elevated soluble interleukin-2 receptor levels in the sera and synovial fluids of patients with rheumatoid arthritis. Arthritis Rheum. 31:844, 1988.
10. Hilliquin, P., Menkes, C. J., Laoussadi, S., et al.: Presence of paf-acether in rheumatic diseases. Ann. Rheum. Dis. 51:29, 1992.
11. Lohmander, L. S., Neame, P. J., and Sandy, I. D.: The structure of aggrecan fragments in human synovial fluid: evidence that aggrecanase mediates cartilage degradation in inflammatory joint disease, joint injury, and osteoarthritis. Arthritis Rheum. 36:1214, 1993.
12. Henderson, E. B., Grootveld, M., Farrell, A., et al.: A pathological role for damaged hyaluronan in synovitis. Ann. Rheum. Dis. 50:196, 1991.
13. Dixon, S. J., Jacoby, R. K., Berry, H., et al.: Clinical trial of intra-articular injection of sodium hyaluronate in patients with osteoarthritis of the knee. Curr. Med. Res. Opin. 11: 205, 1988.
14. Belcher, C., Fawthrop, F., Bunning, R., Doherty, M.: Plasminogen activators and their inhibitors in synovial fluids from normal, osteoarthritis, and rheumatoid arthritis knees. Ann. Rheum. Dis. 55:230, 1996.
15. Waggett, A. D., Kielty, C. M., and Shuttleworth, C. A.: Micrifibrillar elements in the synovial joint: presence of type VI collagen and fibrillin-containing microfibrils. Ann. Rheum. Dis. 52:449, 1993.
16. Garcia, J. G. N., James, H. L., Zinkgraf, S., et al.: Lower respiratory tract abnormalities in rheumatoid interstitial lung disease: potential role of neutrophils in lung injury. Am. Rev. Resp. Dis. 136:811, 1987.
17. Kitsis, E., and Weissmann, G.: The role of the neutrophil in rheumatoid arthritis. Clin. Orthop. Rel. Res. 265:63, 1991.
18. Weissmann, G., Zurier, R. B., Spieler, P. J., et al.: Mechanisms of lysosomal enzyme release from leukocytes exposed to immune complexes and other particles. J. Exp. Med. 134:149, 1971.
19. Goetzl, E. J., and Pickett, W. C.: The human PMN leukocyte chemotactic activity of complex hydroxyeicosatetraenoic acids (HETEs). J. Immunol. 125:1789, 1980.
20. Bellavite, P.: The superoxide forming enzymatic system of phagocytes. Free Radic. Biol. Med. 4:225, 1988.

21. Berger, M., O'Shea, J., Cross, A. S., et al.: Human neutrophils increase expression of C3bi as well as C3b receptors upon activation. J. Clin. Invest. 74:1566, 1984.

22. Watson, F., Robinson, J. J., Phelan, M., et al.: Receptor expression in synovial fluid neutrophils from patients with rheumatoid arthritis. Ann. Rheum. Dis. 52:354,1993.

23. Jones, J., Laffafian, I., Lawson, T., et al.: Signalling through neutrophil Fc RIII, Fc RII, and CD59 is not impaired in active rheumatoid arthritis. Ann Rheum. Dis. 55:294, 1996.

24. Robinson, J. J., Watson, F., Bucknall, R. C., et al.: Role of Fcγ receptors in the activation of neutrophils by soluble and insoluble immunoglobulin aggregates isolated from the synovial fluid of patients with rheumatoid arthritis. Ann. Rheum. Dis. 53:515, 1994.

25. Perussia, B., Dayton, E., Lazarus, R., et al.: Immune interferon induces the receptor for monomeric IgG1 on human monocyte and myeloid cells. J. Exp. Med. 158:1092, 1985.

26. Felzmann, T., Gadd, S., Majdic, O., et al.: Analysis of function-associated receptor molecules on peripheral blood and synovial fluid granulocytes from patients with rheumatoid and reactive arthritis. J. Clin. Immunol. 11:205, 1991.

27. Nurcombe, H. L., Bucknall, R. C., and Edwards, S. W.: Neutrophils isolated from the synovial fluid of patients with rheumatoid arthritis: priming and activation *in vivo*. Ann. Rheum. Dis. 50:147, 1991.

28. Beaulieu, A. D., Lang, F., Belles-Isles, M., et al.: Protein biosynthetic activity of polymorphonuclear leukocytes in inflammatory arthropathies: increased synthesis and release of fibronectin. J. Rheumatol. 14:656, 1987.

28a. Quayle, J. A., Adams, S., Bucknall, R. C., and Edwards, S. W.: Interleukin-1 expression by neutrophils in rheumatoid arthritis. Ann. Rheum. Dis. 54:930, 1995.

29. Bomalaski, J. S., Fallon, M., Turner, R. A., et al.: Identification and isolation of a phospholipase A$_2$ activating protein in human rheumatoid arthritis synovial fluid: induction of eicosanoid synthesis and an inflammatory response in joints injected *in vivo*. J. Lab. Clin. Med. 116:814, 1990.

30. Zurier, R. B.: Prostaglandins, leukotrienes, and related compounds. *In* Kelley, W. N., Harris, E. D. Jr., Ruddy, S., and Sledge, C. B. (eds.): Textbook of Rheumatology, 4th ed., Vol. 1. Philadelphia, W. B. Saunders, 1993, pp. 201–212.

31. Kremer, J. M., Lawrence, D. A., Jubiz, W., et al.: Dietary fish oil and olive oil supplementation in patients with rheumatoid arthritis: clinical and immunological effects. Arthritis Rheum. 33:810, 1990.

32. Abramson, S., Korchak, J., Ludewig, R., et al.: The modes of action of aspirin-like drugs. Proc. Natl. Acad. Sci. U.S.A. 82:7227, 1985.

33. Mohr, W., Wild, A., and Wolf, H. P.: Role of polymorphs

34. Ugai, K., Ishikawa, H., Hirohata, K., et al.: Interaction of polymorphonuclear leukocytes with immune complexes trapped in rheumatoid articular cartilage. Arthritis Rheum. 26:1434, 1983.

35. Greenwald, R. A.: Oxygen radicals, inflammation, and arthritis: pathophysiological considerations and implications for treatment. Semin. Arthritis Rheum. 20:219, 1991.

36. Weiss, S. J.: Tissue destruction by neutrophils. N. Engl. J. Med. 320:365, 1989.

37. Robinson, J. J., Watson, F., Phelan, M., et al.: Activation of neutrophils by soluble and insoluble immunoglobulin aggregates from synovial fluid of patients with rheumatoid arthritis. Ann. Rheum. Dis. 52:347, 1993.

38. Blake, D. R., Unsworth, J., Outhwaite, J. M., et al.: Hypoxic reperfusion injury in the inflamed human joint. Lancet 1:289,1989.

39. Nurcombe, H. L., Bucknall, R. C., and Edwards, S. W.: Activation of the neutrophil myeloperoxidase-H$_2$O$_2$ system by synovial fluid isolated from patients with rheumatoid arthritis. Ann. Rheum. Dis. 50:237, 1991.

40. Gutteridge, J. C.: Bleomycin detectable iron in knee-joint synovial fluid from arthritic patients and its relationship to the extracellular oxidant activities of ceruloplasmin, transferrin, and lactoferrin. Biochem. J. 245:415, 1987.

41. Halliwell, B.: Superoxide-induced generation of hydroxyl radicals in the presence of iron salts: its role in degradation of hyaluronic acid by a superoxide-generating system. FEBS Lett. 96:238, 1978.

42. Davies, J. M. S., Horwitz, D. A., and Davies, K. J. A.: Potential role of hypochlorous acid and N-chloroamines in collagen breakdown by phagocytic cells in synovitis. Free Radic. Biol. Med. 15:637, 1993.

43. Weiss, S. J., Peppin, G. J., Ortiz, X., et al.: Oxidative autoactivation of latent collagenase by human neutrophils. Science 227:747, 1985.

44. Bates, J., Johnson, C. C., and Lowther, D. A.: Inhibition of proteoglycan synthesis by hydrogen peroxide in cultured bovine articular cartilage. Biochim. Biophys. Acta 838:221, 1985.

45. Singh, D., Nazhat, N. B., Fairburn, K., et al.: Electron spin resonance spectroscopic demonstration of the generation of reactive oxygen species by diseased human synovial tissue following *ex vivo* hypoxia-reoxygenation. Ann. Rheum. Dis. 5:94, 1995.

46. Eggleton, P., Wang, L., Penhallow, J., et al.: Differences in oxidative response of subpopulations of neutrophils from healthy subjects and patients with rheumatoid arthritis. Ann. Rheum. Dis. 54:916, 1995.

47. Gutteridge, J. M. C.: Antioxidant properties of the proteins ceruloplasmin, albumin, and transferrin: a study of their activity in serum and synovial fluid from patients with rheumatoid arthritis. Biochim. Biophys. Acta 869:119, 1986.

SECTION VI

IMPORTANT SECONDARY FACTORS IN THE PATHOGENESIS OF RHEUMATOID ARTHRITIS

It would have been reasonable to include discussions of nitric oxide, neuropeptides, arachidonic acid metabolites, and the kinin/complement/clotting and fibrinolysin systems that are activated in rheumatoid arthritis in a discussion of rheumatoid synovium or synovial fluid. After all, it is in these sites that these pathways have their expression in the disease. However, each of these pathogenic pathways is gaining in importance in pathogenesis with each month of newly published data. Thus it is appropriate to include them in separate chapters. Each of them mediates inflammation or proliferation in different ways, but each contributes substantially to the progression and cyclic amplification of the rheumatoid process. By ''cyclic amplification'' is meant the interactive process among pathogenic pathways within a rheumatoid joint that may make it possible for synovitis to sustain itself without the presence of the originating immune stimulus. These secondary factors should be considered as crucial cofactors in development of rheumatoid arthritis.

15

Nitric Oxide: Messenger for Modulation of Inflammation

Nitric oxide, a noxious by-product of automobile exhaust and power stations, is now known to be an important biologic messenger. It has profound effects upon blood vessels, neurotransmission, and the immune system. Because it is an uncharged molecule with an unpaired electron, it diffuses easily across cell membranes, and having an unpaired electron, it is highly reactive. Its half-life is less than 30 seconds.

NITRIC OXIDE SYNTHASE—CONSTITUTIVE AND INDUCIBLE

Nitric oxide is generated by nitric oxide synthase in a reaction that catalyzes conversion of L-arginine and oxygen into citrulline and nitric oxide[1] (Fig. 15–1). The mechanism involves a complicated cascade of electron transfer between various cofactors, including tetrahydrobiopterin and heme.

Nitric oxide synthase is a constitutive product of neuronal and endothelial cells but must be induced in macrophages, chondrocytes, and synovial cells. It has been shown that nitric oxide synthase is induced by cytokines in synovial fibroblasts[2] and in neutrophils by PAF and LTB$_4$.[3] In most systems, IL-1 and TNFα have similar effects. However, IL-1 induces nitric oxide synthesis in articular chondrocytes, whereas TNFα does not, a finding consistent with others indicating that, whereas IL-1β and TNFα are often synergistic in their actions on synovial cells, IL-1β has a much greater effect upon cartilage. Chondrocytes in cell culture appear to produce three to four times more nitric oxide per cell than do synovial fibroblasts,[4] and nitric oxide appears to decrease prostaglandin and type II collagen production by chondrocytes in culture and increase metalloprotease as well as aggrecan production by these cells.

Whereas the constitutive isoforms of nitric oxide are inactive until cellular calcium levels increase

and a calcium-calmodulin complex activates the enzyme, the role of calmodulin in activation of the inducible form is not well defined.[1] Induction of nitric oxide synthase in macrophages by IFNγ, IL-1, and TNFα has been demonstrated in rodent cells, and probably is accomplished by their stimulation of formation of one of the crucial cofactors, tetrahydrobiopterin.[5] It is clear that production of angiogenic activity by human monocytes requires a L-arginine–nitric oxide synthase-dependent effector mechanism.[6] Patients given IL-2 in therapeutic trials excrete nitric oxide by-products in their urine; from these data it has been inferred that the cytokine-activated macrophages are producing the nitric oxide.[7] Once nitric oxide synthase is produced, it always synthesizes large amounts of nitric oxide when abundant cofactors are present.

EFFECTS OF NITRIC OXIDE ON TARGET CELLS

Once it is generated, nitric oxide diffuses out of the cell and into nearby target cells, where it interacts with specific molecules. Among these are heme iron and iron-sulfur in iron-dependent enzymes. In smooth muscle cells, for example, nitric oxide activates guanylate cyclase, leading to an increase in cGMP that leads to arteriole dilation; indeed, nitric oxide is now known to be ''endothelial-derived relaxation factor,'' first described physiologically in the 1980s.[8]

POTENTIAL ROLE FOR NITRIC OXIDE IN RHEUMATOID SYNOVITIS

Unlike many mediators, nitric oxide appears to have *both* phlogistic and anti-inflammatory potential in the synovium. For example, the neuropeptide substance P promotes generation of nitric oxide that

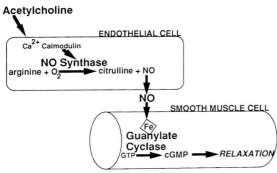

Acetylcholine

FIGURE 15–1. Effect of nitric oxide on arterial smooth muscle. A messenger molecule such as acetylcholine binds to the acetylcholine receptor on an endothelial cell, activating inward calcium currents. Calcium binds to calmodulin and activates endothelial cell nitric oxide synthase, which converts arginine plus oxygen into citrulline and nitric oxide. Nitric oxide diffuses out of the endothelial cell into an adjacent smooth muscle cell and activates guanylate cyclase by binding to the iron in its heme group. The increase in cGMP causes smooth muscle relaxation, and thus vasodilation. (From Lowenstein C. J., Dinerman, J. L., and Snyder, S. H.: Nitric oxide: a physiologic messenger. Ann. Intern. Med. 120:227, 1994. Used by permission.)

mediates angiogenesis in vivo (rabbit cornea) and the migration and proliferation of endothelial cells in cultures.[9] Interestingly, one major stimulus of angiogenesis—bFGF—does not use the nitric oxide pathway to induce new capillary formation.

Nitric oxide inhibits expression by human endothelial cells of cytokine-induced adhesion molecules, such as VCAM-1 and E-selectin. This could down-regulate synovitis. Data suggest that this effect is on gene transcription, in part, by inhibiting NF-$\kappa\beta$. Experiments suggest that, in addition to being antiatherogenic, nitric oxide is anti-inflammatory within the vessel wall.[10]

In contrast, although nitric oxide itself does not affect T-cell proliferation, one of its derivatives—*S*-nitrosoglutathione—inhibits DNA synthesis by activated lymphocytes.[11] This inhibition may be related to inactivation by the nitric oxide derivative of ribonucleotide reductase required for DNA synthesis in activated T cells. There is evidence that *S*-nitrosoglutathione is formed intracellularly within neutrophils in response to nitric oxide interacting with glutathione, and that this thiol can inhibit superoxide production within the cytosol.[12] Activated neutrophils have the capability to degrade *S*-nitrosothiols however,[13] and it is not clear whether the net effect in synovial cells is inflammatory or anti-inflammatory.

It has also been suggested that the interaction of superoxide and nitric oxide (also a free radical) could be dangerous to tissues. A preliminary product of their combination, peroxynitrite ($ONOO^-$),

can oxidize methionine and sulfhydryl groups of proteins. Peroxynitrite breaks down to multiple toxic products, including nitrogen dioxide and the hydroxyl radical (see review in ref. 14). One study has determined that nitric oxide produced by human endothelial cells interacts with neutrophils to produce lipoxin A_4 and superoxide radicals, leading to significant toxicity to the endothelial cells.[15]

On histologic examination of rheumatoid synovium, synovial endothelial cells appear luxuriant and healthy, and there is little suggestion that they are being damaged. However, particularly at the ends of synovial fronds, there are areas of infarction and necrosis of synovium; perhaps nitric oxide or its metabolites have a role in causing this terminal vasculitis.

Certain NSAIDs appear to block inducible nitrogen oxide synthase independently of their effects on cyclo-oxygenase (Amin et al. Abstract 1144). It is possible that this has an impact on the activity in rheumatoid arthritis of these drugs.

A recently developed and relatively simple assay for endogenous nitric oxide production should make more clinical studies of this substance possible. Instead of the use of chemiluminescence as a detection system, or assaying its breakdown products, nitrate and nitrite, after dietary restriction, there is evidence that the nitrate-creatinine ratio in a morning urine specimen obtained after an overnight fast provides a robust and sensitive assay system.[16] This urinary nitrate-creatinine ratio is elevated in patients with rheumatoid arthritis, and is more sensitive than serum nitrate concentrations. Unanswered remain the questions of which tissues are contributing to the nitrate production, and whether the net effect of increased nitric oxide is proinflammatory or anti-inflammatory.

Although there is no way to be sure, on balance, the effects of nitric oxide would be more in favor of down-regulation of lymphocyte and neutrophil function than upgrading of the immunoproliferative disease in rheumatoid arthritis. It is not unrealistic to suggest that trials of large amounts of L-arginine, to drive production of more nitric oxide, would be interesting to pursue.

REFERENCES

1. Lowenstein, C. J., Dinerman, J. L., and Snyder, S. H.: Nitric oxide: a physiologic messenger. Ann. Intern. Med. 120: 227, 1994.
2. Stefanovic-Racic, M., Stadler, J., Georgescu, H., et al.: Nitric oxide production by cytokine stimulated synovial fibroblasts. Trans. Orthop. Res. Soc. 17:228, 1992.
3. Schmidt, H. H. H. W., Seifer, R., and Bohme, E.: Formation and release of nitric oxide from human neutrophils and HL-60 c induced by a chemotactic peptide, platelet acti-

vating factor, and leukotriene B_4. FEBS Lett. 244:357, 1989.

4. Stefanovic-Racic, M., Stadler, J., and Evans, C. H.: Nitric oxide and arthritis. Arthritis Rheum. 36:1036, 1993.

5. Rosenkranz-Weiss, P., Sessa W. C., Milstien, S., et al.: Regulation of nitric oxide synthesis by proinflammatory cytokines in human umbilical vein endothelial cells: elevation in tetrahydrobiopterin levels enhance endothelial nitric oxide synthase specific activity. J. Clin. Invest. 93:2236, 1994.

6. Leibovich, S. J., Polverini, P. J., Fong, T. W., et al.: Production of angiogenic activity by human monocytes requires an L-arginine/nitric oxide-synthase-dependent effector mechanism. Proc. Natl. Acad. Sci. U.S.A. 91:4190, 1994.

7. Hibbs, J. B. Jr., Westenfelder, C., Taintor, et al.: Evidence for cytokine-inducible nitric oxide synthesis from L-arginine in patients receiving interleukin-2 therapy. J. Clin. Invest. 89:867, 1992.

8. Palmer, R. M., Ferrige, A. G., and Moncada, S.: Nitric oxide release accounts for the biological activity of endothelium-derived relaxing factor. Nature 327:524, 1987.

9. Ziche, M., Morbidelli, L., Masini, E., et al.: Nitric oxide mediates angiogenesis *in vivo* and endothelial cell growth and migration *in vitro* promoted by substance P. J. Clin. Invest. 94:2036, 1994.

10. de Caterina, R., Libby, P., Peng, H.-B., et al.: Nitric oxide decreases cytokine-induced endothelial activation: nitric oxide selectively reduces endothelial expression of adhesion molecules and proinflammatory cytokines. J. Clin. Invest. 96:60, 1995.

11. Meryman, P. F., Clancy, R. M., Xy, H. E. et al.: Modulation of human T cell responses by nitric oxide and its derivative, *S*-nitrosoglutathione. Arthritis Rheum. 10:1414, 1993.

12. Clancy, R. M., Levartovsky, D., Leszczynska-Piziak, J., et al.: Nitric oxide reacts with intracellular glutathione and activates the hexose monophosphate shunt in human neutrophils: evidence for *S*-nitrosoglutathione as a bioactive intermediary. Proc. Natl. Acad. Sci. U.S.A. 91:3680, 1994.

13. Clancy, R. M., and Abramson, S. B.: *De novo* synthesis of *S*-nitroglutathione and degradation by human neutrophils. Anal. Biochem. 204:365, 1992.

14. Halliwell, B.: Oxygen radicals, nitric oxide and human inflammatory disease. Arthritis Rheum. 54:505, 1995.

15. Bratt, J., and Gyllenhammar, H.: The role of nitric oxide in lipoxin Af-induced polymorphonuclear neutrophil-dependent cytotoxicity to human vascular endothelium *in vitro*. Arthritis Rheum. 38:768, 1995.

16. Grabowski, P. S., England, A. J., Dykhuizen, R., et al.: Elevated nitric oxide production in rheumatoid arthritis: Detection using the fasting urinary nitrate: creatinine ratio. Arthritis Rheum. 39:643, 1996.

16

The Pain of Arthritis—Neuroendocrine Associations

It is interesting, and somewhat ironic, that articular cartilage—the tissue targeted for destruction in rheumatoid arthritis—has no afferent or efferent innervation from the nervous system. Thus, the pain that patients have is not directly related to ongoing loss of cartilage. It is of equal interest that, although the pathology of osteoarthritis begins in cartilage, it is not until periosteal tissues, subchondral bone, or synovium are secondarily involved in the degradative process that these individuals have pain.

The pain of arthritis can be severe, and has been the topic of novels and the catch phrase of advertisements for analgesics. An understanding of the origins of this pain is now possible by the realization that fixed, simple neural pathways do not explain pain in and around inflamed joints. The interlinking nerve networks are flexible, involve spinal circuits, and are both triggered and amplified by many cytokines, neuropeptides, and other inflammatory mediators.

The striking symmetry of joint involvement in rheumatoid arthritis in most if not all patients with the disease has intrigued students and investigators for many years, and has stimulated the search for links of joint inflammation to the central nervous system. Such connections have been found, and may have important bearing on why rheumatoid arthritis is symmetrical, why some individuals are more susceptible to developing inflammation than others, why inflammation subsides in limbs that become paralyzed, and, perhaps, how emotions can influence the activity of disease.

THE PAIN OF ARTHRITIS

Synovial joints are innervated by all three groups of fibers found within afferent peripheral nerves: heavily myelinated $A\beta$ fibers, thinly myelinated $A\delta$ fibers and unmyelinated C fibers. C fibers comprise the vast majority. Some of the unmyelinated

nerves are sympathetic postganglionic fibers. The tissues innervated by these groups of fibers include the synovium, tendons, ligaments, and periosteum. Heavily myelinated $A\beta$ fibers detect movement within the normal range (proprioception); noxious stimuli are carried centrally by $A\delta$ and C fibers.

When sustained inflammation develops in a rheumatoid joint, several mechanisms of pain amplification come into play (this topic is reviewed well in ref. 1):

- Inflammatory mediators released by cells in the synovium and synovial fluid have direct effects on afferent nerves. PGE_2, PGD_2, and PGI_2 activate sensory fibers directly and also sensitize nerve endings to chemicals such as bradykinin.
- Protons, increased in inflamed joints during relative ischemia and acidosis (see Chapter 13), have an excitatory effect on nerve endings.
- C fibers become sensitized to noradrenaline and sympathetic nerve ending discharges.
- Neurogenic inflammation is mediated through biologically active peptides such as substance P. These are synthesized in dorsal root ganglion cell bodies; from there they are transported both to peripheral tissues by unmyelinated fibers and to synaptic terminals within the spinal cord. Substance P and other neuropeptides are found in increased concentrations in nerves around inflamed joints (see following section).
- A strong contribution by interconnections in the spinal cord to pain perceived in and around inflamed joints is now recognized. Of particular importance is the *N*-methyl-D-aspartate (NDMA) receptor in spinal neurons that is activated by "excitatory" amino acids, including glutamate and aspartate delivered by C fibers. C fiber activity appears to "unmask" receptors in spinal neurons, and the subsequent NDMA receptor activation maintains a central hyperexcitability. The net effect, as summarized by Woolf,[2] is that re-

sponses to normal stimuli are increased; the size of the receptive field is increased from, for example, inflamed synovium to surrounding ligaments, muscle, and even skin; and the threshold for activation is reduced.

This is an active field for research, particularly because recognition of these multiple pathways in generation of the pain of arthritis may lead to new modalities of reducing pain.

SUBSTANCE P AND RELATED NEUROPEPTIDES

Substance P is a neuropeptide stored in secretory granules of sensory neurons such as unmyelinated C fibers. Once released, substance P has been linked to the following activity in tissues (see ref. 3–6 and references therein):

- Activation of macrophages
- Stimulation of human B lymphocyte differentiation
- Degranulation of mast cells, with release of histamine
- Proliferation of fibroblasts
- Increase in expression of cytokines, prostaglandins, and metalloproteases
- Increase in microvascular permeability
- Chemotaxis and activation of neutrophils
- Stimulation of mononuclear leukocyte chemotaxis

Substance P and Joint Innervation

Substance P is an undecapeptide member of the tachykinin family, and therefore related to neurokinins A and B, sharing a common carboxyl-terminal sequence (Phe-X-Gly-Leu-Met). After synthesis in dorsal root ganglia substance P is distributed to peripheral nerve terminals. It is also the central neurotransmitter in afferent C fibers that have a nociceptive function. In addition, it is established that substance P has an efferent action, when sensory nerve activation causes reverse (antidromic) transmission in these same peripheral C fibers. Thus antidromic stimulation of a peripheral sensory nerve causes vasodilation, plasma extravasation into tissues, and increased vascular permeability.[7] This phenomenon is referred to as neurogenic inflammation; it can be prevented by denervation and by pretreatment with capsaicin.

Careful studies have shown that, in experimental arthritis, joints that have a higher density of inner-

vation develop a more severe arthritis than other joints with fewer Aδ or C fiber nerve endings.[8]

In rheumatoid joints, nerve fibers reactive with substance P are found around small blood vessels deep in the synovium, but in lesser density in superficial synovial layers than is found in normal synovium.[9]

Neuropeptides and Rheumatoid Arthritis

Studies of experimental arthritis have emphasized that a decrease in peripheral sympathetic activity may have a beneficial effect on arthritis. To test this, a double-blind trial with regional sympathetic blockade using guanethidine has been tried[10]; in short-term trials, the guanethidine-treated group had better clinical outcome.

Measurements of substance P–like immunoreactivity have been performed on patients with rheumatoid arthritis and osteoarthritis. Higher levels were found in synovial fluid of rheumatoid patients than in the patients with osteoarthritis, but the content in the synovium was higher in osteoarthritis than in rheumatoid arthritis, suggesting that there is a secretory process of substance P into the fluid in rheumatoid arthritis.[4]

It is of interest that another neuropeptide stored in secretory granules of sensory neurons and released upon axonal stimulation is **somatostatin**. Unlike substance P, which has inflammatory activity, somatostatin appears to have actions that downregulate synovitis. In vitro, somatostatin was found to be a selective antagonist of substance P on human neutrophils,[5] setting it up as an endogenous inhibitor of ''neurogenic inflammation.'' In contrast, a similar neuropeptide, **calcitonin gene-related peptide,** may be synergistic as a phlogistic agent with substance P.

Capsaicin—Experimental and Therapeutic Uses

Capsaicin is the active ingredient in chili peppers. It has been incorporated into cremes that can be applied to skin. After initial application, small sensory fibers are activated, neuropeptides are released, and the skin becomes hyperalgesic. Continued application blocks conduction in C fibers and depletes neuropeptides from terminal axons, thereby suppressing neurogenic inflammation. Used regularly in patients who have exquisite sensitivity to pressure or temperature over inflamed joints, capsaicin may block one or more components of the spinal neuron amplification of referred pain from inflamed joints.

THE HYPOTHALAMIC-PITUITARY-ADRENAL AXIS IN RHEUMATOID ARTHRITIS

The hypothalamus and paraventricular nucleus, and their secretion of corticotropin-releasing hormone (CRH), are affected by many different stimuli[11] (Table 16–1). CRH regulates many adaptive responses, including

- Mood
- Food intake
- Behavior
- Reproductive function
- Immune and inflammatory responses

Large amounts of CRH have been found in rheumatoid synovial fluid and synovial tissue. It is of great potential importance that differences in the CRH responsiveness of animals—and perhaps humans—may affect inflammation. The complexity of the neuroendocrine system is illustrated by the fact that CRH has both stimulatory and suppressive effects upon inflammation. As a coordinator of the stress response, it sets off a cascade resulting in increased synthesis and release of glucocorticoids. In contrast, in the periphery (e.g., joints) it acts as an autocrine or paracrine inflammatory cytokine[12] (Fig. 16–1).

TABLE 16–1. Stimuli Affecting Secretion of CRH

UP-REGULATORS	DOWN-REGULATORS
Acetylcholine	γ-Aminobutyric acid
Norepinephrine	Opioids
Serotonin	Corticosteroids
IL-1	IL-1ra
TNFα	
IL-6	
IL-2	
PAF	

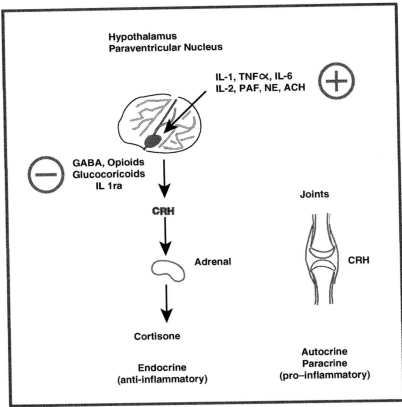

FIGURE 16–1. The regulation and effects of CRH. Released from the hypothalamus, it is anti-inflammatory through its enhancement of cortisol secretion. In joints, however, it has proinflammatory qualities. NE, norepinephrine; ACH, acetylcholine; GABA, γ-aminobutyric acid.

In the streptococcal cell wall arthritis model in rats, which has many similarities to rheumatoid arthritis, there is a remarkable difference between Fischer rats that are resistant to the streptococcal cell wall stimulus and the susceptible Lewis rats. The data show that Lewis rats do not secrete significant amounts of CRH, and thus do not have an adrenal response of cortisone to inflammatory stimuli. When IL-1β is applied directly to the hypothalamus of Lewis rats, there is neither a CRH release nor a cortisol response.[13,14] Thus, the susceptibility of the Lewis rats to arthritis may be due to a hypothalamic defect in synthesis and secretion of CRH. Is it possible that rheumatoid patients have a similar defect, an inability to muster sufficient glucocorticoids to suppress the initial inflammation that, unchecked, goes on to active and chronic synovitis?

These studies have led to the hypothesis that rheumatoid patients produce less cortisol than normal patients.[15] To support this, it has been shown that, despite being treated with low-dose steroids, the ratio of corticotropin to cortisol in rheumatoid patients is much increased,[16,17] and that rheumatoid patients have a profoundly blunted response of cortisol to surgery versus controls, in spite of increased plasma concentrations of IL-1β and IL-6. Treatment of rheumatoid patients with NSAIDs reduced plasma corticotropin levels to normal but did not affect the serum cortisol levels significantly.[17] Many further studies are needed to determine whether there are pathogenetic or therapeutic implications to these studies.

Another interesting finding relating to the neuroendocrine system is that patients with rheumatoid arthritis have less bioreactive **prolactin** than do control patients.[18] Conditions that have high levels of prolactin (e.g., pregnancy) are inversely associated with rheumatoid arthritis, but it remains to be determined whether variations in prolactin synthesis have a bioactive effect upon the immune system in rheumatoid arthritis.

REFERENCES

1. Kidd, B. L., Morris, V. H., and Urban, L.: Pathophysiology of joint pain. Ann. Rheum. Dis. 55:276, 1996.
2. Wolff, C. J.: Generation of acute pain: Central mechanisms. Br. Med. J. 47:523, 1991.
3. Garrett, N. E., Mapp, P. I., Cruwys, S. C., et al.: Role of substance P in inflammatory arthritis. Ann Rheum Dis 51:1014, 1992.
4. Menkes, C. J., Renoux, M., Laoussadi, S., et al.: Substance P levels in the synovium and synovial fluid from patients with rheumatoid arthritis and osteoarthritis. J. Rheumatol. 20:714, 1993.
5. Kolasinski, S. L., Haines, K. A., Siegel, E. L., et al.: Neuropeptides and inflammation: a somatostatin analog as a selective antagonist of neutrophil activation by substance P. Arthritis Rheum. 35:369, 1992.
6. Levine, J. D., Goetzl, E. J., and Basbaum, A. I.: Contribution of the nervous system to the pathophysiology of rheumatoid arthritis and other polyarthritides. Rheum. Dis. Clin. North Am. 13:369, 1987.
7. Jansco, N., Jansco-Gabor, A., and Szolcsanyi, I.: Direct evidence for neurogenic inflammation and its prevention by denervation and by pretreatment with capsaicin. Br. J. Pharmacol. 31:138, 1967.
8. Levine, J. D., Collier, D. H., Basbaum, A. I., et al.: The nervous system may contribute to the pathophysiology of rheumatoid arthritis. J. Rheumatol. 12:406, 1985.
9. Mapp, P. I., Kidd, B. L., Gibson, S. J., et al.: Substance P-, calcitonin gene-related peptide-, and c-flanking peptide of neuropeptide Y-immunoreactive fibres are present in normal synovium but depleted in patients with rheumatoid arthritis. Neuroscience 37:143, 1990.
10. Herfort, R. A.: Extended sympathectomy in the treatment of advanced rheumatoid arthritis. N. Y. J. Med. 56:1292, 1956.
11. Reichlin, S.: Neuroendocrine-immune interactions. N. Engl. J. Med. 329:1246, 1993.
12. Karalis, K., Sano, H., Redwine, J., et al.: Autocrine or paracrine inflammatory actions of corticotropin-releasing hormone *in vivo*. Science 254:421, 1991.
13. Sternberg, E. M., Hill, J. M., Chrousos, G. P., et al.: Inflammatory mediator-induced hypothalamic–pituitary–adrenal axis activation is defective in streptococcal cell wall arthritis-susceptible Lewis rats. Proc. Natl. Acad. Sci. U.S.A. 86:2374, 1989.
14. Sternberg, E. M., Young, W. S. III, Bernardini, R., et al.: A central nervous system defect in biosynthesis of corticotropin-releasing hormone is associated with susceptibility to streptococcal cell wall-induced arthritis in Lewis rats. Proc. Natl. Acad. Sci. U.S.A. 86:4771, 1989.
15. Neeck, G., Federlin, K., Graef, V., et al.: Adrenal secretion of cortisol in patients with rheumatoid arthritis. J. Rheumatol. 17:24, 1990.
16. Chikanza, I. C., Petrou, P., Kingsley, G., et al.: Defective hypothalamic response to immune and inflammatory stimuli in patients with rheumatoid arthritis. Arthritis Rheum. 35:1281, 1992.
17. Hall, J., Morand, E. F., Medbak, S., et al.: Abnormal hypothalamic-pituitary-adrenal axis function in rheumatoid arthritis. Arthritis Rheum. 37:1132, 1994.
18. Nagy, E., Chalmers, I. M., Baragar, F. D., et al.: Prolactin deficiency in rheumatoid arthritis. J. Rheumatol. 18:1662, 1991.

17

Phospholipase A$_2$, Cyclo-oxygenase, Prostaglandins, and Leukotrienes

Arachidonic acid is a nonesterified fatty acid that, when released from cell membranes, is oxygenated to several classes of eicosanoids, including (1) the prostaglandins, thromboxanes, and prostacyclin; (2) leukotrienes; and (3) lipoxins.

Phospholipase A$_2$ (PLA$_2$) is the enzyme responsible for releasing arachidonic acid from membrane phospholipids. PLA$_2$ is elevated in rheumatoid synovial fluids and blood, and is identical to the PLA$_2$ found in human platelets (for review, see ref. 1). In addition to hydrolyzing phospholipids, PLA$_2$ has inflammatory activity of its own. When injected into rabbit joints, recombinant human PLA$_2$ causes a marked inflammatory and proliferative arthritis. IL-1 and TNFα both can induce mRNA for chondrocyte PLA$_2$, so that this enzyme joins the ranks of those factors triggered by these cytokines.

Cyclo-oxygenase (COX) is the enzyme that oxygenates arachidonic acid, leading to formation of PGH$_2$, from which the biologically active prostanoids evolve[2] (Fig. 17–1). The discovery that COX was inhibited by aspirin led to the development of many NSAIDs based on the information that prostaglandins were major mediators of fever, pain, and inflammation. Prostaglandins are produced in large quantities by rheumatoid synovial tissue and have a major potential role in depletion of bone in rheumatoid arthritis[3,4] and possibly in the enhancement of erosions of bone by the invasive pannus.

It is now established that there are two forms of COX. **COX-1** is constitutively expressed by cells, but **COX-2** is inducible and regulated by many extracellular stimuli. COX-2 is present in vivo in synovial tissues from patients with rheumatoid arthritis. COX-2 biosynthesis is markedly increased by IL-1β and is suppressed by dexamethasone in tissue cultures and cell cultures of rheumatoid synoviocytes.[5] IL-1 also increases the COX-2 activity in cultures of rheumatoid synovial microvessel endothelial cells.[6]

NSAIDs such as indomethacin and piroxicam are much more potent inhibitors of COX-1 than of COX-2.[7] A logical next objective for the pharmaceutical industry is to develop specific inhibitors of human COX-2 in order to selectively suppress this inducible isoform. One such selective COX-2 inhibitor is **flosulide**. This compound (Bjarnason et al., Abstract 761) is much better tolerated in the gastrointestinal tract than the NSAID naproxen. IL-4, the anti-inflammatory cytokine, inhibits biosynthesis of COX-2, but not COX-1, in cultures of rheumatoid synovial cells (Sugiyama et al., Abstract 1193).

RELEVANCE TO RHEUMATOID ARTHRITIS OF PROSTAGLANDINS AND LEUKOTRIENES

With the discovery in the 1960s that aspirin could inhibit COX, a new era of pharmaceutical development began. Beginning with indomethacin, many new drugs designed or exploited for their capacity to inhibit COX were produced and marketed as "nonsteroidal anti-inflammatory drugs." Concurrently, more was learned about the pathways initiated in prostaglandin and leukotriene metabolism by the activation of COX and 5-lipoxygenase and the biologic effects that they mediate.[8,9] It is now appreciated that the effects of NSAIDs may be more related to inhibition of neutrophil activation than to inhibition of prostaglandin synthesis (see Chapter 28), but it is important to recognize the roles that these eicosanoids do have in inflammation.

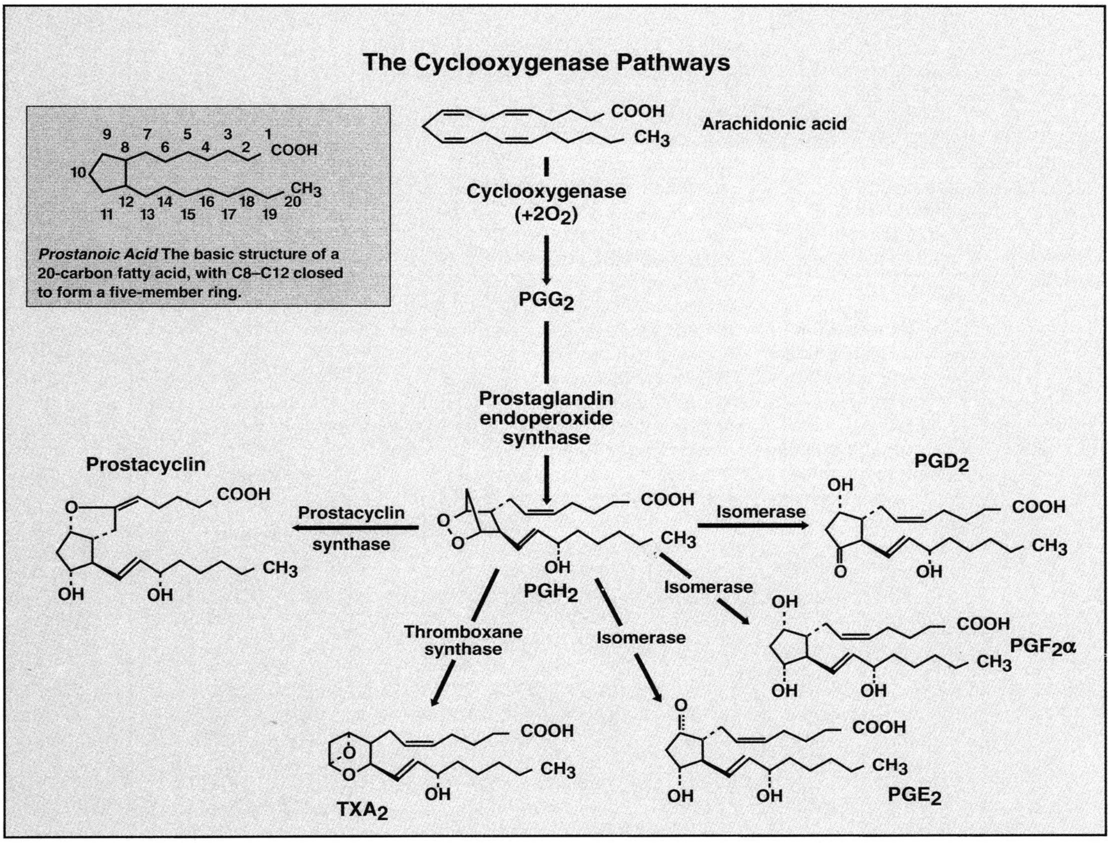

FIGURE 17–1. The cyclo-oxygenase pathways. (From Zurier, R. B.: Prostaglandins in rheumatologic diseases. Cliniguide Rheum. Dis. 2[4]:17, 1992. Used by permission.)

Prostaglandins

The structure common to all prostaglandins is a chain of 20 carbons with a five-component ring at C8 through C12. Figure 17–1 describes the derivation of the five principal biologically active compounds. Prostaglandins are produced in joints by neutrophils, macrophages, and synovial fibroblasts in response to activating agents such as IL-1 and TNFα. Pain and increased vascular permeability are associated with their appearance in tissues. A major role for the inflammatory prostaglandins is in potentiating the inflammatory effects of other mediators. For example, PGE$_2$ enhances the chemotactic responsiveness of monocytes to bioactive complement components. A major effect of PGE$_2$ in rheumatoid arthritis is in stimulating bone resorption locally around inflamed joints. A good case can be made for the argument that PGE$_2$ is responsible for the first radiographic bone sign of rheumatoid arthritis, periarticular osteopenia.

Another product of COX activity is thrombox-ane, and its inflammatory effects appear to relate to activation of platelets. Platelets not only aggregate to initiate clotting, but also release growth factors and proteases.

Leukotrienes

Human neutrophils and macrophages synthesize 5-hydroperoxy-eicosatetraenoic acid (5-HPETE; see Fig. 17–2), an unstable compound that can be converted to LTB$_4$. 5-HPETE also stimulates the generation of ODFRs in human neutrophils. LTB$_4$ is a potent chemoattractant for neutrophils and, along with C5a and PAF, forms a potent gradient that draws neutrophils from the circulation to the joint fluid in rheumatoid arthritis. LTB$_4$ and products of glutathione-S-transferase may affect growth and differentiation pathways of synovial fibroblasts, enhancing proliferation of these cells, especially when prostaglandin synthesis is inhibited. LTB$_4$ also stimulates IL-2 and IFNγ production by

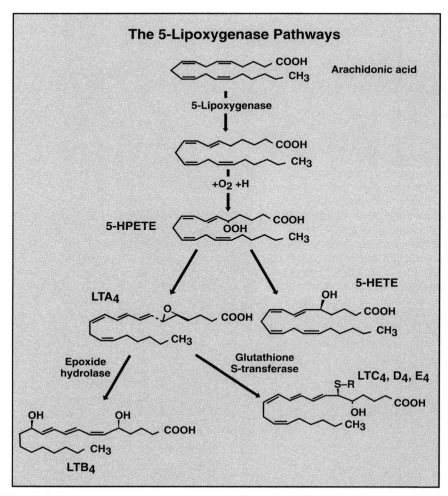

FIGURE 17–2. The 5-lipoxygenase pathways. (From Zurier, R. B.: Prostaglandins in rheumatologic diseases. Cliniguide Rheum. Dis. 2[4]:17, 1992. Used by permission.)

T cells and adds enhancement to agents that trigger IL-1 production by macrophages.

Anti-inflammatory Effects of Prostaglandin E₁ and Its Derivatives

It is appreciated more and more that PGE_1 has beneficial effects on inflammation when given exogenously in sufficient concentrations. PGE_1 and its derivative, 15-S-15-methyl-PGE, which is active when given orally, suppress immune complex–induced vasculitis and inflammation in different animal models, diminish T-cell reactivity, and may protect against degranulation of neutrophils. Misoprostol, the PGE_1 analogue that is used in patients with NSAID-associated peptic ulcer, has immunosuppressive effects when used in synchrony with other immunosuppressive agents. Data in Chapter 27, reviews the evidence that fish oils, particularly the ω-3 fatty acids, diminish formation of COX and lipoxygenase products produced in vivo, and have a demonstrated therapeutic benefit. The challenge for drug development is to create specific inhibitors of the inflammatory products of arachidonic acid metabolism but not suppress synthesis or activity of those products that have, overall, beneficial effects in inflammation.[10]

REFERENCES

1. Bomalaski, J. S., and Clark, M. A.: Phospholipase A_2 and arthritis. Arthritis Rheum. 36:190, 1993.
2. Zurier, R. B.: Prostaglandins in rheumatologic diseases. Cliniguide Rheum. Dis. 2(4):17, 1992.

3. Robinson D. R., Tashijian H. J., and Levine, L.: Prostaglandin-stimulated bone resorption by rheumatoid synovia: a possible mechanism for bone destruction in rheumatoid arthritis. J. Clin. Invest. 56:1181, 1975.

4. Dayer, J.-M., Krane, S. M., Russell, R. G. G., et al.: Production of collagenase and prostaglandins by isolated adherent rheumatoid synovial cells. Proc. Natl. Acad. Sci. U.S.A. 73:945, 1976.

5. Crofford, L. J., Wilder, R. L., Ristimäki, A. P., et al.: Cyclooxygenase-1 and -2 expression in rheumatoid synovial tissues: effects of interleukin-1β, phorbol ester, and corticosteroids. J. Clin. Invest. 93:1095, 1994.

6. Szczepanski, A., Moatter, T., Carley, W. W., et al.: Induction of cyclooxygenase II in human synovial microvessel endothelial cells by interleukin-1: inhibition by glucocorticoids. Arthritis Rheum. 37:495, 1994.

7. Meade, E. A., Smith, W. L., and DeWitt, D. L.: Differential inhibition of prostaglandin endoperoxide synthase (cyclooxygenase) isozymes by aspirin and other non-steroidal anti-inflammatory drugs. J. Biol. Chem. 268:6610, 1993.

8. Fantone, J. C., Kunkel, S. L., and Zurier, R. B.: Effects of prostaglandins on *in vivo* immune and inflammatory reactions. *In* Goodwin, J. S. (ed.): Prostaglandins and Immunity. Boston, Martinus Nijhoff, 1985, pp. 123–146.

9. Lewis, R. A., Fitzgerald. G., Branch R. A., et al.: Leukotrienes and other products of the 5-lipoxygenase pathway. N. Engl. J. Med. 323:645, 1990.

10. Zurier, R. B.: Prostaglandins, leukotrienes, and related compounds. *In* Kelley, W. N., Harris, E. D. Jr. Ruddy, S., and Sledge, C. B. (eds.): Textbook of Rheumatology, 4th ed., Vol. 1. Philadelphia, W. B. Saunders, 1993, pp. 201–212.

18

Immune Complexes, Complement, Kinins, Clot Formation, and Fibrinolysis

Those who do surgery on rheumatoid joints are often impressed with the amount of evidence for clot formation within rheumatoid joints. Fibrin clots are found free in the joint space as rice bodies, or overlying cartilage and synovium, or replacing normal cells and matrix within the villous strands of synovium on histologic examination.

As with most systems within biology, clotting and fibrinolysis are related not only to each other but to other inflammatory and proliferative pathways, including the complement and kinin systems. This may be especially true within closed spaces such as the joint.[1]

IMMUNE COMPLEXES AND THE COMPLEMENT CASCADE IN RHEUMATOID SYNOVIUM

The physical nature of the immune complexes formed between antigens and antibodies has much influence on the subsequent biologic effects of those immune complexes. A few of the most important effects that immune complexes stimulate are the following:

- Development of secondary antibody responses toward T-cell–dependent antigens
- Activation of memory B cells and plasma cells
- Activation of the complement cascade

As an example, follicular dendritic cells in germinal centers display immune complexes for long periods of time and can activate continuous streams of B cells.

Receptors for the Fc portion of IgG (FcγR) mediate cellular effects of immune complexes by activating expressive functions of these cells. As mentioned in Chapter 14, three species of FcγR are recognized[2]:

1. **FcγRI**—bind monomeric IgG with high affinity. They are found on monocyte-macrophages and can be induced to appear on neutrophils.
2. **FcγRII**—have a low affinity for IgG, are expressed on all inflammatory and immune cells, and bind immune complexes.
3. **FcγRIII**—expressed on most cells (except neutrophils) and bind both monomeric IgE and immune complexes with low to moderate affinity.

The Fc receptors clear imune complexes from serum particularly well after the complexes have induced activation and fixation of complement. They are aided in this process by complement receptors on red blood cells (**CR1**) and, to a lesser degree, platelets (**CR2 and CR3**). In rheumatoid arthritis, there is little doubt that immune complexes are being formed but, consistent with our understanding of the pathophysiology, which centers on synovitis, it is accepted that assays for immune complexes in plasma or serum are not sensitive or specific enough to use for either diagnosis or management. Perhaps the most important role for immune complexes in rheumatoid arthritis may be their apparent chemoattractant power for invasive pannus when they lodge with complement in the superficial layers of articular cartilage.

Considering the large amount of immunoglobulin aggregates within rheumatoid tissues, synovial fluid, and blood, it is not surprising that many studies have indicated that activation of the complement system can be demonstrated in these compartments in rheumatoid arthritis, particularly in the context of extra-articular vasculitis.[3] In patients with relatively little extra-articular disease, C3, C4, and CH50 levels are usually normal or even high. Low levels of total hemolytic complement, C4, or C2 are found in synovial fluid of patients with active disease, and these levels have a general inverse correlation with levels of rheumatoid factor. It is of interest that some of the early components of the complement system—C1q, C1r/C1s, and the inhibitor of the first component of complement, C1 INH—are synthesized by the lining cells of rheumatoid synovium.[4] In this and other systems, conformational changes in C1q result in activation of C1r and C1s. C1 INH binds and dissociates C1r/C1s to inactive forms. Only B-type synoviocytes (fibroblast-like) produce C1r, whereas macrophages generate C1q. After biosynthesis, all three components are found in a thin film covering the synovial lining, and perhaps interact there with immune complexes within the synovial fluid, although there is no proof that the C1q or C1r/C1s components are active in this locus.

Another consequence of complement activation in rheumatoid synovitis is that many different inflammatory components of the complement system are produced as by-products of complement activation. The major ones are[5]

C3a (C3 anaphylotoxin): Increases capillary permeability

C3b: Liberates histamine from mast cells and is chemotactic for leukocytes

C5a: A major chemotactic peptide; along with LTB_4 and PAF, it provides the majority of chemotactic attraction in synovial fluid for neutrophils

C567: Sensitizes innocent bystander cells for lysis by the components of complement

C3b also enhances binding of immune complexes to leukocytes, leading to phagocytosis and activation. Certain B cells have C3b receptors on their surfaces, and ligand binding may trigger antibody formation. Synovial fluid from rheumatoid patients frequently contains neutrophils with intracytoplasmic inclusions that contain IgG, IgM, and the C3 and C4 components of complement. A correlation has been found between the depressions of synovial fluid complement levels and the frequency of these intracellular inclusions.[6]

C3a is inactivated by a serum carboxypeptidase that removes the carboxyl-terminal arginine to form C3a desArg. C3a and C3a desArg levels are more than seven times higher in joint fluids of rheumatoid patients than in patients with degenerative arthritis, and these levels correlate well with C-reactive protein, the ESR, and disease activity indices.[7]

Other studies have confirmed that the entire complement cascade is activated in rheumatoid arthritis. For example, levels of C3d (an indicator of C3 activation) parallel those in the terminal complement complex (C5b, C6, C7, C8, and C9). Both are elevated in most rheumatoid synovial fluids.[8]

The activators of the complement cascade in rheumatoid arthritis can include rheumatoid factor, immune complexes, plasmin, and C-reactive protein itself.[9] In addition, some of the same cytokines that fuel the inflammatory and proliferative lesions in rheumatoid synovitis enhance the biosynthesis of complement proteins. Addition of IL-13 (see Chapter 8) to fibroblast cultures primed with TNFα, IL-1, or IFNγ resulted in a dose-dependent increase in C3 protein biosynthesis and a concomitant downregulation of factor B biosynthesis.[10] IL-13 is a product of activated T cells. IL-4 has similar effects that are independent of IL-13–induced responses.

Immunostains of rheumatoid synovium showed C3 and C4 throughout the synovial vessels, interstitium, and lining layers in patients, similar to the distribution of IgG.[11] The significance of complement proteins bound to immunoglobulins in cartilage in rheumatoid patients is discussed in Chapter 11.

THE KININ SYSTEM IN RHEUMATOID ARTHRITIS

Kinins are a group of polypeptides that can produce the cardinal signs of inflammation. They are formed from α_2-globulin substrates (**kininogens**) found in excess in plasma by the **kallikrein** enzymes. Plasma kallikrein, activated from a latent form by many diverse stimuli, forms **bradykinin** from kininogen.

In rheumatoid arthritis, it is likely that immune complexes (rheumatoid factor IgG) can activate kallikrein.[12]

PLATELETS

Platelets are of particular interest because of their wide variety of cellular reactions, including adhesion, aggregation, protease and cytokine production, and degranulation. Although they pass without notice through intact vessels, they adhere quickly to components of the subepithelial matrix in synovium when capillaries are injured, and immediately have actions in addition to facilitating the clotting of blood. They **adhere** to types I, III, and IV collagens, fibronectin, vitronectin, and laminin.[13] Adhesion of these matrix components to the platelet receptor (glycoprotein IIb/IIIa) is promoted by von Willebrand factor. Additional platelets are recruited to stick specifically to the adherent platelets in a process of **aggregation**. Activators of platelets

TABLE 18–1. Activators of Platelets during Hemotastasis and Inflammatory Reactions

MECHANISM	ACTIVATOR
Adhesion	Collagen
	Microfilaments
	Fibronectin
	Laminin
	Vitronectin
	Urate crystals
Fluid phase	
Nonimmunologic	
Hemostatic	Thrombin
	Collagen
	ADP
	Epinephrine
	Arachidonic acid metabolites
	(e.g., PGG_2, PGH_2,
	thromboxane A_2)
Other	Serotonin
	Vasopressin
	Double-stranded DNA
Immunologic	PAF
	Immune complexes
	Antibodies to drugs
	Micro-organisms
	Substance P
Enhancers of	Complement
activation	Single-stranded DNA
	Lipopolysaccharides (endotoxin)

From Valone, F. H.: Platelets. *In* Kelley, W. N., Harris, E. D. Jr., Ruddy, S., and Sledge, C. B. (eds.): Textbook of Rheumatology, 4th ed., Vol. 1. Philadelphia, W. B. Saunders, 1993, pp. 319–326. Used by permission.

(Table 18–1)[13] cause degranulation in a **release reaction**. Aspirin and other NSAIDs inhibit platelet activation by effects upon platelet COX; the acetylation by aspirin is permanent and irreversible, whereas the other nonsteroidal drugs only incapacitate the enzyme for several days.

Platelet-derived mediators of inflammation are many in number[13] (Table 18–2). The lipid factors prostaglandins, leukotrienes, and PAF are the best studied of these. A special note about PAF is in order: Platelets synthesize and release an inactive precursor, lyso-PAF, which is converted to PAF by neutrophils. Active PAF is a very potent chemoattractant for neutrophils in synovial fluid.

Proteins and peptides from platelet granules activate many subsequent pathways in synovial cells. Among these active substances released by platelets are PGDF, TGFβ, CTAP III, IL-1, and endothelial growth factor. It is possible that CTAP III and platelet factor 4 are derived from a single precursor molecule, platelet basic protein.[14] The functions of each of these cytokines have been reviewed in Chapter 8.

In considering rheumatoid arthritis, there are many circumstantial data to implicate overexpression of numbers and function of platelets in this disease. It has been observed, for example, that the thrombocytosis seen in rheumatoid arthritis correlates roughly with disease activity. Circulating antibodies that stimulate platelet secretion are found frequently in patients with rheumatoid arthritis.[15] The platelet counts in rheumatoid synovial fluid range from 1 to 10 per cent of circulating levels, so that there are ample numbers for activation of platelet functions within the confines of a particular joint.[16]

THE CLOTTING CASCADE IN RHEUMATOID ARTHRITIS

Thrombin (factor IIa in the coagulation cascade) catalyzes the conversion of fibrinogen into fibrin, aiding in the formation of a blood clot. In addition, thrombin initiates a number of proinflammatory and mitogenic effects generated by cleavage by thrombin of a G-protein–coupled transmembrane receptor.

Generation and Regulation of Thrombin

Thrombin is generated by actions of factor Xa and Va that form a "prothrombinase" complex catalyzing cleavage of prothrombin. This process has feedback inhibition; thrombomodulin binds to thrombin, altering thrombin from an inducer of clot formation to an efficient activator of protein C, a serine protease that inactivates factor Va. Thrombomodulin levels in rheumatoid arthritis synovial fluid have been reported to be elevated[17] (Fig. 18–1).

The thrombin receptor on cells is a member of the seven transmembrane domain receptor family. Its activation requires cleavage by thrombin of an arginine-serine bond within the receptor's amino-terminal extracellular region on platelets.[18] It is likely that an identical receptor is present on synovial fibroblasts.

Endogenous thrombin inhibitors include members of the serine protease (serpin) superfamily, such as plasminogen activator inhibitor 1 (PAI-1), α_2-antiplasmin, and the principal thrombin inhibitor, antithrombin III.[19] Protease nexin 1 is another serpin that controls thrombin action at the cell sur-

TABLE 18–2. Platelet-Derived Mediators of Inflammation

CLASS	MEDIATOR	ACTIONS
LIPID		
Cyclo-oxygenase dependent	Thromboxane A_2	Vasoconstrictor; proaggregant; increases neutrophil adherence
	Thromboxane B_2	More stable thromboxane A_2 derivative
	Prostaglandins D_2, E_2, F_2	Vasoactive; modulates hemostasis and leukocyte function
	HHT	Chemotactic
Lipoxygenase dependent	12-HPETE	Vasoconstrictor; cyclooxygenase inhibitor; stimulates leukocyte LTB_4 synthesis
	12-HETE	Chemotactic
Phospholipid	PAF	Proaggregant; increases vascular permeability; neutrophil and monocyte activation
PROTEIN/PEPTIDE		
Dense body	Serotonin	Vasoconstrictor; increases vascular permeability; fibrogenic
Alpha granule	PDGF	Chemotactic
	PF4	Proaggregant; chemotactic; induces basophil histamine release
	TGF-β	Neutrophil and monocyte activation
"Granule" contents	IL-1β	Pyrogen; tissue inflammation
	Cationic permeability factor	Stimulates mast cell histamine; chemotactic
	Elastase	Neutral proteinase
	Collagenase	Neutral proteinase
	α_1-Antitrypsin	Protease inhibitor
	α_2-Macroglobulin	Protease inhibitor
	α_2-Antiplasmin	Primary plasmin inhibitor
	Plasminogen activator inhibitor-1	Inhibits plasminogen activators

From Valone, F. H.: Platelets. *In* Kelley, W. N., Harris, E. D. Jr., Ruddy, S., and Sledge, C. B. (eds.): Textbook of Rheumatology, 4th ed., Vol. 1. Philadelphia, W. B. Saunders, 1993, pp. 319–326. Used by permission.

face, as is heparin cofactor II. During inflammation in mesenchymal tissues, such as a joint, both oxygen radicals and metalloproteases such as stromelysin can inactivate serpins.[20,21]

Possible Roles for Thrombin in Rheumatoid Arthritis[19]

A Mediator of Inflammation

In the coagulation cascade, in addition to its major role in catalyzing the fibrinogen-to-fibrin sequence, thrombin acts directly on platelets to facilitate their aggregation. Thrombin up-regulates arachidonic acid synthesis, an action that drives generation of prostaglandins and leukotrienes. To facilitate neutrophil and monocyte transendothelial migration, thrombin up-regulates expression of P-selectin and ICAM-1 on endothelium in rheumatoid synovial vasculature.[22]

A Cell Growth Factor

Thrombin, added to cell cultures, is mitogenic for virtually all cells found in synovial inflammation. It also acts indirectly by stimulating release of cytokines such as PDGF. Activation of the thrombin receptor enhances proliferation of new capillaries in tissues.[23]

Pathologic Effects of Synovial Microhemorrhage

Microhemorrhage is very common in the proliferative synovium. These little bleeds are caused by microtrauma when joints move and synovial fronds are crushed between cartilage-on-cartilage contact. This activates the coagulation cascade. In addition to fibrin formation, thrombin can accelerate the entry of neutrophils and monocytes into the joint and can facilitate angiogenesis and the profusion of synovial lining cells; in histopathologic studies,

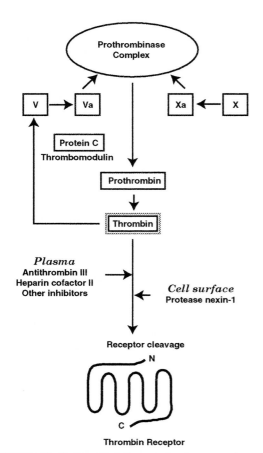

FIGURE 18–1. Simplified diagram showing generation, action, and inhibition of thrombin. Solid arrows, activation mechanisms; dotted arrows, inhibitory mechanisms. (From Morris, R., Winyard, P. G., Blake, D. R., et al.: Thrombin in inflammation and healing: relevance to rheumatoid arthritis. Ann. Rheum. Dis. 53:72, 1994. Used by permission.)

capillary proliferation, synovial hyperplasia, and infiltration by mononuclear cells are in striking parallel.[24]

THE PLASMINOGEN ACTIVATOR/PLASMIN SYSTEM IN RHEUMATOID ARTHRITIS

Just as thrombin has many more biologic actions than those involved in producing fibrin, it is apparent that the fibrinolytic system does more than break up fibrin clots.

Plasminogen Activators

These enzymes are serine proteases, like trypsin. The two mammalian forms of plasminogen activa-

tor are a urokinase type (uPA) and a tissue type (tPA) uPA is the type expressed by rheumatoid synovium, not tPA.[25] uPA binds to a plasma membrane receptor, whereas tPA is targeted by structure to fibrin and other components of the extracellular matrix.[26] The preferred substrate for plasminogen activator is plasminogen, but it may affect other molecules as well. PAI-1 is the major arginine-specific serine protease inhibitor (Arg-serpin) of tPA in plasma. Another inhibitor, PAI-2, is largely bound to cell membranes, is a less effective inhibitor of tPA than of uPA, and is weaker than PAI-1 against both.

Virtually all cell types produce plasminogen activator, but of particular relevance is its synthesis by isolated, adherent rheumatoid synovial lining cells. In this system, the same nuclear factor that activates biosynthesis of uPA also increases expression of procollagenase,[27] and synthesis of both is inhibited by glucocorticoids. Similar to thrombin, there is a receptor for uPA on monocyte-macrophages, neutrophils, fibroblasts, and endothelial cells. Plasminogen binds to cell surfaces as well, and the plasminogen activator–plasminogen interaction is believed to be protected there from natural inhibitors.

Plasmin

Under physiologic conditions, only tPA and uPA activate plasmin (also a serine protease) from plasminogen, which is present in plasma in abundant quantity. Unlike plasminogen activators, plasmin has a wide substrate specificity. It is the most efficient co-activator of tissue metalloproteases, activates latent growth factors, and has some catalytic effect upon degradation of most extracellular matrix proteins and glycoproteins. α_2-Antiplasmin is the primary plasmin inhibitor in plasma, but protease nexin 1 inhibits it as well.

Clotting and Fibrinolysis in Rheumatoid Arthritis

Levels of plasminogen activator in synovial fluids of rheumatoid patients are substantially higher than those in fluid from patients with osteoarthritis.[28] IL-1 inhibits biosynthesis of PAI-1 in cultures of cartilage or chondrocytes; thus it can be inferred that in rheumatoid arthritis, dominated as it is by inflammatory cytokines, the balance is tipped in favor of plasminogen activator rather than PAI. The discovery that plasminogen activator (uPA) was produced by rheumatoid synovial tissue provided data for a pathway for activation of stromelysin, which, in turn, activates procollagenase and enables matrix destruction to occur. Plasmin is

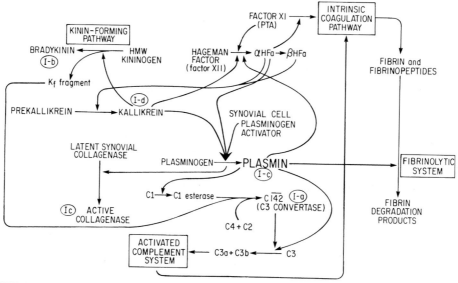

FIGURE 18–2. In this schematic representation, plasmin I-c is placed at the center of an activation network. Plasmin can degrade fibrin, initiate conversion of C1 to the active C3 convertase (I-a), activate factor XII, and (in the presence of stromelysin) activate collagenase. Kallikrein (I-d) also contributes activation capabilities by converting high-molecular-weight kininogen to bradykinin (I-b), helping to convert plasminogen to plasmin, and activating Hageman factor. Not drawn here is the capability of kallikrein to combine with stromelysin in activation of procollagenase.

a very effective activator of metalloproteases, especially in the presence of stromelysin itself.

INTERACTION AMONG THE INFLAMMATORY CASCADES

Within synovial fluid, there is opportunity for much interaction among various inflammatory cascades. The interconnections of the coagulation, fibrinolytic, complement, and kinin systems are diagrammed in Figure 8–2.

REFERENCES

1. Henson, P. M., and Gordon, J. L.: Cellular components of inflammation: platelets. In Kelley, W. N., Harris, E. D. Jr., Ruddy, S., and Sledge, C. B. (eds.): Textbook of Rheumatology, 2nd ed. Philadelphia, W. B. Saunders, 1985, pp. 169–179.
2. Moxley, G., and Ruddy, S.: Immune complexes and complement. In Kelley, W. N., Harris, E. D. Jr., Ruddy, S., and Sledge, C. B. (eds.): Textbook of Rheumatology, 5th ed., Vol. 1. Philadelphia, W. B. Saunders, 1996 (in press).
3. Moxley, G., and Ruddy, S.: Immune complexes and complement. In Kelley, W. N., Harris, E. D. Jr., Ruddy, S., and Sledge, C. B. (eds.): Textbook of Rheumatology, 4th ed., Vol. 1. Philadelphia, W. B. Saunders, 1993, pp. 188–200.
4. Breitner, S., Storkel, S., Reichel, W., et al.: Complement components C1q, C1r/C1s, and C1 INH in rheumatoid arthritis. Arthritis Rheum. 38:492, 1995.
5. Ruddy, S.: Synovial fluid: Mirror of the inflammatory lesion in rheumatoid arthritis. In Harris, E. D. Jr. (ed.) Rheumatoid Arthritis. New York, Medcom Press, 1974, pp. 58–72.
6. Winchester, R. J., Agnello, V., and Kunkel, H. G.: Gamma globulin complexes in synovial fluids of patients with rheumatoid arthritis: partial characterization and relationship to lowered complement levels. Clin. Exp. Immunol. 6:689, 1970.
7. Moxley, G., and Ruddy, S.: Elevated plasma C3 anaphylotoxin levels in rheumatoid arthritis patients. Arthritis Rheum. 30:1097, 1978.
8. Mollnes, T. E., Lea, T., Mellbye, O. J., et al.: Complement activation in rheumatoid arthritis evaluated by C3dg and the terminal complement complex. Arthritis Rheum. 29:715, 1986.
9. Kaplan, M. H., and Volanakis, J. E.: Interaction of C-reactive protein complexes with the complement system. I. Consumption of human complement associated with the reaction of C-reactive protein with pneumococcal C-polysaccharide and with the choline phosphatides, lecithin and sphingomyelin. J. Immunol. 112:2135, 1974.
10. Katz, Y., Stav, D., Barr, J., and Passwell, J. H.: IL-13 results in differential regulation of the complement proteins C3 and factor B in tumour necrosis factor (TNF)-stimulated fibroblasts. Clin. Exp. Immunol. 101:150, 1995.
11. Rodman, W. S., Williams, R. C. Jr., Bilka, P. J., et al.: Immunofluorescent localization of the third and fourth component of complement in synovial tissue from patients with rheumatoid arthritis. J. Lab. Clin. Med. 69:141, 1967.
12. Nies, A. S., and Melmon, K. L.: Kinins and arthritis. Bull. Rheum. Dis. 19:512, 1968.
13. Valone, F. H.: Platelets. In Kelley, W. N., Harris, E. D. Jr., Ruddy, S., and Sledge, C. B. (eds.): Textbook of Rheumatology, 4th ed., Vol. 1. Philadelphia, W. B. Saunders, 1993, pp. 319–326.

14. Harrison, P., Savidge, G. F., and Cramer, E. M.: The origin and physiological relevance of alpha granule adhesive proteins. Br. J. Haematol. 74:125, 1990.

15. Weissbarth, E., Baruth, B., Mielke, H., et al.: Platelets as target cells in rheumatoid arthritis and systemic lupus erythematosus: a platelet specific immunoglobulin inducing the release reaction. Rheumatol. Int. 2:67, 1982.

16. Farr, M., Wainwright, A., Salmon, M., et al.: Platelets in the synovial fluid of patients with rheumatoid arthritis. Rheumatol. Int. 4:13, 1984.

17. Conway, E. M., and Nowakowski, B.: Biologically active thrombomodulin is synthesized by adherent synovial fluid cells and is elevated in synovial fluid of patients with rheumatoid arthritis. Blood 81:726, 1993.

18. Vu, T.-K. H., Hung, D. T., Wheaton, V. I., et al.: Molecular cloning of a functional thrombin receptor reveals a novel proteolytic mechanism of receptor activation. Cell 64:1057, 1991.

19. Morris, R., Winyard, P. G., Blake, D. R., et al.: Thrombin in inflammation and healing: relevance to rheumatoid arthritis. Ann. Rheum. Dis. 53:72, 1994.

20. Docherty, A. J. P., and Murphy, G.: The tissue metalloproteinase family and the inhibitor TIMP: a study using cDNAs and recombinant proteins. Ann. Rheum. Dis. 49:469, 1990.

21. Mast, A. E., Enghild, J. J., Nagase, H., et al.: Kinetics and physiologic relevance of the inactivation of α_1-proteinase inhibitor, α_1-antichymotrypsin, and antithrombin III by matrix metalloproteinases-1 (tissue collagenase), -2 (72-kDa gelatinase/type IV collagenase), and -3 (stromelysin). J. Biol. Chem. 266:15810, 1991.

22. Grober, J. S., Bowen, B. L., Ebling, H., et al.: Monocyte-endothelial adhesion in chronic rheumatoid arthritis. J. Clin. Invest. 91:2609, 1993.

23. Carney, D. H., Mann, R., Redlin, W. R., et al.: Enhancement of incisional wound healing and neovascularisation in normal rats by thrombin receptor-activating peptide. J. Clin. Invest. 89:1469, 1992.

24. Rooney, M., Condell, D., Quinlan, W., et al.: Analysis of the histologic variation of synovitis in rheumatoid arthritis. Arthritis Rheum. 31:956, 1988.

25. Busso, N., Péclat, V., Sappino, A.-P., et al.: Plasminogen activation system in synovial tissue: difference between normal osteoarthritis, and rheumatoid arthritis joints. Arthritis Rheum. 39:S198, 1996.

26. Vassalli, J.-D., Sappino, A.-P., and Belin, D.: The plasminogen activator/plasmin system. J. Clin. Invest. 88:1067, 1991.

27. Rorth, P., Nerlov, C., Blasi, F., et al.: Transcription factor PEA3 participates in the induction of urokinase plasminogen activator transcription in murine keratinocytes stimulated with epidermal growth factor or phorbol ester. Nucleic Acids Res. 18:5009, 1990.

28. Kikuchi, H., Tanaka, S., and Matsuo, O.: Plasminogen activator in synovial fluid from patients with rheumatoid arthritis. J. Rheumatol. 14:439, 1987.

SECTION VII

CLINICAL MANIFESTATIONS OF RHEUMATOID ARTHRITIS

With these chapters, we begin the clinical and therapeutic sections in this book on rheumatoid arthritis. The two components, pathophysiology and clinical aspects, are inextricably linked, however. One component should never be analyzed without being in the context of the other. Understanding of the clinical manifestations allows one to ask the right questions about pathogenesis, and a comprehension of the phases of pathogenesis allows a much more intelligent approach to therapy in this complex disease. Previous sections, have covered history and epidemiology, and in subsequent ones the instruments for assessment, prognosis, and treatment are covered in detail.

Clinical Features and Differential Diagnosis

CRITERIA FOR DIAGNOSIS

The diagnosis of rheumatoid arthritis is primarily based on clinical grounds. Despite the usefulness of tests for rheumatoid factor in both diagnosis and understanding of the pathophysiology of the disease, the presence of neither anti-IgG nor any other laboratory variable is specific for rheumatoid arthritis. For epidemiologic studies, several sets of criteria have been developed for classification of adult rheumatoid arthritis by the ACR (formerly the American Rheumatism Association). The most recent of these was published in 1988[1] and was constructed using data from 262 rheumatoid patients and the same number of controls from varied groups of other connective tissue diseases (Table 19–1).

These criteria are widely used. They are relatively simple and have no exclusion diagnoses. They have been compared with the Rome criteria (Table 19–2) in a Pima Indian population. The major classification difference is that the cutoff for diagnosis is shifted toward a higher specificity and a lower sensitivity with the ACR 1987 criteria. Both sets of criteria have the shortcoming of being unable to diagnose inactive disease.[2]

CLINICAL SYNDROME OF EARLY RHEUMATOID ARTHRITIS

In the northern hemisphere, the onset of rheumatoid arthritis is more frequent in winter than in summer. In several series, the onset of rheumatoid arthritis from October to March is twice as frequent as in the other 6 months,[3,4] and exacerbations of the disease are more common in winter.[5] Comparable data from the southern hemisphere are not available.

Some data suggest that the appearance of rheumatoid factor may precede symptoms of arthritis in more patients than was previously recognized. In 30 patients from whom frozen sera were available from a time before symptoms of rheumatoid arthritis began, half had a positive latex fixation test[6] and, unlike the male-female prevalence of disease, many more of these were men than women.

Much more diffuse, subjective, and difficult to study are *precipitating factors* of arthritis. There is no evidence that any have a direct cause-and-effect relationship. Trauma is one of the most common preludes to arthritis; this can include surgery. Other stimuli, including infections, vaccine inoculations, and emotional trauma, have been implicated by many patients as the cause of their rheumatoid arthritis, but none has been substantiated. However, the increasing awareness of the effects of the central nervous system on arthritis make it essential to be aware of these ''nonscientific'' associations, and be sensitive to patients' concerns about them.

Patterns of Onset

Rheumatoid arthritis develops in varying locations and has different patterns of joint involvement[7] (Table 19–3). The onset may be acute, occurring within only a few days, or insidious, the most common mode of onset; some studies describe an ''intermediate'' onset over a few weeks.

Insidious Onset

Rheumatoid arthritis usually has an insidious, slow onset over weeks to months. Fifty-five to 70 per cent of cases begin this way.[3,8] The initial symptoms may be systemic or articular. In some patients, fatigue, malaise, or diffuse musculoskeletal pain may be the first nonspecific complaint, with joints becoming involved later. Although symmetric involvement is common, asymmetric presentation (often developing more symmetry later in the course of disease) is not unusual. The reason for symmetry of joint involvement may be related to release of phlogistic neuropeptides at terminal nerve endings in joints (see Chapter 16).

TABLE 19–1. 1988 Revised ACR Criteria for Classification of Rheumatoid Arthritis (RA)*

CRITERIA	DEFINITION
1. Morning stiffness	Morning stiffness in and around the joints lasting at least 1 hour before maximal improvement
2. Arthritis of three or more joint areas	At least three joint areas have simultaneously had soft tissue swelling or fluid (not bony overgrowth alone) observed by a physician. The 14 possible joint areas are (right or left): PIP, MCP, wrist, elbow, knee, ankle, and MTP joints
3. Arthritis of hand joints	At least one joint area swollen as above in wrist, MCP, or PIP joint
4. Symmetric arthritis	Simultaneous involvement of the same joint areas (as in 2) on both sides of the body (bilateral involvement of PIP, MCP, or MTP joints is acceptable without absolute symmetry)
5. Rheumatoid nodules	Subcutaneous nodules, over bony prominences or extensor surfaces or in juxta-articular regions, observed by a physician
6. Serum rheumatoid factor	Demonstration of abnormal amounts of serum ''rheumatoid factor'' by any method that has been positive in less than 5 per cent of normal control subjects
7. Radiographic changes	Radiographic changes typical of RA on PA hand and wrist x-rays, which must include erosions or unequivocal bony decalcification localized to or most marked adjacent to the involved joints (osteoarthritis changes alone do not qualify)

* For classification purposes, a patient is said to have RA if he or she has satisfied at least four of the above seven criteria. Criteria 1 through 4 must be present for at least 6 weeks. Patients with two clinical diagnoses are not excluded. Designation as classic, definite, or probable rheumatoid arthritis is *not* to be made.

Morning stiffness may be the first symptom, appearing even before pain. This phenomenon is probably related to accumulation of edema fluid within inflamed tissues during sleep, and it improves as edema and products of inflammation are absorbed by lymphatics and venules and returned to the circulation by motion accompanying use of muscles (Fig. 19–1). Pain and stiffness may develop in other joints, but it is rare for symptoms to remit completely in one set of joints while developing in another. This quality sets rheumatoid arthritis apart from rheumatic fever, in which a true migratory pattern of arthritis is common.

A subtle, early change in rheumatoid arthritis is development of muscle atrophy around affected joints. This decreases efficiency and strength, and weakness develops that is out of proportion to pain.

TABLE 19–2. New York Criteria for the Diagnosis of Rheumatoid Arthritis (RA)

RA is present if criteria 1 and 2 plus either 3 or 4 are met:
1. History of an episode of three painful limb joints. Each group of joints (e.g., proximal interphalangeal joint) is counted as one joint, scoring each side separately
2. Swelling, limitation of motion, subluxation, and/or ankylosis of three limb joints. *Necessary inclusions:* (1) at least one hand, wrist, or foot; (2) symmetry of one joint pair. *Exclusions:* (1) distal interphalangeal joints; (2) fifth proximal interphalangeal joints; (3) first metatarsophalangeal joints; (4) hips
3. Radiographic changes (erosions)
4. Serum positive for rheumatoid factors

From Jacobsson, L. T. H., Knowler, W. C., Pillemer, S., et al.: A cross-sectional and longitudinal comparison of the Rome criteria for active rheumatoid arthritis and the American College of Rheumatology 1987 criteria for rheumatoid arthritis. Arthritis Rheum. 37:1479, 1994. Used by permission.

TABLE 19–3. Onset of Rheumatoid Arthritis in 300 Patients with Definite or Classic Disease

CHARACTERISTIC		PERCENTAGE
1. Mode of onset	Rapid* (days or weeks)	46
	Insidious	54
2. Site of onset	Small joints	32
	Medium-sized joints	16
	Large joints	29
	Combined	26
3. Pattern of onset	Monarticular	21
	Oligoarticular	44
	Polyarticular	35

From Fahalli, S., Halla, J. T., and Hardin, J. G.: Onset patterns of rheumatoid arthritis. Clin. Res. 31:650A, 1983. Used by permission.

* This time frame includes patients described in other studies as having ''intermediate'' onset.

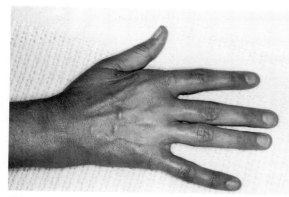

FIGURE 19–1. Hand of a young man several weeks into an illness that was diagnosed 2 months later as definite rheumatoid arthritis. His principal symptoms were morning stiffness in the hands. The only objective abnormalities were a mild diffuse swelling of the dorsum of the hand, prominent veins, and slight swelling of the fourth PIP and second MCP joints.

Opening doors, climbing stairs, and doing repetitive work become more demanding.

A low-grade fever without chills is not uncommon. Depression and both focused and nonspecific anxiety affect the patient and accentuate symptoms. Weight loss is not unusual, and anorexia contributes to this.

Acute Onset

Eight to 15 per cent of patients have an acute onset of symptoms that develop within a few days. Rarely, a patient will pinpoint onset of disease to a specific time or activity, such as opening a door or driving a golf ball. Pain in muscles can be severe and mimic that accompanying muscle necrosis from ischemia. Diagnosis of rheumatoid arthritis when it presents acutely may be difficult to make, and sepsis or vasculitis must be ruled out.

Intermediate Onset

Fifteen to 20 per cent of patients have an intermediate type of onset. Symptoms develop over days or weeks. Systemic complaints are more noticeable than in the insidious type of onset.

Joint Involvement in Early Rheumatoid Arthritis

The joints most commonly involved first in rheumatoid arthritis are the metacarpophalangeal (MCP) joints, proximal interphalangeal (PIP) joints, and wrists[9,10] (Table 19–4). Larger joints generally become symptomatic after smaller joints. This raises the question of whether early disease in large joints remains asymptomatic for a longer time. The answer was sought in one study by performing xenon clearances on clinically normal knees of patients with early rheumatoid arthritis.[11] Seven of 22 had abnormally high perfusion, supporting this hypothesis. An anatomic study has correlated the area in square centimeters of synovial membrane with that of hyaline cartilage in each joint. The joints with the highest ratio of synovium to articular cartilage correlated positively with the joints most frequently involved in the disease.[12]

Unusual Patterns of Early Disease

Adult-Onset Still's Disease

Still's disease appears in adults, usually in the third or fourth decade, as a syndrome similar to that seen in children with the acute, febrile onset of juvenile arthritis. Still's disease was first described by Bywaters in 14 patients.[13] Women are more commonly affected than are men. Serologic studies (rheumatoid factor and antinuclear antibody [ANA]) are negative, and patients do not have subcutaneous nodules.[14] Most are febrile. Fever patterns in these patients are usually quotidian (i.e., reaching normal levels at least once each day). The skin often has salmon-colored or pink macules that are evanescent and become more prominent when patients are febrile, usually in the afternoon. The cervical spine is involved, and loss of neck motion may be striking. Pericarditis, pleural effusions, and severe abdominal pain may be present and confound attempts at diagnosis.[15] Unlike systemic lupus erythematosus (SLE), serum complement level is normal or high.[16]

In one series, 11 patients (all of whom were white women) followed for a mean of 20.2 years after disease onset had the following characteristics[17]:

- Ten had a polycyclic pattern (characterized by remissions and exacerbations).
- Patterns of exacerbations were similar to but less severe than the original presentations.
- Loss of wrist extension was the most common clinical abnormality, and carpal ankylosis was present in 10 patients.
- Five of 11 patients developed distal interphalangeal (DIP) joint involvement.
- Biopsy of the characteristic skin rashes of Still's disease and juvenile rheumatoid arthritis showed

TABLE 19–4. Joints Involved in Rheumatoid Arthritis*

	PERCENTAGE INITIALLY INVOLVED[9]			PERCENTAGE ULTIMATELY INVOLVED[3]
	RIGHT	LEFT	BILATERAL	
Metacarpophalangeal	65	58	52	87
Wrist	60	57	48	82
Proximal interphalangeal	63	53	45	63
Metatarsophalangeal	48	47	43	48
Shoulder	37	42	30	47
Knee	35	30	24	56
Ankle	25	23	18	53
Elbow	20	15	14	21

From Harris, E. D. Jr.: Clinical features of rheumatoid arthritis. *In* Kelley, W. N., Harris, E. D. Jr., Ruddy, S., and Sledge, C. B. (eds.): Textbook of Rheumatology, 4th ed., Vol. 1. Philadelphia, W. B. Saunders, 1993, pp. 874–911. Used by permission.

* Other joints (e.g., distal interphalangeal joints) are involved in rheumatoid arthritis but are not tabulated here.

perivascular infiltrate of neutrophils in the superficial dermis.

Within another group,[18] 20 per cent showed significant functional deterioration from erosive joint disease. Functional class III/IV (Steinbrocker's classification) was usually related to hip disease. As in classical rheumatoid arthritis in adults, polyarticular disease was more often associated with a poor functional outcome than was oligoarticular disease. Individuals with monocyclic or polycyclic systemic disease, no arthritis at presentation, or oligoarticular presentation and progression tended to have a considerably better outcome. The occurrence of amyloidosis may be as high as 30 per cent within 10 years of onset of the illness.[19,20]

Classification criteria have been developed for adult Still's disease through a Japanese study of 90 patients compared with 267 control.[21] The proposed criteria are fever, arthralgia, typical rash, and leukocytosis as major criteria, and sore throat, lymphadenopathy and/or splenomegaly, liver dysfunction, and the absence of rheumatoid factor as minor ones. Five or more criteria (including two major ones) yielded 96.2 per cent sensitivity and 92.1 per cent specificity.

Despite the chronic and recurrent nature of adult Still's disease, the need for continuing medication, higher levels of pain, and physical and psychological disability, these patients have been found in a same-sex matched sibling study to have equal educational achievement, occupational prestige, social functioning, and family income.[22]

Palindromic Pattern of Onset

Palindromic rheumatism[23] was first described by Hench and Rosenberg in 1941. Like many other clinical complexes in rheumatology, it should be considered a syndrome that can be the initial manifestation of many different organic processes, or one that never evolves into anything more. Pain usually begins in one joint; symptoms worsen for several hours and are associated with swelling and erythema. The joints that were involved in a series of 227 patients are listed in Table 19–5.[24]

An intercritical period, as in gout, is asymptomatic. It is likely that 20 to 40 per cent of patients

TABLE 19–5. Distribution of Joints Involved in Attacks Based upon Cumulative Experience with 227 Patients

JOINT INVOLVEMENT	MEAN % OF PATIENTS	RANGE OF % OF PATIENTS
MCP and PIP	91	74–100
Wrists	78	54–82
Knees	64	41–94
Shoulders	65	33–75
Ankles	50	10–67
Feet	43	15–73
Elbows	38	13–60
Hips	17	0–40
Temporomandibular	8	0–28
Spine	4	0–11
Sternoclavicular	2	0–6
Para-articular sites	27	20–29

From Guerne, P.-A., and Weisman, M. H.: Palindromic rheumatism: part of or apart from the spectrum of rheumatoid arthritis? Am. J. Med. 93:451, 1992. Used by permission. Copyright 1992 by Excerpta Medica Inc.

with palindromic rheumatism go on to develop rheumatoid arthritis, particularly those with HLA-DR4. It is significant that, in a compilation of 653 patients from nine series, only 15 per cent became asymptomatic after at least 5 years with a palindromic syndrome.[24] In patients progressing to rheumatoid arthritis, multiple joints become involved, swelling does not subside completely between attacks, and tests become positive for rheumatoid factor. Neither the characteristics of joint fluid nor the pathologic findings of synovial biopsies allow the prediction that rheumatoid arthritis will evolve from palindromic rheumatism.[25] Of 51 patients with palindromic rheumatism, 41 experienced marked improvement in frequency and duration of attacks during treatment with antimalarials.[26]

Effects of Age on Onset

Rheumatoid arthritis developing in older persons, more often men than women (60 years of age and older), is often dominated by stiffness, limb girdle pain, and diffuse boggy swelling of the hands, wrists, and forearms. One study has emphasized that an initial clinical onset resembling polymyalgia rheumatica occurs four times more frequently in the elderly than in younger patients.[27] Those with an age of onset greater than 60 years are less likely to have subcutaneous nodules or rheumatoid factor at the onset of disease, despite the high prevalence of rheumatoid factor in the general population in this age group. In general, elderly individuals who develop rheumatoid arthritis tend to have a more benign course than do younger patients; there is a lower frequency of positive tests for rheumatoid factor, but there is a strong association with HLA-DR4.[28] Onset is slow, but the stiffness often is incapacitating. In other respects, the disease is similar to other forms of adult rheumatoid arthritis. NSAIDs are rarely effective, but low-dose glucocorticoids (<7.5 mg of prednisone per day) may be helpful in reducing edema and increasing motion and function.

Rheumatoid Arthritis and Paralysis: Asymmetric Disease

Being relatively common, rheumatoid arthritis is likely to occur with many other types of chronic disease. A striking asymmetry or even unilateral involvement has been described in patients with poliomyelitis, meningioma, encephalitis, neurovascular syphilis, strokes, and cerebral palsy.[29,30] Joints are spared on the paralyzed side, and the degree of protection demonstrates a rough correlation with the extent of paralysis.[31] The protective effect on the affected side is less if a neurologic deficit develops in a patient who already has rheumatoid arthritis.[32]

Arthritis Robustus

Arthritis robustus is not so much an unusual presentation of disease as an unusual reaction of patients to the disease.[33,34] Men usually form this group, although notable exceptions occur in women. Their disease is characterized by a proliferative synovitis that appears to cause little pain and even less disability. These patients are athletic and invariably keep working (often at physical labor). Osteopenia is less severe, and new bone proliferation at joint margins is common. Bulky subcutaneous nodules develop. Subchondral cysts develop, presumably from the excessive pressure developed from synovial fluid within a thick joint capsule during muscular effort.

THE COURSE OF RHEUMATOID ARTHRITIS

Long Clinical Remissions

In one study of 250 patients receiving only simple medical and orthopedic treatment, almost 10 per cent were in clinical remission for 12 to 31 years (mean, 22 years).[5] Many of these patients had an acute onset of symptoms with marked fever and severe joint pain and inflammation, raising the question (in retrospect) of whether they indeed had rheumatoid arthritis. Nevertheless, some sign of disease activity (e.g., an elevated ESR) persisted in many throughout the "clinical remission," and occasional patients had brief but true flares of disease in one or a few joints. Rheumatoid factor tests that are positive initially may become negative; this is an excellent prognostic sign. The criteria for a complete clinical remission are, appropriately, very stringent[35] (Table 19–6).

Intermittent Course

An intermittent course, noted in 15 to 30 per cent of patients, is marked by partial to complete remissions without need for continuous therapy. It is a mild disease initially, and only a few joints are involved. Insidious return of disease is often marked by involvement of more joints than during the first episode.[36,37] Within this group, it is reported that approximately half had remissions lasting more than 1 year, and in the entire group remissions lasted longer than exacerbations.

TABLE 19–6. Criteria for Complete Clinical Remission in Rheumatoid Arthritis*

A minimum of five of the following requirements must be fulfilled for at least 2 consecutive months in a patient with definite or classical rheumatoid arthritis:

1. Morning stiffness not to exceed 15 minutes
2. No fatigue
3. No joint pain
4. No joint tenderness or pain on motion
5. No soft tissue swelling in joints or tendon sheaths
6. ESR (Westergren) less than 30 mm/hr (women) or 20 mm/hr (men)

Exclusions: Clinical manifestations of active vasculitis, pericarditis, pleuritis, or myositis and/or unexplained recent weight loss or fever secondary to rheumatoid arthritis prohibit a designation of complete clinical remission.

Modified from Harris, E. D. Jr.: Clinical features of rheumatoid arthritis. *In* Kelley, W. N., Harris E. D. Jr., Ruddy, S., and Sledge, C. B. (eds.): Textbook of Rheumatology, 4th ed., Vol. 1. Philadelphia, W. B. Saunders, 1993, pp. 874–911. Used by permission.
* Data from Pinals et al.[35]

Progressive Disease

The 55 to 70 per cent of patients who have progressive rheumatoid arthritis but the end-point is usually the same: disabling, destructive disease. In assessing symptoms in rheumatoid arthritis, both patients and their physicians must be aware of environmental factors that may accentuate symptoms. One of these, the weather, has a strong base in folklore as a major determinant of symptom severity in rheumatoid arthritis and other rheumatic diseases. Using a climate-controlled chamber for patients, early data suggested that symptoms worsened if humidity was raised and barometric pressure lowered simultaneously,[38] and another study showed that pain in patients with rheumatoid arthritis increased significantly as temperature and vapor pressure increased.[39] The folklore may be accurate; a consistent dry and temperate climate appears to alleviate symptoms in rheumatoid arthritis.

DIAGNOSIS OF RHEUMATOID ARTHRITIS

Diagnosis of rheumatoid arthritis must be by established criteria that are based on effective clinical history and examination, laboratory tests, and diagnoses that exclude it (see earlier). There is no single feature that makes a definite diagnosis. The ACR criteria for classification need not be used in individual cases for diagnosis; however, the requirement that objective evidence for synovitis must be present for at least 6 weeks is an important one. A physician should not make a premature diagnosis of rheumatoid arthritis in a patient who may have a self-limited synovitis; however, in order to prevent irreversible damage to joints, the diagnosis of rheumatoid arthritis should be ruled in or out within 2 months after the onset of synovitis.

The characteristic patient with rheumatoid arthritis complains of pain and stiffness in multiple joints. The joint swelling is boggy and includes both soft tissue and synovial fluid. These joints are tender to touch, especially the small joints of the hands and feet. Palmar erythema and prominent veins on the dorsum of the hand and wrist indicate an increase in blood flow to the joint areas. DIP joints rarely are involved. Temperature over the involved joints (except the hip) is elevated, but the joints are not usually red. Range of motion is limited, and muscle strength and function around inflamed joints are diminished. Soft, poorly delineated subcutaneous nodules are often found in the extensor surface of the forearm. Findings on general physical examination are normal, except for a possible low-grade fever (38° C); soft, small lymph nodes are found occasionally in epitracheal, axillary, and cervical areas. Movement is guarded, and apprehension often dominates the facial expression. Initial laboratory tests often show the following:

- A slight leukocytosis with normal differential WBC count
- Thrombocytosis
- Slight anemia ($\geq$10g of hemoglobin/dl), normochromic and either normocytic or microcytic
- Normal urinalysis
- ESR (Westergren method) of 30 mm or more per hour
- Normal renal, hepatic, and metabolic function
- Normal serum uric acid level (before initiation of salicylate therapy)
- Positive rheumatoid factor test and negative ANA test
- Elevated levels of α_2 globulins and α_1 globulins
- Normal or elevated serum complement level

It is important to emphasize that these diagnostic guidelines are just that, and, as with all such lists, are subject to a wide standard deviation from the mean. A clear example of this is the wide variation in serologic manifestations of rheumatoid arthritis among different American Indian groups in Oklahoma. In a group of patients with homogeneous clinical findings, 9 of 12 from the Kiowa tribe had positive fluorescent ANA tests, and 4 of these had anti-Ro precipitins (Ro are small nuclear ribonuclear proteins; autoantibodies against them are common in Sjögren's syndrome and frequent in SLE). In contrast, among 33 patients from other tribes, only 9 were fluorescent ANA positive and only one had anti-Ro.[40]

A "typical" arthrocentesis in early rheumatoid arthritis reveals the following. Joint fluid is straw-colored and slightly cloudy, and contains many flecks of fibrin. Within the fluid, a clot forms on standing at room temperature. There are 3,500 to 25,000 WBC/mm^3, and at least 85 per cent of these are polymorphonuclear (PMN) leukocytes. Other findings in rheumatoid joint fluid have been reviewed in Chapter 14.

Differential Diagnosis of Rheumatoid Arthritis

It is important to exclude many other diseases before making a diagnosis of rheumatoid arthritis.[41] One of the most difficult challenges is the patient with polyarthritis and fever; these patients deserve a full work-up to define the underlying cause, which often may be more life-threatening than rheumatoid arthritis itself.[42] The relative frequency of the entities discussed here is recorded as common, uncommon, or rare; they are listed in alphabetical order, not in an order of likely diagnoses.

Amyloidosis (Rare)

Deposits of the glycoprotein amyloid can be found in synovial and periarticular tissues[43] and are, presumably, responsible for the joint complaints that these patients often have. The synovial fluid in amyloid arthropathy is noninflammatory, and, on occasion, particulate material with apple-green fluorescence after Congo red staining may be found in the fluid. Amyloid formed of β_2-microglobulin is found in joints of patients with chronic renal failure, usually those who are on dialysis.

Angioimmunoblastic Lymphadenopathy (Rare)

Nonerosive, symmetric, seronegative polyarthritis involving large joints can be an initial complaint in this unusual disease.[44] Typical clinical features are lymphadenopathy, hepatosplenomegaly, rash, and hypergammaglobulinemia. It can resemble Still's disease in adults if the arthritis precedes other manifestations. Diagnosis is made by the characteristic appearance of a lymph node or skin biopsy specimen: effacement of lymph node architecture, proliferation of small vessels, and a cellular infiltrate (immunoblasts, plasma cells, T lymphocytes, and histiocytes) within amorphous acidophilic interstitial material. It is believed that symptoms may be related to excessive production of IL-2 by T-helper cells in this process.

Ankylosing Spondylitis, Seronegative Spondyloarthropathy, and Reactive Arthritis (Common)

These are often referred to as the "B27-associated diseases." The problem in differentiating them from rheumatoid arthritis arises with the patient (particularly a woman) who has minimal back pain and definite peripheral joint involvement. Suspicion that this is not rheumatoid arthritis is generated when small joints are not involved, when joint disease is asymmetric, and when the lumbar spine is involved. In some cases, the conclusion is inescapable that rheumatoid arthritis and ankylosing spondylitis are present in the same patient. In one series, nine patients with rheumatoid factor in serum had spinal ankylosis and symmetric erosive polyarthritis; eight of the nine carried HLA-B27.[19] If one assumes that these two diseases occur completely independently of each other, simultaneous occurrence in the same patient should occur once in every 50,000 to 200,000 members of the adult population.

In distinguishing patients with *Reiter's syndrome* from those with rheumatoid arthritis, a careful search for heel pain or tenderness and ocular or urethral symptoms is of great importance. Polyarthritis persists chronically in over 80 per cent of patients with Reiter's syndrome. The characteristics of enthesopathy (i.e., sausage digits indicating periarticular soft tissue inflammation), insertional tendinitis, periostitis, and peri-insertional osteoporosis or erosions in patients with Reiter's syndrome may point to the diagnosis.

The differential diagnosis between rheumatoid arthritis with psoriasis and *psoriatic arthritis* may be artificial. Some patients with DIP joint involvement and severe skin involvement obviously have a disease that is not rheumatoid arthritis. Others, however, have a seropositive symmetric polyarthritis that appears to be rheumatoid arthritis, yet they also have psoriasis. These patients can be treated with the same disease-modifying drugs as those with progressive rheumatoid arthritis.

A syndrome described extensively in the French literature, *acne-pustulosis-hyperostosis-osteitis*,[45] may resemble psoriatic arthritis and, occasionally, when peripheral arthritis is present, rheumatoid arthritis. As implied in the name, these patients variably express severe acne, palmar and plantar pustules, hyperostotic reactions (particularly in the clavicles and sternum), sacroiliitis, and peripheral inflammatory arthritis.

Inflammatory bowel disease (ulcerative colitis and Crohn's disease) is associated with arthritis in 20 per cent of cases.[46] Peripheral arthritis occurs more commonly than spondylitis in many series.[47] Ankles, knees, and elbows are the most often involved peripheral joints, with PIP joints and wrists next in frequency. Simultaneous attacks of arthritis and development of erythema nodosum are not uncommon. Only two or three joints are affected at once. Involvement is usually asymmetric, and erosions are uncommon. The occurrence of peripheral arthritis in inflammatory bowel disease is not related to HLA-B27.

Behçet's syndrome is marked by an asymmetric polyarthritis in 50 to 60 per cent of cases.[48] It is rare, with a prevalence of less than 1:25,000 in the United States. In more than in half of the cases, the attacks of arthritis are monarticular.[49] Knees, ankles, and wrists are affected most often; synovial fluid usually contains less than 5,000 but more than 30,000 WBC/mm³. Joint deformity is unusual. The painful oral and genital ulcers and central nervous system involvement are characteristic. Uveal tract involvement seen in Behçet's syndrome must be differentiated from scleritis characteristic of rheumatoid arthritis in patients with ocular and joint disease. Methotrexate and cyclosporine A are currently favored as therapy for this debilitating syndrome (G. V. Ball, personal communication).

Enteric infections are complicated occasionally by inflammatory joint disease resembling rheumatoid arthritis. The joint disease associated with *Yersinia enterocolitica* infections occur several weeks after the gastrointestinal illness.[50] Knees and ankles are the joints most commonly involved, and the majority of patients (even those with peripheral arthritis and no spondylitis) have HLA-B27.[51] Reactive arthritis also has been reported after *Salmonella, Shigella*, and *Campylobacter (Helicobacter) jejuni* infections.

Arthropathy may precede other findings of *Whipple's disease*. The pattern is that of a migratory poly- or oligoarthritis involving ankles, knees, shoulders, elbows, and fingers, as with inflammatory bowel disease. Remission may occur when diarrhea begins. Joint destruction in Whipple's disease is rare,[52] presumably because the synovitis lacks sustained chronicity.

Arthritis Associated with Oral Contraceptives (Uncommon)

A syndrome of persistent arthralgias, myalgias, and morning stiffness with occasional development of polyarticular synovitis has been described in women, usually in their 20s, who have been taking oral contraceptives (estrogens and progestins).[53] Positive tests for ANA are common, and several patients have had circulating rheumatoid factor. Symptoms resolve after the contraceptive is discontinued.

Arthritis of Thyroid Disease (Uncommon)

In hypothyroidism, synovial effusions and synovial thickening simulating rheumatoid arthritis have been described.[54] The ESR may be elevated because of hypergammaglobulinemia. Joint fluid is noninflammatory and may have an increased viscosity. Knees, wrists, hands, and feet are involved most often, and not infrequently coexisting calcium pyrophosphate dihydrate (CPPD) deposition disease is found.

The syndrome of thyroid acropachy complicates less than 1 per cent of cases of hyperthyroidism.[55] This represents periosteal new bone formation, which may be associated with a low-grade synovitis similar to hypertrophic osteoarthropathy. Although impossible to quantitate, patients with coexisting rheumatoid arthritis and hyperthyroidism have pain from their arthritis that appears to exceed that expected from the degree of inflammation.

Bacterial Endocarditis (Uncommon)

Arthralgias, arthritis, and myalgias occur in approximately 30 per cent of patients with subacute bacterial endocarditis.[56] The joint symptoms are usually in one or several joints, usually large proximal ones. It is probable that this synovitis is caused by circulating immune complexes.[57] Fever out of proportion to joint findings in the setting of leukocytosis should lead to consideration of infective endocarditis as a diagnostic possibility, even in the absence of a significant heart murmur. It is wise to obtain blood cultures in all patients with polyarthritis and significant fever. Embolic phenomena with constitutional symptoms, including arthralgias, can be presenting symptoms of atrial myxoma, but this process usually mimics systemic vasculitis or subacute bacterial endocarditis more than it does rheumatoid arthritis.[58]

Calcific Periarthritis (Uncommon)

Although usually involving single joints, calcific periarthritis can be confused occasionally with polyarthritis.[59] The skin is red over and around the affected joints; the tissues are boggy and tender, but no joint effusion is present. Passive motion is easier than active motion. Periarticular calcification is visible on radiographs. Unless the periarthritis can be differentiated from true arthritis, the findings may mimic palindromic rheumatism or early monarticular rheumatoid arthritis.

Calcium Pyrophosphate Dihydrate Deposition Disease (Common)

CPPD deposition disease, a crystal-induced synovitis, has many different forms, ranging from a syndrome of indolent osteoarthrosis to that of an acute, hot joint. About 5 per cent of patients have a chronic polyarthritis (sometimes referred to as pseudorheumatoid arthritis) associated with proliferative erosions at subchondral bone.[60] Although radiographs are of great help when chondrocalcinosis is present, CPPD deposition may be present in the absence of calcification on radiographs.[61] Diagnosis then can be made only by arthrocentesis. One of the radiographic signs of CPPD deposition that helps differentiate it from rheumatoid arthritis is the presence of unicompartmental disease in the wrists.

Chronic Fatigue Syndrome (Common)

Although numerous physicians prefer to separate this syndrome away from fibromyalgia because of the possibility that it is caused by a slow virus infection (e.g., EBV), there is such a great overlap between the two that the best approach is to consider both as forms of ''generalized rheumatism'' and to approach management in the same way. The finding of true synovitis essentially rules out the diagnosis of either chronic fatigue syndrome or fibromyalgia.

Congenital Camptodactyly and Arthropathy (Rare)

Congenital camptodactyly and arthropathy[62] begins in utero and produces synovial cell hypertrophy and hyperplasia without inflammatory cells. Clinical manifestations include contractures of the fingers, flattening of the metacarpals, and short, thick femoral neck. This deformity can present as would oligoarticular seronegative rheumatoid arthritis.

Diffuse Connective Tissue Disease (Common)

Connective tissue diseases such as SLE, scleroderma, dermatomyositis/polymyositis, vasculitis, and mixed connective tissue disease (MCTD) may begin with a syndrome of mild systemic symptoms and minimal polyarthritis involving the PIP and MCP joints. It is not uncommon for one of these illnesses, diagnosed at one point in time, to evolve into another as years go by. There are rules of thumb for characterizing joint disease of the various entities:

1. In **SLE**, an organized synovitis that causes erosions is rare. Soft tissue and muscle inflammation may lead to dislocation of normal tendon alignment, resulting in ulnar deviation similar to Jaccoud's arthropathy.

2. Limitation of joint motion in **scleroderma** is due to taut skin bound down to underlying fascia. The same considerations hold for **dermatomyositis/polymyositis**; proliferative synovitis is rarely sustained in these processes.

3. In **MCTD** (i.e., arthralgias, arthritis, hand swelling, sclerodactyly, Raynaud's phenomenon, esophageal hypomotility, and myositis with circulating antibody to ribonucleoprotein), 60 to 70 per cent of patients have arthritis. Few have significant titers of rheumatoid factor in their serum. Many are given an initial diagnosis of rheumatoid arthritis, and numerous studies of MCTD have shown deforming, erosive arthritis. In one series, for example, 8 of 17 patients had presentations similar to that of rheumatoid arthritis.[63] Articular and periarticular osteopenia alone was found in eight. Six had loss of joint space, and five had erosions typical of rheumatoid arthritis. Although MCTD is a different diagnosis, there are few differences in therapy between these patients with aggressive joint disease and those with rheumatoid arthritis.

Familial Mediterranean Fever (Uncommon)

The articular syndrome in this disease is an episodic monarthritis or oligoarthritis of the large joints that appears in childhood or adolescence, mimicking oligoarthritic forms of juvenile rheumatoid arthritis.[64] Sephardic Jews comprise up to 60 per cent of reported cases. Episodes of arthritis come on acutely with fever and other signs of inflammation (e.g., peritonitis or pleuritis) and can precede other manifestations of the disease. Although usually self-limited (days to weeks), attacks occasionally will last for months and be associated with radiographic changes of periarticular osteopenia without erosions. The abdominal pain these patients experience can be a key to diagnosis. Amyloidosis (type AA) is a late complication of this syndrome in a number of patients. Regular doses of colchicine (0.5–2.0 mg/day) have been effective in decreasing the frequency of attacks, and also may prevent development of amyloidosis.

Fibromyalgia (Fibrositis) (Common)

In fibromyalgia there is rarely evidence of synovitis. Although there are no specific diagnostic tests that define fibromyalgia, there are certain recurrent nonarticular locations for pain that are seen in different patients. In an analysis of the pain properties[65] contrasted with those of rheumatoid arthritis, the fibromyalgia patients used diverse modifiers to describe their pain, the most common adjectives being pricking, pressing, shooting, gnawing, cramping, splitting, and crushing. A majority of both groups defined the pain as aching and exhausting. Evidence is accumulating that some patients with rheumatoid arthritis may develop a superimposed fibromyalgia. Rheumatoid patients have fewer psychological disturbances than patients with primary fibromyalgia, but patients with both syndromes score higher on testing scales for hypochondriasis, depression, and hysteria than those with rheumatoid arthritis who do not have fibrositis. Indeed, there has been a study of 67 rheumatoid patients in which emotion and mood were recorded every day for 75 days and matched with both joint tenderness and the "tender point count" characteristically found in fibromyalgia. The tender point count correlated extremely well with patients' reports of daily stress.[66] Interestingly, joint tenderness and fibromyalgia symptoms were not well associated, raising the possibility that patients with rheumatoid arthritis and concomitant fibromyalgia are at risk for overtreatment of their arthritis.

Glucocorticoid Withdrawal Syndrome (Common)

Often confused with rheumatoid arthritis are the symptoms of glucocorticoid withdrawal. These patients, treated for nonrheumatic diseases, may have diffuse polyarticular pain, particularly in the hands, if the glucocorticoid dose is tapered too rapidly. Although glucocorticoids suppress inflammation and pain, there is an arthropathy associated with their use[67] that resembles avascular necrosis.

Gout (Common)

Before a diagnosis of chronic erosive rheumatoid arthritis is made, chronic tophaceous gout must be ruled out. The reverse applies as well. Features of gouty arthritis that can mimic those of rheumatoid arthritis include polyarthritis, symmetric involvement, fusiform swelling of joints, subcutaneous nodules, and subacute presentation of attacks. Conversely, certain aspects of rheumatoid arthritis that suggest gouty arthritis include hyperuricemia (after treatment with low doses of aspirin), periarticular nodules, and seronegative disease (particularly in men).[68] Radiographic findings may be similar, with appearance of the subcortical erosions of rheumatoid arthritis resembling the small osseous tophi in gout.[69] Although large asymmetric erosions with ballooning of the cortex are more likely to be gout than rheumatoid arthritis, this is not always the case.[70] Serologic test results may be misleading as well; rheumatoid factor has been found in as many as 30 per cent of patients with chronic tophaceous gout,[71] and these patients have had no clinical or radiographic signs of rheumatoid arthritis.

The coexistence of rheumatoid arthritis and gout is rare, and curiously so. Only 10 cases of gout coexisting with rheumatoid arthritis have been reported in the medical literature since 1881, even though many more could have been anticipated considering the combined prevalence of the two diseases. Wallace and associates have calculated that, considering the prevalence of the two diseases, gout and rheumatoid arthritis should be anticipated to coexist in 10,617 cases in the United States.[72] In several patients with definite rheumatoid arthritis and persistent hyperuricemia, flares of the rheumatoid process coincided with normalization of the uric acid level.[73] Several other case reports have noted this, and the possibility that the hyperuricemic state is anti-inflammatory must be investigated further.

Hemochromatosis (Uncommon)

The characteristic articular feature of hemochromatosis that is almost diagnostic is firm bony enlargement of the MCP joints, particularly the second and third, with associated cystic degenerative disease on radiographs and, not infrequently, chondrocalcinosis.[74] Marginal erosions, juxta-articular osteoporosis, synovial proliferation, and ulnar deviation are not seen in the arthropathy of hemochromatosis but are common in rheumatoid arthritis. Wrists, shoulders, elbows, hips, and knees are involved less often than the MCP joints. More than one third of patients with this iron overload syndrome have an arthropathy.[75]

Hemoglobinopathies (Uncommon)

In homozygous (SS) sickle cell disease, the most common arthropathy is associated with crises and is believed to be a result of microvascular occlusion in articular tissues.[76] However, in some cases a destructive arthritis with loss of articular cartilage has been defined,[77] and this resembles severe rheumatoid arthritis. In most patients with sickle cell disease and joint complaints, periosteal elevation, bone infarcts, fish mouth vertebrae, and avascular necrosis can be found on radiographs.[77] In a series of 37 patients with sickle cell anemia from which those with gout or avascular necrosis of the femoral head were excluded, 12 complained of a monarthritis or oligoarthritis associated with painful crises; tenderness was most marked over the epiphyses rather than the joint space, and synovial fluid was noninflammatory. Another 12 patients had arthritis of the ankle associated with a malleolar ulcer; this arthritis was chronic and resolved with improvement of the leg ulcer.[78] Episodic polyarthritis and noninflammatory synovial effusions are also found in sickle cell/β-thalassemia.[79]

Hemophilic Arthropathy (Uncommon)

A deficiency of factor VIII or, less frequently, factor IX sufficient to produce clinical bleeding frequently results in hemarthroses. The iron overload in the joint generates a proliferative synovitis that often leads to joint destruction. The clotting abnormality rarely is overlooked, however, and it is unlikely that a diagnosis of rheumatoid arthritis would be made in the setting of hemophilia A or B.

Hepatitis C (Common)

Several patients have been described with joint inflammation and positive serum tests for hepatitis C viral antigens. Acute-phase reactants were markedly elevated, and complement levels were normal. Cryoglobulins were present in two of three patients. The arthritis was not erosive, but it was unresponsive to NSAIDs.[80] α-Interferon therapy for the hepatitis was associated with clinical improvement of the arthritis in two of three patients.

Human Immunodeficiency Virus Infection (Common)

Several types of arthropathy have been described in association with HIV infection[81]:

- Acute arthralgias concurrent with the initial HIV viremia lasting for a few days.
- AIDS-associated arthritis, lower extremity oligoarthritis, or a persistent polyarthritis.
- Seronegative spondyloarthropathy, resembling Reiter's syndrome, psoriatic arthritis or reactive

arthritis; symptoms and signs are often more severe than in patients without HIV infection.[82]

The importance of ruling out HIV in any patient with an acute polyarthritis and fever is crucial; HIV-positive patients do not do well when treated with immunosuppressive drugs!

Hyperlipoproteinemia (Uncommon)

Achilles tendinitis and tenosynovitis can be presenting symptoms in familial type II hyperlipoproteinemia and may be accompanied by arthritis.[83] Synovial fluid findings may resemble those of mild rheumatoid arthritis, and the tendon xanthomas may be mistaken for rheumatoid nodules or gouty tophi. Similarly, bilateral pseudoxanthomatous rheumatoid nodules have been described.[84]

Asymmetric and oligoarticular synovitis has been described in type IV hyperlipoproteinemia.[85] The absence of morning stiffness in the presence of noninflammatory synovial effusions helps rule out rheumatoid arthritis. The treatment of hyperlipoproteinemia with clofibrate may cause an acute muscular syndrome[86] that resembles myositis or polymyalgia rheumatica more than it does rheumatoid arthritis.

Hypertrophic Osteoarthropathy (Uncommon)

Hypertrophic osteoarthropathy may present as oligoarthritis involving knees, ankles, or wrists. The synovial inflammation accompanies periosteal new bone formation that can be seen on radiographs. Correction of the inciting factor (e.g., cure of pneumonia in a child with cystic fibrosis) will likely alleviate the synovitis. The synovium is characterized primarily by an increased blood supply and synovial cell proliferation. Little infiltration by mononuclear cells is seen.[87] Pain, which increases when extremities are dependent, is characteristic, although not always present. If clubbing is not present or is not noticed, this entity is easily confused with rheumatoid arthritis.

Idiopathic Hypereosinophilic Syndrome with Arthritis (Rare)

This poorly defined syndrome often presents with myalgias and arthralgias, and evolves into a clinical picture of hepatomegaly with or without pericarditis, pulmonary hypertension, subcutaneous nodules, and cardiomyopathy. Synovitis, characterized by inflammatory joint fluid, rarely is erosive or deforming.[88] The similarities between this and **toxic oil syndrome** and **eosinophilia-myalgia syndrome**, both of which were caused by ingestion of toxic substances, suggests a basic hypersensitivity reaction.

Infectious Arthritis (Common)

Bacterial sepsis may be superimposed on rheumatoid arthritis. Viral infections, however, may present as arthritis, with many characteristics of rheumatoid arthritis. Rubella arthritis occurs more often in adults than in children and often affects small joints of the hands.[89] Lymphocytes predominate in synovial effusions. Arthritis often precedes viral hepatitis and is associated with the presence of circulating hepatitis B surface antigen (HBsAg) and hypocomplementemia.[90] HBsAg has been found in synovial tissues by direct immunofluorescence, supporting the concept that this synovitis is mediated by immune complexes.[91] A relatively acute onset of diffuse polyarthritis with small joint effusions and minimal synovial swelling should prompt the physician to obtain liver function tests in the patient with a history of exposure to hepatitis. With the onset of icterus, the arthritis usually resolves without a trace.

Fever, sore throat, and cervical adenopathy followed by symmetric polyarthritis are compatible with infection caused by hepatitis B, rubella, adenovirus type 7, echovirus type 9, *Mycoplasma pneumoniae*, or EBV,[92] as well as acute rheumatic fever or adult-onset Still's disease.

A chronic polyarthritis resembling rheumatoid arthritis has been described following serologic proof of parvovirus infection. Usually the process is self-limited and has not progressed to a destructive synovitis.

Intermittent Hydrarthrosis (Common)

Intermittent hydrarthrosis is a syndrome of periodic attacks of benign synovitis in one or a few joints, usually the knee, beginning in adolescence.[93] The difference between this and oligoarticular juvenile rheumatoid arthritis or rheumatoid arthritis is one of degree, not kind. In contrast to palindromic rheumatism, in which acute synovitis often may occur in different joints during successive attacks,[94] the same joint or joints are affected during each attack in intermittent hydrarthrosis.[95] Joint destruction does not occur because there is no proliferative synovitis.

Lyme Disease (Common in Endemic Areas)

Lyme disease can closely stimulate rheumatoid arthritis in adults or children by having an intermittent course with development of chronic synovitis.[96] A proliferative, erosive synovitis necessitating synovectomy has evolved in several cases. Histopathology of the proliferative synovium is not different from that of rheumatoid arthritis.

Malignancy (Uncommon)

Direct involvement by cancer of the synovium usually presents as a monarthritis.[97] However, non-Hodgkin's lymphoma can occur as seronegative polyarthritis without hepatomegaly or lymphadenopathy.[98] In children, acute lymphocytic leukemia can present as a polyarticular arthritis.[99] T-lymphocyte malignancy has been associated with arthritis; several patients with a seronegative, erosive arthritis have been described who evolved mycosis fungoides more than 4 years after the presentation of synovitis.[100]

Multicentric Reticulohistiocytosis (Rare)

Multicentric reticulohistiocytosis is particularly interesting because it causes severe arthritis mutilans with an opera-glass hand (*main en lorgnette*).[101] Other causes of arthritis mutilans are rheumatoid arthritis, psoriatic arthritis, erosive osteoarthritis treated with glucocorticoids, and gout (after treatment with allopurinol). The cell that damages tissues is the multinucleate lipid-laden histiocyte, which appears to release degradative enzymes sufficient to destroy connective tissue.

Osteoarthritis (Common)

Although osteoarthritis begins as a degeneration of articular cartilage, and rheumatoid arthritis begins as inflammation in the synovium, each process approaches the other as the diseases progress. In osteoarthritis, as cartilage deteriorates and joint congruence is altered, a reactive synovitis often develops. Conversely, as the rheumatoid pannus erodes cartilage, secondary osteoarthritic changes in bone and cartilage develop. At the end stages of both degenerative joint disease and rheumatoid arthritis, the involved joints appear the same. To differentiate clearly between the two, therefore, the physician must delve into the early history and functional abnormalities of the disease (Table 19–7). Erosive osteoarthritis occurs frequently in middle-aged women (more frequently than in men) and is characterized by inflammatory changes in PIP joints with destruction and functional ankylosis of the joints. The PIP joints can appear red and hot, yet there is almost no synovial proliferation or effusion. Joint swelling is hard, bony tissue, not

TABLE 19–7. Factors Useful for Differentiating Early Rheumatoid Arthritis from Osteoarthrosis (Osteoarthritis)

	RHEUMATOID ARTHRITIS	OSTEOARTHRITIS
Age at onset	Childhood and adults; peak incidence in 50s	Increases with age
Predisposing factors	HLA-DR4, -DR1	Trauma, congenital abnormalities (e.g., shallow acetabulum)
Symptoms, early	Morning stiffness	Pain increases through the day and with use
Joints involved	MCP joints, wrists, PIP joints most often; DIP joints almost never	DIP joints (Heberden's nodes), weight-bearing joints (hips, knees)
Physical findings	Soft tissue swelling, warmth	Bony osteophytes, minimal soft tissue swelling early
Radiologic findings	Periarticular osteopenia, marginal erosions	Subchondral sclerosis, osteophytes
Laboratory findings	Increased ESR, rheumatoid factor, anemia, leukocytosis	Normal

From Harris, E. D. Jr.: Clinical features of rheumatoid arthritis. *In* Kelley, W. N., Harris, E. D. Jr., Ruddy, S., and Sledge, C. B. (eds.): Textbook of Rheumatology, 4th ed., Vol. 1. Philadelphia, W. B. Saunders, 1993, pp. 874–911. Used by permission.

synovium. The ESR may be slightly elevated, but rheumatoid factor is not present.[102]

Parkinson's Disease (Common)

Although the tremor and/or rigidity of Parkinson's disease is rarely confused with rheumatoid arthritis, Parkinson's disease patients have a predilection for developing swan-neck deformities of the hands, a phenomenon generally unappreciated by rheumatologists. This abnormality, the pathogenesis of which still is unknown, was first described in 1864 (Fig. 19–2).[103]

Pigmented Villonodular Synovitis (Rare)

Pigmented nodular synovitis is a nonmalignant but proliferative disease of synovial tissue that has many functional characteristics similar to those of rheumatoid arthritis and usually involves only one joint. The histopathology is characterized by proliferation of histiocytes, multinucleate giant cells, and hemosiderin and lipid-laden macrophages. Clinically, this is a relatively painless chronic synovitis (most often of the knee) with joint effusions and greatly thickened synovium.[104] Subchondral bone cysts and cartilage erosion may be associated with the bulky tissue. It is not clear whether this should be classified as an inflammation or a neoplasm of the synovium. Its tendency to recur after surgical removal necessitates a guarded prognosis.

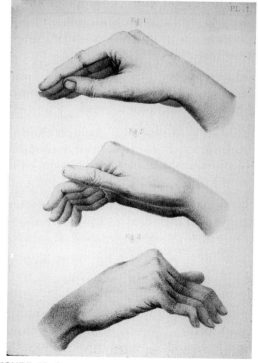

FIGURE 19–2. These swan-neck deformities are a result of Parkinson's disease, not rheumatoid arthritis. (From Ordenstein, L.: Sur la Paralysie Agitante et la Sclerose en Plaques Generalisée. Paris, Imprimerie de E. Martinet, 1864.)

Polychondritis (Uncommon)

Polychondritis can mimic infectious processes, vasculitis, granulomatous disease, or rheumatoid arthritis. Patients with rheumatoid arthritis and ocular inflammation (e.g., scleritis) usually have active joint disease before ocular problems develop; the reverse is true in polychondritis. In addition, polychondritis is not associated with rheumatoid factor. The joint disease is usually episodic. Nevertheless, erosions can develop that are not unlike those of rheumatoid arthritis. In affecting cartilage of the external ears, nose, larynx, trachea, and costochondral areas, this disease may represent a true immune response against cartilage.

Polymyalgia Rheumatica and/or Giant Cell Arteritis (Common)

Although joint radionuclide imaging studies have indicated increased vascular flow in synovium of patients with classic polymyalgia rheumatica, it remains appropriate to exclude this as a diagnosis if significant synovitis (soft tissue proliferation or effusions) can be detected. Otherwise, many patients who actually have rheumatoid arthritis would be diagnosed as having polymyalgia rheumatica and treated with potentially harmful doses of glucocorticoids. A careful history will usually differentiate shoulder or hip girdle muscle pain from shoulder or hip joint pain. Examination of synovial biopsies from polymyalgia rheumatica patients indicates that the synovitis is more mild than that found in rheumatoid arthritis.[105] It is probable that rheumatoid arthritis and polymyalgia rheumatica coexist in numerous patients, but careful descriptions of such patients are rare.

Several patients have been described whose initial symptom of GCA was a peripheral polyarthritis clinically indistinguishable from rheumatoid arthritis.[106] In 19 such patients found in a group of 522 with biopsy-proven GCA, however, only 3 were positive for rheumatoid factor. The interval between onset of each of symptoms was 3 years or less in 15 of the 19, which also suggests a relationship between the two diseases.

Rheumatic Fever (Uncommon)

Rheumatic fever is much less common than it was previously but still must be considered in adults with polyarthritis. In adults, the arthritis is the most prominent clinical finding of rheumatic fever; carditis is less frequent than it is in children, and erythema marginatum, subcutaneous nodules, and chorea are rare.[107,108] The presentation is often that of an additive, symmetric, large-joint polyarthritis (involving lower extremities in 85 per cent of patients), developing within a week and associated with a severe tenosynovitis.[107] This extremely painful process is dramatically responsive to salicylates.[109] Unlike Still's disease in the adult, rheumatic fever generally has no remittent or quotidian fevers, has a less protracted course, and shows evidence of antecedent streptococcal infection. There are many similarities between rheumatic fever in adults and ''reactive'' postinfectious synovitis developing from *Shigella, Salmonella, Brucella, Neisseria,* or *Yersinia* infections. These latter processes do not respond well to salicylates, however. As rheumatic fever becomes less frequent, and as penicillin prophylaxis effectively prevents recurrences of the disease, Jaccoud's arthritis (chronic postrheumatic fever arthritis) is becoming rare. This entity, described first by Bywaters in 1950,[110] results from severe and repeated bouts of rheumatic fever and synovitis, which stretch joint capsules and produce ulnar deformity of the hands without erosions.[111] The same deformity can develop in SLE, characterized by recurrent synovitis and soft tissue inflammation, or in Parkinson's disease. Differentiating rheumatic fever from rheumatoid arthritis is particularly difficult when subcutaneous nodules associated with rheumatic fever are present.[112]

Sarcoidosis (Uncommon)

The two most frequent forms of sarcoid arthritis are usually easily differentiated from rheumatoid arthritis. In the acute form with erythema nodosum and hilar adenopathy (Lofgren's syndrome), the articular complaints usually are related to periarthritis affecting large joints of the lower extremities. Differential diagnosis may be confused because many of these patients have rheumatoid factor in serum.[113] Joint erosions and proliferative synovitis do not occur in this form of sarcoidosis.

In chronic granulomatous sarcoidosis, cyst-like areas of bone destruction, mottled rarefaction of bone, and a reticular pattern of bone destruction giving a lacy appearance on radiographs may simulate destructive rheumatoid arthritis. This form of sarcoid is often polyarticular, and biopsy of bone or synovium for diagnosis may be essential because there is often no correlation between joint disease and clinical evidence for sarcoid involvement of other organ systems.[114] It is likely that Poncet's disease or tuberculous rheumatism[115] actually represents granulomatous ''idiopathic'' arthritis (i.e., sarcoidosis).

Sweet's Syndrome (Rare)

Sweet's syndrome is also called acute febrile neutrophilic dermatosis.[116,117] It has been described in adults, often following an influenza-like illness. The three major features are an acute illness with fever, leukocytosis, and raised painful plaques on the skin that show neutrophilic infiltration of the dermis on biopsy. Joint disease occurs in 20 to 25 per cent of cases and is characterized by acute, self-limited polyarthritis. Because of the skin lesions, Sweet's syndrome is confused with SLE, erythema nodosum, and erythema elevatum diutinum more often than with rheumatoid arthritis. It has been treated effectively with indomethacin[117] and glucocorticoids.

Thiemann's Disease (Rare)

Thiemann's disease is a rare form of idiopathic vascular necrosis of the PIP joints of the hands with occasional involvement of other joints.[118,119] Bony enlargement begins relatively painlessly, and the digits (one or more may be involved) become fixed in flexion. The primary lesion is in the region of the epiphysis, and the lesion begins most often before puberty, distinguishing it from erosive osteoarthritis, which it resembles radiographically. It is clearly a heritable disease, but the genetic factors have not been defined.

REFERENCES

1. Arnett, F. C., Edworthy, S. M., Bloch, D. A., et al.: The American Rheumatism Association 1987 revised criteria for the classification of rheumatoid arthritis. Arthritis Rheum. 31:315, 1988.
2. Jacobsson, L. T. H., Knowler, W. C., Pillemer, S., et al.: A cross-sectional and longitudinal comparison of the Rome criteria for active rheumatoid arthritis and the American College of Rheumatology 1987 criteria for rheumatoid arthritis. Arthritis Rheum. 37:1479, 1994.
3. Jacoby, R. K., Jayson, M. I., and Cosh, J. A.: Onset, early stages, and prognosis of rheumatoid arthritis: a clinical study of 100 patients with 11-year follow-up. Br. Med. J. 2:96, 1973.
4. Lawrence, J. S.: Surveys of rheumatic complaints in the population. In Dixon, A. St. J. (ed.): Progress in Clinical Rheumatology. London, Churchill Livingstone, 1965, p. 1.
5. Short, C. L., and Bauer, W.: The course of rheumatoid arthritis in patients receiving simple medical and orthopedic measures. N. Engl. J. Med. 238:142, 1948.
6. Aho, K., Palosuo, T., Raunio, V., et al.: When does rheumatoid disease start? Arthritis Rheum. 28:485, 1985.
7. Fallahi, S., Halla, J. T., and Hardin, J. G.: Onset patterns of rheumatoid arthritis. Clin. Res. 31:650A, 1983.
8. Fleming, A., Crown, J. M., and Corbett, M.: Early rheumatoid disease. 1. Onset. Ann. Rheum. Dis. 35:357, 1976.
9. Ritchie, D. M., Boyle, J. A., McInnes, J. M., et al.: Clinical studies with an articular index for the assessment of joint tenderness in patients with rheumatoid arthritis. Q. J. Med. 37:393, 1968.
10. Fleming, A., Benn, R. T., Corbett, M., et al.: Early rheumatoid disease. II. Patterns of joint involvement. Ann. Rheum. Dis. 35:361, 1976.
11. Dick, W. C., Grayson, M. F., Woodburn, A., et al.: Indices of inflammatory activity: relationship between isotope studies and clinical methods. Ann. Rheum. Dis. 29:643, 1970.
12. Mens, J. M.: Correlation of joint involvement in rheumatoid arthritis and in ankylosing spondylitis with the synovial: cartilagenous surface ratio of various joints [Letter]. Arthritis Rheum. 30:359, 1987.
13. Bywaters, E. G. L.: Still's disease in the adult. Ann. Rheum. Dis. 30:121, 1971.
14. Gupta, R. C., and Mills, D. M.: Still's disease in an adult: a link between juvenile and adult rheumatoid arthritis. Am. J. Med. Sci. 269:137, 1975.
15. Aptekar, R. G., Decker, J. L., Bujak, J. S., et al.: Adult onset juvenile rheumatoid arthritis. Arthritis Rheum. 16:715, 1973.
16. Strampl, I. J., and Lozar, J. D.: Adult-onset Still's disease: variant of rheumatoid arthritis. Postgrad. Med. 58:175, 1975.
17. Elkon, K. B., Hughes, G. R., Bywaters, E. G., et al.: Adult-onset Still's disease: twenty-year followup and further studies of patients with active disease. Arthritis Rheum. 25:647, 1982.
18. Cush, J. J., Medsger, T. A. Jr., Christy, W. C., et al.: Adult-onset Still's disease: clinical course and outcome. Arthritis Rheum. 30:186, 1987.
19. Fallet, G. H., Mason, M., Berry, H., et al.: Rheumatoid arthritis and ankylosing spondylitis occurring together. Br. Med. J. 1:804, 1976.
20. Cabane, J., Michon, A., Ziza, J. M., et al.: Comparison of long term evolution of adult onset and juvenile onset Still's disease, both followed up for more than 10 years. Ann. Rheum. Dis. 49:283, 1990.
21. Yamaguchi, M., Ohta, A., Tsunematsu, T., et al.: Preliminary criteria for classification of adult Still's disease. J. Rheumatol. 19:424, 1992.
22. Sampalis, J. S., Esdaile, J. M., Medsger, T. A., et al.: A controlled study of the long-term prognosis of adult Still's disease. Am. J. Med. 98:384, 1995.
23. Hench, P. S., and Rosenberg, E. F.: Palindromic rheumatism: New oft-recurring disease of joints (arthritis, periarthritis, para-arthritis) apparently producing no articular residues; report of 34 cases. Proc. Mayo Clin. 16:808, 1942.
24. Guerne, P.-A., and Weisman, M. H.: Palindromic rheumatism: part of or apart from the spectrum of rheumatoid arthritis? Am. J. Med. 93:451, 1992.
25. Schumacher, H. R.: Palindromic onset of rheumatoid arthritis: clinical, synovial fluid, and biopsy studies. Arthritis Rheum. 25:361, 1982.
26. Youssef, W., Yan, A., and Russell, A. S.: Palindromic rheumatism: a response to chloroquine. J. Rheumatol. 18:35, 1991.
27. Deal, C. L., Meenan, R. F., Goldenberg, D. L., et al.: The clinical features of elderly-onset rheumatoid arthritis: a comparison with younger-onset disease of similar duration. Arthritis Rheum. 28:987, 1985.
28. Terkeltaub, R., Decary, F., and Esdaile, J.: An immunogenetic study of older age onset rheumatoid arthritis. J. Rheumatol. 11:147, 1984.
29. Yoghmai, I., Rooholamini, S. M., and Faunce, H. F.: Unilateral rheumatoid arthritis: protective effects of neurologic deficits. Am. J. Roentgenol. 128:299, 1977.
30. Bland, J., and Eddy, W.: Hemiplegia and rheumatoid hemiarthritis. Arthritis Rheum. 11:72, 1968.
31. Glick, E. N.: Asymmetrical rheumatoid arthritis after poliomyelitis. Br. Med. J. 3:26, 1967.
32. Thompson, M., and Bywaters, E. G. L.: Unilateral rheuma-

toid arthritis following hemiplegia. Ann. Rheum. Dis. 21:370, 1961.

33. Bywaters, E. G. L.: The hand. *In* Radiological Aspects of Rheumatoid Arthritis, No. 64. Amsterdam, Excerpta Medica Foundation, 1964, p. 43.

34. de Haas, W. H. D., de Boer, W., Griffioen, F., et al.: Rheumatoid arthritis of the robust reaction type. Ann. Rheum. Dis. 33:81, 1974.

35. Pinals, R. S., Masi, A. T., and Larsen, R. A.: Preliminary criteria for clinical remission in rheumatoid arthritis. Arthritis Rheum. 24:1308, 1981.

36. Short, C. L., Bauer, W., and Reynolds, W. E.: Rheumatoid Arthritis: A Definition of the Disease and a Clinical Description Based on a Numerical Study of 293 Patients and Controls. Cambridge, MA, Harvard University Press, 1957.

37. Short, C. L.: Rheumatoid arthritis: types of course and prognosis. Med. Clin. North Am. 52:549, 1968.

38. Hollander, J. L., and Yeostros, S. J.: The effects of simultaneous variations of humidity and barometric pressure on arthritis. Bull. Am. Meteorol. Soc. 44:389, 1963.

39. Patberg, W. R., Nienhuis, R. L., and Veringa, F.: Relation between meteorological factors and pain in rheumatoid arthritis in a marine climate. J. Rheumatol. 12:711, 1985.

40. Scofield, R. H., Fogel, M., Rhoades, E. R., and Harley, J. B.: Rheumatoid arthritis in a United States Public Health Service hospital in Oklahoma: Serologic manifestations in rheumatoid arthritis vary among tribal groups. Arthritis Rheum. 39:283, 1996.

41. Hoffman, G. S.: Polyarthritis: the differential diagnosis of rheumatoid arthritis. Semin. Arthritis Rheum. 8:115, 1978.

42. Pinals, R. S.: Polyarthritis and fever. N. Engl. J. Med. 330: 769, 1994.

43. Gordon, D. A., Pruzanski, W., Ogryzlo, M. A., et al.: Amyloid arthritis simulating rheumatoid disease in five patients with multiple myeloma. Am. J. Med. 55:142, 1973.

44. Davies, P. G., and Fordham, J. N.: Arthritis and angioimmunoblastic lymphadenopathy. Ann. Rheum. Dis. 42: 516, 1983.

45. Chamot, A. M., Benhamou, C. L., Kahn, M. F., et al.: Le syndrome acne pustulose hyperostose osteite (SAPHO)—85 observations. Rev. Rhum. Mal. Osteo-Articulaires 54:187, 1987..

46. Morris, R. I., Metzger, A. L., Bluestone, R., et al.: HLA B27—a useful discriminator in arthropathies of inflammatory bowel disease. N. Engl. J. Med. 290:1117, 1974.

47. McEwen, C., Lingg, C., and Kirsner, J. B.: Arthritis accompanying ulcerative colitis. Am. J. Med. 33:923, 1962.

48. Zizic, T. M., and Stevens, M. B. The arthropathy of Behçet's disease. Johns Hopkins Med. J. 136:243, 1975.

49. Yurdakul, S., Yazici, H., Tuzuir, Y., et al.: The arthritis of Behçet's disease: a prospective study, in press.

50. Ahvonen, P., Sievers, K., and Ano, K.: Arthritis associated with *Yersinia enterocolitica* infection. Acta Rheumatol. Scand. 15:232, 1969.

51. Aho, K., Ahvonen, P., Lassus, A., et al.: HLA-B27 in reactive arthritis: a study of *Yersinia* arthritis and Reiter's disease. Arthritis Rheum. 17:521, 1974.

52. Hawkins, C. F., Farr, M., Morris, C. J., et al.: Detection by electron microscope of rod-shaped organisms in synovial membrane from a patient with the arthritis of Whipple's disease. Ann. Rheum. Dis. 35:502, 1976.

53. Bole, G. G. Jr., Friedlaender, M. H., and Smith, C. K.: Rheumatic symptoms and serological abnormalities induced by oral contraceptives. Lancet 1:323, 1969.

54. Bland, J. H., and Frymoyer, J. W.: Rheumatic syndromes of myxedema. N. Engl. J. Med. 282:1171, 1970.

55. Gimlette, T. M. D.: Thyroid acropathy. Lancet 1:22, 1960.

56. Churchill, M. D. Jr., Geraci, J. E., and Hunder, G. G.: Musculoskeletal manifestations of bacterial endocarditis. Ann. Intern. Med. 87:754, 1977.

57. Bayer, A. S., Theofilopoulos, A. N., Eisenberg, R., et al.: Circulating immune complexes in infective endocarditis. N. Engl. J. Med. 295:1500, 1976.

58. Bulkley, B. H., and Hutchins, G. M.: Atrial myxomas: a fifty year review. Am. Heart J. 97:639, 1979.

59. Pinals, R. S., and Short, C. L.: Calcific periarthritis involving multiple sites. Arthritis Rheum. 9:566, 1966.

60. McCarty, D. J.: Diagnostic mimicry in arthritis—patterns of joint involvement associated with calcium pyrophosphate dihydrate crystal deposits. Bull. Rheum. Dis. 25: 804, 1975.

61. Utsinger, P. D., Zvaifler, N. J., and Resnick, D.: Calcium pyrophosphate dihydrate deposition disease without chondrocalcinosis. J. Rheumatol. 2:258, 1975.

62. Martin, J. R., Huang, S. N., Lacson, A., et al.: Congenital contractural deformities of the fingers and arthropathy. Ann. Rheum. Dis. 44:826, 1985.

63. Halla, J. T., and Hardin, I. G.: Clinical features of the arthritis of mixed connective tissue disease. Arthritis Rheum. 21:497, 1978.

64. Heller, H., Gafni, J., Michaeli, D., et al.: Arthritis of familial Mediterranean fever (FMF). Arthritis Rheum. 9:1, 1966.

65. Wolfe, F., Cathey, M. A., Kleinkeksel, S. M., et al.: Psychological status in primary fibrositis and fibrositis associated with rheumatoid arthritis. J. Rheumatol. 11:500, 1984.

66. Urrows, S., Affleck, G., Tennen, H., et al.: Unique clinical and psychological correlates of fibromyalgia tender points and joint tenderness in rheumatoid arthritis. Arthritis Rheum. 37:1513, 1994.

67. Velayos, E. E., Leidholt, J. D., Smyth, C. J., et al.: Arthropathy associated with steroid therapy. Ann. Intern. Med. 64:759, 1966.

68. Talbott, J. H., Altman, R. D., and Yu, T. F.: Gouty arthritis masquerading as rheumatoid arthritis or vice versa. Semin. Arthritis Rheum. 8:77, 1978.

69. Resnick, D.: Gout-like lesions in rheumatoid arthritis. Am. J. Roentgenol. 127:1062, 1976.

70. Rappoport, A. S., Sosman, J. L., and Weissman, B. N.: Lesions resembling gout in patients with rheumatoid arthritis. Am. J. Roentgenol. 126:41, 1976.

71. Kozin, F., and McCarty, D. J.: Rheumatoid factor in the serum of gouty patients. Arthritis Rheum. 20:1559, 1977.

72. Wallace, D. J., Klinenberg, J. R., Morham, D., et al.: Coexistent gout and rheumatoid arthritis: case report and literature review. Arthritis Rheum. 22:81, 1979.

73. Agudelo, C. A., Turner, R. A., Panetti, M., et al.: Does hyperuricemia protect from rheumatoid inflammation? A clinical study. Arthritis Rheum. 27:443, 1984.

74. Hirsch, J. H., Killien, F. C., and Troupin, R. H.: The arthropathy of hemochromatosis. Radiology 118:591, 1976.

75. Dymock, I. W., Hamilton, E. B. D., Laws, J. W., et al.: Arthropathy of hemochromatosis: clinical and radiological analysis of 63 patients with iron overload. Ann. Rheum. Dis. 29:469, 1970.

76. Schumacher, H. R., Andrews, R., and McLaughlin, G.: Arthropathy in sickle-cell disease. Ann. Intern. Med. 78: 203, 1973.

77. Schumacher, H. R., Dorwart, B. B., Bond, J., et al.: Chronic

synovitis with early cartilage destruction in sickle cell disease. Ann. Rheum. Dis. 36:413, 1977.

78. deCeulaer, K., Forbes, M., Roper, D., et al.: Non-gouty arthritis in sickle cell disease: report of 37 consecutive cases. Ann. Rheum. Dis. 43:599, 1984.

79. Crout, J. E., McKenna, C. H., and Petitt, R. M.: Symptomatic joint effusions in sickle cell–beta-thalassemia disease: report of a case. JAMA 235:1878, 1976.

80. Rosner, I., Rozenbaum, M., Zuckerman, E., et al.: Rheumatoid-like arthritis associated with hepatitis. C. J. Clin. Rheumatol. 1:182, 1995.

81. Calabrese, L. H.: Human immunodeficiency virus infection and arthritis. Rheum. Dis. Clin. North Am. 19:477, 1993.

82. Solomon, G., Brancato, L., and Winchester, R.: An approach to the human immunodeficiency virus-positive patient with a spondyloarthropathic disease. Rheum. Dis. Clin. North Am. 17:43, 1991.

83. Glueck, C. J., Levy, R. I., and Fredickson, D. S.: Acute tendinitis and arthritis: a presenting symptom of familial type II hyperlipoproteinemia. JAMA 206:2895, 1968.

84. Watt, T. L., and Baumann, R. R.: Pseudoxanthomatous rheumatoid nodules. Arch. Dermatol. 95:156, 1967.

85. Buckingham, R. B., Bole, G. G., and Bassett, D. R.: Polyarthritis associated with type IV hyperlipoproteinemia. Arch. Intern. Med. 135:286, 1975.

86. Langer, T., and Levy, R. I.: Acute muscular syndrome associated with administration of clofibrate. N. Engl. J. Med. 279:856, 1968.

87. Schumacher, H. R. Jr.: Articular manifestations of hypertropic pulmonary osteoarthropathy in bronchogenic carcinoma. Arthritis Rheum. 19:629, 1976.

88. Brogadir, S. P., Goldwein, M. I., and Schumacher, H. R.: A hypereosinophilic syndrome mimicking rheumatoid arthritis. Am. J. Med. 69:799, 1980.

89. Yanez, J. E., Thompson, G. R., Mikkelsen, W. M., et al.: Rubella arthritis. Ann. Intern. Med. 64:772, 1966.

90. Alpert, E., Isselbacher, K. J., and Schur, P. H.: The pathogenesis of arthritis associated with viral hepatitis: complement component studies. N. Engl. J. Med. 285:185, 1971.

91. Schumacher, H. R., and Gall, E. P.: Arthritis in acute hepatitis and chronic active hepatitis: pathology of the synovial membrane with evidence for the presence of Australia antigen in synovial membranes. Am. J. Med. 57:655, 1974.

92. Sigal, L. H., Steere, A. C., and Niederman, J. C.: Symmetric polyarthritis associated with heterophile-negative infectious mononucleosis. Arthritis Rheum. 26:553, 1983.

93. Weiner, A. D., and Ghormley, R. K.: Periodic benign synovitis: idiopathic intermittent hydrarthrosis. J. Bone Joint Surg. Am. 38:1039, 1956.

94. Williams, M. H., Sheldon, P. J., Torrigiani, G., et al.: Palindromic rheumatism: clinical and immunological studies. Ann. Rheum. Dis. 30:375, 1971.

95. Ehrlich, G. E.: Intermittent and periodic rheumatic syndromes. Bull. Rheum. Dis. 24:746, 1974.

96. Steere, A. C., Malawista, S. E., Hardin, J. A., et al.: Erythema chronicum migrans and Lyme arthritis: the enlarging clinical spectrum. Ann. Intern. Med. 86:685, 1977.

97. Moutsopoulos, H. M., Fye, K. H., Pugay, P. I., et al.: Monarthritic arthritis caused by metastatic breast carcinoma: value of cytologic study of synovial fluid. JAMA 234:75, 1975.

98. Dorfman, H. D., Siegel, H. L., Perry, M. C., et al.: Non-Hodgkin's lymphoma of the synovium simulating rheumatoid arthritis. Arthritis Rheum. 30:155, 1987.

99. Emkey, R. D., Ragsdale, B. D., Ropes, M. W., et al.: A case of lymphoproliferative disease presenting as juvenile rheumatoid arthritis: diagnosis by synovial fluid examination. Am. J. Med. 54:825, 1973.

100. Schapira, D., Kerner, H., and Scharf, Y.: Erosive arthritis in a patient with mycosis fungoides. J. R. Soc. Med. 86:176, 1993.

101. Gold, R. H., Metzger, A. L., Mirra, J. M., et al.: Multicentric reticulohistiocytosis (lipoid dermato-arthritis): an erosive polyarthritis with distinctive clinical, roentgenographic and pathological features. Am. J. Roentgenol. 124:610, 1975.

102. Ehrlich, G. E.: Inflammatory osteoarthritis. I. The clinical syndrome. J. Chron. Dis. 25:317, 1972.

103. Ordenstein, L.: Sur la Paralysie Agitante et la Sclérose en Plaques Generalisée. Paris, Imprimerie de E. Martinet, 1864. (original in the Library of the New York Academy of Medicine)

104. Granowitz, S. P., and Mankin, H. J.: Localized pigmented villonodular synovitis of knee: report of five cases. J. Bone Joint Surg. Am. 49:122, 1967.

105. Chou, C.-T., and Schumacher, H. R. Jr.: Clinical and pathological studies of synovitis in polymyalgia rheumatica. Arthritis Rheum. 27:1107, 1984.

106. Ginsburg, W. W., Cohen, M. D., Hall, S. B., et al.: Seronegative polyarthritis in giant cell arteritis. Arthritis Rheum. 28:1362, 1985.

107. McDonald, E. C., and Weisman, M. H.: Articular manifestations of rheumatic fever in adults. Ann. Intern. Med. 89:917, 1978.

108. Barnett, A. L., Terry, E. E., and Persellin, R. H.: Acute rheumatic fever in adults. JAMA 232:925, 1975.

109. Stollerman, G. H., Markowitz, M., Tarania, A., et al.: Jones' criteria (revised) for guidance in the diagnosis of rheumatic fever. Circulation 32:664, 1965.

110. Bywaters, E. G. L.: Relation between heart and joint disease including ''rheumatoid heart disease'' and chronic post-rheumatic arthritis (type Jaccoud). Br. Heart J. 12:101, 1950.

111. Zvaifler, N. J.: Chronic postrheumatic-fever (Jaccoud's) arthritis. N. Engl. J. Med. 267:10, 1962.

112. Ruderman, J. E., and Abruzzo, J. L.: Chronic post rheumatic-fever arthritis (Jaccoud's): report of a case with subcutaneous nodules. Arthritis Rheum. 9:640, 1966.

113. Spilberg, I., Siltzbach, L. E., and McEwen, C.: The arthritis of sarcoidosis. Arthritis Rheum. 12:126, 1969.

114. Kaplan, H.: Sarcoid arthritis: a review. Arch. Intern. Med. 112:162, 1963.

115. Poncet, A.: Address to the Congress Francais de Chirurgie, 1897. Bull. Acad. Med. Paris 46:194, 1901.

116. Krauser, R. E., and Schumacher, H. R.: The arthritis of Sweet's syndrome. Arthritis Rheum. 18:35, 1975.

117. Hoffman, G. S.: Treatment of Sweet's syndrome (acute febrile neutrophilic dermatosis) with indomethacin. J. Rheumatol. 4:201, 1977.

118. Thiemann, H.: Juvenile epiphysenstorungen. Fortschr. Geb. Rontgenstr. Nuklearmed. 14:79, 1909–10.

119. Rubinstein, H. M.: Thiemann's disease: a brief reminder. Arthritis Rheum. 18:357, 1975.

20

Course and Complications of Established Rheumatoid Arthritis

INVOLVEMENT OF SPECIFIC JOINTS: EFFECTS OF DISEASE ON FORM AND FUNCTION

When rheumatoid synovitis is established in joints, the effects that the process has on those joints are a complex function of the intensity of the underlying disease, its chronicity, and the stress put on individual involved joints by the patient.

Joints of the Spine

Cervical Spine

Unlike other nonsynovial joints, such as the sternomanubrial joint or symphysis pubis, the discovertebral joints in the cervical spine often manifest osteochondral destruction in rheumatoid arthritis,[1,2] and on lateral radiographs may be found narrowed to less than 5 mm. There is significant pain, but passive range of motion may be normal in the absence of muscle spasm. There are two possible mechanisms for this process: (1) extension of the inflammatory process from adjacent neurocentral joints—the joints of Luschka, which are lined by synovium—into the discovertebral area[1,2] and (2) chronic cervical instability initiated by apophyseal joint destruction leading to vertebral malalignment or subluxation.[3] This may produce microfractures of the vertebral end-plates, disc herniation, and degeneration of disc cartilage.

The atlantoaxial joint is prone to subluxation in several directions:

- The atlas moves *anteriorly* on the axis (most common). This results from laxity of the ligaments induced by proliferative synovial tissue developing in an adjacent synovial bursa.
- The atlas moves *posteriorly* on the axis. This can occur only if the odontoid peg has been fractured from the axis or destroyed.

- The *vertical* subluxation of the atlas is in relation to the axis (least common). This results from destruction of the lateral atlantoaxial joints or of bone around the foramen magnum. It is apparent now that vertical (superior) migration of the odontoid can develop from progressive anteriorposterior subluxation.

The earliest and most common symptom of cervical subluxation is pain radiating up into the occiput.[4] Two other less common clinical patterns are

- Slowly progressive spastic quadriparesis, frequently with painless sensory loss in the hands.
- Transient episodes of medullary dysfunction associated with vertical penetration of the dens and probable vertebral artery compression.[5] Paresthesias in the shoulders or arms may occur during movement of the head.

Recent histopathologic studies of brain stems and spinal cords of nine patients with end-stage rheumatoid arthritis have revealed significant subaxial degenerative changes in the cervical spine related directly to spinal cord pathology. Thus, it is not surprising that, in severe rheumatoid disease, craniocervical decompression alone may not alleviate neurologic signs.[6]

Physical findings suggestive of atlantoaxial subluxation include loss of occipitocervical lordosis, resistance to passive spine motion, and abnormal protrusion of the axial arch felt by the examining finger on the posterior pharyngeal wall. Radiographic views (lateral, with the neck in flexion) reveal more than 3 mm of separation between the odontoid peg and the axial arch.[5,7] In symptomatic patients, the films in flexion should be taken only after radiographs (including an open-mouth posteroanterior view) have ruled out an odontoid fracture or severe atlantoaxial subluxation. Studies have indicated that computed tomography (CT) is useful for demonstrating spinal cord compression by loss of posterior subarachnoid space in patients with C1–C2 subluxation.[8] Magnetic resonance imaging (MRI) will be valuable in the future in determining pathologic anatomy in this syndrome.[9]

Neurologic symptoms often have little relationship to the degree of subluxation and may be related to individual variations in diameter of the spinal canal. Symptoms of spinal cord compression that demand intervention include[10]

- A sensation of the head falling forward on flexion of the cervical spine
- Changes in levels of consciousness
- ''Drop'' attacks
- Loss of sphincter control
- Dysphagia, vertigo, convulsions, hemiplegia, dysarthria, or nystagmus
- Peripheral paresthesias without evidence of peripheral nerve disease or compression

Some of these symptoms may be related to compression of the vertebral arteries, which must wind through foramina in the transverse process of C1 and C2, rather than to compression of the spinal cord.

The progression of peripheral joint erosions parallels cervical spine disease in rheumatoid arthritis. The two coincide in severity and timing; development of cervical subluxation is more likely in patients with erosion of the hands and feet.[11] In a series of 113 patients with rheumatoid arthritis referred for hip or knee arthroplasty, 61 percent had roentgenographic evidence of cervical spine instability[12]

Is mortality increased in patients with atlantoaxial subluxation? It has been shown in a 5-year follow-up that neurologic signs do not develop inevitably in patients with large subluxations.[13] However, when signs of cervical cord compression do appear, myelopathy progresses rapidly and 50 per cent of the patients die within 1 year.[14,15] In one series of 104 consecutive autopsies of patients with rheumatoid arthritis, 11 cases of severe dislocation were found.[16] In all 11 cases the odontoid protruded posterosuperiorly and impinged on the medulla within the foramen magnum. In five, spinal cord compression was determined to be the only cause of death. These patients are at risk during even small falls, whiplash injuries, and general anesthesia with intubation. Cervical collars should be prescribed for stability.

Surgery should be considered very carefully and on an individualized basis. Operative stabilization may be considered if symptoms are progressive. In a series of 84 patients with some form of subluxation but without cord or brain stem lesions, one

fourth worsened and one fourth improved without surgery over 5 to 14 years of follow-up.[17] Some data support the hypothesis that early C1–C2 fusion for atlantoaxial subluxation before development of superior migration of the odontoid decreases the risk of further progression of cervical spine instability.[18] However, the incidence of sustained neurologic deterioration related to surgery may be as high as 6 per cent,[19] emphasizing the importance of having a skilled surgical team and a careful assessment of each patient.

Vertical atlantoaxial subluxation is important, and as mentioned earlier, may follow upon anterior-posterior subluxation. It was noted in one study in 13 of 476 (3.7 per cent) hospitalized patients with rheumatoid arthritis.[20] Neurologic findings have included decreased sensation in the distribution of cranial nerve V and sensory loss in the C2 area, nystagmus, and pyramidal lesions. Vertical subluxations are believed to have a worse prognosis than the other varieties.[15]

Bywaters has demonstrated bursal spaces between the cervical interspinous processes in autopsies of patients without joint disease; in rheumatoid patients, bursal proliferation led in several cases to radiographically demonstrated destruction of the spinous processes.[21]

MRI is particularly valuable in assessment of cervical spine disease in rheumatoid arthritis because the spinal cord as well as bone can be visualized.[9] This technology has enabled new diagnoses, including rheumatoid pannus–induced syringomyelia, to be made[22] (see Chapter 21).

Thoracic, Lumbar, and Sacral Spine

These portions of the spine usually are spared in rheumatoid arthritis. The exceptions are the apophyseal joints; rarely, synovial cysts at the apophyseal joint can impinge as an epidural mass on the spinal cord, causing pain and/or neurologic deficits.[23]

Joints of the Head and Neck

Temporomandibular Joints

The temporomandibular joints (TMJs) are commonly involved in rheumatoid arthritis. A careful history reveals that 55 per cent of patients have jaw symptoms at some time during the course of their disease.[24] Radiographic examination reveals structural alterations in 78 per cent of the joints examined. An overbite may develop[25] as the mandibular condyle and the corresponding surface of the temporal bone, the *eminentia articularis*, are eroded. Physical examination of the rheumatoid patient should include palpation for tenderness and auscultation for crepitus. Occasionally patients will have acute pain and an inability to close the mouth, necessitating intra-articular glucocorticoids to suppress the acute process. It is important to remember that TMJ abnormalities are very common in nonrheumatoid populations. The only specific findings for rheumatoid arthritis in the TMJ are erosions and cysts of the mandibular condyle detected by CT or MRI, and there is no correlation between clinical and CT findings of TMJ involvement in rheumatoid arthritis.[26]

Cricoarytenoid Joints

These small diarthrodial joints have an important function; they rotate with the vocal cords as they abduct and adduct to vary pitch and tone of the voice. A careful history may reveal hoarseness in up to 30 per cent of rheumatoid patients.[27] This is not disabling in itself, but there is a danger that the cricoarytenoid joints may become inflamed and immobilized, with the vocal cords adducted to the midline, causing inspiratory stridor.[28] Autopsy examinations have demonstrated cricoarytenoid arthritis in almost half the patients with rheumatoid arthritis, suggesting that much significant disease of the larynx may be asymptomatic.[29] This is borne out by the finding that, although CT scans detected laryngeal abnormalities in 54 per cent of patients with moderately severe rheumatoid arthritis, no symptoms predicted these abnormalities.[30] In contrast, indirect laryngoscopy, which detected mucosal and gross functional abnormalities (including rheumatoid nodules), was abnormal in 32 per cent of the same patients and correlated with symptoms of sore throat and difficult inspiration. It follows that the latter examination should be obtained in symptomatic rheumatoid patients. Asymptomatic cricoarytenoid synovitis may occasionally lead to aspiration of pharyngeal contents, particularly at night.

Ossicles of the Ear

Many rheumatoid patients experience a decrease in hearing. In general, this has been ascribed to salicylate toxicity, and it is believed to be reversible when the drug is discontinued. However, conductive hearing loss in patients not taking salicylates was reported by Copeman.[31] Studies using otoadmittance measurements have been carried out in patients with rheumatoid arthritis in an attempt to determine whether the interossicle joints were involved.[32] The data showed that 38 per cent of ''rheumatoid ears'' and only 8 per cent of controls demonstrated a pattern characteristic of an increase in the flacidity of a clinically normal tympanic membrane. This is consistent with erosions and shortening of the ossicles produced by the erosive synovitis, not with ankylosis.

Sternoclavicular and Manubriosternal Joints

These joints, both possessing synovium and a large cartilaginous disc, are often involved in rheumatoid arthritis.[33] Because of their relative immobility, there are few symptoms; however, patients occasionally complain of pain in sternoclavicular joints while lying on their sides in bed. When symptoms do occur, the physician must be concerned about superimposed sepsis. CT or MRI is useful for careful delineation of the sternoclavicular joint. Manubriosternal involvement is almost never clinically important, although by tomographic criteria it is common in rheumatoid arthritis.[34] Some patients develop manubriosternal joint subluxation.

Joints of the Upper Limb

Shoulder

Rheumatoid arthritis of the shoulder not only affects synovium within the glenohumeral joint but also involves the distal third of the clavicle, various bursae and the rotator cuff, and multiple muscles around the neck and chest wall.

In recent years, it has been appreciated that involvement of the rotator cuff in rheumatoid arthritis is a principal cause of morbidity. The function of the rotator cuff is to stabilize the humeral head in the glenoid. Weakness of the cuff results in superior subluxation. Rotator cuff tears or insufficiency for other reasons can be demonstrated by shoulder arthrogram. In a series of 200 consecutive patients with rheumatoid arthritis studied by arthrography, 21 per cent had rotator cuff tears and an additional 24 per cent had evidence of frayed tendons.[35] One likely mechanism for tears is that the rotator cuff tendon insertion into the greater tuberosity is vulnerable to erosion by the proliferative synovitis that develops there.[36] Previous injury and aging may predispose to the development of tears.[37] Sudden tears may be accompanied by pain and inflammation so great as to suggest sepsis.

Standard radiographic examinations of the shoulder in rheumatoid arthritis reveal erosion (69 per cent) and superior subluxation (31 per cent).[38] Arthrograms, in addition to showing tears of the rotator cuff, can demonstrate (1) diffuse nodular filling defects, (2) irregular capsular attachment, (3) bursal filling defects, (4) adhesive capsulitis, and (5) dilation of the biceps tendon sheath (perhaps unique to rheumatoid arthritis).[39] High-resolution CT or MRI may provide much of this information without invasive techniques. Marked tissue swelling of the anterolateral aspect of the shoulders in rheumatoid arthritis may be caused by chronic subacromial bursitis rather than by glenohumeral joint effusions.[40] In contrast to rotator cuff tears, bursal swelling is not necessarily associated with decreased range of motion or pain. Synovial proliferation within the subdeltoid bursa may explain resorption of the undersurface of the distal clavicle seen in this disease.[41] Rarely, the shoulder joint may rupture, with symptoms resembling those of obstruction of venous return from the arm.[42]

Elbow

Perhaps because it is a stable hinge joint, severe pain in the elbow rarely is manifested early in rheumatoid arthritis. Nevertheless, involvement of the elbow is common and, if lateral stability at the elbow is lost as the disease progresses, disability can be severe.

The frequency of elbow involvement varies from 20 to 65 per cent, depending on the severity of disease in the patient populations studied. One of the earliest findings, often unnoticed by the patient, is loss of full extension. Because the elbow is principally a connecting joint between the hand and trunk, the shoulder and wrists can compensate for the loss of elbow motion.[43] With progressive disease, severe elbow pain may be noted during pronation and sapination the wrist.

Hand and Wrist

The hand and wrist should be considered together because they form a functional unit. There are data, for example, linking disease of the wrist to ulnar deviation of the MCP joints[44,45]; the hypothesis is that weakening of the extensor carpi ulnaris muscle leads to radial deviation of the wrist as the carpal bones rotate (the proximal row in an ulnar direction, the distal ones in a radial direction).[44] Ulnar deviation of the fingers (a "zigzag" deformity) occurs in response to this in order to keep the tendons to the phalanges in a normal line with the radius. Other factors, including the tendency for power grasp to pull the fingers into an ulnar attitude[46] and inappropriate intrinsic muscle action,[47] are involved[48–52] (Figs. 20–1 and 20–2). It is important to note that erosion of bone or articular cartilage is not essential for development of ulnar deviation. Significant although reducible ulnar deviation can result from repeated synovitis or muscle weakness in the hands (e.g., in SLE).

Wrist. Dorsal swelling on the wrist within the tendon sheaths of the extensor muscles is one of the earliest signs of disease. Typically, the extensor carpi ulnaris and extensor digitorum communis sheaths are involved. Rarely, cystic structures resembling ganglia will be early findings of rheumatoid arthritis.[53,54] Rupture of extensor tendons of the ingers is an unfortunate result of tenosynovitis in the wrist.

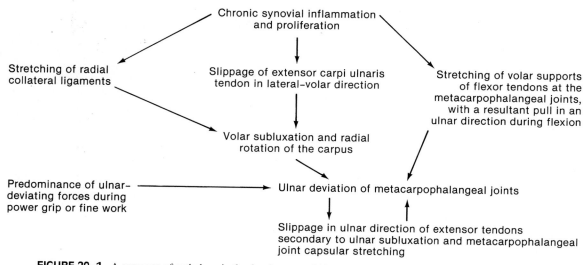

FIGURE 20–1. A sequence of pathology in the development of ulnar deviation at MCP joints. (From Harris, E. D. Jr.: Clinical features of rheumatoid arthritis. *In* Kelley, W. N., Harris, E. D. Jr., Ruddy, S., and Sledge, C. B. [eds.]: Textbook of Rheumatology, 4th ed., Vol. 1. Philadelphia, W. B. Saunders, 1993, pp. 874–911. Used by permission.)

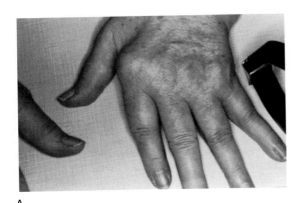

A

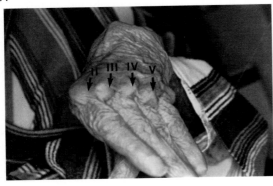

B

FIGURE 20–2. *A*, Early ulnar deviation of the MCP joints without subluxation. Extensor tendons have slipped to the ulnar side. The fifth finger, in particular, is compromised with weak flexion, causing loss of power grip. *B*, Complete subluxation with marked ulnar deviation at the MCP joints of a 90-year-old woman with rheumatoid arthritis. Arrows mark the heads of the metacarpals, now in direct contact with the joint capsule instead of the proximal phalanges. (Courtesy of James L. McGuire, M.D.) (From Harris, E. D. Jr.: Clinical features of rheumatoid arthritis. *In* Kelley, W. N., Harris, E. D. Jr., Ruddy, S., and Sledge, C. B. [eds.]: Textbook of Rheumatology, 4th ed., Vol. 1. Philadelphia, W. B. Saunders, 1993, pp. 874–911. Used by permission.)

As the synovial proliferation develops within the wrist, pressure increases within the relatively non-distensible joint spaces. Proliferative synovium develops enzymatic machinery sufficient to destroy ligaments, tendons, and the articular disc distal to the ulnar head. Pressure and enzymes combine to produce communications among radiocarpal, radioulnar, and midcarpal joints.[47,55] Integrity of the distal radioulnar joint is lost. The ulnar collateral ligament, stretched by the proliferative synovium of the radioulnar joint, finally either ruptures or is destroyed, and the ulnar head springs up into dorsal prominence, where it ''floats'' and can easily be depressed by the examiner's fingers (Fig. 20–3).

On the volar side of the wrist, synovial protrusion cysts develop; they can be palpated, and their origins can be confirmed by arthrography.[56] The thick transverse carpal ligament prevents significant resistance to decompression, however, and the hyperplastic synovium compressing the median nerve can cause carpal tunnel syndrome.

Progression of disease in the wrist is characterized either by loss of joint space and loss of bone or by ankylosis. Disintegration of the carpus has been quantitated as a carpal-to-metacarpal (C:MC) ratio (length of the carpus divided by that of the third metacarpal). There is a linear decrease in the C:MC ratio with progressive disease[57] caused by compaction of bone at the radiolunate, lunate-capitate, and capitate–third metacarpal joints. One study has confirmed the usefulness of the C:MC ratio for quantitating joint destruction and making correlations with anatomic progression over time.[50] Early detection of carpal bone involvement by rheumatoid arthritis is possible using MRI, which can define early synovial proliferation and carpal bone erosions. Bony ankylosis is associated with both duration and severity of disease,[59] and probably is found in joints that have been relatively immobilized by pain, inflammation, treatment, or all of these.

Hand. The hand often has many joints involved in rheumatoid arthritis. A sensitive index of hand involvement is grip strength. The act of squeezing brings stress on all hand joints. Muscular contraction causes ligamentous tightening around joints, compressing inflamed synovium. The immediate result is weakness, with or without pain; the reflex inhibition of muscular contraction as a result

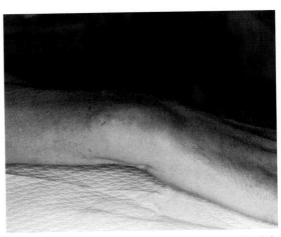

FIGURE 20–3. A 37-year-old woman with rheumatoid arthritis principally involving both wrists. Although she has no fixed deformities, she has bilateral swelling around both ulnar heads, which are easily depressed by an examiner's fingers, implying stretching of ligaments by synovitis.

of pain may be a primary factor in this weakness. Quantitative radiographic scores for joint space narrowing, erosion, and malalignment correlate well with loss of motion but do not correlate with joint count tenderness scores[60]; these data support the concept that inflammatory synovitis and the erosive/destructive potential of proliferative synovitis in rheumatoid arthritis are not one and the same, but rather reflect different aspects of the same disease.

The *swan-neck deformity* is one of flexion of the DIP and MCP joints, with hyperextension of the PIP joint. The lesion probably begins with shortening of the interosseous muscles and tendons. Shortening of the intrinsic muscles exerts tension on the dorsal tendon sheath, leading to hyperextension of the PIP joint.[61] Deep tendon contracture or, rarely, DIP joint involvement with rheumatoid arthritis leads to DIP joint flexion.[62] Rupture of the sublimis tendon, which would reduce capacity to flex the PIP joint, can lead to the same deformity.[63] Marginal erosive changes in the DIP joints occur more often in patients with rheumatoid arthritis who have co-existing osteoarthritis[64] (Fig. 20–4A).

If, during chronic inflammation of a PIP joint, the extensor hood stretches or is avulsed, the PIP joint may pop up into flexion, producing a *boutonnière deformity*[49,63] (Fig. 20–4B, C). The DIP joint remains in hyperextension. Without either of these deformities, limitation of movement develops at the PIP and DIP joints. Limitation of full flexion of the DIP joint is common in rheumatoid arthritis and represents incomplete profundus contraction. Similarly, tight intrinsic muscles may prevent full flexion of PIP joints when the MCP joints are in full extension.

The most serious result of rheumatoid involvement of the hand is *resorptive arthropathy*, defined as severe resorption of bone that begins at the articular cartilage and spreads along the diaphysis of the involved phalanges. Digits appear shortened, excess skin folds are present, and phalanges can be retracted (telescoped) into one another and then pulled out into abnormally long extension, often without pain. Resorptive arthropathy occurs in about 5 per cent of rheumatoid patients,[65] and is associated with longer duration of aggressive synovitis.

Three types of deformity have been described for the *thumb*:[66]

Type I: MCP inflammation leads to stretching of the joint capsule and a boutonnière-like deformity.

Type II: inflammation of the carpometacarpal

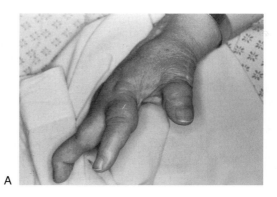

A

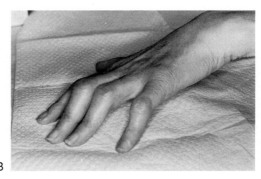

B

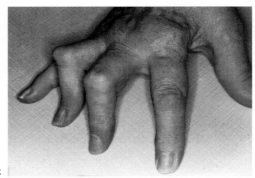

C

FIGURE 20–4. *A,* Hand of a patient with severe and deforming rheumatoid arthritis. The typical swan-neck deformity is seen in the third finger. She has had thumb surgery. She progressed to a classical resorptive arthropathy. *B* and *C,* Early (*B*) and late (*C*) boutonnière deformity of the phalanges in rheumatoid arthritis. In *C,* moderate soft tissue swelling at the second and third MCP joints is visible. (*B* and *C* from Harris, E. D. Jr.: Clinical features of rheumatoid arthritis. *In* Kelley, W. N., Harris, E. D. Jr., Ruddy, S., and Sledge, C. B. [eds.]: Textbook of Rheumatology, 4th ed., Vol. 1. Philadelphia, W. B. Saunders, 1993, pp. 874–911. Used by permission.)

(CMC) joint leads to volar subluxation as a result of contracture of the adductor hallucis.

Type III: after prolonged disease of both the CMC and MCP joints, exaggerated adduction of the first metacarpus, flexion of the MCP joint, and hyperextension of the DIP joint result from the patient's need to provide a means to pinch.

The DIP joints have less synovial membrane than the PIP joints; perhaps because of this and lower intra-articular temperatures protecting them, DIP joints are less often involved in rheumatoid arthritis. However, in one study using DIP joints as a primary focus, radiographic abnormalities (surface erosions and joint space narrowing) were observed in 37 per cent of 62 rheumatoid arthritis patients and only 14 per cent of control. The DIP joint changes were not related to duration or overall severity of the rheumatoid arthritis.[67]

One of the most common manifestations of rheumatoid arthritis in hands is *tenosynovitis* in flexor tendon sheaths; this can be a major cause of hand weakness.[56] (Table 20–1). It is manifested on the volar surfaces of the phalanges as diffuse swelling between joints or a palpable grating within flexor tendon sheaths in the palm, and may occur in up to 55 per cent of patients.[68] Although hand flexor tenosynovitis is not associated with more prolonged or severe disease, there is an association with a number of para-articular manifestations (distinct from extra-articular manifestations).[69] It is particularly important to diagnose *de Quervain's tenosynovitis* because it causes severe discomfort and yet is relatively easily treated; it represents tenosynovitis in the extensors of the thumb. Pain originating from these sheaths can be demonstrated by Finklestein's test demonstrating pain on ulnar flexion at the wrist after the thumb is maximally flexed and adducted.

Not infrequently, rheumatoid nodules will develop within tendon sheaths, and they may "lock" the finger painfully into flexion, necessitating surgical excision or glucocorticoid injections when they become chronic and recurrent.

Joints of the Lower Limb

Hip

The hip is less frequently involved early in rheumatoid arthritis than in juvenile rheumatoid arthritis. Hip joint involvement must be ascertained by a careful clinical examination. Pain on the lateral aspect of the hip is often a manifestation of trochanteric bursitis rather than of synovitis.

About half of the patients with established rheumatoid arthritis will have radiographic evidence of hip disease.[70] The femoral head may collapse and be resorbed, while the acetabulum often remodels as it is pushed medially, leading to protrusio acetabuli. Significant protrusion occurs in about 5 per cent of all patients with rheumatoid arthritis.[71] Loss of internal rotation on physical examination correlates best with radiographic findings. Similar to the situation in other weight-bearing joints, the femoral head may develop cystic lesions. Communication of these lesions with the joint space can often be demonstrated on surgically resected femoral heads.[72]

Knee

In contrast to the hips, synovial inflammation and proliferation are readily demonstrated in the knees. Early in synovitis of the knee, often within 1 week after onset of symptoms, quadriceps atrophy is noticeable and leads to the application of more force than usual through the patella to the femoral surface. Another early manifestation of knee disease in rheumatoid arthritis is loss of full extension, a functional loss that can become a fixed flexion contracture unless corrective measures are undertaken.[73]

Full flexion of the knee markedly increases the intra-articular pressure and may produce an outpouching of posterior components of the joint space creating a popliteal or Baker's cyst. Fluid from the anterior compartments of the knee may enter the popliteal portion but does not readily return.[74] This one-way valve may produce pressures so high in the popliteal space that it may rupture down into the calf or, rarely, superiorly into the posterior thigh. Rupture occurs posteriorly between the medial head of the gastrocnemius and the tendinous insertion of the biceps. Clinically, popliteal cysts and complications of them have several manifestations. The intact popliteal cyst may compress superficial venous flow to the upper part of the leg, producing dilation of superficial veins and/or edema.[75] Rupture of the

---

TABLE 20–1. Factors Diminishing Hand Grasp Strength in Rheumatoid Arthritis

1. Synovitis in joints
2. Reflex inhibition of muscular contraction secondary to pain
3. Altered kinesiology; distorted relation of joint, bones, and tendons during motion
4. Flexor tenosynovitis, with or without rheumatoid nodules on tendons
5. Vascular ischemia leading to pain, from altered sympathetic tone
6. Edema of all structures, from inflammation and perhaps altered lymphatic drainage
7. Intrinsic muscle atrophy and/or fibrosis

Modified from Harris, E. D. Jr.: Clinical features of rheumatoid arthritis. *In* Kelley, W. N., Harris, E. D. Jr., Ruddy, S., and Sledge, C. B. (eds.): Textbook of Rheumatology, 4th ed., Vol. 1. Philadelphia, W. B. Saunders, 1993, pp. 874–911. Used by permission.

TABLE 20–2. Differential Diagnosis of Popliteal Cysts

Lipoma	Hemangioma
Xanthoma	Lymphadenopathy
Fibrosarcoma	Charcot joint
Vascular tumor	Thrombophlebitis
Varicose veins	

From Harris, E. D. Jr.: Clinical features of rheumatoid arthritis. *In* Kelley, W. N., Harris, E. D. Jr., Ruddy, S., and Sledge, C. B. (eds.): Textbook of Rheumatology, 4th ed., Vol. 1. Philadelphia, W. B. Saunders, 1993, pp. 874–911. Used by permission.

joint posteriorly with dissection of joint fluid into the calf may resemble acute thrombophlebitis, with swelling and tenderness as well as systemic signs of fever and leukocytosis.[76,77] (Table 20–2). One helpful sign in identifying joint rupture may be the appearance of a crescentic hematoma beneath one of the malleoli.[78] Although arthrography will clearly define the abnormal anatomy of a Baker's cyst, this invasive procedure has been replaced by ultrasound[79] and, when necessary, MRI.

It has been well documented that high-resolution MRI accurately portrays the gross state of articular cartilage in the knee, including its precise thickness, erosions or thinning, and irregularities.[80]

Ankle and Foot

The ankle rarely is involved in mild or oligoarticular rheumatoid arthritis but often is damaged in severe progressive forms of the disease. Clinical evidence for ankle involvement is a cystic swelling anterior and posterior to the malleoli. Much of the stability of the ankle depends on integrity of ligaments holding the fibula to the tibia and these two bones to the talus. In rheumatoid arthritis, inflammatory and proliferative disease may loosen these connections by stretching and eroding the collagenous ligaments. The result is incongruity, which, once initiated, progresses to pronation deformities and eversion of the foot.

The Achilles tendon is a major structural component and generator of kinetic force in the foot and ankle. Rheumatoid nodules develop in this collagenous structure, and spontaneous rupture of the tendon has been reported when diffuse granulomatous inflammation is present.[81]

The subtalar joint controls eversion and inversion of the foot on the talus; patients with rheumatoid arthritis invariably have more pain while walking on uneven ground, and this is related to the relatively common subtalar joint involvement in rheumatoid arthritis.[82]

More than one third of patients with rheumatoid arthritis have significant disease in the feet.[83] Metatarsophalangeal (MTP) joints are involved early, and gait is altered as pain develops during push-off in striding. It is of interest that downward subluxation of the metatarsal heads occurs soon after the MTP synovitis develop, producing "cock-up" toe deformities of the PIP joints. Hallux valgus and bunion/callus formation appear if disease continues. Cystic collections representing outpouchings of flexor tendon sheaths often develop under the MTP joints.[84] Patients with subluxation of the metatarsal heads to the subcutaneous area may develop pressure necrosis. Alternatively, patients who have subluxation of MTP joints often develop pressure necrosis over the PIP joints that protrude dorsally (hammer toes).

The sequence of changes as disease progresses in the foot is as follows[82,85]:

1. Intermetatarsal joint ligaments stretch.
2. Spread of the forefoot occurs.
3. The fibrofatty cushion on the plantar surface migrates anteriorly.
4. There is subluxation of toes dorsally, and extensor tendons shorten.
5. Subluxation of metatarsal heads to a subcutaneous site on the plantar surface occurs (Fig. 20–5).
6. Development of hallux valgus results in "stacking" of the second and third toes on top of the great toe.

It is important to note that DIP joints of the foot rarely are affected in rheumatoid arthritis. A functional rigid hallux caused by muscle spasm of the great toe intrinsic muscles in an effort to relieve

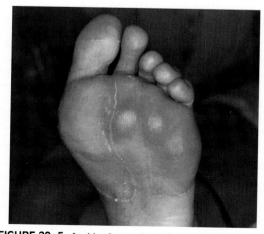

FIGURE 20–5. In this plantar view of a rheumatoid foot, the shiny, thickened calluses over the depressed and subluxed metatarsal heads of the second, fourth, and (to a lesser extent) fifth metatarsal are apparent. The toes are in a "cock-up" deformity. (Courtesy of James L. McGuire, M.D.)

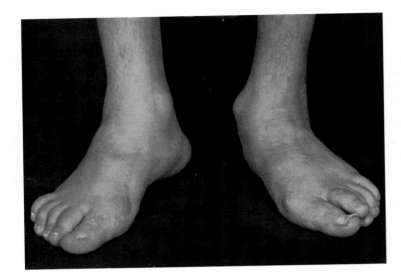

FIGURE 20–6. This patient (a 26-year-old man) had more pain and inflammation in the left foot than in the right. He began to evert his foot, pushing off in a skating motion as he walked. This eventually led to a rocker-bottom foot with a convex rather than concave plantar arch. (From Harris, E. D. Jr.: Clinical features of rheumatoid arthritis. *In* Kelley, W. N., Harris, E. D. Jr., Ruddy, S., and Sledge, C. B. [eds.]: Textbook of Rheumatology, 4th ed., Vol. 1. Philadelphia, W. B. Saunders, 1993, pp. 874–911. Used by permission.)

pressure on the lesser metatarsal heads can be very painful and require surgical intervention.[86]

An alternative abnormality in the foot of rheumatoid patients is the development of progressive eversion associated with tarsal joint inflammation. Weight is borne on the medial aspect and hammer toes do not necessarily develop (Fig. 20–6).

Another cause of foot pain in rheumatoid patients is the tarsal tunnel syndrome. In a group of 30 patients with rheumatoid arthritis, radiographically demonstrated erosions in the feet, and foot pain, 4 (13 per cent) were shown by electrodiagnostic techniques to have slowing of medial and/or lateral plantar nerve latency.[87]

Involvement of the Skeleton Distant from Joints

The skeleton has two anatomically and functionally separate components—cortical and trabecular bone—that respond differently to systemic and local diseases and to drugs. There are three questions about bones that are of great interest to those studying and caring for patients with rheumatoid arthritis:

1. Does rheumatoid arthritis produce a generalized osteopenia?

2. What are the influences of sex and age on the skeleton in patients with rheumatoid arthritis?

3. What are the effects of low-dose glucocorticoids on bone in rheumatoid arthritis and, if deleterious, can they be prevented or treated?

The available data on these topics are reviewed in Chapter 30.

The diffuse loss of bone in rheumatoid arthritis, whether or not it is related to glucocorticoid therapy, leads to the high incidence of stress fractures of long bones in rheumatoid arthritis.[88,89] The fibula is the most common fracture site. Acute leg pain in the thin, elderly rheumatoid patient, even without a history of trauma, should generate suspicion of a stress fracture. Geodes (i.e., subchondral cysts developed by synovial penetration of the cortex or subchondral plate and subsequent proliferation) produce weak bone and can predispose to fracture, even in phalanges.[90]

Muscle Involvement

Clinical weakness is common in rheumatoid arthritis, but is it caused by muscle involvement in the rheumatoid inflammation or is it a reflex weakness response to pain? Most rheumatoid patients have muscle weakness but few have muscle tenderness. An exception to this is the occasional patient with a severe flare of active disease; such a patient may cry out in severe pain, unable to move either muscles or joints. These symptoms resemble those of vascular insufficiency (ischemic pain) in their intensity.

In an autopsy series, focal accumulations of lymphocytes and plasma cells with some contiguous degeneration of muscle fibers were found in all rheumatoid patients and named *nodular myositis.*[91] More recent studies have pointed to at least five different types of muscle disease in rheumatoid arthritis[92,93]:

Type I: diminution of muscle bulk with atrophy of type II fibers

Type II: peripheral neuromyopathy, usually caused by mononeuritis multiplex

Type III: steroid myopathy

Type IV: active myositis and muscle necrosis with foci of endomysial mononuclear cell infiltration

Type V: chronic myopathy resembling a dystrophic process, probably the end stage of inflammatory myositis

Active myositis and focal necrosis are not uncommonly noted on biopsy specimens of patients with active disease, particularly in an interesting subset with mild synovitis and a disproportionately high ESR.[93] To emphasize the systemic nature of rheumatoid arthritis, in some patients the lymphocytes in biopsied muscle have been shown to synthesize IgM rheumatic factor. Thus the ''nodules of myositis'' contain plasma cells as well as lymphocytes. Unlike polymyositis/dermatomyositis, myositis in rheumatoid arthritis is patchy, and the weakness experienced by these patients responds readily to low-dose prednisone.

Involvement of the Skin

The most frequently recognized skin lesion found in rheumatoid arthritis is the rheumatoid nodule (see later), but there are several other manifestations as well. Perhaps related to the underlying synovitis, skin—particularly over the hands and fingers—becomes thin and atrophic. Palmar erythema is common, but Raynaud's syndrome is rarely found. Manifestations of vasculitis can range from occasional nail-fold infarcts to a deep, erosive, scarring pyoderma gangrenosa. Palpable purpura in rheumatoid patients often is related to a reaction to one or another drug that the patient is taking, but can be primary and correlated with the severity of articular disease.[94]

Involvement of the Eye

Virtually all ocular manifestations of rheumatoid arthritis can be considered complications of the disease. **Keratoconjunctivitis sicca** is a component of Sjögren's syndrome, and is discussed later in the section on that entity. More of a direct extension of the rheumatoid process seen in the synovium and within rheumatoid nodules are **scleritis** and **episcleritis**. The highly differentiated connective tissues in the eye make rheumatoid manifestations particularly interesting and, when they occur as aggressive forms, very serious.[95]

The episclera of the eye is highly vascular in comparison with the dense, relatively avascular sclera. Either scleritis or episcleritis or both occur in less than 1 per cent of rheumatoid patients.[96] In episcleritis, the eye becomes red quickly. Unlike conjunctivitis, there is no discharge other than tearing in response to the gritty discomfort. Loss of vision as a direct result of the episcleritis does not occur, but a keratitis or cataract developing secondarily can cause visual loss. Scleritis causes severe ocular pain, and a dark red discoloration, no discharge is present. Depending on the intensity of the process, scleritis can be localized and superficial or generalized, with or without granulomatous resorption of the sclera down to the uveal layer. This latter complication is known as **scleromalacia perforans**.

EXTRA-ARTICULAR COMPLICATIONS OF RHEUMATOID ARTHRITIS

The complications of rheumatoid arthritis may be fatal. In general, the number and severity of extra-articular features vary with the duration and severity[97,98] of the disease. A number of these may be related to extra-articular foci of an immune response,[99] with evidence for independent and qualitatively different production of rheumatoid factor in the pleural space, pericardium, muscle, and even meninges. These patients with ''spillover'' immune responses have true rheumatoid disease, not just rheumatoid arthritis.

Rheumatoid Nodules

The pathologic findings in rheumatoid nodules are well documented[100,101] and have been reviewed in Chapter 9. In the well-formed nodule, there is a central area of necrosis rimmed by a corona of palisading fibroblasts that is surrounded by a collagenous capsule with perivascular collections of chronic inflammatory cells. The earliest nodules, a nest of granulation tissue, have been identified at a size less than 4 mm (for review, see ref. 102). The nodules grow by accumulating cells that expand centrifugally, leaving behind central necrosis initiated by vasculopathy and contributed to by protease destruction of the connective tissue matrix.

Occurring in 20 to 35 per cent of patients with definite or classical rheumatoid arthritis, nodules are found most easily on extensor surfaces such as the olecranon process and the proximal ulna. They are subcutaneous and vary in consistency from a soft, amorphous, entirely mobile mass to hard, rubbery masses attached firmly to the periosteum.

Rheumatoid factor is almost always found in the serum of patients with rheumatoid nodules. Rarely, such nodules are present without obvious arthritis.[103] Multiple nodules on the hands and a positive test for rheumatoid factor associated with episodes of acute intermittent synovitis and subchondral cystic lesions of small bones of the hands and feet has been called *rheumatoid nodulosis*.[104,105] Aggressive therapy with second-line drugs helped induce complete resolution of all nodules in one patient.[106] Rheumatoid nodules may grow in patients treated with methotrexate even as disease activity subsides.

The *differential diagnosis* of rheumatoid nodules includes the following:

- *"Benign" nodules:* These usually are found in healthy children without rheumatoid factor or arthritis. They are nontender; appear often on the pretibial regions, feet, and scalp; increase rapidly in size; and are histologically identical to rheumatoid nodules.[107] They usually resolve spontaneously, although in one case classical rheumatoid arthritis developed 50 years after the first appearance of "benign" olecranon nodules.[108]

- *Granuloma annulare:* These nodules are intracutaneous but histologically identical to rheumatoid nodules. They slowly resolve and are not associated with other disease.[109]

- *Xanthomatosis:* These nodules usually have a yellow tinge, and patients have abnormally high plasma lipoprotein and cholesterol levels. There is no underlying bone involvement.[110]

- *Tophi:* These collections of monosodium urate crystals in patients with gout are associated with small, punched-out bone lesions and are rarely found in patients with a normal serum urate concentration. A search for crystals with a polarizing microscope will reveal the classical needle-shaped, negatively birefringent crystals.

- *Miscellaneous nodules:* The nodules of multicentric reticulohistiocytosis have been described earlier. Numerous proliferative disorders affecting cutaneous tissue, including erythema elevatum diutinum, acrodermatitis chronica atrophicans, bejel, yaws, pinta, and leprosy, can resemble rheumatoid nodules. A rheumatoid nodule, particularly when it occurs on the face, may simulate basal cell carcinoma.[111]

Appearance of nodules in unusual sites may lead to confusion in diagnosis. Sacral nodules may be mistaken for bedsores if the overlying skin breaks down.[112] Occipital nodules also occur in bedridden patients. In the larynx, rheumatoid nodules on the vocal cords may cause progressive hoarseness.[113] Nodules found in the heart and lungs are discussed later. Nodules on the sclera can produce perforation

of this collagenous tissue (Fig. 20–7). There have been at least 14 reports of rheumatoid nodule formation within the central nervous system (reviewed in ref. 114), involving leptomeninges more than parenchyma. Occasional patients develop rheumatoid nodules within vertebral bodies, resulting in bone destruction and signs of myelopathy.[115]

Fistula Development

Cutaneous sinuses near joints develop rarely in seropositive patients with longstanding disease and positive tests for rheumatoid factor.[116] These fistulas can be either sterile or septic and connect the skin surface with a joint, with a para-articular cyst in bone or soft tissues,[117] or with a bursa.[118] The pathogenesis of fistulas without a septic origin is particularly difficult to understand because the rheumatoid process usually is so clearly centripetal in nature (i.e., progressing toward the center of the joint).

Infection

Neither before nor after onset of joint disease has a higher frequency of genitourinary or bronchopulmonary infections been reported in rheumatoid patients compared with osteoarthritic patients.[119] Thus, the increased mortality in rheumatoid arthritis from infection appears related to factors that evolve during the course (and treatment) of the disease and not to any predisposition to infection. The incidence of infections as a complication of rheumatoid arthritis has paralleled the use of glucocorticoids and immunosuppressive agents.[120] Pulmonary infections, skin sepsis, and pyarthrosis are most common.[121,122] In addition to the presence of drugs that suppress host resistance, the phagocytic capacity of leukocytes in rheumatoid arthritis may be less than normal.[123] Difficulty in diagnosis is accentuated by the similarity of aggressive rheumatoid arthritis to infection, particularly in joints; a "pseudoseptic" arthritis in rheumatoid patients, associated with fever, chills, and grossly purulent synovial fluid, can be part of a severe exacerbation of rheumatoid arthritis and clearly must be distinguished from infection.[124]

Cancer

It is very difficult to tease out the influence of rheumatoid arthritis associations with malignancy when there are such strong oncogenic influences from the immunosuppressive treatments used in the disease, each of which can be shown to lead to neoplasms of the immune system. Indeed, there is

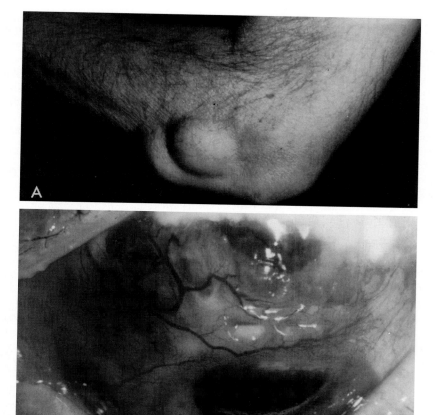

FIGURE 20–7. Manifestations of increased reactivity of mesenchymal tissue in rheumatoid arthritis appearing (*A*) as nodules on the elbow and (*B*) within the sclera of the eye. The eye lesion represents scleral perforation associated with a granulomatous scleral reaction. Treatment was placement of a scleral patch graft. Note the increase in vascularity of the sclera. The dark areas represent scleral thinning with exposure of uveal pigment. (Eye patient of Drs. S. Arthur Bouchoff and G. N. Fouhls; photograph courtesy of Marty Schener.) (From Harris, E. D. Jr.: Clinical features of rheumatoid arthritis. *In* Kelley, W. N., Harris, E. D. Jr., Ruddy, S., and Sledge, C. B. [eds.]: Textbook of Rheumatology, 4th ed., Vol. 1. Philadelphia, W. B. Saunders, 1993, pp. 874–911. Used by permission.)

justified debate about whether to think of cancer occurring in rheumatoid patients as a complication or an association. With these reservations in mind, there appears to be an increased risk for malignancy occurring in all rheumatoid arthritis patients, with marked increased risk in certain subsets of patients.[125] The exception to this is cancer of the gastrointestinal tract, for which there appears to be a reduced risk for patients with rheumatoid arthritis.[126] Is it possible that NSAIDs lower the risk of cancer of the gastrointestinal tract? Evidence that these drugs can diminish numbers and occurrences of colonic polyps gives this some credence.

There is a relative risk of Hodgkin's disease, non-Hodgkin's lymphoma, and leukemia in rheumatoid arthritis of 2 to 3; this is independent of immunosuppressive therapy.[127,128] Of the lymphomas arising in rheumatoid arthritis, about half are low grade and the remainder high grade; most of these are B-cell lymphomas, although there is no evidence that these originated from clonally proliferated lymphocytes associated with rheumatoid arthritis. In contrast, although the relative risk for total cancer in patients with Felty's syndrome is only 2, the relative risk for non-Hodgkin's lymphoma is near 13,[129] similar to that associated with Sjögren's syndrome.[130]

Hematologic Abnormalities

The majority of patients with rheumatoid arthritis have a mild normocytic hypochromic anemia that correlates with the ESR elevation and with activity of the disease.[131,132] Anemia is often of mixed causes in rheumatoid arthritis. One deficiency may mask evidence for others, resulting in ineffective therapy. In a European series[133] of 25 patients, iron deficiency (assessed by bone marrow iron content) was present in 52 per cent, vitamin B_{12} deficiency in 29 per cent, and folate deficiency in 21 per cent. All patients with rheumatoid arthritis are likely to have anemia of chronic disease. The following guidelines may be helpful in sorting out anemia in the rheumatoid patient:

- Anemia of chronic disease has significantly higher serum ferritin concentration than does iron-deficiency anemia.
- Folate and B_{12} deficiency may mask iron deficiency by increasing the mean cell volume and mean cell hemoglobin of erythrocytes.
- The ESR correlates inversely with hemoglobin in rheumatoid arthritis, as expected in anemia of chronic disease.[134]
- Erythropoietin levels are elevated more in patients with iron-deficiency anemia than in those with the anemia of chronic disease; rheumatoid patients also have a diminished response to erythropoietin.[133]

In patients with the anemia of chronic disease, total erythroid heme turnover is slightly reduced, and ineffective erythropoiesis accounts for a much greater than normal percentage of total heme turnover.[135–137] The pathogenesis of impaired hemoglobin synthesis in these patients may be related in part to a significantly low δ-aminolevulinic acid synthase deficiency compared with controls.[138] These patients also may demonstrate a diminished ability to absorb iron through the gastrointestinal tract, usually related to the irritative presence of one or another anti-inflammatory medication.[139] The ineffective erythropoiesis will return to normal if remission can be induced in rheumatoid arthritis.[140] Red blood cell aplasia, immunologically mediated, is a rare finding in rheumatoid arthritis. However, because erythropoiesis in animals has been shown to be dependent on T lymphocytes, it is logical to search for immunologic factors that can induce anemia in rheumatoid arthritis. Serum from rheumatoid arthritis patients profoundly suppresses erythroid colony formation,[141] but T lymphocytes from bone marrow of rheumatoid patients have not been shown to inhibit erythroid development in vitro as do T cells from certain patients with aplastic anemia or pure red blood cell aplasia.[142]

Eosinophilia and *thrombocytosis* are often associated with rheumatoid arthritis. Eosinophilia (eosinophils ≥ 5 per cent of total WBCs) was observed in 40 per cent of patients with severe seropositive disease.[143] Similarly, there is a significant relationship between thrombocytosis and extra-articular manifestations of rheumatoid disease[144] and disease activity.[145]

Large Granular Lymphocyte Syndrome

There is an interesting subset of patients with rheumatoid arthritis who have increased numbers of large granular lymphocytes (LGLs) in the peripheral blood, bone marrow, and liver. The lymphocytes contain many azurophilic granules in the cytoplasm and may account for more than 90 per cent of mononuclear cells in blood. They are increased in certain viral infections. The cells are E rosette positive, are Fc receptor positive, do not produce IL-2, respond poorly to mitogens, and have either antibody-dependent cell-mediated cytotoxic activity (expressing CD3, CD8, and CD57) or are NK cells (expressing CD16 and CD56).[146,147] Of previously described patients with LGL proliferation, almost one third have had rheumatoid arthritis.[148] Because the LGL syndrome in patients with rheumatoid arthritis has the same HLA-DR4 association seen in Felty's syndrome, the proposal has been made that both Felty's and the LGL syndrome represent different variants of a broader syndrome comprising rheumatoid arthritis, neutropenia, LGL expansions, HLA-DR4 positivity, and variable splenomegaly (see later section on Felty's syndrome).[146]

Vasculitis

In one sense, it is redundant to think of vasculitis as a complication of rheumatoid arthritis, because the initial pathologic change in rheumatoid arthritis is believed to rest in small blood vessels. However, it is useful to use the term "vasculitis" to group those extra-articular complications related not to proliferative granulomas but rather to inflammatory vascular disease. Clinical vasculitis usually takes one of the following forms:

- Distal arteritis (ranging from splinter hemorrhages to gangrene)
- Cutaneous ulceration (including pyoderma gangrenosum)
- Peripheral neuropathy
- Pericarditis

- Arteritis of viscera, including heart, lungs, bowel, kidney, liver, spleen, pancreas, lymph nodes, and testis
- Palpable purpura

The pathologic findings in rheumatoid vasculitis are those of a panarteritis. All layers of the vessel wall are infiltrated with mononuclear cells. Fibrinoid necrosis is seen in active lesions. Intimal proliferation may predispose to thrombosis. Obliterative endarteritis of the finger is one of the most frequent manifestations of vasculitis, and immune complex deposits have been demonstrated in those vessels.[149,150] When larger vessels are involved, the pathologic changes resemble those of polyarteritis nodosa.[151] In addition, a venulitis associated with rheumatoid arthritis has been described.[152,153] In patients with hypocomplementemia, the cellular infiltrate around the vessels contains neutrophils; in normocomplementemic patients, lymphocytes predominate. Uninvolved skin from rheumatoid patients is positive for immunoglobulin and complement when sections for histpathology are stained with fluorescein-labeled antibodies. The presence of IgG correlates directly with circulating immune complexes, vasculitic skin lesions, subcutaneous nodules, and a high titer of rheumatoid factor.[154]

Biopsy of skin or muscle reveals changes ranging from mild (perivascular infiltration with inflammatory cells) to more severe (fibrinoid necrosis with immunoglobulin deposits in the vessel walls, and infarctions within the distal vascular beds) abnormalities. Labial salivary gland biopsy, used for many years for diagnosis and classification of Sjögren's syndrome, is also a good technique for finding immunopathologic and histologic evidence for rheumatoid vasculitis, especially when skin lesions are absent.[155]

It is unusual for vasculitis to be active in any but the sickest patients, those with severe deforming arthritis and high titers of rheumatoid factor; this subgroup represents fewer than 1 per cent of patients with rheumatoid arthritis. Although rheumatoid arthritis is more common in women than in men, vasculitis is more often seen in men with rheumatoid arthritis. Evidence supporting the hypothesis that vascular injury is mediated by deposition of circulating immune complexes includes (1) depressed levels of C2 and C4[156]; (2) hypercatabolism of C3[157]; (3) deposition of IgG, IgM, and C3 in involved arteries[158]; and (4) the presence of large amounts of cryoimmunoglobulin in serum of patients with vasculitis.[159]

Neurovascular disease may be the only manifestation of vasculitis. The two common clinical patterns are a mild distal sensory neuropathy and a severe sensorimotor neuropathy (mononeuritis multiplex).[160] The latter form is characterized by severe arterial damage on nerve biopsy specimens. Symptoms of the milder form may be paresthesias or "burning feet" in association with decreased touch and pin sensation distally. Patients with mononeuritis multiplex have weakness (e.g., footdrop) in addition to sensory abnormalities. Symptoms and signs are identical to those found in polyarteritis. Rheumatoid pachymeningitis is a rare complication of rheumatoid arthritis; confined to the dura and pia mater, this process may be limited to certain areas (e.g., lumbar cord and/or cisternae).[161] Elevated levels of IgG (including IgM and IgG rheumatoid factors and low-molecular-weight IgM) and immune complexes are found in the cerebrospinal fluid. Although there is a possible negative association between psychosis and rheumatoid arthritis, organic brain syndromes may be related to rheumatoid arthritis in patients not taking glucocorticoids or indomethacin,[162] and it is presumed that these manifestations are caused by small-vessel disease. In addition, there appears to be a real entity of autonomic nervous system disease in rheumatoid arthritis that is isolated from other peripheral or central nervous system damage.[163]

Visceral lesions occur generally as claudication or infarction of the organ supplied by the involved arteries. Intestinal involvement with vasculitis presents as abdominal pain, at first intermittent, progressing often to continuous pain and a tender, quiet belly on examination. If infarction develops, resection must be accomplished promptly.[164]

The presence of gangrene of digits and extremities, the development of intestinal lesions with bleeding or perforation, cardiac or renal involvement, and mononeuritis multiplex indicates extensive vasculitis and is associated with a poor prognosis.[165,166]

Renal Disease

The kidney is an organ that is rarely involved directly in rheumatoid arthritis but often is compromised indirectly. Amyloidosis is a complication of chronic rheumatoid arthritis and particularly of Still's disease. Another indirect cause of renal disease is toxicity from therapy. Phenacetin abuse causes renal papillary necrosis, and salicylates and other NSAIDs cause abnormalities as well[167] (see Chapter 29). A membranous nephropathy is the pathologic lesion related to therapy with gold salts and D-penicillamine. Rarely, a focal necrotizing glomerulitis is seen in patients dying from rheumatoid arthritis and disseminated vasculitis.[168] The major reason that cyclosporin is not used as much as physicians would prefer in rheumatoid arthritis is its depressive effect upon glomerular filtration (see Chapter 33).

Pulmonary Disease

There are at least six forms of lung disease in rheumatoid arthritis: pleural disease, interstitial fibrosis, nodular lung disease, bronchiolitis, arteritis with pulmonary hypertension, and "airways" disease.

Pleural Disease

Pleural inflammation is found in approximately 70 per cent of rheumatoid patients at the time of autopsy, but clinical disease during life is seen less frequently.[169] In about 20 per cent of patients it develops concurrent with onset of the arthritis, and, in some, pleurisy precedes arthritis. Male sex, positive tests for rheumatoid factor, and subcutaneous nodules or other extra-articular disease are risk factors.

Pleuritic pain is not usually major, perhaps because effusions can be large, sometimes enough to cause dyspnea. Pleurisy and effusions more commonly affect the left hemithorax. Characteristics of the exudative rheumatoid effusions are as follows: glucose, 10 to 50 mg/dl; protein, greater than 4 g/dl; mononuclear cells, 100 to 3,500/mm^3; lactic dehydrogenase, elevated; and CH_{50}, depressed. The low glucose concentrations are of interest. Sepsis (particularly tuberculosis) is the only other condition that commonly has such a low pleural fluid glucose level. An impaired transport of glucose into the pleural space—an "entrance block"—appears to be the cause.[170]

Interstitial Fibrosis

The increased reactivity of mesenchymal cells in rheumatoid arthritis is believed to be the cause of pulmonary fibrosis in this disease. Similar to findings in scleroderma, auscultation reveals fine, diffuse, dry rales. Radiographs show a diffuse reticular (interstitial) or reticulonodular pattern in both lung fields[171,172]; these can progress to a honeycomb appearance on plain radiographs and a characteristic lattice net shown on high-resolution CT. The pathologic findings are those of diffuse fibrosis in the midst of a mononuclear cell infiltrate.[171] The principal functional defect is impairment of alveolocapillary gas exchange with decreased diffusion capacity, best measured utilizing single-breath carbon monoxide diffusion capacities.[173,174] It is likely that rheumatoid arthritis patients who smoke are at a

higher risk for fibrotic complications in the lungs than are those in the general population. However, never-smoking rheumatoid patients have a significant prevalence of basal bronchiectasis as diagnosed by high-resolution CT.[175] It has been reported that bronchoalveolar lavage may reveal increased numbers of lymphocytes, even in patients with only mildly abnormal chest radiographs and normal pulmonary function test results.[176]

Nodular Lung Disease

Pulmonary nodules may appear singly or in clusters that coalesce. Single ones appear as a coin lesion and, when significant peripheral arthritis and nodules are present, can be diagnosed by needle biopsy without thoracotomy. Caplan's syndrome,[177] in which pneumoconiosis and rheumatoid arthritis are synergistic and produce a violent fibroblastic reaction with obliterative granulomatous fibrosis, is a rare occurrence because the respiratory environment in mining operations has improved. Nodules may cavitate and create a bronchopleural fistula[178] and may precede arthritis.[179] In several cases, solitary pulmonary nodules in rheumatoid arthritis patients have proved to be both a rheumatoid nodule and a coexistent bronchogenic carcinoma,[180] a finding that suggests caution in interpreting "benign" results from fine-needle aspiration biopsy in such patients.

Bronchiolitis

A rare finding is an interstitial pneumonitis that progresses to alveolar involvement and bronchiolitis; respiratory insufficiency, and death. Pathologic studies show a cellular loose fibrosis and proteinaceous exudate in bronchioles and alveoli; interstitial infiltrations of lymphocytes attest to the immunogenic aspects of the disease. It must be emphasized that this pathology is separate from the obliterative pneumonitis seen with opportunistic infections from immunosuppressive therapy.

Arteritis

Pulmonary hypertension from arteritis of the pulmonary vasculature is rare and is occasionally associated with digital arteritis.[181] One patient with pleuritis, interstitial lymphocytic infiltrate, pulmonary arterial hypertension, and venous sclerosis has been described.[182]

Airways Disease

Defined by a reduced maximal midexpiratory flow rate and maximal expiratory flow rate at 50 per cent of functional vital capacity, small airways disease was observed in 50 per cent of 30 rheumatoid arthritis patients, compared with 22 per cent of a control population.[183] The study was adjusted for pulmonary infections, α_1-antitrypsin deficiency, penicillamine treatment, environmental pollution, and smoking. Other investigations have not found small airways dysfunction in rheumatoid arthritis and have suggested that, if it is present, it probably is related to factors other than rheumatoid arthritis.[184] If real, this phenomenon may be part of a generalized exocrinopathic process in the disease, expressed most flagrantly, of course, in Sjögren's syndrome.

Cardiac Complications

Cardiac disease in rheumatoid arthritis can take many forms related to granulomatous proliferation or vasculitis. Advances in echocardiography have made diagnosis of pericarditis and endocardial inflammation easier and more specific.[185] Myocardial biopsy through vascular catheters has facilitated diagnosis and classification of myocarditis.

Pericarditis

Infrequently diagnosed by history and physical examination in rheumatoid arthritis, pericarditis is present in up to 50 per cent of patients at autopsy.[186,187] In one study, 31 per cent of ambulatory patients with rheumatoid arthritis had echocardiographic evidence of pericardial effusion. The same study revealed only rare evidence of impaired left ventricular function in prospectively studied outpatients.[188] Although unusual, cardiac tamponade with constrictive pericarditis develops in rheumatoid arthritis and may require pericardectomy.[189,190] Most patients have a positive test for rheumatoid factor, and half will have nodules.

Myocarditis

Myocarditis can take the form of either granulomatous disease or interstitial myocarditis. The granulomatous process resembles subcutaneous nodules and could be considered specific for the disease. Diffuse infiltration of the myocardium by mononuclear cells, in contrast, may involve the entire myocardium and yet have no clinical manifestations.[190]

Endocardial Inflammation

Echocardiographic studies have reported evidence of previously unrecognized mitral valve disease diagnosed by a reduced E-to-F slope of the anterior leaflet of the mitral valve.[191,192] Although aortic valve disease and arthritis are generally associated through ankylosing spondylitis, a number of granulomatous nodules in the valve have been reported.[193]

Conduction Defects

Atrioventricular block is unusual in rheumatoid arthritis but is probably related to direct granulomatous involvement. Pathologic examination may reveal proliferative lesions[194,195] or healed scars.[196] Complete heart block has been described in more than 30 patients with rheumatoid arthritis. It generally occurs in patients with established erosive nodular disease.[196] It usually is permanent and is caused by rheumatoid granulomas in or near the atrioventricular node or bundle of His. Rarely, amyloidosis is responsible for heart block.

Coronary Arteritis

Patients with severe rheumatoid arthritis and active vasculitis who develop a myocardial infarction are likely to have coronary arteritis as a basis for the process.[197]

Granulomatous Aortitis/Valvular Disease

In severe rheumatoid heart disease, granulomatous disease can spread to involve even the base of the aorta.[198] Occasionally, granulomatous disease associated with rheumatoid arthritis necessitates urgent valve replacement for aortic incompetence.[199]

FELTY'S SYNDROME AND SJÖGREN'S SYNDROME

Felty's and Sjögren's syndromes are relatively unusual complications of rheumatoid arthritis. Both can readily become the dominant problem in individual patients. Sjögren's syndrome develops independently of rheumatoid arthritis, sometimes in association with other immune-based diseases such as SLE, and sometimes as a primary process with no recognized associated illness. Both syndromes involve special disorders of the immune system.

Felty's Syndrome

Patients with Felty's syndrome have seropositive rheumatoid arthritis and neutropenia.[200,201] In most patients the arthritis is moderate to severe, and many have an associated anemia or thrombocytopenia. Splenomegaly is usually present, although not a constant feature. Felty's syndrome is uncommon, found in no more than 1 per cent of all rheumatoid patients. In most patients, it is of concern primarily to their physicians, who are understandably concerned about the low neutrophil counts. In occasional patients, however, the neutropenia is associated directly with recurrent and occasionally life-threatening infections.

Clinical Features

Two thirds of these patients are women, and most are older than 50 years of age. Only one third will have inactive synovitis, and most of these have had previously active arthritis and continue to have an elevated Westergren sedimentation rate, often greater than 85 mm/hr.[202] The spleen size is variable, ranging from massive splenomegaly in a few patients to normal size in up to 10 per cent of patients. Associated symptoms and signs indicative of active and extra-articular rheumatoid disease, usually with vasculitis as a basis, are shown in Table 20–3.[200]

Infections, often concurrent with development of mouth ulcers secondary to microhemophilic streptococcal infections, generally do not correlate well with neutropenia until the granulocytes dip below 500/mm[3]. *Staphylococcus aureus* and streptococcal species are the most common organisms causing skin and respiratory tract infections, although, consonant with changing patterns of infections in chronic diseases, gram-negative infections are becoming more prominent.[202]

An unusual feature is nodular regenerative hyperplasia in the liver,[203] which, although it does not histologically resemble cirrhosis, can lead to

TABLE 20–3. Frequency of Extra-articular Manifestations in Felty's Syndrome*

Rheumatoid nodules	76%
Weight loss	68%
Sjögren's syndrome[†]	56%
Lymphadenopathy	34%
Leg ulcers	25%
Pleuritis	19%
Skin pigmentation	17%
Neuropathy	17%
Episcleritis	8%

From Pinals, R. S.: Felty's syndrome. *In* Kelley, W. A., Harris, E. D. Jr., Ruddy, S., and Sledge, C. B. (eds.): Textbook of Rheumatology, 4th ed., Vol. 1. Philadelphia, W. B. Saunders, 1993, pp. 924–930. Used by permission.

* From a review of 10 reports since 1962.
† Determined by positive Schirmer's test.

obliteration of portal venules, portal hypertension, and esophageal variceal bleeding.

The examination of bone marrow in these patients generally shows a myeloid hyperplasia with a relative excess of immature forms consistent with a maturation arrest. In addition to the anemia of chronic disease that most rheumatoid arthritis patients have, Felty's syndrome patients often have a decreased red blood cell survival related to splenic sequestration. The thrombocytopenia rarely is severe enough to cause bleeding into the skin, mucosal surfaces, or other organs.

As an indication of immune abnormalities, 98 per cent of Felty's syndrome patients have a positive test for rheumatoid factor, and tests for ANA are positive in two thirds of the patients, usually directed against DNA/histone complexes.[204] Serum immunoglobulin levels are elevated. Anti-neutrophil cytoplasmic antibodies directed against lactoferrin are positive in more than 75 per cent of patients.[205]

Although the diagnosis is an easy one to suspect when the classical signs are present in an active rheumatoid patient, it is very important to rule out infection with organisms such as tuberculosis, and lymphoproliferative malignancies.

One clinical association with rheumatoid arthritis that can resemble Felty's syndrome is the LGL syndrome or "pseudo-Felty's syndrome."[201] These patients have an abnormal proliferation of LGLs, a neutropenia, splenomegaly, and susceptibility to infection. The syndrome often is associated with a chronic polyarticular arthritis and a high prevalence of HLA-DR4. These LGLs are probably cytotoxic T cells or NK cells. A comparison between Felty's syndrome and the LGL syndrome with rheumatoid arthritis is shown in Table 20–4. In rheumatoid patients with neutropenia, one third are likely to have the LGL syndrome and the remainder will have true Felty's syndrome.[206] The distinction between the LGL syndrome and Felty's syndrome may be blurring, however, as these cells become recognized as a marker for a broader definition of Felty's syndrome.[146] Specific therapy of LGL syndrome, other than that for the arthritis, is rarely needed. Splenectomy in these patients may be less often corrective of neutropenia than in "true" Felty's syndrome. The coexistence of Felty's syndrome and palindromic rheumatism, rather than rheumatoid arthritis, has been described.[207]

Pathogenesis

The most logical explanation for the neutropenia—splenic sequestration—is not the whole story. Patients who have splenectomy improve tran-

TABLE 20–4. Comparison of Felty's Syndrome and LGL Syndrome with Rheumatoid Arthritis (Pseudo-Felty's Syndrome)

	FELTY'S SYNDROME	LGL SYNDROME
Duration of neutropenia (yr)	10–15	0–3
Extra-articular manifestations	Common	Rare
Erosive disease	Common	Rare
Recurrent infections	Common	Common
Splenomegaly	Common	Common
Progression to leukemia	Rare	3%–14%
Spontaneous remission	0%–22%	0%–14%
Total WBC	Low	Normal/elevated
Lymphocytosis	Absent	Present
CD3+, CD16+, CD57+ cells	Absent	Present
CD4:CD8 ratio	Normal	Low
TCR gene abnormalities	Absent	Present
RF*	+ + +	+ + +
ANA	+ +	+ +
Neutrophil-associated Ig	+ +	+ +
Bone marrow histology	Normal or reactive	LGL infiltration
Response to splenectomy	Improvement	Exacerbation

From Rosenstein, E. D., and Kramer, N.: Felty's and pseudo-Felty's syndromes. Semin. Arthritis Rheum. 21:129, 1991. Used by permission.

* Rheumatoid factor.

siently, but in many the neutrophil count begins to drop again, sometimes reaching nadirs lower than those before surgery. The best data suggest that Felty's syndrome is multifactorial in its genesis. In any given patient, one or all of the following mechanisms may be active:

- Development of granulocyte-specific antibodies that bind neutrophils, resulting in their sequestration and destruction by the spleen.[208]
- Splenic production of a humoral inhibitor of granulocyte production.
- Phagocytosis of immune complexes by neutrophils and their subsequent removal from the circulation in an enlarged spleen.
- Margination of neutrophils by adherence to activated endothelial cells.
- Decreased stimuli for granulocyte colony-forming units in the bone marrow.

It is very likely that each, some, or all of these mechanisms may be involved in different patients, and that the same syndrome may result from multiple mechanisms.[209,210]

Management

The rheumatoid arthritis in these patients is managed as is any other, as detailed in later chapters in this book. The exception is the need to avoid additional granulocytopenia that could exacerbate the patient's risk for infection. Felty's syndrome patients have a 20-fold greater risk of developing significant infection than do rheumatoid patients without neutropenia.[211] Splenectomy is the oldest therapy, and almost 90 per cent of patients have an early short-term response with increase in neutrophil counts in the blood.[209] Neutropenia recurs in about 25 per cent, however, focusing attention on the fact that the splenomegaly itself is not the full story in pathogenesis. An alternative to surgical splenectomy is partial splenic embolization by interventional radiology, a procedure that has a promising 10-year follow-up.[212] Gold salt injections have provided a complete hematologic response in 60 per cent of patients and a partial response in 20 per cent, supporting the hypothesis that suppressing macrophages and immune function will reverse the neutropenia.[213] Lithium salts may transiently elevate cell counts. Use of G-CSF is a logical therapy for the infected and neutropenic patient as a way to forestall splenectomy.[214] However, use of GM-CSF has exacerbated the arthritis, and was associated with an increase in IL-6 levels in blood.[215]

Sjögren's Syndrome

Sjögren's syndrome exists in primary and secondary forms. Although they are related closely, only the secondary form associated with rheumatoid arthritis is considered here. Appropriately stringent diagnostic criteria for Sjögren's syndrome associated with rheumatoid arthritis are

1. Objective evidence of keratoconjunctivitis sicca
2. Objective evidence of diminished salivary gland flow
3. Positive rheumatoid factor and a firm diagnosis of rheumatoid arthritis

Techniques for assaying tears and saliva are time consuming[216] but, to avoid possible toxic therapies, the diagnosis should be a definite one, not based primarily on a rheumatoid patient's complaint that he or she has "dry eyes" or a "dry mouth." If diminished salivary flow is demonstrated, a minor salivary gland biopsy can be obtained to confirm the presence of CD4[+] T cells and a B-cell lymphocytic infiltrate in the gland.[217] This also helps rule out lymphoma or other tumors, sarcoidosis, amyloidosis, and other known causes of keratitis and salivary gland enlargement. A strong association with keratoconjunctivitis was found in patients whose labial salivary gland inflammation showed focal lymphocytic sialadenitis, but not chronic sialadenitis.[218]

Clinical Features

When these patients present to the physician with eye symptoms, they complain most often of a foreign body sensation. Gross examination may be normal, but a rose bengal/fluorescein test shows filamentary keratitis in almost every patient. In patients complaining of oral symptoms, the usual pool of saliva near the frenulum attachment may be gone, and the mucosa appears dull and gray.

Other sites are occasionally involved in Sjögren's syndrome, resulting in the following clinical findings:

- Pulmonary abnormalities, including tenacious secretions, pleurisy, and interstitial fibrosis[219]
- Gastrointestinal tract symptoms, most often dysphagia and atrophic gastritis
- Vaginal dryness
- Thyroiditis, with antibodies to thyroglobulin and thyroid microsomal antigens[220] in patients with no endocrine symptoms
- An inability to acidify the urine, related to a distal nephron defect[221]
- Hyperglobulinemia, sometimes with cryoglobulins and hypergammaglobulinemic purpura

It must be emphasized that primary Sjögren's syndrome and Sjögren's syndrome secondary to rheumatoid arthritis are very different processes. The primary variety is characterized by antibodies against ANAs (SS-A, SS-B), primary biliary cirrhosis, central nervous system manifestations, pseudolymphoma, and lymphomatous degeneration—few of which are seen in rheumatoid patients with the ocular and oral symptoms. An exception to this may be paraproteinemia, which has been described in rheumatoid patients and occasionally transforms to a malignancy.[222]

Pathogenesis

The same factors have been implicated in secondary Sjögren's syndrome as in rheumatoid arthritis itself. EBV, a polyclonal B-cell activator, has been implicated, as have retroviruses.[223]

Treatment

Effective management of the sicca syndrome is challenging. The keratoconjunctivitis can be very bothersome, and associated (see earlier) with scleritis in rheumatoid patients. Effective artificial tears are the best symptomatic therapy. Special gels and toothpastes are available, and attention to oral hygiene is essential to prevent dental caries and gum disease.[216] Details of therapy of the immunologic abnormalities, which can range from meningoencephalitis to pseudolymphoma, are beyond the scope of this book.

REFERENCES

1. Bland, J.: Rheumatoid arthritis of the cervical spine. J. Rheumatol. 1:319, 1974.
2. Ball, J.: Enthesopathy of rheumatoid and ankylosing spondylitis. Ann. Rheum. Dis. 30:213, 1971.
3. Martel, W.: Pathogenesis of cervical discovertebral destruction in rheumatoid arthritis. Arthritis Rheum. 20: 1217, 1977.
4. Stevens, J. C., Cartlidge, N. E., Saunders, M., et al.: Atlanto-axial subluxation and cervical myelopathy in rheumatoid arthritis. Q. J. Med. 40:391, 1971.
5. Nakano, K. K., Schoene, W. C., Baker, R. A., et al.: The cervical myelopathy associated with rheumatoid arthritis: analysis of patients, with 2 postmortem cases. Ann. Neurol. 3:144, 1978.
6. Henderson, F. C., Geddes, J. F., and Crockard, H. A.: Neuropathy of the brainstem and spinal cord in end stage rheumatoid arthritis: implications for treatment. Ann. Rheum. Dis. 52:629, 1993.
7. Martel, W.: The occipito-atlanto-axial joints in rheumatoid arthritis and ankylosing spondylitis. Am. J. Roentgenol. 86:223, 1961.
8. Raskin, R. J., Schnapf, D. J., Wolf, C. R., et al.: Computerized tomography in evaluation of atlantoaxial subluxation in rheumatoid arthritis. J. Rheumatol. 10:33, 1983.
9. Breedveld, F. C., Algra, P. R., Veilvoye, C. J., et al.: Magnetic resonance imaging in the evaluation of patients

with rheumatoid arthritis and subluxations of the cervical spine. Arthritis Rheum. 30:624, 1987.

10. Mayer, J. W., Messner, R. P., and Kaplan, R. J.: Brain stem compression in rheumatoid arthritis. JAMA 236:2094, 1976.

11. Winfield, J., Young, A., Williams, P., et al.: Prospective study of the radiological changes in hands, feet, and cervical spine in adult rheumatoid disease. Ann. Rheum. Dis. 42:613, 1983.

12. Collins, D. N., Barnes, C. L., and FitzRandolph, R. L.: Cervical spine instability in rheumatoid patients having total hip or knee arthroplasty. Clin. Orthop. Rel. Res. 272:127, 1991.

13. Pellicci, P. M., Ranawat, C. S., Tsairis, P., et al.: A prospective study of the progression of rheumatoid arthritis of the cervical spine. J. Bone Joint Surg. Am. 65:342, 1981.

14. Meijers, K. A., Cats, A., Kremer, H. P. H., et al.: Cervical myelopathy in rheumatoid arthritis. Clin. Exp. Rheumatol. 2:239, 1984.

15. Davidson, R. C., Horn, J. R., Herndon, J. H., et al.: Brainstem compression in rheumatoid arthritis. JAMA 238:2633, 1977.

16. Mikulowski, P., Wollheim, F. A., Rotmil, P., et al.: Sudden death in rheumatoid arthritis with atlanto-axial dislocation. Acta Med. Scand. 198:445, 1975.

17. Smith, P. H., Benn, R. T., and Sharp, J.: Natural history of rheumatoid cervical luxations. Ann. Rheum. Dis. 31:431, 1972.

18. Agarwal, A. K., Peppelman, W. C., Kraus, D. R., et al.: Recurrence of cervical spine instability in rheumatoid arthritis following previous fusion: can disease progression be prevented by early surgery? J. Rheumatol. 19:1364, 1992.

19. Yonenobu, K., Hosono, N., Iwasaki, M., et al.: Neurologic complications of surgery for cervical compression myelopathy. Spine 16:1277, 1991.

20. Henderson, D. R.: Vertical atlanto-axial subluxation in rheumatoid arthritis. Rheumatol. Rehab. 14:31, 1975.

21. Bywaters, E. G.: Rheumatoid and other diseases of the cervical interspinous bursae, and changes in the spinous process. Ann. Rheum. Dis. 41:360, 1982.

22. Tumiati, B., and Casoli, P.: Syringomyelia in a patient with rheumatoid subluxation of the cervical spine. J. Rheumatol. 18:1403, 1991.

23. Jacob, J. R., Weisman, M. H., Mink, J. H., et al.: Reversible cause of back pain and sciatica in rheumatoid arthritis: an apophyseal joint cyst. Arthritis Rheum. 29:431, 1986.

24. Ericson, S., and Lundberg, M.: Alterations in the temporomandibular joint at various stages of rheumatoid arthritis. Acta Rheumatol. Scand. 13:257, 1967.

25. Marbach, J. J., and Spiera, H.: Rheumatoid arthritis of the temporomandibular joints. Ann. Rheum. Dis. 26:538, 1967.

26. Goupille, P., Fouquet, B., Cotty, P., et al.: The temporomandibular joint in rheumatoid arthritis: correlations between clinical and computed tomography features. J. Rheumatol. 17:1285, 1990.

27. Lofgren, R. H., and Montgomery, W. W.: Incidence of laryngeal involvement in rheumatoid arthritis. N. Engl. J. Med. 267:193, 1962.

28. Polisar, I. A., Burbank, B., Levitt, L. M., et al.: Bilateral midline fixation of cricoarytenoid joints as serious medical emergency. JAMA 172:901, 1960.

29. Bienenstock, H., Ehrich, G. E., and Freyberg, R. H.: Rheumatoid arthritis of the cricoarytenoid joint: a clinicopathologic study. Arthritis Rheum. 6:48, 1963.

30. Lawry, G. V., Finerman, M. L., Hanafee, W. N., et al.: Laryngeal involvement in rheumatoid arthritis: a clinical, laryngoscopic, and computerized tomographic study. Arthritis Rheum. 27:873, 1984.

31. Copeman, W. S. C.: Rheumatoid oto-arthritis. Br. Med. J. 2:1536, 1963.

32. Moffat, D. A., Ramsden, R. T., Rosenberg, J. N., et al.: Otoadmittance measurements in patients with rheumatoid arthritis. J. Laryngol. Otol. 91:917, 1977.

33. Kalliomaki, J. L., Viitanen, S. M., and Virtama, P.: Radiological findings of sternoclavicular joints in rheumatoid arthritis. Acta Rheumatol. Scand. 14:233, 1968.

34. Kormano, M.: A microradiographic and histological study of the manubrio-sternal joint in rheumatoid arthritis. Acta Rheumatol. Scand. 16:47, 1970.

35. Ennevaara, K.: Painful shoulder joint in rheumatoid arthritis: a clinical and radiological study of 200 cases, with special reference to arthrography of the glenohumeral joint. Acta Rheumatol. Scand. 11:1, 1967.

36. Weiss, J. J., Thompson, G. R., Doust, V., et al.: Rotator cuff tears in rheumatoid arthritis. Arch. Intern. Med. 135:521, 1975.

37. Mosley, H. F.: Ruptures of the rotator cuff—shoulder lesions. 3rd ed. Edinburgh, E & S Livingston Ltd., 1969, p. 73.

38. Edeiken, J., and Hodes, P. J.: Roentgen diagnosis of disease of bone. 2nd ed. Baltimore, Williams & Wilkins, 1978, pp. 690–709.

39. DeSmet, A. A., Ting, Y. M., and Weis, J. J.: Shoulder arthrography in rheumatoid arthritis. Radiology 116:601, 1975.

40. Huston, K. A., Nelson, A. M., and Hunder, G. G.: Shoulder swelling in rheumatoid arthritis secondary to subacromial bursitis. Arthritis Rheum. 21:145, 1978.

41. Resnick, D., and Niwayama, G.: Resorption of the undersurface of the distal clavicle in rheumatoid arthritis. Radiology 120:75, 1976.

42. de Jager, J. P., and Fleming, A.: Shoulder joint rupture and pseudothrombosis in rheumatoid arthritis. Ann. Rheum. Dis. 43:503, 1984.

43. Peterson, L. F., and Janes, J. M.: Surgery of the rheumatoid elbow. Orthop. Clin. North Am. 2:667, 1971.

44. Shapiro, J. S.: A new factor in the etiology of ulnar drift. Clin. Orthop. Rel. Res. 68:32, 1970.

45. Hastings, D. E., and Evans, J. A.: Rheumatoid wrist deformities and their relation to ulnar drift. J. Bone Joint Surg. Am. 57:930, 1975.

46. Inglis, A. E.: Rheumatoid arthritis in the hand. Am. J. Surg. 109:368, 1965.

47. Swezey, R. L., and Fiegenberg, D. S.: Inappropriate intrinsic muscle action in the rheumatoid hand. Ann. Rheum. Dis. 30:619, 1971.

48. Fearnley, G. R.: Ulnar deviation of the fingers. Ann. Rheum. Dis. 10:126, 1951.

49. Flatt, A. E.: Surgical rehabilitation of the arthritic hand. Arthritis Rheum. 11:278, 1959.

50. Hakstian, R. W., and Tubiana, R.: Ulnar deviation of the fingers: the role of joint structure and function. J. Bone Joint Surg. Am. 49:299, 1967.

51. Snorrason, E.: The problem of ulnar deviation of the fingers in rheumatoid arthritis. Acta Med. Scand. 140:359, 1951.

52. Vainio, K., and Oka, M.: Ulnar deviation of the fingers. Ann. Rheum. Dis. 12:122, 1953.

53. Martin, L. F., and Bensen, W. G.: An unusual synovial cyst in rheumatoid arthritis. J. Rheumatol. 14:139, 1987.

54. Croft, J. D. Jr.: Rheumatoid "ganglion" as an unusual presenting sign of rheumatoid arthritis. JAMA 203:144, 1968.

55. Harrison, M. O., Freiberger, R. H., and Ranawat, C. S.: Arthrography of the rheumatoid wrist joint. Am. J. Roentgenol. 112:480, 1971.

56. Iveson, J. M., Hill, A. G., and Wright, V.: Wrist cysts and fistulae: an arthrographic study of the rheumatoid wrist. Ann. Rheum. Dis. 34:388, 1975.

57. Trentham, D. E., and Masi, A. T.: Carpo:metacarpal ratio: a new quantitative measure of radiologic progression of wrist involvement in rheumatoid arthritis. Arthritis Rheum. 19:939, 1976.

58. Alarcon, G. S., and Koopman, W. J.: The carpometacarpal ratio: a useful method for assessing disease progression in rheumatoid arthritis. J. Rheumatol. 12:846, 1985.

59. Kaye, J. J., Callahan, L. F., Nance, E. P. Jr., et al.: Bony ankylosis in rheumatoid arthritis: associations with longer duration and greater severity of disease. Invest. Radiol. 22:303, 1987.

60. Fuchs, H. A., Callahan, L. F., Kaye, J. J., et al.: Radiographic and joint count findings of the hand in rheumatoid arthritis: related and unrelated findings. Arthritis Rheum. 31:44, 1988.

61. Brewerton, D. A.: Hand deformities in rheumatoid disease. Ann. Rheum. Dis. 16:183, 1957.

62. McCarty, D. J., and Gatter, R. A.: A study of distal interphalangeal joint tenderness in rheumatoid arthritis. Arthritis Rheum. 9:325, 1966.

63. Vaughan-Jackson, O. J.: Rheumatoid hand deformities considered in the light of tendon imbalance. J. Bone Joint Surg. Br. 44:764, 1962.

64. Abbott, G. T., Bucknall, R. C., and Whitehouse, G. H.: Osteoarthritis associated with distal interphalangeal joint involvement in rheumatoid arthritis. Skeletal Radiol. 20:495, 1991.

65. Mody, G. M., and Meyers, O. L.: Resorptive arthropathy in rheumatoid arthritis. J. Rheumatol. 15:1075, 1988.

66. Nalebuff, E. A.: Diagnosis, classification, and management of rheumatoid thumb deformities. Bull. Hosp. Joint Dis. 29:119, 1968.

67. Jacob, J., Sartoris, D., Kursunoglu, S., et al.: Distal interphalangeal joint involvement in rheumatoid arthritis. Arthritis Rheum. 29:10, 1986.

68. Kellgren, J. H., and Ball, J.: Tendon lesions in rheumatoid arthritis: a clinicopathological study. Ann. Rheum. Dis. 9:48, 1950.

69. Gray, R. G., and Gottlieb, N. L.: Hand flexor tenosynovitis in rheumatoid arthritis: prevalence, distribution, and associated rheumatic features. Arthritis Rheum. 20:1003, 1977.

70. Duthie, R. B., and Harris, C. M.: A radiographic and clinical survey of the hip joint in sero-positive rheumatoid arthritis. Acta Orthop. Scand. 40:346, 1969.

71. Hastings, D. E., and Parker, S. M.: Protrusio acetabuli in rheumatoid arthritis. Clin. Orthop. Rel. Res. 108:76, 1975.

72. Colton, C., and Darby, A.: Giant granulomatous lesions of the femoral head and neck in rheumatoid arthritis. Ann. Rheum. Dis. 29:626, 1970.

73. Gupta, P. J.: Physical examination of the arthritis patient. Bull. Rheum. Dis. 20:596, 1970.

74. Jayson, M. I. V., and Dixon, A. St. I.: Valvular mechanisms in juxta-articular cysts. Ann. Rheum. Dis. 29:415, 1970.

75. Hench, P. K., Reid, R. T., and Reames, P. M.: Dissecting popliteal cyst stimulating thrombophlebitis. Ann. Intern. Med. 64:1259, 1966.

76. Hall, A. P., and Scott, J. T.: Synovial cysts and rupture of the knee joint in rheumatoid arthritis. Ann. Rheum. Dis. 25:32, 1966.

77. Tait, G. B. W., Bach, F., and Dixon, A. St. J.: Acute synovial rupture. Ann. Rheum. Dis. 24:273, 1965.

78. Kraag, G., Thevathasan, E. M., Gordon, D. A., et al.: The hemorrhagic crescent sign of acute synovial rupture [Letter]. Ann. Intern. Med. 85:477, 1976.

79. Gordon, G. V., and Edell, S.: Ultrasound evaluation of popliteal cysts. Arch. Intern. Med. 140:1453, 1980.

80. Karvonen, R. L., Negendank, W. G., Fraser, S. M., et al.: Articular cartilage defects of the knee: correlation between magnetic resonance imaging and gross pathology. Ann. Rheum. Dis. 49:672, 1990.

81. Rask, M. R.: Achilles tendon rupture owing to rheumatoid disease: case report with a nine-year follow-up. JAMA 239:435, 1978.

82. Dixon, A. St. J.: The rheumatoid foot. In Hill, A. G. S. (ed.): Modern Trends in Rheumatology. London, Butterworths, 1971, pp. 158–173.

83. Vidigal, E., Jacoby, R., Dixon, A. St. J., et al.: The foot in chronic rheumatoid arthritis. Ann. Rheum. Dis. 34:292, 1975.

84. Bienenstock, H.: Rheumatoid plantar synovial cysts. Ann. Rheum. Dis. 34:98, 1975.

85. Calabro, J. J.: A critical evaluation of the diagnostic features of the feet in rheumatoid arthritis. Arthritis Rheum. 5:19, 1962.

86. Clayton, M. L., and Ries, M. D.: Functional hallux rigidus in the rheumatoid foot. Clin. Orthop. Rel. Res. 271:233, 1991.

87. McGuigan, L., Burke, D., and Fleming, A.: Tarsal tunnel syndrome and peripheral neuropathy in rheumatoid disease. Ann. Rheum. Dis. 42:128, 1983.

88. Maddison, P. J., and Bacon, P. A.: Vitamin D deficiency, spontaneous fractures and osteopenia in rheumatoid arthritis. Br. Med. J. 4:433, 1974.

89. Schneider, R., and Kaye, J. J.: Insufficiency and stress fractures of the long bones occurring in patients with rheumatoid arthritis. Radiology 116:595, 1975.

90. Lowthian, P. J., and Calin, A.: Geode development and multiple fractures in rheumatoid arthritis. Ann. Rheum. Dis. 44:130, 1985.

91. Steiner, G., Freund, H. A., Leichtentritt, B., et al.: Lesion of skeletal muscles in rheumatoid arthritis. Am. J. Pathol. 22:103, 1946.

92. Haslock, D. I., Wright, V., and Harriman, D. G. F.: Neuromuscular disorders in rheumatoid arthritis: a motorpoint muscle biopsy study. Q. J. Med. 39:335, 1970.

93. Halla, J. T., Koopman, W. J., Fallahi, S., et al.: Rheumatoid myositis: clinical and histologic features and possible pathogenesis. Arthritis Rheum. 27:737, 1984.

94. Soter, N. A., and Franks, A. G. Jr.: The skin and rheumatic diseases. In Kelley, W. N., Harris, E. D. Jr., Ruddy, S., and Sledge, C. B. (eds.): Textbook of Rheumatology, 4th ed., Vol. 1. Philadelphia, W. B. Saunders, 1993, pp. 519–534.

95. Ferry, A. P.: The eye and rheumatic diseases. In Kelley, W. N., Harris, E. D. Jr., Ruddy, S., and Sledge, C. B. (eds.): Textbook of Rheumatology, 4th ed., Vol. 1. Philadelphia, W. B. Saunders, 1993, pp. 507–518.

96. Watson, P. G., and Hayreh, S. S.: Scleritis and episcleritis. Br. J. Ophthalmol. 60:163, 1976.

97. Hurd, E. R.: Extra-articular manifestations of rheumatoid arthritis. Semin. Arthritis Rheum. 8:151, 1979.

98. Hart, F. D.: Rheumatoid arthritis: extra-articular manifestations. Br. Med. J. 3:131, 1969.

99. Halla, J. T., Schrohenloher, R. E., and Koopman, W. J.: Local immune responses in certain extra-articular manifestations of rheumatoid arthritis. Ann. Rheum. Dis. 51:698, 1992.

100. Collins, D. H.: The subcutaneous nodule of rheumatoid arthritis. J. Pathol. Bacteriol. 45:97, 1937.
101. Bennett, G. A., Zeller, J. W., and Bauer, W.: Subcutaneous nodules of rheumatoid arthritis and rheumatic fever: a pathologic study. Arch. Pathol. 30:70, 1940.
102. Ziff, M.: The rheumatoid nodule. Arthritis Rheum. 33:761, 1990.
103. Ganda, O. P., and Caplan, H. I.: Rheumatoid disease without joint involvement. JAMA 2281:338, 1974.
104. Ginsberg, M. H., Genant, H. K., Yu, T. F., et al.: Rheumatoid nodulosis: an unusual variant of rheumatoid disease. Arthritis Rheum. 18:49, 1975.
105. Brower, A. C., NaPombejara, C., Stechschulte, D. J., et al.: Rheumatoid nodulosis: another cause of juxta-articular nodules. Radiology 125:669, 1977.
106. McCarty, D. J.: Complete reversal of rheumatoid nodulosis. J. Rheumatol. 18:736, 1991.
107. Simons, F. E., and Schaller, J. G.: Benign rheumatoid nodules. Pediatrics 56:29, 1975.
108. Olive, A., Maymo, J., Lloreta, J., et al.: Evolution of benign rheumatoid nodules into rheumatoid arthritis after 50 years. Ann. Rheum. Dis. 46:624, 1987.
109. Wood, M. G., and Beerman, H.: Necrosiosis lipoidica, granuloma annulare: report of a case with lesions in the galea aponeurotica of a child. Am. J. Dis. Child. 96:720, 1958.
110. Watt, T. L., and Baumann, R. R.: Pseudoxanthomatous rheumatoid nodules. Arch. Dermatol. 95:156, 1967.
111. Healey, L. A., Wilske, K. R., and Sagebiel, R. W.: Rheumatoid nodules simulating basal-cell carcinoma. N. Engl. J. Med. 277:7, 1967.
112. Sturrock, R. D., Cowden, E. A., Howie, E., et al.: The forgotten nodule: complications of sacral nodules in rheumatoid arthritis. Br. Med. J. 4:92, 1975.
113. Friedman, B. A.: Rheumatoid nodules of the larynx. Arch. Otolaryngol. 101:361, 1975.
114. Jackson, C. G., Chess, R. L., and Ward, J. R.: A case of rheumatoid nodule formation within the central nervous system and review of the literature. J. Rheumatol. 11:237, 1984.
115. Pearson, M. E., Kosco, M., Huffer, W., et al.: Rheumatoid nodules of the spine: case report and review of the literature. Arthritis Rheum. 30:709, 1987.
116. Bywaters, E. G. L.: Fistulous rheumatism: a manifestation of rheumatoid arthritis. Ann. Rheum. Dis. 12:114, 1953.
117. Shapiro, R. F., Resnick, D., Castles, J. J., et al.: Fistulization of rheumatoid joints: spectrum of identifiable syndromes. Ann. Rheum. Dis. 34:489, 1975.
118. Bassett, L. W., Gold, R. H., and Mirra, J. M.: Rheumatoid bursitis extending into the clavicle and to the skin surface. Ann. Rheum. Dis. 44:336, 1985.
119. Vandenbroucke, J. P., Kaaks, R., Valkenburg, H. A., et al.: Frequency of infections among rheumatoid arthritis patients, before and after disease onset. Arthritis Rheum. 30:810, 1987.
120. Baum, J.: Infection in rheumatoid arthritis. Arthritis Rheum. 14:135, 1971.
121. Gaulhofer de Klerch, E. H., and Van Dam, G.: Septic complications in rheumatoid arthritis. Acta Rheumatol. Scand. 9:254, 1963.
122. Huskisson, E. C., and Hart, F. D.: Severe, unusual and recurrent infections in rheumatoid arthritis. Ann. Rheum. Dis. 31:118, 1972.
123. Bodel, P. T., and Hollingsworth, J. W.: Comparative morphology, respiration, and phagocytic function of leukocytes from blood and joint fluid in rheumatoid arthritis. J. Clin. Invest. 45:580, 1966.
124. Singleton, J. D., West, S. G., and Nordstrom, D. M.:

"Pseudoseptic" arthritis complicating rheumatoid arthritis: a report of six cases. J. Rheumatol. 18:1319, 1991.
125. Cash, J. M., and Klippel, J. H.: Second-line drug therapy for rheumatoid arthritis. N. Engl. J. Med. 330:1368, 1994.
126. Gridley, G., McLaughlin, J. K., Ekbom, A., et al.: Incidence of cancer among patients with rheumatoid arthritis. J. Natl. Cancer Inst. 85:307, 1993.
127. Hakulinen, T., Isomaki, H., and Knekt, P.: Rheumatoid arthritis and cancer studies based on linking nationwide registries in Finland. Am. J. Med. 78:29, 1985.
128. Prior, P., Symmons, D. P., Hawkins, C. F., et al.: Cancer morbidity in rheumatoid arthritis. Ann. Rheum. Dis. 43:128, 1984.
129. Gridley, G., Klippel, J. H., Hoover, R. N., et al.: Incidence of cancer among men with the Felty syndrome. Ann. Intern. Med. 120:35, 1994.
130. Kassan, S. S., Thomas, T. L., Moutsopoulos, H. M., et al.: Increased risk of lymphoma in sicca syndrome. Ann. Intern. Med. 89:888, 1978.
131. Mowat, A. G.: Hematologic abnormalities in rheumatoid arthritis. Semin. Arthritis Rheum. 1:195, 1971.
132. Engstedt, L., and Strandberg, O.: Haematological data and clinical activity of the rheumatoid diseases. Acta Med. Scand. 180:13, 1966.
133. Vreugdenhil, G., Wognum, A. W., van Eijk, H. G., et al.: Anaemia in rheumatoid arthritis: the role of iron, vitamin B_{12}, and folic acid deficiency, and erythropoietin responsiveness. Ann. Rheum. Dis. 49:93, 1990.
134. Beck, J. R., Cornwell, G. G., and Rawnsley, H. M.: Multivariate approach to predictive diagnosis of bone-marrow iron stores. Am. J. Clin. Pathol. 70:665, 1978.
135. Samson, D., Halliday, D., and Gumpel, J. M.: Role of ineffective erythropoiesis in the anaemia of rheumatoid arthritis. Ann. Rheum. Dis. 36:181, 1977.
136. Cartwright, G. E.: The anemia of chronic disorders. Semin. Hematol. 3:351, 1966.
137. Raymond, F. D., Bowie, M. A., and Dugan, A.: Iron metabolism in rheumatoid arthritis. Arthritis Rheum. 8:233, 1965.
138. Houston, T., Moore, M., Porter, D., et al.: Abnormal haem biosynthesis in the chronic anaemia of rheumatoid arthritis. Ann. Rheum. Dis. 53:167, 1994.
139. Ridolfo, A. S., Rubin, A., Crabtree, R. E., et al.: Effects of fenoprofen and aspirin on gastrointestinal microbleeding in man. Clin. Pharmacol. Ther. 14:226, 1973.
140. Williams, R. A., Samson, D., Tikerpae, J., et al.: In-vitro studies of ineffective erythropoiesis in rheumatoid arthritis. Am. J. Rheum. Dis. 41:502, 1982.
141. Reid, C. D., Prouse, P. J., Baptista, L. C., et al.: The mechanism of anaemia in rheumatoid arthritis: effects of bone marrow adherent cells and of serum on in vivo erythropoiesis. Br. J. Haematol. 58:607, 1984.
142. Prouse, P. J., Bonner, B., Gumpel, J. M., et al.: Stimulation of bone marrow erythropoiesis by T lymphocytes of anaemic patients with rheumatoid arthritis. Ann. Rheum. Dis. 44:220, 1985.
143. Winchester, R. J., Koffler, D., Litwin, S. D., et al.: Observations on the eosinophilia of certain patients with rheumatoid arthritis. Arthritis Rheum. 14:650, 1971.
144. Hutchinson, R. M., Davis, P., and Jayson, M. I.: Thrombocytosis in rheumatoid arthritis. Ann. Rheum. Dis. 35:138, 1976.
145. Farr, M., Scott, D. L., Constable, T. J., et al.: Thrombocytosis of active rheumatoid disease. Ann. Rheum. Dis. 42:545, 1983.
146. Bowman, S. J., Sivakumaran, M., Snowden, N., et al.: The

large granular lymphocyte syndrome with rheumatoid arthritis: immunogenetic evidence for a broader definition of Felty's syndrome. Arthritis Rheum. 37:1326, 1994.

147. Combe, B., Andary, M., Caraux, J., et al.: Characterization of an expanded subpopulation of large granular lymphocytes in a patient with rheumatoid arthritis. Arthritis Rheum. 29:675, 1986.

148. Loughran, T. P. Jr.: Clonal diseases of large granular lymphocytes. Blood 82:1, 1993.

149. Wittenborg, A., Gille, J., Ostertag, H., et al.: Die dugitalartritis bei chronischer polyarthritis. Folia Angiol. 22:409, 1974.

150. Fischer, M., Mielke, H., Glaefke, S., et al.: Generalized vasculopathy and finger blood flow abnormalities in rheumatoid arthritis. J. Rheumatol. 11:33, 1984.

151. Sokoloff, L., and Bunin, J. J.: Vascular lesions in rheumatoid arthritis. J. Chron. Dis. 5:668, 1957.

152. Kulka, J. P., Bocking, D., Ropes, M. W., et al.: Early joint lesions of rheumatoid arthritis: report of 8 cases with knee biopsies of less than one year's duration. Arch. Pathol. 59:129, 1955.

153. Soter, N. A., Mihm, M. C. Jr., Gigli, I., et al.: Two distinct cellular patterns in cutaneous necrotizing angiitis. J. Invest. Dermatol. 66:344, 1976.

154. Rapoport, R. J., Kozin, F., Mackel, S. E., et al.: Cutaneous vascular immunofluorescence in rheumatoid arthritis. Am. J. Med. 68:344, 1976.

155. Flipo, R. -M., Janin, A., Hachulla, E., et al.: Labial salivary gland biopsy assessment in rheumatoid vasculitis. Ann. Rheum. Dis. 53:648, 1994.

156. Mongan, E. S., Cass, R. M., Jacox, R. F., et al.: A study of the relation of seronegative and seropositive rheumatoid arthritis to each other and to necrotizing vasculitis. Am. J. Med. 47:23, 1969.

157. Weinstein, A., Peters, K., Brown, D., et al.: Metabolism of the third component of complement (C3) in patients with rheumatoid arthritis. Arthritis Rheum. 15:49, 1972.

158. Conn, D. L., McDuffie, F. C., and Dyck, P. I.: Immunopathologic study of sural nerves in rheumatoid arthritis. Arthritis Rheum. 15:135, 1972.

159. Weisman, M., and Zvaifler, N.: Cryoimmunoglobulinemia in rheumatoid arthritis: significance in serum of patients with rheumatoid vasculitis. J. Clin. Invest. 56:725, 1975.

160. Schmid, F. R., Cooper, N. S., Ziff, M., et al.: Arteritis in rheumatoid arthritis. Am. J. Med. 30:56, 1961.

161. Markenson, J. A., McDougal, J. S., Tsairis, P., et al.: Rheumatoid meningitis: a localized immune process. Ann. Intern. Med. 119:359, 1967.

162. Siomopoulos, V., and Shah, N.: Acute organic brain syndrome associated with rheumatoid arthritis. J. Clin. Psychol. 40:46, 1979.

163. Toussirot, E., Serratrice, G., and Valentin, P.: Autonomic nervous system involvement in rheumatoid arthritis: 50 cases. J. Rheumatol. 20:1508, 1993.

164. Bienenstock, H., Minick, C. R., and Rogoff, B.: Mesenteric arteritis and intestinal infarction in rheumatoid disease. Arch. Intern. Med. 119:359, 1967.

165. Geirsson, A. J., Sturfelt, G., and Truedsson, L.: Clinical and serological features of severe vasculitis in rheumatoid arthritis: prognostic implications. Ann. Rheum. Dis. 46:727, 1987.

166. Scott, D. G., Bacon, P. A., Elliott, P. J., et al.: Systemic vasculitis in a district general hospital 1972–80: clinical and laboratory features, classification and prognosis of 80 cases. Q. J. Med. 51:292, 1982.

167. Lawson, A. A., and MacLean, N.: Renal disease and drug therapy in rheumatoid arthritis. Ann. Rheum. Dis. 25:441, 1966.

168. Via, C. S., Hasbargen, J. A., Moore, J. Jr., et al.: Rheumatoid arthritis and membranous glomerulonephritis: a role for immune complex dissociative techniques. J. Rheumatol. 11:342, 1984.

169. Walker, W. C., and Wright, V.: Pulmonary lesions and rheumatoid arthritis. Medicine 47:501, 1968.

170. Dodson, W. H., and Hollingsworth, J. W.: Pleural effusion in rheumatoid arthritis: impaired transport of glucose. N. Engl. J. Med. 275:1337, 1966.

171. Walker, W. C., and Wright, V.: Diffuse interstitial pulmonary fibrosis and rheumatoid arthritis. Ann. Rheum. Dis. 28:252, 1969.

172. Dixon, A. St. J., and Ball, J.: Honeycomb lung and chronic rheumatoid arthritis: a case report. Ann. Rheum. Dis. 16:241, 1957.

173. Stack, B. H. R., and Grant, I. W. B.: Rheumatoid interstitial lung disease. Br. J. Dis. Chest 59:202, 1965.

174. Frank, S. T., Weg, J. G., Harkleroad, L. E., et al.: Pulmonary dysfunction in rheumatoid disease. Chest 63:27, 1973.

175. Hassan, W. U., Keaney, N. P., and Holland, C. D.: High resolution computed tomography of the lung in lifelong non-smoking patients with rheumatoid arthritis. Ann. Rheum. Dis. 54:308, 1995.

176. Tishler, M., Grief, J., Fireman, E., et al.: Bronchoalveolar lavage—a sensitive tool for early diagnosis of pulmonary involvement in rheumatoid arthritis. J. Rheumatol. 13:547, 1986.

177. Caplan, A.: Certain unusual radiographic appearances in the chest of coal miners suffering from RA. Thorax 8:29, 1953.

178. Portner, M. M., and Gracie, W. A. Jr.: Rheumatoid lung disease with cavitary nodules, pneumothorax and eosinophilia. N. Engl. J. Med. 275:697, 1966.

179. Hull, S., and Mathews, J. A.: Pulmonary necrobiotic nodules as a presenting feature of rheumatoid arthritis. Ann. Rheum. 41:21, 1982.

180. Shenberger, K. N., Schned, A. R., and Taylor, T. H.: Rheumatoid disease and bronchogenic carcinoma—case report and review of the literature. J. Rheumatol. 11:226, 1984.

181. Gardner, D. L., Duthie, J. R., MacLeod, J., et al.: Pulmonary hypertension in RA: report of a case study with intimal sclerosis of pulmonary and digital arteries. Scott. Med. J. 2:183, 1957.

182. Scully, R. E., Mark, E. J., McNeely, W. F., et al.: Case 37–1992: presentation of case. N. Engl. J. Med. 327:873, 1992.

183. Radoux, V., Menard, H. A., Begin, R., et al.: Airways disease in rheumatoid arthritis patients: one element of a general exocrine dysfunction. Arthritis Rheum. 30:249, 1987.

184. Sassoon, C. S., McAlpine, S. W., Tashkin, D. P., et al.: Small airways function in non-smokers with rheumatoid arthritis. Arthritis Rheum. 27:1218, 1984.

185. Popp, R. L.: Echocardiography (first of two parts). N. Engl. J. Med. 323:101, 1990.

186. Bonfiglio, T. A., and Atwater, E. C.: Heart disease in patients with seropositive rheumatoid arthritis: a controlled autopsy study and review. Arch. Intern. Med. 124:714, 1969.

187. Lebowitz, W. B.: The heart in rheumatoid arthritis: a clinical and pathological study of 62 cases. Ann. Intern. Med. 58:102, 1963.

188. MacDonald, W. J. Jr., Crawford, M. H., Klippel, J. H., et al.: Echocardiographic assessment of cardiac structure

and function in patients with rheumatoid arthritis. Am. J. Med. 63:890, 1977.

189. Lange, R. K., Weiss, T. E., and Ochsner, J. L.: Rheumatoid arthritis and constrictive pericarditis: a patient benefited by pericardectomy. Arthritis Rheum. 8:403, 1965.

190. Thadini, U., Iveson, J. M., and Wright, V.: Cardiac tamponade, constrictive pericarditis and pericardial resection in rheumatoid arthritis. Medicine 54:261, 1975.

191. Prakash, R., Atassi, A., Poske, R., et al.: Prevalence of pericardial effusion and mitral-valve involvement in patients with rheumatoid arthritis without cardiac symptoms. N. Engl. J. Med. 289:597, 1975.

192. Weintraub, A. M., and Zvaifler, N. J.: The occurrence of valvular and myocardial disease in patients with chronic joint disease. Am. J. Med. 35:145, 1963.

193. Iveson, J. M., Thadani, U., Ionescu, M., et al.: Aortic valve incompetence and replacement in rheumatoid arthritis. Ann. Rheum. Dis. 34:312, 1975.

194. Gowans, J. D. C.: Complete heart block with Stokes-Adams syndrome due to rheumatoid heart disease. N. Engl. J. Med. 262:1012, 1960.

195. Lev, M., Bharati, S., Hoffman, F. G., et al.: The conduction system in rheumatoid arthritis with complete atrioventricular block. Am. Heart J. 90:78, 1975.

196. Ahern, M., Lever, J. V., and Cosh, J.: Complete heart block in rheumatoid arthritis. Ann. Rheum. Dis. 42:389, 1983.

197. Swezey, R. L.: Myocardial infarction due to rheumatoid arteritis: an antemortem diagnosis. JAMA 199:855, 1967.

198. Reimer, K. A., Rodgers, R. F., and Oyasu, R.: Rheumatoid arthritis with rheumatoid heart disease and granulomatous aortitis. JAMA 235:2510, 1976.

199. Camilleri, J. P., Douglas-Jones, A. G., and Pritchard, M. H.: Rapidly progressive aortic valve incompetence in a patient with rheumatoid arthritis. Br. J. Rheumatol. 30:379, 1991.

200. Pinals, R. S.: Felty's syndrome. In Kelley, W. N., Harris, E. D. Jr., Ruddy, S., and Sledge, C. B. (eds.): Textbook of Rheumatology, 4th ed., Vol. 1. Philadelphia, W. B. Saunders, 1993, pp. 924–930.

201. Rosenstein, E. D., and Kramer, N.: Felty's and pseudo-Felty's syndromes. Semin. Arthritis Rheum. 21:129, 1991.

202. Sienknecht, C. W., Urowitz, M. B., Pruzanski, W., et al.: Felty's syndrome: clinical and serological analysis of 34 cases. Ann. Rheum. Dis. 36:500, 1977.

203. Ruiz, F. P., Martinez, J. J. O., Mendoza, A. C. Z., et al.: Nodular regenerative hyperplasia of the liver in rheumatic diseases: report of seven cases and review of the literature. Semin. Arthritis Rheum. 21:47, 1991.

204. Cohen, M. G., and Webb, J.: Antihistone antibodies in rheumatoid arthritis and Felty's syndrome. Arthritis Rheum. 32:1319, 1989.

205. Coremans, I. E. M., Hagen, E. C., van der Voort, E. A. M., et al.: Autoantibodies to neutrophil cytoplasmic enzymes in Felty's syndrome. Clin. Exp. Rheumatol. 11:255, 1993.

206. Saway, P. A., Prasthofer, E. F., and Barton, I. C.: Prevalence of granular lymphocyte proliferation in patients with rheumatoid arthritis and neutropenia. Am. J. Med. 86:303, 1989.

207. Alvillar, R. E., O'Grady, L., and Robbins, D.: Coexistent Felty's syndrome and palindromic rheumatism. Ann. Rheum. Dis. 50:953, 1991.

208. Wright, C. S., Doan, C. A., Bouroncle, B. A., et al.: Direct splenic arterial and venous blood studies in the hypersplenic syndromes before and after epinephrine. Blood 6:195, 1951.

209. Breedveld, F. C., Fibbe, W. E., and Cats, A.: Neutropenia and infections in Felty's syndrome. Br. J. Rheumatol. 27:191, 1988.

210. Abdou, N. L.: Heterogeneity of bone marrow-directed immune mechanisms in the pathogenesis of neutropenia of Felty's syndrome. Arthritis Rheum. 26:947, 1983.

211. Campion, G., Maddison, P. J., Goulding, N., et al.: The Felty syndrome: a case-matched study of clinical manifestations and outcome, serologic features and immunogenetic associations. Medicine 69:69, 1990.

212. Nakamura, H., Ohishi, A., Asano, K., et al.: Partial splenic embolization for Felty's syndrome: a 10-year follow-up. J. Rheumatol. 21:1964, 1994.

213. Khan, M. A., and Kushner, I.: Improvement in rheumatoid arthritis following splenectomy for Felty's syndrome. JAMA 237:116, 1977.

214. Jakubowski, A. A., Souza, L., Kelly, F., et al.: Effects of human granulocyte colony-stimulating factor in a patient with idiopathic neutropenia. N. Engl. J. Med. 320:38, 1989.

215. Hazenberg, B. P. C., VanLeewen, M. A., Van Rijswijk, M. H., et al.: Correction of granulocytopenia in Felty's syndrome by granulocyte-macrophage colony-stimulating factor: simultaneous induction of interleukin-6 release and flare-up of the arthritis. Blood 74:2769, 1989.

216. Fox, R. I., and Kang, H.-I.: Sjögren's syndrome. In Kelley, W. N., Harris, E. D. Jr., Ruddy, S., and Sledge, C. B. (eds.): Textbook of Rheumatology, 4th ed., Vol. 1. Philadelphia, W. B. Saunders, 1993, pp. 931–942.

217. Daniels, T. E.: Labial salivary gland biopsy in Sjögren's syndrome. Arthritis Rheum. 27:147, 1984.

218. Daniels, T. E., and Whitcher, J. P.: Association of patterns of labial salivary gland inflammation with ketoconjunctivitis sicca. Arthritis Rheum. 37:869, 1994.

219. Hunninghake, G., and Fauci, A.: Pulmonary involvement in the collagen vascular diseases. Am. Rev. Resp. Dis. 119:471, 1979.

220. Whaley, K., Webb, J., McAvoy, B., et al.: Sjögren's syndrome. 2. Clinical associations and immunological phenomena. Q. J. Med. 66:513, 1973.

221. Talal, N., Zisman, E., and Schur, P.: Renal tubular acidosis, glomerulonephritis and immunologic factors in Sjögren's syndrome. Arthritis Rheum. 11:774, 1968.

222. Kelly, C., Baird, G., Foster, H., et al.: Prognostic significance of paraproteinaemia in rheumatoid arthritis. Ann. Rheum. Dis. 50:290, 1991.

223. Talal, N., Dauphinée, M. J., Dang, H., et al.: Detection of serum antibodies to retroviral proteins in patients with primary Sjögren's syndrome (autoimmune exocrinopathy). Arthritis Rheum. 33:774, 1990.

Section VIII

EVALUATION, ASSESSMENT, AND PROGNOSIS

Earlier chapters have stressed the importance of early diagnosis of rheumatoid arthritis. This may be the physician's easiest task. Much more difficult is attempting to estimate the extent of disease activity and the rate at which it is progressing, and to then recommend the most effective therapy.

Although there are some fascinating associations of certain laboratory tests with radiographic evidence of connective tissue remodeling in rheumatoid arthritis, none of these is available on a routine basis. Similarly, articular cartilage is invisible to standard X-ray beams; loss of proteoglycans and the burrowing of invasive fingers of synovial pannus happen long before the apparent joint space is narrowed on radiographic films. Magnetic resonance imaging gives accurate views of cartilage and pannus, but its use is appropriately restricted by cost.

The challenge of assessing disease activity over time and in response to therapy is the single most important therapeutic challenge. For each patient there must be a real or virtual graph in the physician's records that plots the baseline intensity of disease activity and the rate of change over time.

Armed with data from longitudinal follow-up of many patients and an accurate assessment of a patient's disease activity, the physician can approach prognosis, predicting for himself or herself and the patient what the outcome, given the current disease activity and rate of progression, will be. Prognosticating is the most difficult challenge, but in many ways the most important, because having a view of the future is the only way that decisions can be made in the present.

21

Diagnostic Imaging in Rheumatoid Arthritis

There is no routine strategy for use of imaging in rheumatoid arthritis. Unlike pulmonary diseases, for which chest radiographs are appropriately obtained as a baseline as well as an adjunct for early diagnosis, it is an unusual patient for whom radiographs of involved joints made shortly after symptoms of polyarthritis begin are useful either for diagnosis or for forming a therapeutic strategy. The reasons for this are that inflamed synovium and an increase in synovial fluid are much more accurately assessed by physical examination than by radiographs, and loss of cartilage sufficient to narrow the joint space would be unusual this early in the disease process. However, most damage to joints occurs within the first 2 years after onset of rheumatoid arthritis. It has been calculated that the square root of the disease duration seems to better fit curves of the development of erosions and joint space narrowing than do linear models[1] (Fig. 21–1). The point is that radiographic changes are not necessary for the clinician to implement second-line therapy, and it must be emphasized that radiographic deterioration can occur in rheumatoid arthritis even when clinical features improve with therapy.[2] One of the principal reasons for this is demonstrated in Figure 21–2, which shows that, if a joint is examined by arthroscopy at stage II of pathologic involvement, when cartilage has been damaged peripherally and proteoglycans depleted from it so that irreversible changes are present, the radiographs may be normal. Conversely, even if the inflammatory process recedes completely at this point, the radiographic changes progress secondary to the irreversible degradation of the cartilage and bone.

IMAGING PLAN FOR RHEUMATOID ARTHRITIS

A useful plan for imaging of patients with rheumatoid arthritis is as follows:

- Unless sepsis is high on the list of differential diagnoses, or unless there already are flexion contractures of subluxations present, routine radiographs are not necessary in the patient who presents with polyarthritis.
- After a month or more of sustained polyarthritis, when a diagnosis of rheumatoid arthritis is definite, baseline imaging is appropriate, but it should be kept simple:
  - posterior-anterior views of both hands and wrists on the same film
  - if knees are involved, views of both knees on the same film with the patient standing, in order to assess width of the apparent joint space (i.e., cartilage thickness)
  - if feet are involved, a view of both forefeet and toes on the same film

  In a regression analysis of ratings of 1-year progression of total radiologic damage, the odds ratios for progressive disease were 12 for the presence of rheumatoid factor, 5 for the presence of damage at baseline, and 2 for cumulative joint inflammation. Each of these factors was independent of the others.[3]
- Six to 8 months after the first set of baseline films, a repeat series on involved joints is appropriate to assess progression of periarticular bone loss and joint space thickness, and to search for early evidence of bone erosions at the cartilage-bone-synovium junction.
- It is primarily in more advanced disease that careful imaging assessments are useful. They should be obtained in consultation with both orthopedic surgeons and radiologists. Good imaging is essential for planning arthroplasty or other surgery designed to enhance function.
- Special imaging studies, including thermography or bone scans, rarely give information that other studies could not, and they are more expensive. There are exceptions to this statement. One is in the rheumatoid patient with long bone or rib pain, when either a fracture or a metastasis from malig-

259

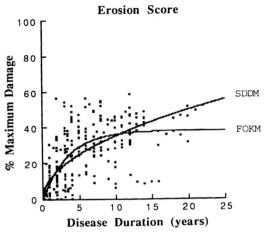

FIGURE 21–1. Scattergram of the plain radiographic scoring values for erosion damage according to the square root of disease duration model (SDDM) and first-order kinetics model (FOKM). (From Salaffi, F., Ferraccioli, G., Peroni, M., et al.: Progression of erosion and joint space narrowing scores in rheumatoid arthritis assessed by nonlinear models. J. Rheumatol. 21: 1626, 1994. Used by permission.)

nancy is among the differential diagnoses; in these cases, a technetium-99m diphosphonate scan may indicate hot spots not in areas containing synovium and indicative of a fine cortical fracture. Another is the use of ultrasound to delineate planes of soft tissue or fluid not seen on radiographs.[4]

- Standard radiographic images are effectively supplemented by quantitation of bone mineral density (BMD) using dual-energy x-ray absorptiometry. This noninvasive technique has a small radiation dose and therefore can safely be repeated to evaluate patients at risk for fracture, particularly those treated with glucocorticoids. It has been adapted for use in rheumatoid hands as well as the spine and long bones[5] and has a reproducibility to 1 per cent in the hand, correlating well with both age and disease activity[6] (Figs. 21–3 and 21–4).

- It is generally accepted that joint space narrowing, erosions, and subluxations of involved joints correlate significantly with duration of disease, and significant findings without evidence for ma-

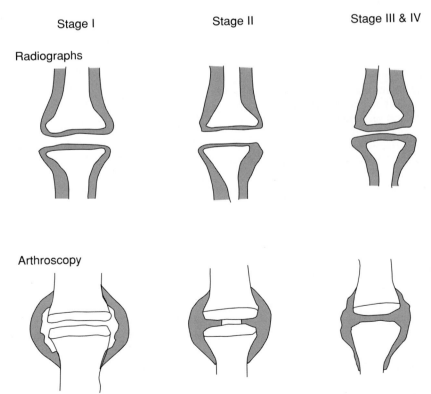

FIGURE 21–2. If a joint is examined by arthroscopy at stage II of pathologic involvement, when cartilage has been damaged peripherally and proteoglycans depleted from it so that irreversible changes are present, the radiographs may be normal. Conversely, even if the inflammatory process recedes completely at this point, the radiographic changes may progress secondary to the irreversible degradation already in development.

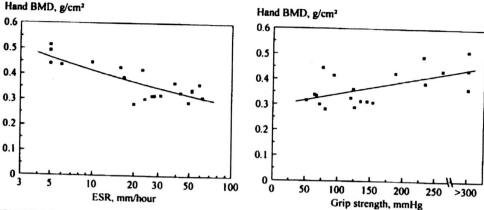

FIGURE 21–3. Relationship between hand BMD and markers of disease severity in 20 patients with early rheumatoid arthritis. For the ESR, $r = -.81$, $p < .0001$; for grip strength, $r = .49$, $p = .03$. (From Peel, N. F. A., Spittlehouse, A. J., Bax, D. E., et al.: Bone mineral density of the hand in rheumatoid arthritis. Arthritis Rheum. 37:983, 1994. Used by permission.)

lalignment or subluxation are the rule, not the exception, in most patients with disease duration of less than 2 years.[7] (Fig. 21–5). 315 patients examined early in the course of their disease, radiologic lesions of the small joints of the hands, feet, and/or wrists were found in 37 per cent with disease duration of up to 4 months; this increased to 91 per cent at 36 months.[8] In another study, 90 patients were followed with biannual plain films for 3 years. At 3 years, radiographic damage was present in 70 per cent of patients, all of whom could be identified after 1 year of study. The rate of progression in the first year was higher than in the subsequent 2 years.[9]

Careful analyses of indices of rheumatoid activity have supported contentions that the inflamma-

tory component of rheumatoid arthritis and the proliferative and destructive component are often dissociated. For example, in patients with *arthritis robustus*, data correlating radiographic and physical findings have shown that joint tenderness counts were independent of radiographic erosion scores (Fig. 21–6).[10]

IMAGING FINDINGS CHARACTERISTIC OF RHEUMATOID ARTHRITIS

Although almost every patient with sustained rheumatoid arthritis has radiographic evidence for *marginal erosions* of bone, *compressive ero-*

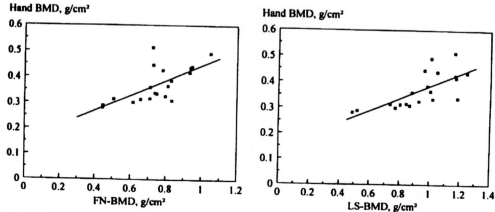

FIGURE 21–4. Relationship between hand BMD and BMD of the femoral neck (FN) ($r = .67$, $p = .002$) and the lumbar spine (LS) ($r = .72$, $p = .0003$) in 20 patients with early rheumatoid arthritis. (From Peel, N. F. A., Spittlehouse, A. J., Bax, D. E., et al.: Bone mineral density of the hand in rheumatoid arthritis. Arthritis Rheum. 37:983, 1994. Used by permission.)

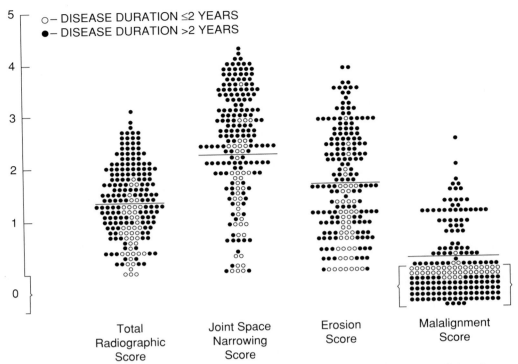

FIGURE 21-5. Frequencies of radiographic scores in 200 patients with rheumatoid arthritis, including total scores and subtotal scores for joint space narrowing, erosion, and malalignment. Open circles, patients with disease duration less than 2 years; closed circles, patients with disease duration 2 years or longer. (From Fuchs, H. A., Kaye, J. J., Callahan, L. F., et al.: Evidence of significant radiographic damage in rheumatoid arthritis within the first 2 years of disease. J. Rheumatol. 16:585, 1989. Used by permission.)

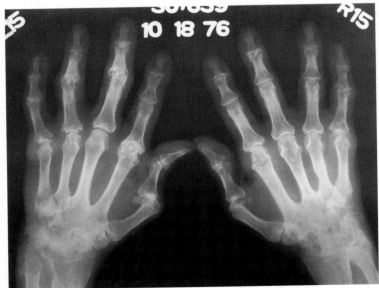

FIGURE 21-6. This patient, a 43-year-old farmer, had active rheumatoid arthritis for 12 years. He had almost no pain, and used his hands vigorously every day. On examination, there was no malalignment or indications of ulnar deviation, even though his wrist joints had been destroyed, the left ulnar head had been erased, and all MCP and PIP joints were affected.

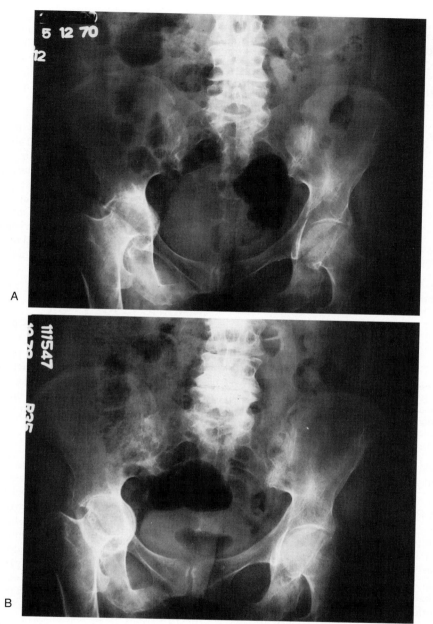

FIGURE 21–7. Right hip of a 57-year-old rheumatoid patient. *A*, In 1970, her pain became so severe that she retired to a wheelchair. This radiograph shows complete loss of the joint space and definite acetabulum protrusion. *B*, In 1978, she had walked or borne weight on the right leg very little during the intervening 8 years. This radiograph shows a remodeled, serviceable hip joint that developed largely because, it is posited, she was bearing no weight.

sions—created when osteoporosis of subchondral bone and subsequent remodeling of the remaining bone lead to invagination of one part of the bone into the other—are seen only in psoriatic and severe rheumatoid arthritis. One site for this is the hip, where the manifestation is *protrusio acetabuli* (Fig. 21–7); another occurs when a phalangeal base col-

lapses within a metacarpal head, producing an apparent ball-and-socket pseudo-joint. *Subchondral cysts* or *geodes* form as destructive proliferative tissue in subchondral areas when the subchondral plate is broken and articular tissue penetrates through. In any rheumatoid patient with disease of many years, the risk of *fracture* is high, particularly

TABLE 21–1. Details of Presentation and Radiologic Findings of Pubic Rami Fractures in 22 Patients with Rheumatoid Arthritis

CHARACTERISTICS	NO. OF PATIENTS
Symptoms	
Low back pain	9
Groin pain	6
Hip pain	4
Pelvic pain	3
Leg pain	2
Knee pain	1
None	3
Onset	
Gradual	7
Acute/spontaneous	12
Precipitating event	
None	12
Fall to ground	7
Getting out of car	2
Getting out of bed	1
Effect on mobility	
None	9
Mild	9
Moderate	2
Immobilized	1*

From Isdale, A. H.: Stress fractures of the pubic rami in rheumatoid arthritis. Ann. Rheum. Dis. 52:681, 1993. Used by permission. Copyright 1993 BMJ Publishing Group.
* Multiple fractures.

along the narrowed cortex of long bones such as the fibula and in the pubic rami[11] (Table 21–1).

Magnetic Resonance Imaging

The evolution of MRI technology has enabled radiologists to delineate many intra-articular structures previously hidden from view within conventional radiographs. Using T_1-weighted imaging, radiologists have been able to develop separate resolution of articular cartilage, synovial fluid, and subchondral bone—all that is needed to demonstrate the stage of invasion by pannus. MRI evaluation analysis is concordant with arthroscopy in being able to identify lesions of articular cartilage.[12]

The drawback of MRI is its expense. However, judicious restraint in obtaining routine radiographs early in disease and in patients without obvious clinical progression can justify appropriate imaging in patients with more aggressive disease. Another benefit of MRI, of course, is that it utilizes nonionizing radiation.

"Dynamic imaging" combines MRI with gado-

linium-diethylenetriamine penta-acetic acid enhancement. Changes in signal intensity have correlated positively with pathologic findings of fibrin exudation, cellular infiltration, villous hypertrophy, vascular proliferation, and granulation formation in synovial biopsy specimens obtained during arthroplasty.[11]

Evidence is substantial that MRI will show more numerous and extensive erosions than will plain films in all stages of arthritis[13] (Table 21–2; Fig. 21–8). This is important for planning more aggressive therapy in the disease, because the window of opportunity for retarding disease progression in bone or cartilage destruction is, in most patients, between 6 months and 2 years. Cartilage remains one of the most difficult tissues to visualize in detail using MRI; improvement in spatial resolution must await an increased strength of gradient magnetic fields.

IMAGING ISSUES FOR INDIVIDUAL JOINT SYSTEMS

This chapter is not intended to provide full descriptions of radiographic and MRI abnormalities peculiar to each joint involved in rheumatoid arthritis, but rather to emphasize certain broad considerations for various areas involved in the disease.

Cervical Spine

Because of the small size of the multiple joints in the cervical spine, the large mass of soft tissue surrounding the spine, and the lower borders of the occipital bones, these structures are difficult to visualize effectively. In advanced disease, for example, the usual landmarks may be obliterated[14] (Fig. 21–9). Although posterior subluxation of the odontoid (so long as it is not eroded away) can be defined on lateral plain radiographs of the cervical spine in a position of flexion, it appears that the information gained from MRI is sufficiently additive and definitive to warrant the increased cost of this procedure, particularly because superior migration of the odontoid can be a cause of sudden death.[15,16] A dynamic (flexion-extension) MRI has been shown to clearly delineate the relationship between the odontoid, foramen magnum, and cervical spinal cord.[14] In addition, gradient-echo MRI pulse sequences provide reliable visualization of the transverse atlantal ligament (Fig. 21–10), enabling the clinician to distinguish rupture from stretching of this important structure,[17] and can identify concurrent cervical spondylosis that could contribute to neurologic signs, particularly in elderly patients.[18]

TABLE 21–2. MRI for the Assessment of Rheumatoid Arthritis: a Comparison with Plain Film Radiographs

	PATIENT NO.	M/F	AGE (YEARS)	RA (YEARS)	X-RAY EROSION NO.	MRI EROSION NO.
Group A	1	F	63	35	3	4
	2	F	54	20	4	5
	3	M	49	19	1	3
Group B	4	F	50	8	3	6
	5	F	25	7	0	5
	6	M	38	5	4	7
	7	F	55	4	0	2
Group C	8	F	49	2	0	1
	9	F	39	2	0	3
	10	M	55	1	0	4
	11	F	52	0.8	0	1

From Foley-Nolan, D., Stack, J. P., Ryan, M., et al.: Magnetic resonance imaging in the assessment of rheumatoid arthritis—a comparison with plain film radiographs. Br. J. Rheumatol. 30:101, 1991. Used by permission.

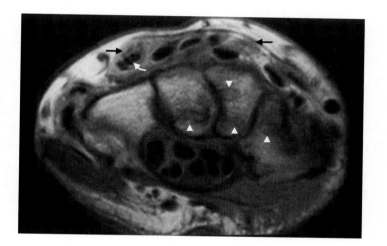

FIGURE 21–8. MRI image (axial plane; proton density weighted) of the wrist in a 40-year-old woman with rheumatoid arthritis. There is extensive soft tissue fullness (arrows) around the extensor tendons, consistent with pannus formation and some fluid within the tendon sheaths. Bony erosions are seen as regions of intermediate gray signal (arrowheads) within the bright signal from marrow fat in the carpal bones. There is fragmentation of the extensor digiti minimi tendon (curved arrow), seen as irregular contour and separate components of the tendon. (Courtesy of A. Gabrielle Bergman, M. D., Stanford University Medical Center.)

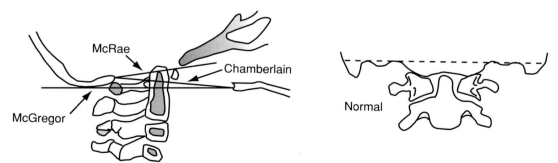

FIGURE 21–9. *A*, Anatomic landmarks normally used for identifying superior odontoid migration. McGregor's line is often the easiest to define, although anatomical variations in the position of the hard palate are difficult visualizing. The posterior edge of the foramen magnum make MRI the imaging procedure of choice to detect superior migration of the odontoid. (From Bell, G. R., and Stearns, K. L.: Flexion-extension MRI of the upper rheumatoid cervical spine. Orthopedics 14:969, 1991. Used by permission.)

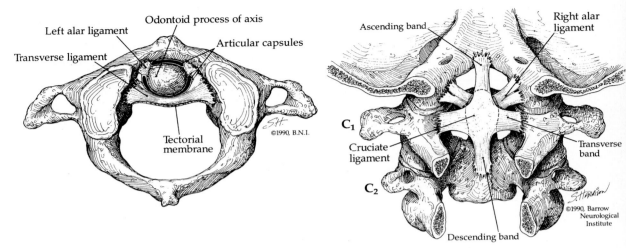

FIGURE 21–10. Illustrations of axial (left) and dorsal (right) views of the atlantoaxial complex depicting the normal anatomic relationships among the cruciate and alar ligaments and the tectorial membrane. (From Dickman, C. A., Mamourian, A., Sonntag, V. K. H., et al.: Magnetic resonance imaging of the transverse atlantal ligament for the evaluation of atlantoaxial instability. J. Neurosurg. 75:221, 1991. Used by permission.)

Temporomandibular Joints

The TMJ is often involved yet often ignored in rheumatoid arthritis. If an overbite develops in a rheumatoid patient, plain radiographs or, if necessary, CT scans, may reveal erosion of the mandibular condyle and the eminentia articularis of the temporal bone.

Sternoclavicular and Manubriosternal Joints

Difficult to visualize by plain films because of the rib cage, these relatively immobile joints are more involved radiographically than symptomatically. It is rare that radiographs of them are truly indicated.

Knee

Physical examination that includes palpation for a popliteal cyst and manipulation tests for range of motion, for patellofemoral grating or malalignment, for lateral and anterior-posterior instability, and for excess synovial fluid is usually sufficient for assessment, when combined with standing radiographic views of both legs to evaluate alignment and the thickness of the apparent joint spaces. There are several exceptions: one is when locking occurs and there is a question of whether synovium or a partially destroyed meniscal cartilage is responsible; another is when therapeutic surgical decisions hinge to some extent on whether the anterior or posterior cruciate ligaments are intact, stretched, thinned, or degraded by the proliferative synovitis. For both of these situations, MRI is appropriate. As shown in Table 21–3, the positive predictive value is often less than 90 per cent, but this procedure has a very high negative predictive value.[19] Thus, if MRI shows intact ligaments and menisci, the chance of significant erosion or fragmentation is minimal.

Ultrasound is particularly useful for detecting popliteal cysts and delineating the extent of dissection into the calf, when that occurs.

In Chapter 11 it is emphasized that, in the knee joint, the functional and anatomic loss of cartilage from peripheral erosions is less than that caused by spread of a fibroblastic pannus over the cartilage surface, which appears to stimulate chondrocyte proliferation and internal destruction of cartilage as well as directly invading it. For this reason, judicious use of MRI or arthroscopy is the best way to determine the state of cartilage in the rheumatoid knee (Fig. 21–11).

Hip

Acetabular protrusio (see earlier) is present if the inner margin of the acetabulum is medial to the ilioischial line by 3 mm or more in men or 6 mm or more in women.[20] Osteonecrosis of the femoral head occurs principally in rheumatoid patients who have been treated with long-term glucocorticoids at doses greater than 15 mg/day. The hip is often one of the last diarthrodial joints to be affected in rheumatoid arthritis. Progression of hip destruction

TABLE 21–3. Measures of Usefulness of MRI of the Knee

	MEDIAL MENISCUS (%)	LATERAL MENISCUS (%)	ACL* (%)
Sensitivity	97	90	87
Specificity	77	87	94
Positive predictive value	85	79	70
Negative predictive value	95	94	98
Accuracy	88	88	93

From Kelly, M. A., Flock, T. J., Kimmel, J. A., et al.: MR imaging of the knee: clarification of its role. Arthroscopy 7:78, 1991. Used by permission.
* ACL, anterior cruciate ligament.

is accelerated by weight bearing and retarded (or reversed) by absence of weight bearing (Fig. 21–7).

Hands and Wrists

Because there is very little soft tissue surrounding the interphalangeal and MCP joints, these are the best ones for detecting marginal erosions on plain radiographs (Figs. 21–12, 21–13, and 21–14). Compressive erosions (see earlier) in se-

vere disease can lead to *main en lorgnette*, a shortening of the phalanges with accordion folds in the overlying skin.

Unlike other diseases, rheumatoid arthritis affects all six compartments of the wrist, although the first CMC compartment occasionally may be spared.[20] In severe active disease, a definite scalloping out of the distal lateral radius by the ulnar

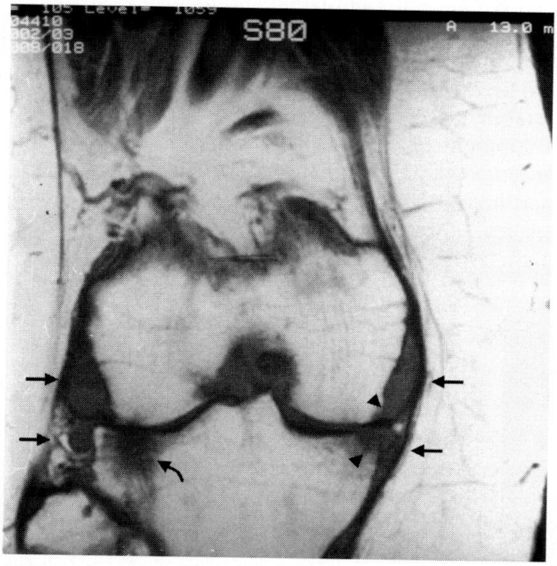

FIGURE 21–11. MRI resonance image (coronal plane; T_1 weighted) of the knee in a 43-year-old woman with rheumatoid arthritis. Abnormal capsular distention is present medially and laterally (arrows), consistent with synovitis or pannus formation and a component of joint effusion. Adjacent bone shows erosive disease (arrowheads), and there is narrowing of the medial and obliteration of the lateral compartment cartilage spaces. The focally abnormal subarticular marrow signal in the lateral tibial plateau (curved arrow) is characteristic of marrow edema or replacement of fatty marrow by pannus or reactive fibrosis. (Courtesy of A. Gabrielle Bergman, M. D., Stanford University Medical Center.)

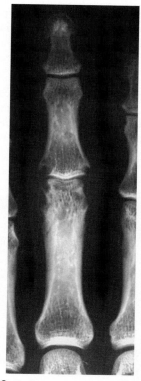

FIGURE 21–12. Radiograph of the long finger in a 42-year-old woman with rheumatoid arthritis. Periarticular soft tissue swelling is present at the PIP joint, with bony erosions on both sides of the joint. There is associated narrowing of the cartilage space, while the cartilage spaces at the MCP and DIP joints are normal. (Courtesy of A. Gabrielle Bergman, M. D., Stanford University Medical Center.)

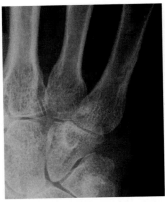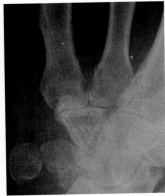

A B

FIGURE 21–13. Two radiographic views of the right wrist in a 57-year-old woman with rheumatoid arthritis: posteroanterior (*A*) and oblique (*B*) (also called Norgaard or Allstate view). Subtle erosive changes are present at the base of the fourth and fifth metacarpals, but because of the location of the erosions, this can be identified only on the oblique view (arrows). If the radiographic exam had been limited to a single posteroanterior view, the presence of erosive disease would not have been known. (Courtesy of A. Gabrielle Bergman, M. D., Stanford University Medical Center.)

head may be seen on radiographs and disease in this area may progress to a whittling away of the entire ulnar head. These defects are examples of the ways in which mechanical stresses and proliferative and destructive synovitis are additive in producing bone and cartilage destruction.

Elbow

Radiographs of the elbow in early rheumatoid arthritis may be normal even though the patient is unable to extend past more than 110 degrees or so because of early soft tissue contractures that prevent full extension. Later, radial head resorption occurs; this may be painless as well.

Foot

Perhaps because of the stress of body weight put on feet, radiographic changes in the multiple joints here are very common. A classical forefoot abnormality consisting of plantar subluxation of metatarsal heads that produces "cock-up" toes, fibular deviation at the MTP joints, and marginal erosions of the first metatarsal head is found relatively early in established disease.[20] These changes precede development of bunions from shoe pressure on the hallux in valgus. Similar to the wrist, the tarsal compartment becomes involved, with loss of joint spaces and sclerosis and flattening of the plantar arch.

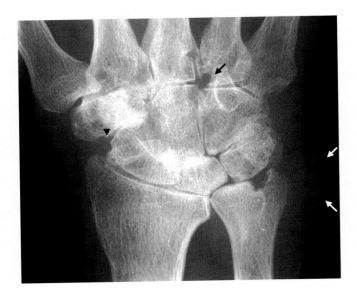

FIGURE 21–14. Wrist radiograph in a 76-year-old woman with advanced changes of rheumatoid arthritis. Prominent soft tissue swelling is present over the ulnar aspect of the wrist, especially over the ulnar styloid process (white arrows). Bony erosions are seen at the base of the fourth metacarpal (black arrow) and at the trapezium (arrowhead), and there is severe cartilage space narrowing at the radiocarpal and midcarpal joints. Bony remodeling (mechanical erosion) with subarticular sclerosis is most advanced at the proximal aspect of the lunate. (Courtesy of A. Gabrielle Bergman, M. D., Stanford University Medical Center.)

Ankle

Marked erosions and joint destruction occur later in the ankle than in other joints, perhaps because this joint and the hip have more limited ranges of motion and less redundant synovium than other diarthrodial joints. Eventually, destruction and ankylosis, with marked eversion of the foot under the ankle, can markedly inhibit walking.

SUMMARY

Developing the proper perspective for use of imaging in rheumatoid arthritis is both important and difficult for the clinician. There should be no ''routine'' radiographs obtained. Initially, radiographs can be useful to affirm clinical impressions that an inflammatory synovitis exists in what have been normal joints. Later in the course of disease, they should be obtained when there is a high likelihood that they will add value by clarifying extent of erosions or cartilage loss or aid in considering specific intrasynovial or orthopedic therapy. Restrained and focused use of MRI will be the clearest way to determine the relationship in a particular joint of synovium, pannus, and cartilage.

REFERENCES

1. Salaffi, F., Ferraccioli, G., Peroni, M., et al.: Progression of erosion and joint space narrowing scores in rheumatoid arthritis assessed by nonlinear models. J. Rheumatol. 21: 1626, 1994.
2. Lopez-Mendeza, A., Daniel, W. W., Reading, J. C., et al.: Radiographic assessment of disease progression in rheumatoid arthritis patients enrolled in the cooperative systematic studies of the rheumatic diseases program randomized clinical trial of methotrexate, auranofin, or a combination of the two. Arthritis Rheum. 36:1364, 1993.
3. van der Heide, A., Remme, C. A., and Hofman, D. M.: Prediction of progression of radiologic damage in newly diagnosed rheumatoid arthritis. Arthritis Rheum. 18: 1466, 1995.
4. Alasaarela, E. M., and Alasaarela, E. L. I.: Ultrasound evaluation of painful rheumatoid shoulders. J. Rheumatol. 21: 1642, 1994.

   Ultrasound examinations were performed bilaterally in 44 rheumatoid patients with shoulder pain. Findings were as follows:

ABNORMALITY	NUMBER POSITIVE
Subacromial-subdeltoid bursitis	35 patients
Glenohumeral synovitis	32 patients
Biceps tendinitis	29 patients

   Sixty-one of the 88 shoulders examined had more than one of these abnormalities. No abnormalities were found in only 10 shoulders. The information provided by ultrasound can be useful before or during injection therapy.

5. Deodhar, A. A., Brabyn, J., Jones, P. W., et al.: Measurement of hand bone mineral content by dual energy X-ray absorptiometry: development of the method, and its application in normal volunteers and in patients with rheumatoid arthritis. Ann. Rheum. Dis. 53:685, 1994.
6. Peel, N. F. A., Spittlehouse, A. J., Bax, D. E., et al.: Bone mineral density of the hand in rheumatoid arthritis. Arthritis Rheum. 37:983, 1994.

   The fascinating finding from this study was that hand BMD was related to BMD at other skeletal sites, giving a good index of rheumatoid activity relatively early in the disease.

7. Fuchs, H. A., Kaye, J, J., Callahan, L. F., et al.: Evidence of significant radiographic damage in rheumatoid arthritis within the first 2 years of disease. J. Rheumatol. 16:585, 1989.

   Quantitative radiographic scores were obtained in hands and wrists of 200 patients with rheumatoid arthritis. The scores correlated well with duration of disease.

8. Caruso, I., Santandrea, S., Puttini, P. S., et al.: Clinical, laboratory and radiographic features in early rheumatoid arthritis. J. Rheumatol. 17:1263, 1990.
9. van der Heijde, D. M. F. M., van Leeuwen, M. A., van Riel, P. L. C. M., et al.: Biannual radiographic assessments of hands and feet in a three-year prospective followup of patients with early rheumatoid arthritis. Arthritis Rheum. 35:26, 1992.
10. Fuchs, H. A., Callahan, L. F., Kaye, J. J., et al.: Radiographic and joint count findings of the hand in rheumatoid arthritis: related and unrelated findings. Arthritis Rheum. 31: 44, 1988.
11. Isdale, A. H. Stress fractures of the pubic rami in rheumatoid arthritis. Ann. Rheum. Dis. 52:681, 1993.

    In this paper, 22 cases of these fractures were collected prospectively from a clinic; the denominator is not given. Presenting clinical features are included in Table 21–1 (see text), in which it can be appreciated that the presenting symptoms were nonspecific and occurred following little or no trauma. All of the pubic rami fractures occurred in women. A total of 86 per cent were receiving prednisolone and all had radiologic evidence of osteoporosis; 63 per cent had vertebral crush fractures.

12. Adams, M. E., Li, D. K. B., McConkey, J. P. et al.: Evaluation of cartilage lesions by magnetic resonance imaging at 0.15 T: comparison with anatomy and concordance with arthroscopy. J. Rheumatol. 18:1573, 1991.
13. Foley-Nolan, D., Stack, J. P., Ryan, M., et al.: Magnetic resonance imaging in the assessment of rheumatoid arthritis—a comparison with plain film radiographs. Br. J. Rheumatol. 30:101, 1991.

    In 11 cases of rheumatoid arthritis involving wrists and carpi and duration of disease from 8 months to 35 years, erosions were more extensive and numerous on MR images compared with plain radiographs.

14. Bell, G. R., and Stearns, K. L.: Flexion-extension MRI of the upper rheumatoid cervical spine. Orthopedics 14:969, 1991.

    The anatomic landmarks and the names associated with them are noted in Figure 21–11 (see text).

15. Davis, F. W., and Markley, H. E.: Rheumatoid arthritis with

death from medullary compression. Ann. Intern. Med. 35:451, 1951.

16. Martel, W. Fatal atlanto-axial luxation in rheumatoid arthritis. Arthritis Rheum. 6:224, 1963.

17. Dickman, C. A., Mamourian, A., Sonntag, V. K. H., et al.: Magnetic resonance imaging of the transverse atlantal ligament for the evaluation of atlantoaxial instability. J. Neurosurg. 75:221, 1991.

18. Glew, D., Watt, I., Dieppe, P. A., et al.: MRI of the cervical spine: rheumatoid arthritis compared with cervical spondylosis. Clin. Radiol. 44:71, 1991.

19. Kelly, M. A., Flock, T. J., Kimmel, J. A., et al.: MR imaging of the knee: clarification of its role. Arthroscopy 7:78, 1991.

20. Resnick, D., Berthiaume, M. -J. and Sartoris, D.: Imaging. *In* Kelley, W. N., Harris, E. D. Jr., Ruddy, S., and Sledge, C. B. (eds.): Textbook of Rhematology, 4th ed., Vol. 1. Philadelphia, W. B. Saunders, 1993, pp. 579–638.

22

Laboratory Assays:
The Acute-Phase Response

There is no specific laboratory test available to diagnose rheumatoid arthritis. As reviewed in detail in early chapters in this book, the pathophysiology of rheumatoid arthritis is extremely complex. The diagnosis is a clinical one, based on symptoms and signs of synovial inflammation. Therefore, an important question is: Are there markers of disease activity that are relatively inexpensive, widely available, accurate, and reproducible?

The answer appears to be a qualified "yes." In the absence of other causes of inflammation, tissue injury, or infection, components of the **acute-phase response** are the most accurate measures for the dollar spent of an active process in patients with this disease. In the presence of a polyarticular synovitis, a number of biologic responses occur that have systemic effects on the patient. These can include fever, malaise, and loss of weight, and are induced by inflammatory cytokines. Numerous hormones, including corticotropin, cortisol, glucagon, insulin, growth hormone, and thyroid-stimulating hormone, are expressed at an increased rate.[1] There also are measurable changes in plasma concentrations of many plasma proteins synthesized by the liver,[2] as noted in Table 22–1.

TABLE 22–1. Plasma Concentration Changes of Plasma Proteins Synthesized by the Liver in Acute-Phase Response

DECREASED CONCENTRATION	INCREASED CONCENTRATION
Albumin	C-reactive protein
Transferrin	Serum amyloid A
α_2-HS glycoprotein	Haptoglobin
	Fibrinogen
	Protease inhibitors

INDUCTION OF THE ACUTE–PHASE RESPONSE

IL-1 and TNFα are the initiators of acute-phase response protein synthesis by the liver. These cytokines induce synthesis of IL-6, which is the major mediator of the acute-phase response.[3] IL-6 can be measured in the synovial fluid and serum from patients with inflammatory arthritis[4] and these levels vary with treatment. In patients with active rheumatoid arthritis being started on intramuscular gold therapy, IL-6 levels correlated directly with a fall in ESR as patients began to improve.[5]

CLINICAL USE OF THE ACUTE–PHASE RESPONSE

Erythrocyte Sedimentation Rate

The ESR is an indirect measure of the acute-phase response, but it is a simple and easily reproducible one that has been in use for more than 65 years. It is based on the effects of changes in plasma proteins on the rate at which red blood cells fall through plasma by the force of gravity. Shortly after inflammation in any tissue begins, increased concentrations of fibrinogen and other acute-phase proteins alter the attraction-repulsion ratio of red blood cells for each other. The red blood cells clump together and fall quickly through plasma, and the result is a high ESR. The problem with an indirect test such as the ESR is that multiple variables affect it; the ESR is very sensitive, but not specific. It is affected by the size, number, and shape of red blood cells; concentration of immunoglobulins; and age and sex of patients. For these reasons, it is more useful for following disease activity in a single patient through the course of disease rather than relating disease in one patient to that in another.[2]

C-Reactive Protein

C-reactive protein (CRP) is synthesized by the liver in response to IL-6 and other cytokines. Liver cells are recruited in an increasing radius around hepatic blood vessels. This geometric consideration leads to a logarithmic increase in CRP in response to linear increases in the inductive stimuli. Measurement of this acute-phase reactant can be quantitative. The techniques used are immunoassay and laser nephelometry. The assays are linear (on a logarithmic scale) through a wide range of concentrations. The following ranges concentration are useful in interpretations of CRP results[6]:

Less than 1 mg/dl:	Normal
Between 1 and 10 mg/dl:	Moderate inflammation
More than 10 mg/dl:	Marked inflammation

When the CRP level is elevated markedly early rheumatoid arthritis, both it and the ESR are useful for predicting severe and erosive disease.[7] In a prospective study of 109 consecutive patients who fulfilled classification criteria for rheumatoid arthritis, the CRP level was found to be a useful short-term correlate with functional outcomes (Devlin et al., Abstract 617). Confounding easy use of the results, however, is the puzzling reality that, in many patients who have a beneficial response to therapy with NSAIDs or methotrexate, the ESR and CRP values do not necessarily fall as one might predict or hope.[8] In addition, there is no convincing evidence that a drug that has the ability to diminish the acute-phase response (i.e., causing a decrease in ESR or CRP) has per se a beneficial influence on the disease process.[9] This dissociation between acute-phase responses and rheumatoid disease activity in certain situations indicates that IL-6 is a secondary, not a primary, mediator of rheumatoid synovitis.

In summary, research on the biology and chemistry of the acute-phase response has given scientific rationale for use of the ESR and CRP in following the activity of synovitis in rheumatoid arthritis.

REFERENCES

1. Dinarello, C. A.: Interleukin-1 and the pathogenesis of the acute-phase response. N. Engl. J. Med. 311:1413, 1984.
2. Kushner, I.: Acute phase response. Clin. Aspects Autoimmun. 3:20, 1989.
3. Castell, J. V., Gomez-Lechon, M. J., David, M., et al.: Recombinant human interleukin-6 (IL-6/BSF-2/HSF) regulates the synthesis of acute phase proteins in human hepatocytes. FEBS Lett. 232:347, 1988.
4. Houssain, F. A., Devogelaer, J. P., Van Damme, J., et al.: Interleukin-6 in synovial fluid and serum of patients with rheumatoid arthritis and other inflammatory arthritides. Arthritis Rheum. 31:784, 1988.
5. Dasgupta, B., Corkill, M., Kirkham, B., et al.: Serial estimation of interleukin 6 as a measure of systemic disease in rheumatoid arthritis. J. Rheumatol. 19:22, 1992.
6. Morley, J. J., and Kushner, I.: C-reactive protein levels in disease. Ann. N. Y. Acad. Sci. 389:406, 1982.
7. Amos, R. S., Constable, T. J., Crockson, R. A., et al.: Rheumatoid arthritis: relation of serum C-reactive protein and erythrocyte sedimentation rates to radiographic changes. Br. Med. J. 1:195, 1977.
8. Forster, P. J. G., and McConkey, B.: The effect of antirheumatic drugs on circulating immune complexes in rheumatoid arthritis. Q. J. Med. 58:29, 1986.
9. Kushner, I.: C-reactive protein in rheumatology. Arthritis Rheum. 34:1065, 1991.

23

Biochemical Markers Associated with Rheumatoid Arthritis

The goal—indeed, the Grail—for many clinical investigators interested in rheumatoid arthritis has been to find a biochemical marker that is specific for rheumatoid arthritis, as well as being sensitive and, at the same time, useful for prognosis. At this time, no successful candidate test has been identified. Certainly, none can compete with the prognostic capability of *HLA-DRB1* genotypes in predicting patients with aggressive disease.

In the quest for the ideal marker, however, numerous interesting associations of various molecules and rheumatoid arthritis have been recognized. A number of these are described in this chapter. Very few are commonly available for diagnosis or prognosis, but each tells us a little more about this disease. In the future, refinements of the tests and cost-effectiveness may bring a number of them into common practice.

The markers discussed are in two groups: those related and those not related to connective tissue destruction.

MARKERS ASSOCIATED WITH CYTOKINES, NUCLEAR PROTEINS, INFLAMMATION, AND IMMUNITY

As can be appreciated from Table 23–1, there are many indices of inflammation and the immune response that can be measured in either serum or synovial fluid that correlate with clinical or radiographic findings in the disease. Several of these (e.g., soluble IL-2R, soluble CD4, IL-6, and IL-1β) would be expected to correlate, given what we know about pathophysiology. Others (e.g., lower selenium and zinc levels in serum of rheumatoid patients) are somewhat surprising. Most intriguing are the positive anti-keratin (filaggrin) and anti-

perinuclear (profilaggrin) antibodies, because of their apparent high specificity. None of these assays is available outside research laboratories, but several must be evaluated carefully for their usefulness for assessment or prognosis.

MARKERS OF INCREASED CONNECTIVE TISSUE TURNOVER

A very readable review of this subject is found in a summary by Poole and Dieppe.[27] A good prognostic measure to predict the rates of joint destruction would be very useful, because radiographic changes lag behind true damage to cartilage in joints.

Whereas propeptides (amino- and carboxyl-terminal propeptides) of collagen type II are indicators in serum of new collagen synthesis in articular cartilage, evidence of type II collagen degradation is demonstrated by assay of collagen cross-links in urine. Bone synthesis is reflected by the presence of excess serum osteocalcin (synthesized by osteoclasts).[28]

From the data summarized in Table 23–2, it is apparent that the **amino-terminal type III procollagen peptide** levels are elevated in proportion to the intensity of synovitis, and that **cartilage oligomeric protein** (COMP) is elevated in patients with rapidly erosive disease. The concentrations of **chondroitin sulfate epitope 846** have an inverse relationship to erosive disease, CRP concentration, and ESR. In the future there may be cost-effective ways to measure COMP and epitope 846 as independent markers of disease activity that can predict prognosis of the proliferative/destructive component of rheumatoid arthritis.

TABLE 23–1. Markers Reflecting Immune and Other Cellular Activity Unrelated to Connective Tissue Destruction

MARKER	COMMENT
Soluble IL-2 receptors (sIL-2R)	Both isoforms have been reported elevated in sera and synovial fluid of patients with rheumatoid arthritis, but neither has correlated with the ESR or with cellular/surface-bound IL-2.[1]
Soluble CD4	Patients with rheumatoid arthritis have increased levels in serum and synovial fluids compared with age-matched healthy controls.[2] Serum levels fell in patients preceding clinical improvement. Synovial fluid levels correlated positively with sIL-2R levels.
Anti-Gm allotypes	These antibodies share with rheumatoid factors reactivity to determinants expressed on the Fc portion of the immunoglobulin molecule. There appears to be a link between antibodies to Gm allotypes and joint destruction in early rheumatoid arthritis.[3]
Agalactosyl IgG	This complicated assay measured the percentage of oligosaccharide chains attached to the $C\gamma2$ domain of IgG that lack galactose (GAL[0]). In one study of 60 consecutive patients presenting with early-onset synovitis, the measure of GAL(0) gave a positive predictive value for a diagnosis of rheumatoid arthritis in 94% of the patients[4] (see Chapter 6).
Interleukin-6	There are increased levels in synovial fluids of rheumatoid arthritis patients; the finding of increased IL-6 in patients who had no measurable rheumatoid factor dissociates the prognostic usefulness of these two proteins.[5]
	There was positive correlation between synovial fluid IL-6 levels and CRP levels, and inverse correlation with the glucocorticoid dose used in therapy.[6] In individual patients, a positive correlation between synovial fluid IL-6 levels and total leukocyte count and a negative correlation with pH was found.[7]
	These and other data help establish IL-6 as a primary mediator for generation of an inflammatory and destructive synovitis. It is activated by IL-1 and then appears to mediate expression of many inflammatory cytokines and other cell-mediated processes.
Interleukin-1β	IL-1β levels in knee joints paralleled inflammation in patients with asymmetric disease.[8] This major cytokine is discussed in detail in Chapter 9.
von Willebrand factor in synovial fluid	There are increased levels in inflammatory synovial fluid, correlating with α_1-antitrypsin and with the WBC count.[9]
Selenium	This is lower in serum of rheumatoid arthritis than in control patients; this essential nutrient is used in systems protecting cells from oxidative damage.[10]
Zinc	Serum and plasma zinc levels are decreased significantly in patients with rheumatoid arthritis,[11] whereas synovial fluid levels in rheumatoid patients have been reported as elevated.[12]
IgA-antitrypsin complex level in serum	In 33 patients, higher levels were the only measured parameter that predicted erosions found on radiographs.[13]
α_1-Antitrypsin phenotypes	A significant increase in the M1M2 phenotype was found in both rheumatoid arthritis and severe rheumatoid arthritis; the M3 phenotype was protective. All three types inhibit proteases equally well.[14]

Table continued on opposite page

TABLE 23–1. *Continued*

MARKER	COMMENT
Serum phospholipase A2	Levels correlated with disease activity ($p < .0001$) assayed by joint scores or by a lab index (hemoglobin, peripheral circulating lymphocytes, platelet count, and ESR.) Phospholipase A2 generates free arachidonic acid; when injected alone into experimental animals, it causes inflammation.[15]
Synovial fluid angiotensin-converting enzyme	Elevated in rheumatoid arthritis more than osteoarthritis; it probably reflects numbers of synovial macrophages.[16]
Complement C3b/C4b receptors (CR1) on erythrocytes	CR1 binds preferentially to the C3b fragment of C3 and to C4b. In blood vessels, 80–90% of CR1 is on erythrocytes; in rheumatoid arthritis, the CR1 sites per erythrocytes are low, as in SLE.[17]
Complement activation products	The C1s:C1-INH complex, C3bp, and the terminal C5b-9 complexes in plasma and synovial fluid are elevated in rheumatoid arthritis and correlate with levels of rheumatoid factor.[18]
	Concentrations of C5a, a potent chemoattractant for neutrophils, were elevated to a mean of 2.5×10^{-9} mol/l in 22 rheumatoid synovial fluids.[19]
	C1q-bearing immune complexes are often found in rheumatoid synovial fluids and sera.[20] Synovial fluid levels of C9- and C3-containing immune complexes were five to eight times those in plasma, implying a local activation of the whole cascade within the joints.[21]
Serum C1q levels in blood	Increased levels in serum suggest that unbound protein is present in excess of the bound complexes.[22]
Anti-keratin antibodies	Serum IgG antibodies that label the stratum corneum of rat esophagus epithelium are reported by a number of investigators to be the most specific serologic criterion for the diagnosis of rheumatoid arthritis. It is projected to allow 44% of rheumatoid arthritis to be diagnosed with a specificity of 99%.[23] In a more refined assay giving the same specificity, 70% sensitivity was achieved in a study of 88 patients using an immunoblot technique.[24] The antigen against which these autoantibodies are binding has been identified is **filaggrin,** a basic intermediate filament–associated protein involved in the aggregation of cytokeratin filaments during terminal differentiation in cells.[25]
Anti-perinuclear factor	The antigen bound by these autoantibodies is a component of human buccal mucosa cells found within keratohyalin granules in the cytoplasm. These granules contain **profilaggrin**. Therefore, the anti-keratin and anti-perinuclear antibodies may be linked to the same or very closely related antigens. In one study, the percentage of serum samples positive for rheumatoid factor among patients with rheumatoid arthritis was 83%, and for anti-perinuclear factor, 81%. However, more than 11% of the sera without anti-perinuclear factor had rheumatoid factor, and 6% without rheumatoid factor contained anti-perinuclear factor.[26]

TABLE 23–2. Markers of Increased Connective Tissue Turnover

MARKER	COMMENT
3-Hydroxypyridinium (pyridinoline and deoxypyridinoline) collagen cross-links (urine)	These are the most common cross-links of cartilage and are significantly elevated in urine in rheumatoid patients, correlating well with the ESR and CRP level.[29,30] In addition, the rates of excretion of these cross-links correlated with appendicular bone loss in early rheumatoid arthritis. Treatment of rheumatoid patients with disease-modifying drugs led to decreased urinary cross-links, although use of glucocorticoids actually increased cross-link excretion, a probable reflection of the catabolic influence of steroids upon bone.[30]
Cartilage oligomeric protein (serum and synovial fluid)	This is an anionic protein found only in cartilage; significant elevations in serum have been found in patients with rapidly progressive erosive rheumatoid arthritis,[31] and serum levels of COMP may reflect those in synovial fluids.[32]
Chondroitin sulfate epitope 846 (serum)	In contrast with COMP (see above), this 846-amino-acid peptide—believed to be preferentially present on newly synthesized aggrecan molecules—was increased in patients with a benign disease course; 846 levels were inversely related to the ESR and CRP level.[33,34] It is possible that increased epitope 846 levels reflect a dominant presence in the joints of reparative cytokines such as TGFβ that stimulate connective tissue matrix biosynthesis.
Hyaluronan (plasma)	In joints, the major producer of hyaluronic acid (hyaluronan) is synovial cells. In rheumatoid arthritis, the level in plasma is elevated,[35] sometimes as high as sevenfold, but does not correlate with joint scores or other laboratory tests.[36] In another study, the serum hyaluronan levels actually increased during periods of clinical improvement.[37]
Keratan sulfate (KS) (serum and synovial fluid)	This is increased in both rheumatoid arthritis and osteoarthritis. The fragments were polydisperse in size, and were largely high-density proteoglycans. No relationship to joint scores or disease duration was found.[38] In another study, more consistent with previous reports, serum KS was reduced in both rheumatoid arthritis and osteoarthritis and in rheumatoid arthritis was inversely related to systemic and joint-involvement markers.[33] The reduced KS may be explained by the finding that, in rheumatoid patients, serum KS correlated *inversely* with circulating levels of both collagenase, stromelysin, and the endogenous inhibitor of these enzymes, TIMP-1.[39] The inference is that up-regulation of TIMP may be suppressing cartilage aggrecan synthesis. Alternatively, the majority of aggrecan may have been depleted before these measurements were made.
Macrophage surface elastolytic activity (synovial fluid)	Using proteoglycan concentration in synovial fluid as a marker for cartilage degradation, there was correlation with elastase activity and with IL-6 levels, but no correlation with elastolytic activity and type III collagen fragments could be found. These findings could be interpreted to mean that this protease activity does not correlate with synovial collagen degradation.[40]
Matrix metalloproteases and tissue inhibitor of metalloproteases 1	Sandwich enzyme immunoassays have detected higher levels of both MMP-3 (stromelysin) and TIMP-1[41] in rheumatoid patients. These correlated well with the ESR, CRP level, and an articular index. The serum levels of stromelysin correlated ($r_s = .588$) with synovial fluid concentration.
Osteocalcin (serum)	This protein is a vitamin K–dependent protein (also known as bone γ-carboxyglutamic acid–containing protein), and is a sensitive and specific serum marker for bone formation. In one series it was elevated only in late-onset rheumatoid arthritis (after age 65).[42] It is decreased in women with postmenopausal osteoporosis.
Procollagen type II C-propeptide (serum and synovial fluid)	The presence of this propeptide in body fluids is indicative of cartilage collagen synthesis; patients with rheumatoid arthritis have abnormally elevated serum levels, and synovial fluid levels are greater than those of serum.[34]
Procollagen type III C-propeptide (serum)	Type III collagen is usually found in more than usual quantity in areas where new collagen formation amid new blood vessels is present. There is a correlation between serum levels of propeptide and the mass of synovitis in rheumatoid arthritis (viz. the Thompson joint score). Thus, the levels are increased in patients who have arthritis in major weight-bearing joints.[43] Another study provided evidence that both serum hyaluronan and amino-terminal type III procollagen peptide are elevated in proportion to the intensity of synovitis in rheumatoid patients.[44]

Table continued on opposite page

TABLE 23–2. *Continued*

MARKER	COMMENT
Procollagen type I C-propeptide (serum)	This peptide is cleaved off the procollagen molecule before fibrils are formed. Using a radioimmunoassay, levels of this peptide in serum were found to correlate strongly with measures of impairment in rheumatoid arthritis, such as function and the number and extent of erosions.[45] It is of interest that the metalloenzyme that cleaves off the C-terminal propeptide of collagen types I, II, and III (procollagen C-proteinase) has a structure and function identical to that of bone morphogenetic protein 1, which can induce bone formation within soft connective tissues and, possibly, contributes to activation of TGFβ.[46]
Procollagen type I and III N-propeptides (pIN-P and pIIIN-P) and cross-linked C-terminal peptide (ITCP)	A recent study has compared pIN-P and pIIIN-P (products of collagen biosynthesis) from synovial fluid and serum with a breakdown product of collagen that has previously been incorporated into fibrils and cross-linked (ITCP). The data showed high synovial fluid–serum ratios for these markers, indicating that there is high turnover of collagen within the joint. Synovial fluid ITDP correlated well with progressive radiographic findings in the corresponding knee joints.[47]

SUMMARY

It is not likely that more complex and expensive assays for purposes of diagnosis and prognosis of rheumatoid arthritis will be necessary or helpful to rheumatologists, because the diagnosis is generally a clinical one, and treatment rarely is determined by one or another test that is oriented toward diagnosis. However, if tests were available and validated to prove an association with erosive destruction of joints better than other available prognostic factors, they could be very useful.

For evaluation of joint destruction, assays for components specific for cartilage are the best to focus on. Elevated COMP and stromelysin levels may be the most sensitive indicators for this, and data now are needed on sensitivity and specificity.

REFERENCES

1. Vaisberg, M., and Scheinberg, M. A.: Simultaneous evaluation of membrane bound and soluble interleukin 2 receptor expression in the blood and synovial fluid of patients with rheumatoid arthritis. Clin. Exp. Rheumatol. 8:579, 1990.
2. Symons, J. A., McCulloch, J. F., Wood, N. C., et al.: Soluble CD4 in patients with rheumatoid arthritis and osteoarthritis. Clin. Immunol. Immunopathol. 60:72, 1991.
3. Eberhardt, K., Grubb, R., Johnson, U., et al.: HLA-DR antigens, Gm allotypes, and anti-allotypes in early rheumatoid arthritis—their relation to disease progression. J. Rheumatol. 20:1825, 1993.
4. Young, A., Sumar, N., Bodman, K., et al.: Agalactosyl IgG: an aid to differential diagnosis in early synovitis. Arthritis Rheum. 34:1425, 1991.
5. Sawada, T., Hirohata, S., Inoue, T., et al.: Correlation between rheumatoid factor and IL-6 activity in synovial fluids from patients with rheumatoid arthritis. Clin. Exp. Rheumatol. 9:363, 1991.
6. Brozik, M., Rosztóczy, I., Merétey, K., et al.: Interleukin 6 levels in synovial fluids of patients with different arthritides: correlation with local IgM rheumatoid factor and systemic acute phase protein production. J. Rheumatol. 19:63, 1992.
7. Miltenburg, A. M. M., van Laar, J. M., de Kuiper, R., et al.: Interleukin-6 activity in paired samples of synovial fluid: correlation of synovial fluid interleukin-6 levels with clinical and laboratory parameters of inflammation. Br. J. Rheumatol. 30:186, 1991.
8. Rooney, M., Symons, J. A., and Duff, G. W.: Interleukin 1 beta in synovial fluid is related to local disease activity in rheumatoid arthritis. Rheumatol. Int. 10:217, 1990.
9. Bolosiu, H. D., Rus, V., Parasca, I., et al.: Von Willebrand factor in synovial fluid. Clin. Exp. Rheumatol. 9:395, 1991.
10. O'Dell, J. R., Lemley-Gillespie, S., Palmer, W. R., et al.: Serum selenium concentrations in rheumatoid arthritis. Ann. Rheum. Dis. 30:376, 1991.
11. Dore-Duffy, P., Peterson, M., Catalanotto, F., et al.: Zinc profiles in rheumatoid arthritis. Clin. Exp. Rheumatol. 8:541, 1990.
12. Neidermeier, W., and Griggs, J. H.: Trace metal composition of synovial fluid and blood serum in patients with rheumatoid arthritis. J. Chron. Dis. 23:527, 1971.
13. Davis, M. J., Dawes, P. T., Fowler, P. D., et al.: The association and predictive value of the complex immunoglobulin A-α_1-antitrypsin in the development of erosions in early rheumatoid arthritis. Scand. J. Rheumatol. 20:23, 1991.
14. Papiha, S. S., Pal, B., Walker, D., et al.: α_1 Antitrypsin (PI) phenotypes in two rheumatic diseases: a reappraisal of the association of PI subtypes in rheumatoid arthritis. Ann. Rheum. Dis. 48:48, 1989.
15. Pruzanski, W., Keystone, E. C., Sternby, B., et al.: Serum phospholipase A_2 correlates with disease activity in rheumatoid arthritis. J. Rheumatol. 15:1351, 1988.
16. Blann, A. D.: von Willebrand factor antigen and angiotensin converting enzyme in synovial fluid. Scand. J. Rheumatol. 20:213, 1991.
17. Corvetta, A., Pomponio, G., Bencivenga, R., et al.: Low number of complement C3b/C4b receptors (CR1) on erythrocytes from patients with essential mixed cryoglobulinemia, systemic lupus erythematosus and rheumatoid arthritis: relationship with disease activity, anticardiolipin antibodies, complement activation and therapy. J. Rheumatol. 18:1021, 1991.

18. Auda, G., Holme, E. R., Davidson, J. E., et al.: Measurement of complement activation products in patients with chronic rheumatic diseases. Rheumatol. Int. 10:185, 1990.

19. Jose, P. J., Moss, I. K., Maini, R. N., et al.: Measurement of the chemotactic complement fragment C5a in rheumatoid synovial fluids by radioimmunoassay: role of C5a in the acute inflammatory phase. Ann. Rheum. Dis. 49:747, 1990.

20. Antes, U., Heinz, H.-P., Schutz, D., et al.: C1q-bearing immune complexes detected by a monoclonal antibody to human C1q in rheumatoid arthritis sera and synovial fluids. Rheumatol. Int. 10:245, 1991.

21. Ölmez, Ü., Garred, P., Mollness, T. E., et al.: C3 activation products, C3 containing immune complexes, the terminal complement complex and native C9 in patients with rheumatoid arthritis. Scand. J. Rheumatol. 20:183, 1991.

22. Olsen, N. J., Ho, E., and Barats, L.: Clinical correlations with serum C1q levels in patients with rheumatoid arthritis. Arthritis Rheum. 34:187, 1991.

23. Vincent, C., Serre, G. G., Lapeyre, F., et al.: High diagnostic value in rheumatoid arthritis of antibodies to the stratum corneum of rat oesophagus epithelium, so-called "anti-keratin antibodies." Ann. Rheum. Dis. 48:712, 1989.

24. Gomes-Daudrix, V., Sebbag, M., Girbal, E., et al.: Immunoblotting detection of so-called "anti-keratin antibodies": a new assay for the diagnosis of rheumatoid arthritis. Ann. Rheum. Dis. 53:735, 1994.

25. Simon, M., Girbal, E., Sebbag, M., et al.: The cytokeratin filament-aggregating protein fillagrin is the target of the so-called "antikeratin antibodies," autoantibodies specific for rheumatoid arthritis. J. Clin. Invest. 92:1387, 1993.

26. Hoet, R. M. A., Boerbooms, A. M. T., Arends, M., et al.: Antiperinuclear factor, a marker autoantibody for rheumatoid arthritis: colocalisation of the perinuclear factor and profilaggrin. Ann. Rheum. Dis. 50:611, 1991.

27. Poole, A. R., and Dieppe, P.: Biological markers in rheumatoid arthritis. Semin. Arthritis Rheum. 23:17, 1994.

28. Poole, A. R.: Immunochemical markers of joint inflammation, skeletal damage and repair: where are we now? Ann. Rheum. Dis. 53:3, 1994.

29. Black, D., Marabani, M., Sturrock, R. D., et al.: Urinary excretion of the hydroxypyridium cross links of collagen in patients with arthritis. Ann. Rheum. Dis. 48:641, 1989.

30. Seibel, M. J., Duncan, A., and Robins, S. P.: Urinary hydroxypyridinium cross links provide indices of cartilage and bone involvement in arthritic disease. J. Rheumatol. 16:964, 1989.

31. Forslind, K., Eberhardt, K., Jonsson, A., et al.: Increased serum concentrations of cartilage oligomeric matrix protein: a prognostic marker in early rheumatoid arthritis. Br. J. Rheumatol. 31:593, 1992.

32. Saxne, T., Glennås A., Kivien, T. K., et al.: Release of cartilage macromolecules into the synovial fluid in patients with acute and prolonged phases of reactive arthritis. Arthritis Rheum. 36:20, 1993.

33. Poole, A. R., Ionescu, M., Swan, A., et al.: Changes in cartilage metabolism in arthritis are reflected by altered serum and synovial fluid levels of the cartilage proteoglycan aggrecan. J. Clin. Invest. 94:25, 1994.

34. Mansson, B., Carey, D., Alini, M., et al.: Cartilage and bone metabolism in rheumatoid arthritis: differences between rapid and slow progression of disease identified by serum markers of cartilage metabolism. J. Clin. Invest. 95:1071, 1995.

35. Engström-Laurent, A., Hällgren, R.: Circulating hyaluronate in rheumatoid arthritis: relationship to inflammatory activity and the effect of corticosteroid therapy. Ann. Rheum. Dis. 44:83, 1985.

36. Goldberg, R. L., Huff, J. P., Lenz, M. E., et al.: Elevated plasma levels of hyaluronate in patients with osteoarthritis and rheumatoid arthritis. Arthritis Rheum. 34:799, 1991.

37. Paimela, L., Heiskanen, A., Kurki, P., et al.: Serum hyaluronate level as a predictor of radiologic progression in early rheumatoid arthritis. Arthritis Rheum. 34:815, 1991.

38. Mehraban, F., Finegan, C. K., and Moskowitz, R. W.: Serum keratan sulfate. Arthritis Rheum. 34:383, 1991.

39. Manicourt, D.-H., Fujimoto, N., Obata, K., et al.: Levels of circulating collagenase, stromelysin, and tissue inhibitor of matrix metalloproteinases 1 in patients with rheumatoid arthritis: relationship to serum levels of antigenic keratan sulfate and systemic parameters of inflammation. Arthritis Rheum. 38:1031, 1995.

40. Jensen, H. S., Jensen, L. T., Saxne, T., et al.: Human monocyte elastolytic activity, the propeptides of types I and III procollagen, proteoglycans, and interleukin-6 in synovial fluid from patients with arthritis. Clin. Exp. Rheumatol. 9:391, 1991.

41. Yoshihara, Y., Obata, K., Fujimoto, N., et al.: Increased levels of stromelysin-1 and tissue inhibitor of metalloproteinases-1 in sera from patients with rheumatoid arthritis. Arthritis Rheum. 38:969, 1995.

42. Marhoffer, W., Schatz, H., Stracke, H., et al.: Serum osteocalcin levels in rheumatoid arthritis: a marker for accelerated bone turnover in late onset rheumatoid arthritis. J. Rheumatol. 18:1158, 1991.

43. Ferraccioli, G. F., Cavalieri, F., Rioda, W. T., et al.: Relationship between procollagen III peptide serum levels, synovitis of weight bearing joints and disability in rheumatoid arthritis. Scand. J. Rheum. 20:314, 1991.

44. Hørslev-Petersen, K., Bentsen, K. D., Engström-Laurent, A., et al.: Serum amino terminal type III procollagen peptide and serum hyaluronan in rheumatoid arthritis: relation to clinical and serological parameters of inflammation during 8 and 24 months' treatment with levamisole, penicillamine, or azathioprine. Ann. Rheum. Dis. 47:116, 1988.

45. Hakala, M., Risteli, L., Manelius, J., et al.: Increased type I collagen degradation correlates with disease severity in rheumatoid arthritis. Ann. Rheum. Dis. 52:866, 1993.

46. Kessler, E., Takahara, K., Biniaminov, L., et al.: Bone morphogenetic protein-1: the type I procollagen C-proteinase. Science 271:360, 1996.

47. Hakala, M., Åman, S., Luukkainen, R., et al.: Application of markers of collagen metabolism in serum and synovial fluid for assessment of disease process in patients with rheumatoid arthritis. Ann. Rheum. Dis. 54:886, 1995.

24

Assessment of Rheumatoid Arthritis

In dealing with rheumatoid arthritis, as with many other chronic diseases, assessment of both progress of the disease and treatment is of vital importance to the individual patient, the physician, and—if one holds the tenet that we learn from both success and failure—other patients. An accurate assessment of how a given patient is faring helps prevent false optimism or inappropriate discouragement for both patient and physician. Similarly, accurate assays for clinical improvement (or the lack of it) are crucial for all clinical trials in rheumatoid arthritis, especially when one considers that death, the principal outcome measurement for more acutely severe diseases, rarely strikes rheumatoid patients early in their clinical course.

The ideal measures for assessment should be "sensible, reliable, accurate, sensitive to change over time, not redundant, and although limited in number, comprehensive."[1] Rheumatoid arthritis is a multidimensional process, not a distinct and focused one, such as an isolated hemolytic anemia. Assessment must be broad enough to encompass all dimensions that have potential for change.

Assessment of progress is different from **prognosis**. Prognosis extrapolates from a known set of severity indices and the degree of measured activity of disease to a prediction of outcome. Assessment is the accurate evaluation of how the disease process is progressing over time.

When more than three or four points in time are captured in assessment of an individual patient, it is possible to derive a prognosis for that person. It is believed that the most sensitive and significant measure of assessment of therapy is fitting a straight line to pretreatment data (at least three points in time) and measuring the difference in slope of that line compared with a similar line connecting two or more time points during treatment.[2] Barring an abrupt change resulting from appearance of a major complication or sudden onset of remission, the lower the slope, the better the prognosis.

ASSESSMENT OF THE INDIVIDUAL PATIENT

Traditionally, accurate assessment of a given patient with rheumatoid arthritis over a period of time was believed to be directly proportional to the number of hard data from joint counts, grip strength, walking time, and laboratory tests, including radiographs. In recent years, however, studies have suggested that there are better ways to assess progress of individual patients.

For most patients, a self-report questionnaire based on degrees of difficulty in performing activities of daily living correlates well with joint count, radiographic score, acute-phase reactants, grip strength, walking time, functional class estimates, and global self-assessment.[3,4] One example of such a form assesses only eight functions[5] (Table 24–1) from a larger array generated at Stanford referred to as the Health Assessment Questionnaire (HAQ).[6,7] (The HAQ is printed in full in the appendix to this chapter.) The modified HAQ[5] although easy to administer and a time saver, has the disadvantage of having a ceiling effect; it fails to detect clinical improvement in patients with relatively few impairments in activities of daily living, whereas the original HAQ had sufficient sensitivity to demonstrate these changes.[8] At this time it seems wise not to use the modified HAQ when one hopes to detect functional changes in early disease.

A few modifications of the full HAQ are appropriate in certain contexts. In patients with progressive articular disease, particularly when orthopedic surgery may be indicated, the physician should take added time to add a joint count to the data at sequential time points. The Thompson index (a modified Lansbury index) uses a relatively small set of joints and weights the data from each joint to reflect joint surface area[9,10] (Table 24–2). This is a useful way to incorporate the "synovitis burden" (akin to the tumor burden for cancer patients) in evaluating an individual patient.

An even simpler joint count (28 joints) has been

TABLE 24–1. Activities of Daily Living and Visual Analogue Questionnaire

A. How often is it PAINFUL for you to:

	Never	Sometimes	Most of the Time	Always
• Dress yourself?	————	————	————	————
• Get in and out of bed?	————	————	————	————
• Lift a cup or glass to your lips?	————	————	————	————
• Walk outdoors on flat ground?	————	————	————	————
• Wash and dry your entire body?	————	————	————	————
• Bend down to pick up clothing from the floor?	————	————	————	————
• Turn faucets on or off?	————	————	————	————
• Get in and out of a car?	————	————	————	————

B. How much pain have you had in the PAST WEEK (mark the scale)

No pain ————————————————————————————— Pain as bad as it could be
0   100

From Callahan, L. F., Brooks, R. H., Summey, J. A., et al.: Quantitative pain assessment for routine care of rheumatoid arthritis patients, using a pain scale based on activities of daily living and a visual analog pain scale. Arthritis Rheum. 30:630, 1987. Used by permission.

generated.[11] The joints evaluated are 10 PIP joints, 10 MCP joints, both wrists, both elbows, both shoulders, and both knees. In studies aiming to validate this reduced joint count using data from a large cohort participating in clinical trials, it was found that most of the joints that are swollen or tender in rheumatoid patients are among those in the 28-joint count, and that changes in joint tenderness and swelling during therapy were measured in this count.[12] There are few indications to use the older version that included 66 or 68 joints, but many rheumatologists add metatarsal joints to the 28 listed above, because the feet are usually involved early in rheumatoid arthritis, especially radiographically.

A number of specific caveats about assessment are appropriate to mention. In almost all patients with rheumatoid arthritis, functional disability and radiographic changes develop very early in the course of disease.[13,14] In many if not most cases of rheumatoid arthritis, it appears that, by the time the patient's disease is taken seriously enough that longitudinal assessment is done, evidence for cartilage damage in the joints has become apparent. Therefore, objective measures (the HAQ and modi-

fied joint counts) should be instituted early, not when deformity or gross loss of function appear.

Radiographic indices are of little use in assessing individual patients on a regular basis, primarily because of documented differences among different physician interpretations of the same films,[15] the lag time between cartilage damage and the appearance of radiographic abnormalities, and a remarkably poor correlation with function of patients.[16] They are essential, however, in assessing clinical trials and for evaluating plans for corrective surgery when synovitis persists and deformity develops.

At present, there are no laboratory tests for monitoring rheumatoid arthritis that are both specific and sensitive in the information they present. For example, the usefulness of a test for rheumatoid factor in diagnosis or assessment is very small[17] (Tables 24–3 and 24–4). As a screening test in patients with poorly focused joint complaints, the predictive value of a rheumatoid factor test is small as well. Changes in titers of rheumatoid factor should not be used to monitor therapy. In rheumatologic practices, where patients are referred with more focused disease patterns, the predictive values for tests for rheumatoid factor are higher.[18] In contrast to its

TABLE 24-2. Weighted and Selective Index for Activity of Synovitis

JOINT	WEIGHTED FACTOR (RELATED TO JOINT SURFACE AREA)	DEGREE OF TENDERNESS *AND* SWELLING (SCALE: 0 to 3)	=	JOINT SCORE
Elbow				
R	48			
L	48			
Wrist				
R	32			
L	32			
MCP (separately)				
R	5			
L	5			
PIP (separately)				
R	5			
L	5			
Knee				
R	95			
L	95			
Ankle (mortise)				
R	32			
L	32			
1st MTP				
R	8			
L	8			
2nd to 5th MTP (separately)				
R	5			
L	5			
	TOTAL			

From Thompson, P. W., Silman, A., Kirwan, J. R., et al.: Articular indices of joint inflammation in rheumatoid arthritis. Arthritis Rheum. 30:618, 1987. Used by permission.

TABLE 24-3. Rheumatic Diseases Associated with a Positive Rheumatoid Factor

DISEASE	FREQUENCY (%)
Rheumatoid arthritis	50–90
Systemic lupus erythematosus	15–35
Sjögren's syndrome	75–95
Systemic sclerosis	20–30
Polymyositis/dermatomyositis	5–10
Cryoglobulinemia	40–100
Mixed connective tissue disease	50–60

From Schmerling, R. H., and Delbanco, T. L.: The rheumatoid factor: an analysis of clinical utility. Am. J. Med. 91:528, 1991. Used by permission. Copyright 1991 by Excerpta Medica Inc.

lack of usefulness in assessment of therapy, rheumatoid factor is useful for prognosis; a positive test is related to increased mortality in both old and young patients.

Objective tests that are useful for assessing progress of individual patients and are not excessively expensive include the following:

- **Accurate patient weight:** The correlation of TNFα levels with loss of body mass and activity of arthritis make this often-ignored measurement useful, particularly in patients with aggressive disease. A therapeutic goal must be to keep patients from developing even mild cachexia.

- **Acute-phase response:** When available at a reasonable cost, the CRP assay gives a wider linear response with less variation than the less expensive Westergren sedimentation rate. The sedimentation rate, nevertheless, is very useful in assessment of an individual patient who has had demonstrably increased test results during phases of active disease.

TABLE 24–4. Nonrheumatic Conditions Associated with a Positive Rheumatoid Factor

CONDITION	FREQUENCY (%)
Aging (>age 70)	10–25
Infection	
Bacterial endocarditis	25–50
Liver disease*	15–40
Tuberculosis	8
Syphilis	Up to 13
Parasitic diseases†	20–90
Leprosy*	5–58
Viral infection†‡	15–65
Pulmonary disease	
Sarcoidosis	3–33
Interstitial pulmonary fibrosis	10–50
Silicosis	30–50
Asbestosis	30
Miscellaneous diseases	
Primary biliary cirrhosis*	45–70
Malignancy*§	10–20

From Schmerling, R. H., and Delbanco, T. L.: The rheumatoid factor: an analysis of clinical utility. Am. J. Med. 91:528, 1991. Used by permission. Copyright 1991 by Excerpta Medica Inc.

* Diseases that may mimic rheumatoid arthritis.

† Chagas' disease, leishmaniasis, onchocerciasis, and schistosomiasis are the best-documented examples.

‡ Rubella, mumps, and influenza are the best-documented examples.

§ Leukemias and colon carcinoma are the best-documented examples.

It has been emphasized appropriately (Pincus et al., Abstract 630) that there are important differences and implications for prognosis between *markers of disease activity* and *damage markers* in rheumatoid arthritis. Whereas the former (e.g., joint counts, pain estimates) may be stable or show improvement, in many of these patients evidence for joint damage that is expressed as loss of function and radiographic deterioration actually worsens. This, as emphasized previously, is due to the inevitable and irreversible deterioration of articular cartilage once proteoglycans are depleted and peripheral invasion by pannocytes begins.

The Core Evaluation recommended by the ACR (see Table 24–5) is very appropriate to use for individual patients as well as groups within clinical trials. Another set of response criteria for rheumatoid arthritis have been developed by the European League Against Rheumatism [EULAR].[19] These are listed in the section on Assessment in Clinical Trials. The EULAR criteria also can be used by practitioners to get an objective reading of whether individual patients are not responding, or are having a moderate or good response, to a specific therapeutic regimen. In recognizing that patients with rheumatoid arthritis can have multiple manifestations of disease, the EULAR study uses a validated index known as the Disease Activity Score (DAS), which incorporates the Ritchie Index (joint count), the number of swollen joints, the ESR, and "general health" quantified on a 100-mm visual analogue scale. The DAS was calculated by the following formula:

$$DAS = 054 (\sqrt{RAI} + 0.065 (SwJ + s) + 0.33 (\ln ESR) + 0.0072 (GH)$$

where

$$
\begin{aligned}
RAI &= \text{Ritchie articular index} \\
ESR &= \text{erythrocyte sedimentation rate in mm/hr} \\
SwJ + s &= \text{number of swollen joints} \\
GH &= \text{General Health Status by 100 mm visual analogue scale}
\end{aligned}
$$

ASSESSMENT IN CLINICAL TRIALS

In contrast to evaluation of individual patients, who are "populations of one" followed longitudinally, the challenge in clinical trials is relating changes in the same criterion in different patients in a significant way. In addition, the outcome of such trials must be related to other trials, and therefore the need for numerical scales of assessment is evident. Finally, except in "postmarketing" trials, most drug trials are planned and executed for approval by the Food and Drug Administration; without that approval, no drug can be marketed.

The ACR has published a "core set" of measures of disease activity in rheumatoid arthritis that are recommended for use in clinical trials of all types of drugs or even nonpharmacologic treatment[20,21] (Table 24–5). Using this core set of outcome measures, a subsequent study has tested 40 different definitions of improvement. After exclusion of 32 definitions, 8 were tested to see which were easiest to use and best in accord with rheumatologists' impressions of improvement. The following definition of improvement for use in clinical trials was selected[22]:

- A 20 per cent improvement in tender and swollen joint counts
- A 20 per cent improvement in three of the five remaining ACR core set measures:
    - Patient assessment of pain
    - Patient global assessment of disease activity
    - Physician global assessment of disease activity
    - Disability
    - ESR or CRP values

TABLE 24–5. American College of Rheumatology Recommendations of Specific Ways to Assess Each Disease Activity Measure in the Core Set

DISEASE ACTIVITY MEASURE	METHOD OF ASSESSMENT*
1. Tender joint count†	ACR tender joint count,[11] an assessment of 28 joints. The joint count should be done by scoring several different aspects of tenderness, as assessed by pressure and joint manipulation on physical examination. The information on various types of tenderness should then be collapsed into a single tender-versus-nontender dichotomy.
2. Swollen joint count‡	ACR swollen joint count, an assessment of 28 or more joints. Joints are classified as either swollen or not swollen.
3. Patient's assessment of pain	A horizontal visual analogue scale (usually 10 cm) or Likert scale assessment of the patient's current level of pain.
4. Patient's global assessment of disease activity	The patient's overall assessment of how the arthritis is doing. One acceptable method for determining this is the question from the AIMS instrument: "Considering all the ways your arthritis affects you, mark 'X' on the scale for how well you are doing." An anchored, horizontal, visual analogue scale (usually 10 cm) should be provided. A Likert scale response is also acceptable.
5. Physician's global assessment of disease activity	A horizontal visual analogue scale (usually 10 cm) or Likert scale measure of the physician's assessment of the patient's current disease activity.
6. Patient's assessment of physical function	Any patient self-assessment instrument that has been validated, has reliability, has been proven in rheumatoid arthritis trials to be sensitive to change, and measures physical function in rheumatoid arthritis patients is acceptable. Instruments that have been demonstrated to be sensitive in rheumatoid arthritis trials include the AIMS, the HAQ, the Quality (or Index) of Well Being, the MHIQ, and the MACTAR.
7. Acute-phase reactant value	A Westergren ESR or a CRP level.

Data from Felson et al.,[20] and Cooperating Clinics Committee of the American Rheumatism Association.[21]

* AIMS, Arthritis Impact Measurement Scales; HAQ, Health Assessment Questionnaire; MHIQ, McMaster Health Index Questionnaire; MACTAR, McMaster Toronto Arthritis Patient Preference Disability Questionnaire.

† The 28 joints to be examined for tenderness are the TMJ ($n = 2$), sternoclavicular ($n = 2$), acromioclavicular ($n = 2$), shoulder ($n = 2$), elbow ($n = 2$), wrist ($n = 2$), MCP ($n = 10$), interphalangeal of thumb ($n = 2$), DIP ($n = 8$), PIP ($n = 8$), hip ($n = 2$), knee ($n = 2$), ankle mortise ($n = 2$), and PIP/DIP of the toes ($n = 8$).

‡ The 26 joints to be examined for swelling are the same as those examined for tenderness, except the hip joints are not included.

In comparative trials this definition was found to be statistically powerful and did not identify a large percentage of improvement in patients given placebos. In addition to being appropriate for clinical trials, this definition should prove useful for practicing physicians as they evaluate therapy in individual patients.

If possible, all clinical assessments should be recorded at roughly the same time of day. Circadian variation in pain and swollen joints of patients can cause wide differences in assessment measures.[23]

An empirical approach to the same task used closely spaced assessments over a prolonged time period to search for differences in relative accuracy and sensitivity to change among 14 measures commonly used to assess arthritis activity in rheumatoid patients.[1] The results showed that the physician global assessment, a functional status questionnaire (e.g., the HAQ or modified versions) and the patient global assessment or pain score should be the principal measures used to assess activity of arthritis in rheumatoid arthritis. The laboratory tests studied were the hemoglobin, platelet count, and ESR; only the ESR reflected change in clinical status demonstrated by other measures.

Using the DAS in a study comparing the response of rheumatoid patients to sulfasalazine versus hydroxychloroquine, the EULAR group[19,19a] set the following numbers for disease activity (see earlier equation):

	DAS
LOW disease activity	≤ 2.4
MODERATE disease activity	2.4 to ≤ 3.7
HIGH disease activity	>3.7

A good response to therapy was a DAS improvement of more than 1.2; a moderate response to therapy was a DAS improvement of 1.2 or less but more than 0.6; and no response was a DAS change of 0.6 or less. The EULAR system showed significant validation of accuracy of the criteria (*criteria validity*), association of the criteria with the expected results (*construct validity*), and the ability of the criteria to detect important differences (*discriminant validity*).

Without accurate assessment of patients, the physician cannot be objective in evaluating responses to therapy or giving patients good advice about whether more or less aggressive therapy is indicated. At present, the best advice for the physician following individual patients or for organizers of clinical trials would be to follow either the ACR or EULAR criteria for improvement using the 28-joint count, a modified HAQ, the visual analogue pain scale, and the physician's assessment of global disease activity.

ASSESSMENT BY IMAGING TECHNIQUES

The issue of whether to include radiographic assay of joints in assessment is largely an economic one; these tests are costly. In addition, rheumatologists have been puzzled by the finding that radiographic progression over time is remarkably constant and correlates poorly with clinical assessment. Studies have shown that, no matter what therapy is given to patients, the radiographic score deteriorates at a disturbingly regular rate for up to 25 years after the onset of disease.[24] It should be the objective of rheumatologists in the 1990s to diminish this deterioration by aggressive, focused early treatment. There are signs of progress, however. As reviewed in the treatment chapters, thorough use of a number of second-line drugs has been associated with a decrease in progression of erosions. This should be a goal of all therapy.

If both cost and invasiveness of evaluation procedures for the condition of cartilage and the proliferation of synovium were *not* crucial factors in disease management, each patient could have high-resolution MRI of involved joints and assays for degradative and synthetic components of collagen as well proteoglycan in joint fluid. At the moment, however, this is an impractical dream.

REFERENCES

1. Ward, M. M.: Clinical measures in rheumatoid arthritis: which are most useful in assessing patients? J. Rheumatol. 21:17, 1993.
2. Edworthy, S. M., Bloch, D. A., Brant, R. F., et al.: Detecting treatment effects in patients with rheumatoid arthritis: the advantage of longitudinal data. J. Rheumatol. 20:40, 1993.

    In this study of different methods of assessment of therapy in patients with rheumatoid arthritis, it was shown that the most sensitive and significant method was fitting a straight line to pretreatment data and measuring the difference in slope from that line.

3. Pincus, T. Callahan, L. F., Brooks, R. H., et al.: Self-report questionnaire scores in rheumatoid arthritis compared with traditional physical, radiographic, and laboratory measures. Ann. Intern. Med. 110:259, 1989.

    A total of 259 patients with definite rheumatoid arthritis were given an extensive evaluation, including joint count, a quantitative radiographic score, ESR and rheumatoid factor titer, grip strength, walking time, and a button test. Data from each of these were compared with results of a self-report questionnaire that gave degrees of difficulty in performing eight activities of daily living. These eight items were modified from the Stanford HAQ. The self-report questionnaire correlated significantly with joint count, radiographic score, ESR, grip strength, button test, walking time, ACR functional class, and global self-assessment. Results did not correlate with rheumatoid factor titers. In these days of managed care and emphasis on cost-effective care, a simple questionnaire has much to recommend it.

4. Fuchs, H. A., Brooks, R. H., Callahan, L. F., et al.: A simplified twenty-eight-joint quantitative articular index in rheumatoid arthritis. Arthritis Rheum. 32:531, 1989.
5. Callahan, L. F., Brooks, R. H., Summey, J. A., et al.: Quantitative pain assessment for routine care of rheumatoid arthritis patients, using a pain scale based on activities of daily living and a visual analog pain scale. Arthritis Rheum. 30:630, 1987.
6. Fries, J. F., Spitz, P. W., and Young, D. Y.: The dimensions of health outcomes: the health assessment questionnaire, disability and pain scales. J. Rheumatol. 9:789, 1982.
7. Fries, J. W., Spitz, P. W., Kraines, R. G., et al.: Measurement of patient outcome in arthritis. Arthritis Rheum. 23:137, 1980.
8. Stucki, G., Stucki, S., Bruhlmann, P., et al.: Ceiling effects of the Health Assessment Questionnaire and its modified version in some ambulatory rheumatoid arthritis patients. Ann. Rheum. Dis. 54:461, 1995.
9. Thompson, P. W., Silman, A., Kirwan, J. R., et al.: Articular indices of joint inflammation in rheumatoid arthritis. Arthritis Rheum. 30:618, 1987.

    Although joint counts are cumbersome and time consuming, for detailed studies on therapy, particularly when orthopedic reconstructive surgery may be indicated, a good articular index is essential. This Thompson Articular Index uses a relatively reduced set of joints from the Ritchie Index, scores joints as abnormal when both pain and swelling are present, and multiplies the joint count by a factor that is proportional to the size of one joint relative to others. This latter analysis makes it possible to incorporate the "synovitis burden" in patients into analysis. Correlations of this index with assays of CRP and joint erosions are higher than with other joint indices.

10. van den Brink, H. R., van der Heide, A., Jacobs, J. W. G., et al.: Evaluation of the Thompson articular index. J. Rheumatol. 20:28, 1993.

    In a cross-sectional study, the Thompson Articular Index correlated better with laboratory variables than did the Ritchie Articular Index or a swollen joint score. In a longitudinal study, it could be demonstrated that the Thompson Articular Index is sensitive to detect changes of disease activity. The ESR correlated well with the Thompson index, better than did CRP values.

11. Fuchs, H. A., and Pincus, T.: Reduced joint counts in con-

trolled clinical trials in rheumatoid arthritis. Arthritis Rheum. 37:470, 1994.

12. Smolen, J. S., Breedveld, F. C., Eberl, G., et al.: Validity and reliability of the twenty-eight-joint count for the assessment of rheumatoid arthritis activity. Arthritis Rheum. 38:38, 1995.

13. Wolfe, F., Hawley, D. J., and Cathey, M. A.: Clinical and health status measures over time: prognosis and outcome assessment in rheumatoid arthritis. J. Rheumatol. 18: 1290, 1991.

A total of 561 patients were evaluated; 264 of these were seen with 2 years of disease onset and followed for an additional 2 years, and some were followed for up to 22 years. Functional disability measured by the HAQ developed very early in the course of rheumatoid arthritis and continued to worsen at an equal rate in subsequent years, as did anxiety, pain scores, and self-assessed severity. ESR, morning stiffness, and joint counts did not change. Functional loss increased in each time period despite treatment.

14. Wolfe, F., and Cathey, M. A.: The assessment and prediction of functional disability in rheumatoid arthritis. J. Rheumatol. 18:1298, 1991.

15. O'Sullivan, M. M., Lewis, P. A., Newcombe, R. G., et al.: Precision of Larsen grading of radiographs in assessing progression of rheumatoid arthritis in individual patients. Ann. Rheum. Dis. 49:286, 1990.

16. Regan-Smith, M. G., O'Connor, G. T., Kwoh, C. K., et al.: Lack of correlation between the Steinbrocker staging of hand radiographs and the functional health status of individuals with rheumatoid arthritis. Arthritis Rheum. 32: 128, 1989.

17. Schmerling, R. H., and Delbanco, T. L.: The rheumatoid factor: an analysis of clinical utility. Am. J. Med. 91:528, 1991.

In the spirit of keeping costs of medical care under control, it is essential to have a concept of the sensitivity, specificity, and predictive value of laboratory tests. For a test such as rheumatoid factor

Sensitivity = true-positive rate

Specificity = 1 − false-positive rate

Predictive value likelihood of disease based on the positive or negative test result.

Because predictive value is markedly affected by disease prevalence, the fact that women in the fourth and fifth decades of life are more likely than others to have rheumatoid arthritis affects the predictions. Tables 4–3 and 4–4 (see text) indicate, in particular, the high frequency of false-positive tests for rheumatoid factor. The existence of seronegative rheumatoid arthritis although its true frequency is probably less than 15 per cent in carefully evaluated patients, affects results as well. Rheumatoid

factor should rarely be used as a screening tool, although it is helpful in evaluation of a patient when the pretest likelihood is neither very low nor very high. It certainly should not be used to monitor therapy. In this study, an analysis of 563 rheumatoid factor tests from a teaching hospital revealed a positive predictive value of only 24 to 34 per cent.

18. Wolfe, F., Cathey, M. A., and Roberts, F. K.: Rheumatoid factor testing in 8,287 rheumatic disease patients. Arthritis Rheum. 34:951, 1991.

In contrast to general medical practice, the predictive values of tests for rheumatoid factor in rheumatologic practices are higher. In this combined series of more than 8,000 patients referred to an outpatient rheumatology practice, the sensitivity and specificity of the rheumatoid factor test were 82 and 97 per cent, respectively, and positive and negative predictive values were 80 and 96 per cent, respectively.

19. van Gestel, A. M., Prevoo, M. L. L., van 't Hof, M. A., et al.: Development and validation of the European League Against Rheumatism response criteria for rheumatoid arthritis: Comparison with the preliminary American College of Rheumatology and the World Health Organization/ International League Against Rheumatism criteria. Athritis Rheum. 39:34, 1996.

19a.van der Heijde, D. M. F. M., van 't Hof, M. A., van Riel, P. L. C. M., et al.: Judging disease activity in clinical practice in rheumatoid arthritis: first step in the development of a disease activity score. Ann. Rheum. Dis. 49: 916, 1990.

20. Felson, D. T., Anderson, J. J. Boers, M., et al.: The American College of Rheumatology preliminary core set of disease activity measures for rheumatoid arthritis clinical trials. Arthritis Rheum. 36:729, 1993.

This paper presents the results of an ACR consensus conference on criteria and standards for clinical trials.

21. Cooperating Clinics Committee of the American Rheumatism Association: A seven-day variability study of 499 patients with peripheral rheumatoid arthritis. Arthritis Rheum. 8:302, 1965.

22. Felson, D. T., Anderson, J. J., Boers, M., et al.: American College of Rheumatology preliminary definition of improvement in rheumatoid arthritis. Arthritis Rheum. 38: 727, 1995.

23. Bellamy, N., Sothern, R. B., Campbell, J., et al.: Circadian rhythm in pain, stiffness, and manual dexterity in rheumatoid arthritis: relation between discomfort and disability. Ann. Rheum. Dis. 50:243, 1991.

24. Sharp, J. T., Wolfe, F., Mitchell, D. M., et al.: The progression of erosion and joint space narrowing scores in rheumatoid arthritis during the first twenty-five years of disease. Arthritis Rheum. 34:660, 1991.

APPENDIX: THE STANFORD HEALTH ASSESSMENT QUESTIONNAIRE

Name_____   Date_____

In this section we are interested in learning how your illness affects your ability to function in daily life. Please feel free to add any comments on the back of this page.

Please check the response which best describes your usual abilities OVER THE PAST WEEK:

	Without ANY Difficulty	With SOME Difficulty	With MUCH Difficulty	UNABLE To Do
DRESSING & GROOMING Are you able to:				
-Dress yourself, including tying shoelaces and doing buttons?	_____	_____	_____	_____
-Shampoo your hair?	_____	_____	_____	_____
ARISING Are you able to:				
-Stand up from a straight chair?	_____	_____	_____	_____
-Get in and out of bed?	_____	_____	_____	_____
EATING Are you able to:				
-Cut your meat?	_____	_____	_____	_____
-Lift a full cup or glass to your mouth?	_____	_____	_____	_____
-Open a new milk carton?	_____	_____	_____	_____
WALKING Are you able to:				
-Walk outdoors on flat ground?	_____	_____	_____	_____
-Climb up five steps?	_____	_____	_____	_____

Please check any AIDS OR DEVICES that you usually use for any of these activities:

_____ Cane	_____ Devices used for dressing (button hook, zipper pull, long-handled shoe horn, etc.)
_____ Walker	_____ Built up or special utensils
_____ Crutches	_____ Special or built up chair
_____ Wheelchair	_____ Other (Specify:_____)

Please check any categories for which you usually need HELP FROM ANOTHER PERSON:

| _____ Dressing and Grooming | _____ Eating |
| _____ Arising | _____ Walking |

PATKEY#_____

QUESTDAT_____

HAQADMIN_____

QUESTYPE___2___

PMSVIS_____1____

RASTUDY_____

QUESTNUM_____

DRESSNEW_____

RISENEW_____

EATNEW_____

WALKNEW_____

DRSGASST_____
RISEASST_____
EATASST_____
WALKASST_____

Please check the response which best describes your usual abilities OVER THE PAST WEEK:

	Without ANY Difficulty	With SOME Difficulty	With MUCH Difficulty	UNABLE To Do	
HYGIENE Are you able to:					
-Wash and dry your body?	_____	_____	_____	_____	
-Take a tub bath?	_____	_____	_____	_____	
-Get on and off the toilet?	_____	_____	_____	_____	HYGNNEW_____
REACH Are you able to:					
-Reach and get down a 5 pound object (such as a bag of sugar) from just above your head?	_____	_____	_____	_____	
-Bend down to pick up clothing from the floor?	_____	_____	_____	_____	REACHNEW_____
GRIP Are you able to:					
-Open car doors?	_____	_____	_____	_____	
-Open jars which have been previously opened?	_____	_____	_____	_____	
-Turn faucets on and off?	_____	_____	_____	_____	GRIPNEW_____
ACTIVITIES Are you able to:					
-Run errands and shop?	_____	_____	_____	_____	
-Get in and out of a car?	_____	_____	_____	_____	
-Do chores such as vacuuming or yardwork?	_____	_____	_____	_____	ACTIVNEW_____

Please check any AIDS OR DEVICES that you usually use for any of these activities:

_____ Raised toilet seat   _____ Bathtub bar
_____ Bathtub seat   _____ Long-handled appliances for reach
_____ Jar opener (for jars   _____ Long-handled appliances in bathroom
         previously opened)   _____ Other (Specify:_____)

Please check any categories for which you usually need HELP FROM ANOTHER PERSON:

_____ Hygiene   _____ Gripping and opening things
_____ Reach   _____ Errands and chores

HYGNASST_____
RCHASST_____
GRIPASST_____
ACTVASST_____

1. How have your physical limitations (such as limitations in walking, standing, climbing stairs, reaching, gripping, lifting, etc.) **changed** in the past 6 months?

Very Much Worse	1	2	3	4 No Change	5	6	7	Very Much Better

PLCHG6MO_____

2. How satisfied are you with the *amount of change* (or lack of change) in your physical limitations (such as limitations in walking, standing, climbing stairs, reaching, gripping, lifting, etc.)?

Not At All Satisfied	1	2	3	4	5	6	7	Extremely Satisfied

PLCHGSAT_____

3. How important to you is the *amount of change* (or lack of change) in your physical limitations (such as in walking, standing, climbing stairs, reaching, gripping, lifting, etc.)?

Not At All Important	1	2	3	4	5	6	7	Extremely Important

PLCHGIMP_____

4. We are also interested in learning whether or not you are affected by pain because of your illness. **How much pain have you had because of your illness IN THE PAST WEEK:**

PLACE A <u>VERTICAL</u> (|) MARK ON THE LINE TO INDICATE THE SEVERITY OF THE PAIN

NO
PAIN
_____

SEVERE
PAIN

0   100   PAINSCAL_____

5. How has your pain **changed** in the past 6 months?

Very Much Worse	1	2	3	4 No Change	5	6	7	Very Much Better

PNCHG6MO_____

6. How satisfied are you with the *amount of change* (or lack of change) in your pain?

Not At All Satisfied	1	2	3	4	5	6	7	Extremely Satisfied

PNCHGSAT_____

7. How important to you is the *amount of change* (or lack of change) in your pain?

Not At All Important	1	2	3	4	5	6	7	Extremely Important

PNCHGIMP_____

SYMPTOMS

Please check any items which apply to your health during the **PAST 7 DAYS**. If "none", check here:_____

HEAD, EYES, EARS, NOSE, MOUTH AND THROAT:

_____Blurred vision
_____Dry eyes
_____Ringing in ears
_____Hearing difficulties
_____Mouth sores
_____Dry mouth
_____Loss, change in taste
_____Headache
_____Dizziness
_____Fever
_____Night sweats

CHEST, LUNGS AND HEART:

_____Chest pain on taking a deep breath
_____Shortness of breath
_____Wheezing (asthma)

GASTROINTESTINAL TRACT:

_____Loss of appetite
_____Difficulty swallowing or feeling
of food getting stuck?
_____Nausea
_____Heartburn, indigestion or belching
_____Vomiting
_____Pain or discomfort in upper abdomen
(stomach)
_____Jaundice
_____Liver problems, kind _____
_____Pain or cramps in lower abdomen (colon)
_____Diarrhea (frequent, explosive watery
bowel movements, severe)
_____Constipation
_____Black or tarry stools (not from iron)

GENITOURINARY:

_____Protein in urine (Confirmed by a doctor)
_____Frequency or burning on urination
_____Kidney problems, kind _____

FEMALES ONLY:

_____Are you pregnant?

OTHER:

_____Any others, (specify)_____

MUSCULOSKELETAL:

_____Joint pain
_____Joint swelling
_____Low back pain
_____Muscle pain
_____Neck pain
_____Numbness/tingling in hands or feet
_____Swelling of legs
_____Weakness of muscles

_____If you are stiff in the morning, about
(hr/min) how long does the stiffness last?

NEUROLOGIC AND PSYCHOLOGIC:

_____Depression
_____Insomnia
_____Nervousness
_____Seizures or convulsions
_____Tiredness (Fatigue)
_____Trouble thinking or remembering

SKIN:

_____Easy bruising
_____Facial skin tightening
_____Hives or welts
_____Loss of hair
_____Itching
_____Rash
_____Rash over cheeks
_____Red, white and blue skin color change
in fingers on exposure to cold or
with emotional upset
_____Sun sensitivity (unusual skin reaction,
not sunburn)

BLOOD:
(Please check only if doctor confirmed results)

_____Low white blood count
_____Low platelets
_____Low red blood count (anemia)

MALES ONLY:

_____Discharge from penis
_____Impotence
_____Rash or ulcers on penis

MEDICATIONS

In the **PAST 6 MONTHS (JULY 1, 1994 through DECEMBER 31, 1994)** have you taken any medications? _____ Yes
_____ No

PLEASE COMPLETE <u>ALL</u> THE BLANKS ON THE LINE FOR ANY MEDICATIONS THAT YOU HAVE TAKEN.

MEDICATIONS FOR YOUR ARTHRITIS

For example: Prednisone, Methotrexate, Plaquenil, and anti-inflammatory drugs such as Aspirin, Naprosyn, Voltaren, Ibuprofen and Feldene. *IF RECORDING ASPIRIN, PLEASE NOTE WHAT TYPE. For example: regular, enteric coated, buffered, etc.*

MEDICATIONS TAKEN BY MOUTH

Medication Name	Months out of Last 6 Months on Drug	Number of Tablets Per Day	Milligrams Per Tablet	Still Taking Circle Yes or No	Month Stopped
_____	_____	_____	_____	Yes No	_____
_____	_____	_____	_____	Yes No	_____
_____	_____	_____	_____	Yes No	_____
_____	_____	_____	_____	Yes No	_____
_____	_____	_____	_____	Yes No	_____
_____	_____	_____	_____	Yes No	_____

If you are taking prednisone, how are you taking it?
(e.g. every other day/once per day/twice per day/other)_____

MEDICATIONS TAKEN BY INJECTION OR IN VEIN (IV)

Medication Name	Months Out of Last 6 Months on Drug	Total Number of Treatments in the Last 6 Months	Still Taking Circle Yes or No	Month Stopped
_____	_____	_____	Yes No	_____
_____	_____	_____	Yes No	_____

Please list all other medications (both prescription and over-the-counter) you have taken in the **PAST 6 MONTHS (JULY 1, 1994 through DECEMBER 31, 1994)** for any other medical condition. Please complete all the blanks on the line for each medication.

OTHER MEDICATIONS

Medication Name	Months out of Last 6 Months on Drug	Number of Tablets Per Day	Milligrams Per Tablet	Still Taking Circle Yes or No	Month Stopped
_____	_____	_____	_____	Yes No	_____
_____	_____	_____	_____	Yes No	_____
_____	_____	_____	_____	Yes No	_____
_____	_____	_____	_____	Yes No	_____
_____	_____	_____	_____	Yes No	_____

DRUG SIDE EFFECTS

Have you had any side effect(s) from your medication in the **PAST 6 MONTHS**   _____ Yes
(JULY 1, 1994 through DECEMBER 31, 1994)?   _____ No

COMPLETE THE REST OF THIS PAGE ONLY IF YOU HAVE SAID "YES".

<u>DIRECTIONS</u>:

1. Write in the name of the drug causing the side effect(s).
2. Indicate whether you stopped the drug.
3. List side effect(s) for each drug. You may want to refer back to page 3.
   Please list any abnormal laboratory findings such as:

   low white blood count   protein in urine
   low platelets   kidney problems
   anemia   liver problems

4. Check the severity of each side effect.
5. If you need more room, please use the back of this page.

SE6MO_____

A.   (1)_____   (2) Did you STOP the drug because of   DRUG1_____

       DRUG NAME   a side effect? _____ Yes _____ No   STOP1_____

                                                                                SE1DRG1_____
   (3) LIST SIDE EFFECT(S)   (4) SEVERITY of each side effect: SEVSE1D1_____

                                                                                SE2DRG1_____
   _____   _____ mild _____ moderate _____ severe SEVSE2D1_____
   _____   _____ mild _____ moderate _____ severe SE3DRG1_____
   _____   _____ mild _____ moderate _____ severe SEVSE3D1_____

B.   (1)_____   (2) Did you STOP the drug because of   DRUG2_____

       DRUG NAME   a side effect? _____ Yes _____ No   STOP2_____

                                                                                SE1DRG2_____
   (3) LIST SIDE EFFECT(S)   (4) SEVERITY of each side effect: SEVSE1D2_____

                                                                                SE2DRG2_____
   _____   _____ mild _____ moderate _____ severe SEVSE2D2_____
   _____   _____ mild _____ moderate _____ severe SE3DRG2_____
   _____   _____ mild _____ moderate _____ severe SEVSE3D2_____

C.   (1)_____   (2) Did you STOP the drug because of   DRUG3_____

       DRUG NAME   a side effect? _____ Yes _____ No   STOP3_____

                                                                                SE1DRG3_____
   (3) LIST SIDE EFFECT(S)   (4) SEVERITY of each side effect: SEVSE1D3_____

                                                                                SE2DRG3_____
   _____   _____ mild _____ moderate _____ severe SEVSE2D3_____
   _____   _____ mild _____ moderate _____ severe SE3DRG3_____
   _____   _____ mild _____ moderate _____ severe SEVSE3D3_____

1. To help you say how good or bad your health state is, we have drawn a scale (rather like a thermometer) on which the best state you can imagine is marked by 100, and the worst state you can imagine is marked by 0.

We would like for you to indicate on this scale how good or bad your own health is today. Please do this by drawing a line from the box to the right to whichever point on the scale indicates how good or bad your current health state is today considering all aspects of your health.

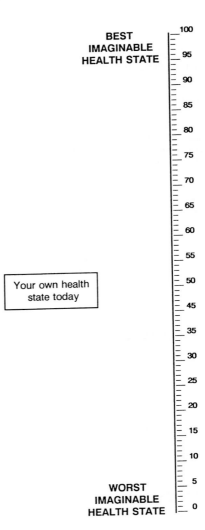

BEST
IMAGINABLE
HEALTH STATE

Your own health state today

WORST
IMAGINABLE
HEALTH STATE

2. Are any of your joints tender? _____ Yes _____ No
    -If "Yes", please circle the tender joints.

    Knuckles   Wrists   Elbows   Shoulders   Hips   Knees   Ankles   Toes

    PTTENJTN_____

3. Are any of your joints swollen? _____ Yes _____ No
    -If "Yes", please circle the swollen joints.

    Knuckles   Wrists   Elbows   Shoulders   Hips   Knees   Ankles   Toes

    PTSWOJTN_____

MEDICAL HISTORY

We are interested in your use of health care providers in the **PAST 6 MONTHS** (JULY 1, 1994 through DECEMBER 31, 1994). Please include **ALL** visits.

1. In the **PAST 6 MONTHS (JULY 1, 1994 through DECEMBER 31, 1994)** did you stay in the hospital overnight <u>or</u> visit an Emergency Room for any reason? _____Yes _____No

    HOSPAUDT_____

    -If "Yes," please describe each hospitalization or emergency room visit:

    ERVISIT_____

Reason	Hospital (City, State)	Admission Date (Month, Year)	Number Of Days in Hospital
_____	_____	_____	_____
_____	_____	_____	_____
_____	_____	_____	_____
_____	_____	_____	_____

2. Were any of these hospitalizations related to a side effect from any of your medications?

    If "Yes", which hospitalization(s) and which medication(s):_____

    _____

3. Did you develop any complications or secondary problems during any of the hospitalizations?

    If "Yes", list hospitalization and problem:_____

    _____

    _____

4. In the **PAST 6 MONTHS (JULY 1, 1994 through DECEMBER 31, 1994)** have you had any outpatient surgery or procedures? _____Yes _____No

    -If "Yes," please list:

Surgery/Procedure	Doctor's Name	Location and Address (Hospital, Doctor's Office)	Date (Month, Year)
_____	_____	_____	_____
_____	_____	_____	_____

5. In the **PAST 6 MONTHS (JULY 1, 1994 through DECEMBER 31, 1994)** were you a patient in a nursing or convalescent home or live-in rehabilitation center? _____Yes _____No

    NURHOMDY_____

    -If "Yes," for how many days? _____Days

6. In the **PAST 6 MONTHS (JULY 1, 1994 through DECEMBER 31, 1994)** have you received care from a doctor, nurse, or other health professional *IN YOUR HOME*? _____Yes _____No

    -If "Yes," how many visits in the PAST 6 MONTHS? _____Visits

    HOMEVSTS_____

7. In the **PAST 6 MONTHS (JULY 1, 1994 through DECEMBER 31, 1994)** have you been told that you have any kind of tumor or cancer? _____Yes _____No

    -If "Yes", was it malignant or benign? (circle one)

    What kind? (for example: leukemia, lymphoma, lung)

    _____

    What treatment was given? (for example: surgery, chemotherapy, radiation therapy)

    _____

    CANCER_____
    BENIGN_____
    CANCTYPE_____
    CANCSURG_____
    CANCCHEM_____
    CANCRAD_____

8. In addition to your arthritis, have you had any medical problems in the **PAST YEAR** (1994)?   _____Yes _____No

    If "Yes", what type(s) of medical problems have you had?

    Vascular problems (e.g., heart attack, angina, coronary artery disease, high blood pressure, stroke, circulatory problems, etc.) _____Yes _____No

    VASPROB_____

    Lung Disease (e.g., emphysema, chronic bronchitis, etc.)   _____Yes _____No

    LUNGPROB_____

    Cancer   _____Yes _____No

    CANCPROB_____

    Skeletal problems (e.g., broken bones or fractures osteoporosis, etc.)   _____Yes _____No

    SKELPROB_____

    Neurological problems (e.g., Parkinson's, Alzheimer's, depression, etc.)   _____Yes _____No

    NEURPROB_____

    Gastrointestinal disease (e.g., ulcer, diverticulitis, gall bladder disease, liver problems, etc.)   _____Yes _____No

    GASTPROB_____

    Other diseases (e.g., diabetes, cataract, kidney disorders, etc.) _____Yes _____No

    MISCDIS_____

9. Have you seen any doctors or any other health workers in the **PAST 6 MONTHS (JULY 1, 1994 through DECEMBER 31, 1994)**? DO NOT INCLUDE ANY WHILE A PATIENT IN THE HOSPITAL. _____Yes _____No

-If "Yes", please complete:

NUMBER of
Visits in
Last 6 Months

Rheumatologist	_____	RHEUMVST_____
Internist	_____	INTERNVT_____
Family physician (General Practitioner)	_____	GPVST_____
General or Orthopedic surgeon	_____	SURGNVT_____
Podiatrist (foot doctor)	_____	PODVST_____
Chiropractor	_____	CHIROVT_____
Physical or occupational therapist	_____	PTOTVST_____

Other doctors (dermatologist or others)

_____   _____

_____   _____   MISCVST_____

Other health workers (Social worker, or others)
(Please DO NOT include any health care workers
who came to your home, they should be recorded
on page 9)

_____   _____

_____   _____   MISCHWVT_____

Diagnostic Procedures

10. Have you had any diagnostic tests or treatments in the **PAST 6 MONTHS (JULY 1, 1994 through DECEMBER 31, 1994)**? DO NOT INCLUDE ANY THAT WERE DONE WHILE YOU WERE A PATIENT IN THE HOSPITAL. _____ Yes _____ No

-If "Yes", please complete the following.

Test	Number of tests	Part of body	
			HDWTXRAY_____
X-Rays (chest, stomach or bowels,	_____	_____	SHLDXY_____
joints, etc.)			HIPXRAY_____
	_____	_____	KNEEXRAY_____
			FEETXRAY_____
	_____	_____	NECKXY_____
			LOBKXY_____
	_____	_____	SPINXY_____
			CHTXY_____
	_____	_____	GIXRAY_____
			MISCXRAY_____
Nuclear Medicine Scans (Bone scan) or			
Magnetic Resonance Imaging (MRI) . . .	_____	_____	NMR_____
CT Scan	_____	_____	CTSCAN_____
Blood tests (Number of times			
blood was drawn)	_____		VENPUNCT_____
Urine tests	_____		URINALYS_____
Endoscopy (Gastroscopy)	_____		ENDOSCOP_____
Colonoscopy	_____		COLONOSC_____
Other tests, please specify	_____	_____	

11. In the **PAST 6 MONTHS (JULY 1, 1994 through DECEMBER 31, 1994)**, have you had any non-traditional treatments?   _____ Yes _____ No

-If "Yes", please complete:

	Number of Visits	
Acupuncturist	_____	ACUPUNNT_____
Acupressurist	_____	ACUPRENT_____
Massage Therapist	_____	MASSAGNT_____
Herbalist	_____	HERBALNT_____
Homeopathic Practitioner	_____	HOPATHNT_____
Other, please specify:		
_____	_____	OTHERNT_____

12. In the **PAST 6 MONTHS (JULY 1, 1994 through DECEMBER 31, 1994)** have you had to pay someone to help in the house or for personal care, or for help in business matters that you are normally able to handle yourself, but could not do because of your health?

_____ Yes _____ No

-If "Yes", please list:

Type of Care	Hours per Month	Number of Months
_____	_____	_____
_____	_____	_____

MISCUNIT_____

H E A L T H   S T A T U S

1. Considering all the ways that your arthritis affects you, rate how you are doing on the following scale by placing a mark on the line.

```
| - - - - | - - - - | - - - - | - - - - | - - - - | - - - - | - - - - | - - - - | - - - - | - - - - |
0              20             40             60             80            100
very                   well            fair           poor                  very
well                                                                        poor
```

GLOBAL_____

2. How much of the time, during the **PAST 4 WEEKS**, has your health limited your social activities (like visiting with friends or close relatives)?

_____ All of the time
_____ Most of the time
_____ A good bit of the time
_____ Some of the time
_____ A little of the time
_____ None of the time

SOCLCHG_____

3. In general, would you say your current health is:

_____Excellent
_____Very Good
_____Good
_____Fair
_____Poor

GLOBALGN_____

4. How satisfied are you with your HEALTH NOW?

_____Very satisfied
_____Somewhat satisfied
_____Neither satisfied or dissatisfied
_____Somewhat dissatisfied
_____Very dissatisfied

GLOBALNW_____

5. For each of the following questions, please circle the number for the one answer that best describes how you have been feeling in the **PAST 4 WEEKS**.

How much of the time did you:	All of the Time	Most of the Time	Some of the Time	Almost Never	Never	
a. Feel full of pep?	1	2	3	4	5	PEPPY_____
b. Feel worn out?	1	2	3	4	5	WORNOUT_____
c. Feel calm and peaceful?	1	2	3	4	5	ATPEACE_____
d. Have enough energy to do the things you want to do?	1	2	3	4	5	ENRGETIC_____
e. Feel downhearted and blue?	1	2	3	4	5	FEELBLUE_____
f. Feel very happy?	1	2	3	4	5	HAPPY_____
g. Feel very nervous?	1	2	3	4	5	NERVOUS_____
h. Feel tired?	1	2	3	4	5	TIRED_____
i. Feel so down in the dumps nothing could cheer you up?	1	2	3	4	5	DOWN_____

We would like to know how your arthritis pain affects you. Please **circle** the number which corresponds to your certainty that you can now perform the following task.

1. How certain are you that you can make a small-to-moderate reduction in your arthritis pain by using methods other than taking extra medication?

SEPS4_____

1	2	3	4	5	6	7	8	9	10
Very Uncertain									Very Certain

In the following questions, we'd like to know how you feel about your ability to control your arthritis. For each of the following questions, please **circle** the number on the scale which corresponds to the certainty that you can <u>now</u> perform the following activities or tasks.

2. <u>How certain</u> are you that you can manage your arthritis symptoms so that you can do the things you enjoy doing?

SESS5_____

```
  1     2     3     4     5     6     7     8     9     10
Very                                              Very
Uncertain                                         Certain
```

3. <u>How certain</u> are you that you can deal with the frustrations of arthritis?

SESS6_____

```
  1     2     3     4     5     6     7     8     9     10
Very                                              Very
Uncertain                                         Certain
```

HEALTH BEHAVIORS

1. Do you regularly drink alcoholic beverages?   _____Yes _____No

   -If "Yes", how many drinks do you usually have in a typical day?

   ___Beer (1 drink = 12 oz. can or bottle)

   ___Wine (1 drink = 6 oz. glass)

   ST_ETHAN_____

   ___Hard liquor, cocktails, or cordial (1 drink = 1 1/2 oz. liquor)

2. Do you smoke cigarettes:

   SMKNOW_____
   SMKPST_____

   Now? _____ Yes _____ No
   In the past? _____ Yes _____ No
   How many years? _____
   How many packs per day? _____

   YRSMOK_____
   SMOKING_____
   PACKYEAR_____

3. Do you presently drink coffee, tea, or soft drinks on a regular basis?   _____Yes _____No

   -If "Yes", how many do you drink on a typical day?
   ___Cups of regular (drip or perk) coffee (1 cup = 5 oz.)
   ___Cups of instant coffee (1 cup = 5 oz.)
   ___Cups of decaffeinated coffee (1 cup = 5 oz.)
   ___Cups of caffeine-containing tea (1 cup = 5 oz.)
   ___Cans of caffeine-containing soft drinks such as regular or diet coke, Pepsi, Dr. Pepper or Mr. Pibb, Tab, or Mountain Dew. (1 can = 12 oz.)

   COFFEE_____
   COFFINST_____
   COFDECAF_____
   TEA_____
   SODA_____

   ___Cans of caffeine-free soft drinks such as regular or diet 7-UP, Sprite, Fanta orange, Fresca, or root beer. (1 can = 12 oz.)

4. How tall are you? _____ Feet _____ Inches.   HGT_HAQ_____

5. How much do you weigh? _____ Pounds.   WGT_HAQ_____

6. Do you participate in exercise specifically for your arthritis (e.g. stretching,
    strenghtening, or range of motion exercises) on a regular basis?   _____Yes _____No

    -If "Yes", how many times per week? _____Times   EXERWEEK_____
    How many minutes per time? _____Minutes

7. Do you participate in exercise for general conditioning (i.e. exercises for
    your heart or lungs) on a regular basis?   _____Yes _____No

    -If "Yes", how many times per week? _____Times   AEROWEEK_____
    How many minutes per time? _____Minutes

E M P L O Y M E N T   S T A T U S

1. Which one of the following categories best describes you at this time?   EMPLOY_____

    _____Working for pay: Occupation_____   OCCUPA_____
                      Job duties_____
                      Hours/week_____   WORKHRS_____
                      Personal yearly earnings - nearest thousand (optional)_____
                      (NOT TOTAL HOUSEHOLD INCOME)   PERINCOM_____

    _____Retired

    _____Homemaker

    _____Student

    _____Disabled

    _____Looking for work

    _____On sick leave: Occupation_____

    _____On vacation: Occupation_____

    _____Other (Specify):_____

2. If you retired or became disabled in **1994**, what was your prior occupation?

       Occupation_____

3. In the **PAST 6 MONTHS (JULY 1, 1994 through DECEMBER 31, 1994)**
    have there been days when you have had to **CUT DOWN** or **LIMIT**
    your usual activities (including housework, school)?   _____Yes _____No   CUTDOWN_____

    If "yes", how many days? _____

IF YOU ARE <u>NOT</u> EMPLOYED, PLEASE ANSWER QUESTION #4.
IF YOU ARE EMPLOYED, PLEASE GO TO QUESTION #5.

4. IN THE **PAST 6 MONTHS**, have there been days when you have
    been COMPLETELY UNABLE to carry out your usual activities
    BECAUSE OF YOUR HEALTH?   _____Yes _____No

    If "yes", how many days? _____

**IF YOU ARE <u>NOT</u> EMPLOYED, PLEASE GO TO THE BACKGROUND INFORMATION SECTION
ON THE NEXT PAGE.**

IF YOU ARE EMPLOYED, PLEASE ANSWER THE FOLLOWING QUESTIONS:

5. IN THE **PAST 6 MONTHS**, have you been unable to work any days
    BECAUSE OF YOUR HEALTH?   _____Yes _____No

    If "Yes", how many days? _____

6. IN THE **PAST 6 MONTHS**, have you stopped or started working
    BECAUSE OF YOUR HEALTH? (Include early retirement)   _____Yes _____No

    If "Yes", please explain:

7. IN THE **PAST 6 MONTHS**, have you changed your HOURS of work
    BECAUSE OF YOUR HEALTH?   _____Yes _____No

    If "Yes", please explain:

8. In the **PAST 6 MONTHS (JULY 1, 1994 through DECEMBER 31, 1994)** have you taken <u>unpaid</u>
    time off from work to visit your doctor, a psychologist, or other health professional?
                                                         _____Yes _____No

    -If "Yes", how many hours have you taken off? _____ hours/past 6 months

DAYSLOST_____

UNABLE_____

CHGWORK_____

CHGAMT_____

HRSLOST_____

BACKGROUND INFORMATION

1. What is your marital status?

    _____ Never married
    _____ Married   _____ Remarried after death of spouse
    _____ Separated   _____ Divorced and remarried
    _____ Divorced
    _____ Widowed   MARITAL_____

2. With whom do you live? Check all that apply.

    _____ Alone   _____ With other relatives
    _____ With spouse or partner _____ With friends or roommates
    _____ With children   _____ Convalescent or Nursing Home
    _____ With parent(s)   _____ Paid live-in help   LVWITH_____

3. Have you taken the Arthritis Self-Management or Arthritis Self-Help course in the past year?
   (A 6-week course where you received a copy of the Arthritis Helpbook)
                                         _____ Yes _____ No   ASMCOURS_____

4. Have you participated in the SMART (Self-Management Arthritis Relief Therapy) Program in the past
   year? (SMART is a series of 3-month questionnaires with personalized feedback and instructional
   materials)
                                         _____ Yes _____ No   SMARTYR_____

       If "Yes", what year?_____

5. Have you received disability payments in the **PAST YEAR** (1994),
   because of your arthritis?   _____ Yes _____ No
   If "Yes", please check who is giving you the payments and complete the rest of the line.

   Payments from who?   Number of months
                                   (Leave blank if not stopped)
   _____ Job   _____   DISPAY1_____

   _____ Workers compensation   _____   DIMO1_____

   _____ State or local government   DISPAY2_____
           disability payments   _____
                                                             DIMO2_____
   _____ Social Security disability payments
           (not retirement Social Security) _____   DISPAY3_____

   _____ Other: _____   DIMO3_____

6. What type(s) of health insurance do you have? Check all that apply.

_____None

_____Medicaid/Medi-Cal (State Assistance)
_____Medicare Part A - (Medicare insurance for hospital care)
_____Medicare Part B - (Medicare insurance for physician visits and other non-hospital care) - Name:_____
_____Medigap Insurance (Additional insurance for people covered by medicare. Medigap insurance covers some services not included under Medicare.)
_____Medicare Disability Insurance
_____Other public assistance

_____Traditional Insurance (Insurance where you may see any physician you choose. Many traditional insurance policies require you to pay coinsurance (a percentage of the charges for each visit) and/or a deductible.) - Name:_____

_____Health Maintenance Organization (HMO) (Insurance where you must see a primary care physician to receive care. In most cases, the primary care physician must authorize visits to specialists or other providers. Primary care physicians are chosen from a list of physicians affiliated with the organization. In most cases, HMOs charge a small copayment for each visit, but have no deductible.) - Name:_____

_____Preferred Provider Organization (PPO) (Insurance where you may see any physician you choose, but you pay a different amount depending on whether or not the physician is affiliated with the organization and whether or not you are referred by your primary care physician) - Name:_____

_____Champus/VA

_____Federal Employees Health Benefit Program (FEHBP)

_____Other - Name:_____

HLTHCAR1_____

HLTHCAR2_____

HLTHCAR3_____

7. If you have private health insurance, an HMO, or PPO plan, how do you obtain your health insurance? Please check the source of your **primary** insurance:

_____Provided through your employer, your spouse's, other family member's, or partner's employer
_____Purchased by you directly from the insurer or from an insurance agent
_____Provided by a union
_____Cobra coverage

HLTHINSR_____

8. Where do you regularly receive your medical care? Please check one.

_____At a hospital outpatient clinic
_____At a private physician's office
_____At a physician's office in a large clinic, not at a hospital
_____At a community-based, publicly financed clinic

MEDCARE_____

9. Which income group below comes closest to your total household income in 1994 from ALL SOURCES BEFORE TAXES?

TOTINCOM_____

_____ Under $10,000	_____ $40,000 - 49,999	_____ $80,000 - 89,999
_____ $10,000 - 19,999	_____ $50,000 - 59,999	_____ $90,000 - 99,999
_____ $20,000 - 29,999	_____ $60,000 - 69,999	_____ $100,000 or more
_____ $30,000 - 39,999	_____ $70,000 - 79,999	

COMMENTS:

_____

_____

_____

_____

_____

_____

_____

_____

_____

_____

_____

_____

_____

_____

_____

_____

_____

_____

_____

_____

_____

_____

_____

This page asks you for permission to allow us to review medical records pertaining to your involvement in this research program. This information will be kept strictly confidential and used for research purposes only.

RELEASE OF MEDICAL INFORMATION

I give permission for the release of information pertaining to my medical care to the Outcome in Rheumatic Disease Study.

<u>PLEASE USE INK</u>

PLEASE PRINT

Name: _____

Address:_____

_____
Postal/Zip Code

Date of Birth: _____

Signature: _____ _____
Date

25

Prognosis for Patients with Rheumatoid Arthritis

The physician can provide for a rheumatoid patient few benefits that are more appreciated than predicting accurately what will happen in the years to come. Will I be disabled? Will I be weak? How long will I be able to take care of myself? Can this disease kill me? All are reasonable questions that every patient asks. Each is difficult to answer.

Giving a prognosis for a chronic and variable disease is particularly difficult because outcome may depend on so many different variables. Laboratory indices can be helpful, but which are independent predictors of disease activity? How does treatment with one or more of the many drugs available affect outcome of rheumatoid arthritis?

In this chapter, the following subgroups of patients are reviewed separately for data available on prognosis:

1. The patient with undifferentiated polyarthritis that could be rheumatoid arthritis.
2. The patient with a firm diagnosis of rheumatoid arthritis made fewer than 2 years after onset of symptoms.
3. The patient with longstanding disease
   a. Risk for disability and joint destruction
   b. Risk for death

UNDIFFERENTIATED POLYARTHRITIS

There is general agreement that rheumatoid arthritis is a more severe process when seen in large specialty clinics at medical centers than it is in community practices. There are several apparent reasons for this, but the principal one is that patients with refractory symptoms and an aggressive course are likely to be referred to medical centers. Most patients with self-limited disease do not appear in university clinics, nor are they grouped in published studies. The exception to this is the growth of treatment trials organized by networks of community physicians.

The earlier a patient with polyarthritis is seen, the more likely it is that the process will be self-limited. Did these patients who get well have another specific but self-limited syndrome, or, as required by Hunter, were they "on the brink of developing rheumatoid arthritis and did not?"[1]

Despite the existence of straightforward criteria for diagnosis of rheumatoid arthritis, there is often a long lag period between the onset of symptoms and the time of diagnosis of this disease. In a retrospective study of 98 patients given a definite diagnosis of rheumatoid arthritis in a multispecialty health maintenance organization in Massachusetts, the median time to diagnosis was 36 weeks (range, 4 weeks to > 10 years).[2] Only half of 26 patients with symmetric joint symptoms and a positive rheumatoid factor test were diagnosed within 10 weeks of the beginning of symptoms. There are many reasons for delays in diagnosis, including reluctance of patients to see physicians and an understandable reluctance of physicians to label a patient with a chronic disease. Nevertheless, if it is an acceptable guideline that the earlier the therapy the more likely it is that joint destruction will be avoided, it is important to make this diagnosis earlier rather than later.

The general internist or family physician is the one likely to see patients with recent onset of an undifferentiated polyarthritis syndrome. These patients most often present with arthralgias, swelling of several joints, and occasionally (22 per cent) a pattern of joint swelling entirely consistent with rheumatoid arthritis.[3] They are less likely than are patients with definite rheumatoid arthritis to have a positive test for rheumatoid factor or a diminished grip strength, although they can have an elevated ESR, morning stiffness, and a perception of disability that is the same as those with definite rheumatoid arthritis.[3] The important point for the internist or family practitioner likely to see these patients first is that more than 50 per cent have complete resolution of symptoms, and fewer than 20 per cent go on to a diagnosis of rheumatoid arthritis.

A patient who presents with oligoarticular arthralgia and joint swelling who does not meet criteria for diagnosis of rheumatoid arthritis, and who has a negative test for rheumatoid factor, has more than a 50 per cent chance of a gradual but complete resolution of symptoms within 6 months.

One recent study has compared the status of patients given a diagnosis of rheumatoid arthritis shortly after becoming sick with a cohort who still were labeled as having "unexplained polyarthritis" up to 1 year after becoming ill.[4] Of 57 patients with a diagnosis of rheumatoid arthritis, 20 had gone into remission at 1 year; of these 20, 9 were in remission at year 5 (20 per cent). In contrast, of 31 who still had active rheumatoid arthritis after 1 year, 21 still had a diagnosis of rheumatoid arthritis at year 5; the other 10 had either died or withdrawn from the study. Conversely, among the 67 patients with unexplained polyarthritis, only 10 were changed to a diagnosis of rheumatoid arthritis at year 1; all but 1 of the 10 kept the diagnosis through year 5. These data leave the physician in a quandary because, although it is appropriate to use aggressive therapy early in those patients with continuous and active disease, one certainly does not want to use toxic drugs on the 20 per cent of patients who will go into remission. These data re-emphasize the importance of finding a specific and sensitive test that portends a poor prognosis in rheumatoid arthritis.

RHEUMATOID ARTHRITIS DIAGNOSED WITHIN 2 YEARS OF ONSET OF SYMPTOMS

The first year of verified rheumatoid arthritis is the most important one in the patient's disease. This is the time that the pace and severity of the process become set, and, at the same time, it is the crucial time for medical intervention if inexorable destruction of joints is to be avoided.

Although difficult to prove, there are suggestions in the literature supporting the belief that early therapy can alter an otherwise progressive course toward death or disability. For example, in a series of 561 patients with definite rheumatoid arthritis followed over 20 years, the patients seen by a rheumatologist during the first 2 years of disease improved significantly compared with others.[5]

In contrast to patients with an undifferentiated polyarthritis syndrome, fewer than 20 per cent of patients with a definite diagnosis of rheumatoid arthritis are likely to have an early true remission or be without erosions (particularly of the metatarsals

and wrist joints) on radiographs[6] after 2 years of disease. A false optimism may surround these patients because their disability indices may remain at a low level even as early loss of cartilage is beginning.

It is important to emphasize that, after the diagnosis is made, the usefulness of a positive test for rheumatoid factor is less than it would have been if the diagnosis were unclear. Instead, the clinical findings that usually are paralleled by a positive test for rheumatoid factor (e.g., nodules, vasculitis) become more important predictive factors. Patients who have had a positive IgM rheumatoid factor early in the course of their disease, and then become rheumatoid factor negative, have a better prognosis than those who remain rheumatoid factor positive. The data suggest that probably fewer 8 per cent of rheumatoid patients become rheumatoid factor negative after being positive.[7]

Although joint swelling has been a useful predictor of radiographic change, joint tenderness and pain are more likely to be associated with disability.[8] This is because patients are understandably loathe to use painful joints.

There are some clinical predictors of more severe disease in patients with definite rheumatoid arthritis of relatively recent onset[9,10]:

- Persistent swelling of the PIP joints
- Flexor tenosynovitis of the hands
- A high CRP level or ESR
- A large number of swollen joints (or a high standard joint score)
- High rheumatoid factor titer

Immunogenetic studies can be helpful as well. As early as 1988, there were indications that there was an association of HLA-DR4 with both rheumatoid factor and radiographic severity in rheumatoid arthritis.[11] Subsequently, it was shown that DR4+ patients had more swollen joints, higher joint scores and disability indices, more radiographic abnormalities, and more use of second-line drugs[12] (see Chapter 3 and below).

HLA-DRB Chains in Prognosis

By use of DNA sequencing at the *HLA-DRB1* locus, with focus on the sequence motif of the amino acid positions 67 to 74 of the third hypervariable region, it has been shown that combinations of *HLA-DRB1* alleles are linked to severity of disease in patients with seropositive rheumatoid arthritis[13] (Table 25–1). (Refer to Chapter 3 for review of the basis for these observations.)

Patients who inherit a disease-linked allele from

TABLE 25–1. Linkage of Combinations of *HLA-DRB1* Alleles with Disease Severity in Seropositive Rheumatoid Arthritis

ALLELIC COMBINATIONS *HLA-DRB1**	RISK TO REQUIRE JOINT SURGERY AFTER 10–15 YEARS OF DISEASE	FORMATION OF RHEUMATOID NODULES	RHEUMATOID ORGAN DISEASE	CATEGORY
04/04 ("double-dose patient")	+ + +	+ + +	+ + +	Nodular and destructive disease High risk for rheumatoid vasculitis
04/01 ("double-dose patient")	+ + +	+ + +	–	Nodular disease High destructive potential
04/x ("single dose patient")	+ +	+ +	(+)	Moderate risk for destructive disease Low risk for rheumatoid organ involvement
01/x ("single-dose patient")	–	–	–	Non-nodular disease ? Low destructive potential
x/x	–	–	–	Non-nodular disease ? Slow progression of joint disease

From Weyand, C. M., and Goronzy, J. J.: Prognosis in rheumatoid arthritis: applying new technologies to old questions. J. Rheumatol. 20:1817, 1993. Used by permission.

both parents are more likely to have aggressive disease than patients with only one disease-linked allele. Patients combining two disease-linked alleles in the form of *HLA-DRB1*0404* and *B1*0401* have a 60 per cent risk of undergoing joint surgery later in the course of their disease, whereas those homozygous for *HLA-DRB1*0401* were more likely to develop Felty's syndrome, rheumatoid vasculitis, and lung disease.[14,15] In a series of 177 patients[16] with early undiagnosed arthritis, serologic tests for rheumatoid factor were done and DNA was typed for presence of the "shared epitope" in the third hypervariable region of the *DRB1* gene. The results were as follows:

- Of the 177 patients, 120 fulfilled the ACR criteria for diagnosis of rheumatoid arthritis.
- Of these, 64 per cent possessed the shared epitope, compared with 45 per cent of healthy controls. Those who went on to develop erosions had a higher prevalence of the shared epitope. These data suggest that milder forms of rheumatoid arthritis are not as strongly associated with the shared epitope, or that the shared epitope encodes for disease severity, not its acquisition. These impressions are supported by the finding that there is no association between *HLA-DRB1*04* and rheumatoid arthritis in newly diagnosed cases from the community.[17]

- The presence of *either* the shared epitope or rheumatoid factor had a relative risk of 13.5 for erosions (specificity, 39 per cent; sensitivity, 95 per cent), whereas the presence of *both* the shared epitope and rheumatoid factor increased the specificity of developing erosions to 88 per cent while reducing the sensitivity to 53 per cent.

At present, of course, it is neither convenient nor financially feasible to assay for *HLA-DRB1* alleles in patients outside of studies in university settings. However, it is possible that, when specific (but expensive) new therapies using targeted biologic agents become available, it may be cost-effective to find out within weeks of establishing a diagnosis of rheumatoid arthritis which patients are at risk, untreated, of developing aggressive disease within the first years of being sick. Despite the HLA class II associations with rheumatoid arthritis, a family history per se is not associated with a poorer prognosis in rheumatoid arthritis.

Other Clinical and Laboratory Assays Used in Prognosis

Summaries of numerous studies indicate that the best signs indicating a poorer prognosis in rheumatoid arthritis during the first several years of disease are the number of swollen joints, limitations of activity, appearance of significant radiographic evidence for disease, and significant titers of rheumatoid factor or CRP and/or and elevated ESR. The combination of a positive test for rheumatoid factor, significant radiographic abnormalities, and either (1) diminished functional activity, (2) elevated ESR or CRP level, or (3) *DRB1* allele assay gives an accuracy of 70 to 80 per cent in predicting a poor prognosis.

A similar example of a test that might be prognostically useful early in disease but is not likely to become available for clinicians in practice at a reasonable cost is proteoglycan concentration in synovial fluid; it has been found that the highest levels of these are from joints that, 10 years later, have undergone the greatest damage[18] (see Chapter 23).

LONGSTANDING JOINT DISEASE

Risk for Disability

Although predicting the future for a rheumatoid patient within the first year of disease is most important for altering the course of the disease, it has been the relatively recent accumulation of data on long-term morbidity and mortality that has given specialists who treat rheumatoid arthritis a sense of urgency. The reason? Rheumatoid arthritis is not a benign process. It generates a great deal of morbidity and is associated with a significant increase in mortality.

In 1987, Scott and his colleagues from London prospectively looked at the outcome in 112 patients with rheumatoid arthritis treated actively for 20 years at one center.[20] The data were not encouraging:

- At 20 years, 35 per cent of patients were dead and an additional 19 per cent were severely disabled.

- Radiographs showed evidence of increasing joint destruction.

- ESR and rheumatoid factor levels changed little.

It was concluded that: "The concept of 'remission-inducing' drugs is fallacious. Early treatment may be advantageous, but the prognosis of rheumatoid arthritis is not good."

It is equally discouraging to learn that, despite multiple different types of therapy for rheumatoid arthritis, the progression of radiographic damage in joints of patients followed for more than 20 years appears to occur at a steady rate with only a moderate decrease over time[21] (Fig. 25–1). The most rapid rates of radiographic score progression occur in the first 3 years of disease. In another study, if there was a marked fall in rheumatoid factor titers, prognosis for the patient was better[22] although in general there has been little agreement that changes in rheumatoid factor have clinical significance.

To supplement the knowledge that there is a general overall deterioration in all patients that is greater than that realized by earlier generations of clinicians, substantial good data have been generated to dissect out factors that increase the likelihood of long-term disability. In one study, using the data bank of the American Rheumatism Association Medical Information System (ARAMIS), which has proved invaluable in such studies, over 400 entry variables in a cohort of patients were followed from 1981 to 1989 in search of those that could predict the severity of rheumatoid arthritis 9 years later.[23] This group of patients had rheumatoid arthritis for an average of 12 years at baseline. The initial level of the disability index of the HAQ was determined to be the strongest predictive variable in these patients with longstanding disease.

Additional studies have added additional items that indicate a poor prognosis. Disability indices worsen more quickly for women than for men, for those with few rather than many years of education, and for older rather than younger persons.[24] As with most chronic diseases, unmarried patients deteriorate faster than their married counterparts.[25]

Interestingly, these longitudinal studies of patients have revealed that the variables most effective in assessing results of controlled clinical trials are not effective in predicting outcome in rheumatoid arthritis.[5] Clinically important and progressive loss of grip strength and function, and worsening of the patients' overall assessment of severity, are significant in assessing patients over time, whereas some of the mainstays of clinical trials (e.g., morning stiffness, ESR, and joint count) are not as useful as outcome measures. Again, the HAQ is sensitive

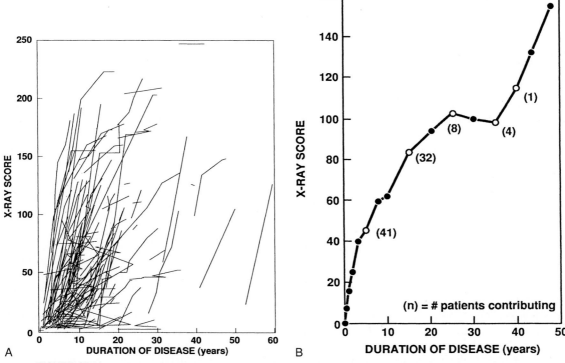

FIGURE 25–1. *A*, Total radiologic scores as a function of disease duration in all patients for whom two or more films were available. *B*, Progression of radiologic scores as illustrated using the averages of constrained cubics at increasing durations of disease. (From Sharp, J. T., Wolfe, F., Mitchell, D. M. et al.: The progression of erosion and joint space narrowing scores in rheumatoid arthritis during the first twenty-five years of disease. Arthritis Rheum. 34:660, 1991. Used by permission.)

to disease progression, even for patients who are "doing well."[5]

One of the components of a good outcome in rheumatoid arthritis is the absence of significant depression. Although it is apparent now that there is not a depressive predisposition for rheumatoid arthritis, the data do suggest that, when patients lose the ability to do valued activities, depression is much more likely to occur.[26] Part of any therapeutic approach should be to help a patient maintain the ability to perform those activities of most value to him or her.

It is of interest to examine follow-up data on relatively homogeneous populations of rheumatoid patients. One such study followed 132 women ages 20 to 25 at onset of disease and seen by a rheumatologist within 5 years after becoming symptomatic. Six years after the diagnosis was made, they had evolved as follows.[7]

- Fifty-one per cent had low activity (<4 swollen joints)
- Seventeen per cent had continually active disease in many joints

- Eight per cent had disease that progressed from high to low activity
- Six per cent progressed from low to high activity
- Eighteen per cent had a fluctuating course

No solid clues were found to distinguish at time zero those who would remain active and those who would not.

Effects of Therapy on Prognosis

Another factor that must be considered in prognosis is the treatment used. It is important to keep in mind, however, that drug therapy can affect data on outcome in two ways:

1. Drugs can suppress or down-regulate disease, or affect outcome adversely by side effects.

2. A particular drug might be used only in more severe disease; data would then show that the drug is associated with increased mortality or morbidity.

One of these caveats applies to use of prednisone in rheumatoid arthritis. For example, in a group of

395 patients with rheumatoid arthritis followed for an average of 6.7 years, the use of corticosteroids in women and a prior diagnosis of osteoporosis were identified as important risk factors for development of fractures. The 5-year probability of a woman taking 5 mg or more of prednisone having a fracture was 34 per cent.[27] Similarly, another study designed to dissect out mortality predictors among 263 patients found that prednisone use was "a strong predictor of impending death."[28] The authors write: "Clearly, this result should not be interpreted as necessarily suggesting that premature death is a side effect of prednisone. Prednisone might be given more frequently to patients who are experiencing severe disease."

The positive and negative aspects of therapy focused on using second-line drugs and cytotoxic agents are highlighted by a report of a cohort followed for 10 years after the time of prescription of their initial second-line agent. Twenty per cent had died, 71 per cent required joint surgery, 36 per cent needed management of peptic ulcer, and 45 per cent had experienced major episodes of sepsis. Seventy-three per cent remained on a second- or "third"-line drug at 10 years. Balancing the complications, those remaining on therapy showed significant improvement in articular index, pain, morning stiffness, hemoglobin value, platelet count, ESR, and IgG and IgM levels. Radiologic changes in the hands correlated best with the area of the curve under the ESR plot over the years.[29] Among other

aspects, this study emphasizes the commitment of time from both patient and physician in managing the disease, its complications, and the toxicity of therapy.

Risk for Death

The disturbingly high death rates suggested by Scott et al.[20] and Reilly et al.[22] have been confirmed by larger studies from detailed data banks. Appreciated long ago, and confirmed by more recent studies,[30] is that, compared with age- and sex-matched control populations, there is an increased risk of death for rheumatoid patients who have cutaneous ulcers, vasculitic rash, neuropathy, or other forms of extra-articular disease.

In a combined study from four centers of collected data in ARAMIS, 3,105 patients were followed for up to 35 years. A total of 922 patients died, for an overall mortality ratio of 2.3 for women and 2.1 for men.[31] This study indicated that there were significant differences among factors that lead to disability and those increasing the likelihood of death. Although joint swelling correlated with development of erosions and joint destruction, it was one of few clinical, laboratory, or radiographic variables not associated with subsequent mortality. In addition, in multivariate analyses, male sex was a prominent predictor of death, whereas being a woman was a predictor for disability. Because

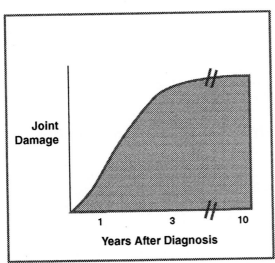 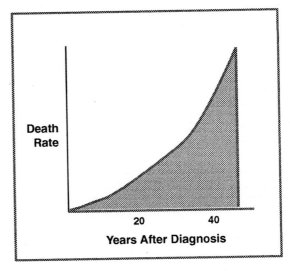

FIGURE 25–2. These two graphs, with very different curve characteristics, illustrate that although joint damage occurs at a maximal rate during the first several years of rheumatoid arthritis, it is the accumulated morbidity from the effects of joint damage, systemic inflammation, toxicity of drugs, and effects of drugs that leads to an accelerated death rate in rheumatoid patients. (Modified from Wolfe, F., Mitchell, D. M., Sibley, J. T., et al.: The mortality of rheumatoid arthritis. Arthritis Rheum. 37-481, 1994. Used by permission.)

being a man was not a risk factor for death in another study,[28] this gender issue remains unsettled.

A very important observation was the gradual increase in the slope of adjusted death rates with time (Fig. 25–2), leading to the insight that the accelerated rate of mortality in rheumatoid arthritis over time *"suggests that it is not merely having rheumatoid arthritis that is bad, but it is the progressive burden of disability, decrepitude, pain, treatment, and treatment side effects, operating over time, that increasingly leads to death in rheumatoid arthritis patients".*[31]

Causes of Death in Rheumatoid Arthritis

If there is indeed an increased mortality associated with having rheumatoid arthritis, what kills these people? A list of such causes matched against those in the U.S. population as a whole is shown in Table 25–2.[32] Unpredicted increases in the rheumatoid arthritis population as causes of death were infection, renal disease, respiratory disease, rheumatoid arthritis, and gastrointestinal disorders. Speculation on the reasons for these numbers includes predisposition to infection by immunosuppression from therapy, amyloidosis (uncommon in the United States), or analgesic abuse for renal disease, rheumatoid lung disease, and ulcerogenic drugs.

In a smaller study at one center of 75 patients followed over 15 years, the mortality rate was 1.62. A principal finding for clinicians was that a modified HAQ that includes only eight items and takes 10 to 15 minutes to administer (see Chapter 24) was as effective a predictor of death risk as were more elaborate, time-consuming, and expensive measures.[33]

Although the HAQ or modified HAQ is inexpensive and easy to perform, there are certain laboratory tests that can predict a poor prognosis for life. One study that, unfortunately, did not plug in simple tests (e.g., ESR and hemoglobin) for comparison, found that patients with raised levels of cryoglobulins and precipitating antibodies to soluble cellular antigens had a substantially increased risk of death[30]; IgM rheumatoid factor levels, ANA, and antibodies against EBV nuclear antigen titers did not predict mortality.

REFERENCES

1. Hunter, T.: The prognosis of early rheumatoid arthritis: how early is early? J. Rheumatol. 20:1999, 1993.
2. Chan, K.-W. A., Felson, D. T., Yood, R. A., et al.: The lag time between onset of symptoms and diagnosis of rheumatoid arthritis. Arthritis Rheum. 37:814, 1994.
3. Wolfe, F., Ross, K., Hawley, D. J., et al.: The prognosis of rheumatoid arthritis and undifferentiated polyarthritis syndrome in the clinic: a study of 1141 patients. J. Rheumatol. 20:2005, 1993.
4. Alarcón, G. S., Willkens, R. F., Ward, J. R., et al.: Early undifferentiated connective tissue disease. IV. Musculoskeletal manifestations in a large cohort of patients with undifferentiated connective tissue diseases compared with cohorts of patients with well-established connective tissue diseases: followup analyses in patients with unexplained polyarthritis and patients with rheumatoid arthritis at baseline. Arthritis Rheum. 39:403, 1996.
5. Wolfe, F., Hawley D. J., and Cathey, M. A.: Clinical and health status measures over time: prognosis and outcome assessment in rheumatoid arthritis. J. Rheumatol. 18:1290, 1991.
6. Eberhardt, K. B., Rydgren, L. C., Pettersson, H., et al.: Early rheumatoid arthritis—onset, course, and outcome over 2 years. Rheumatol. Int. 10:135, 1990.
7. van Zeben, D., Hazes, J. M. W., and Zwinderman, A. H.: The severity of rheumatoid arthritis: a 6-year followup study of younger women with symptoms of recent onset. J. Rheumatol. 21:1620, 1994.
8. van Leeuwen, M. A., van der Heijde, D. M. F. M., van Rijswijk, M. H., et al.: Interrelationship of outcome measures and process variables in early rheumatoid arthritis: a comparison of radiologic damage, physical disability, joint counts, and acute phase reactants. J. Rheumatol. 21:425, 1994.
9. Amos, R. S., Constable, T. J., Crockson, R. A., et al.: Rheumatoid arthritis: relation of serum C-reactive protein and erythrocyte sedimentation rates to radiographic changes. Br. Med. J. 1:196, 1977.
10. Van Leeuwen, M. A., Van Rijswijk, M. H., Van Der Heijde, D. M. F. M., et al.: The acute phase response in relation to radiographic progression in early rheumatoid arthritis: a prospective study during the first three years of the disease. Br. J. Rheumatol. 32:9, 1993.
11. Olsen, N. J., Callahan, L. F., Brooks, R. H., et al.: Associations of HLA-DR4 with rheumatoid factor and radiographic severity in rheumatoid arthritis. Am. J. Med. 84:257, 1988.
12. van Zeben, D., Hazes, J. M. W., Zwinderman, A. H., et al.: Association of HLA-DR4 with a more progressive

TABLE 25–2. Attributed Causes of Death in 2,262 Rheumatoid Arthritis Patients in 13 Series

	% DEATHS	
	RHEUMATOID ARTHRITIS	U.S. POPULATION
Cardiovascular disease	42	41
Cancer	14	20
Infection	9.4	1.0
Renal disease	7.8	1.1
Respiratory disease	7.2	3.9
Rheumatoid arthritis	5.3	Not listed
Gastrointestinal disease	4.2	2.4
Accidents	1.0	5.4

Data from Pincus and Griffin.[32]

disease course in patients with rheumatoid arthritis. Arthritis Rheum. 34:822, 1991.

13. Weyand, C. M., and Goronzy, J. J.: Prognosis in rheumatoid arthritis: applying new technologies to old questions. J. Rheumatol. 20:1817, 1993.

14. Weyand, C. M., Hicok, K. C., Conn, D., et al.: The influence of HLA-DRB1 genes on disease severity in rheumatoid arthritis. Ann. Intern. Med. 117:801, 1992.

15. Weyand, C. M., Xie, C., and Goronzy, J. J.: Homozygosity for the HLA-DRB1 allele selects for extra-articular manifestations in rheumatoid arthritis. J. Clin. Invest. 89:2033, 1992.

16. Gough, A., Faint, J., and Salmon, M.: Genetic typing of patients with inflammatory arthritis at presentation can be used to predict outcome. Arthritis Rheum. 37:1166, 1994.

17. Thompson, W., Pepper, L., Payton, A., et al.: Absence of an association between HLA-DRB1*04 and rheumatoid arthritis in newly diagnosed cases from the community. Ann. Rheum. Dis. 52:539, 1993.

18. Saxne, T., Wolheim, F. A., Petersson, H., et al.: Proteoglycan concentration in synovial fluid: predictor of future cartilage destruction in rheumatoid arthritis. Br. Med. J. 295:1447, 1987.

The highest levels of proteoglycan fragments in synovial fluid are from joints that, after 10 years, have undergone the greatest damage.

19. Ward, M. M., Leigh, P., and Fries J. F.: Progression of functional disability in patients with rheumatoid arthritis: associations with rheumatology subspecialty care. Arch. Intern. Med. 153:2229, 1993.

20. Scott, D. L., Symmons, D. P. M., Coulton, B. L., et al.: Long-term outcome of treating rheumatoid arthritis: results after 20 years. Lancet 1:1108, 1987.

21. Sharp, J. T., Wolfe, F., Mitchell, D. M., et al.: The progression of erosion and joint space narrowing scores in rheumatoid arthritis during the first twenty-five years of disease. Arthritis Rheum. 34:660, 1991.

22. Reilly, P. A., Cosh, J. A., Maddison, P. J., et al.: Mortality and survival in rheumatoid arthritis: a 25 year prospective study of 100 patients. Ann. Rheum. Dis. 49:363, 1990.

23. Leigh, J. P., and Fries, J. F.: Predictors of disability in a longitudinal sample of patients with rheumatoid arthritis. Ann. Rheum. Dis. 51:581, 1992.

24. Leigh, J. P., Fries, J. F., and Parikh, N.: Severity of disability and duration of disease in rheumatoid arthritis. J. Rheumatol. 19:1906, 1992.

25. Ward, M. M., and Leigh, J. P.: Marital status and the progression of functional disability in patients with rheumatoid arthritis. Arthritis Rheum. 36:581, 1993.

26. Katz, P. A., and Yelin, E. H.: The development of depressive symptoms among women with rheumatoid arthritis. Arthritis Rheum. 38:49, 1995.

27. Michel, B. A., Bloch, D. A., and Fries, J. F.: Predictors of fractures in early rheumatoid arthritis. J. Rheumatol. 18:804, 1991.

28. Leigh, J. P., and Fries J. F.: Mortality predictors among 263 patients with rheumatoid arthritis. J. Rheumatol. 18:1307, 1991.

29. Capell, H. A., Murphy, E. A., and Hunter, J. A.: Rheumatoid arthritis: workload and outcome over 10 years. Q. J. Med. 79:461, 1991.

30. Eberhardt, C. C., Mumford, P. A., Venables, P. J. W., et al.: Factors predicting a poor life prognosis in rheumatoid arthritis: an eight year prospective study. Ann. Rheum. Dis. 48:7, 1989.

31. Wolfe, F., Mitchell, D. M., Sibley, J. T., et al.: The mortality

of rheumatoid arthritis. Arthritis Rheum. 37:481, 1994.

In this study combining 3,105 patients from four centers in ARAMIS followed for up to 35 years, 922 patients died. The overall standardized mortality ratio (SMR) was 2.26 to 2.36 in women and 2.14 in men—and it increased with time. Using univariate analyses to test whether a variable present at the first clinic visit was associated with subsequent mortality, only two clinical, laboratory, or radiographic variables were not associated with subsequent mortality: joint swelling and hematocrit. Of demographic variables, family history of rheumatoid arthritis, body mass index, and alcohol use were not associated with subsequent mortality, nor were treatment with hydroxychloroquine, auranofin, and azathioprine treatment. Prednisone therapy generally increased mortality risk.

In multivariate analyses, simultaneous effects of multiple factors on the hazard of death were calculated, and the effect of individual covariates on the hazard of death were identified. In patients from all three centers analyzed in this way, age and male sex were the most prominent associations; in descending order after that were disability measured by HAQ, joint count, rheumatoid factor titers, prednisone therapy, hypertension, rales, nodules, ESR, and education. As examples, a patient 1 year older in age had a 6.6% increased hazard of death and, after controlling for their covariates, the hazard of death was 43.4% higher for men than women. At one center, receiving prednisone at the first visit was associated with a 60.6% increase compared with not taking prednisone at the first visit. The data did not answer the question of whether prednisone is merely a marker of rheumatoid arthritis severity or is, in and of itself, deleterious.

Observed versus expected death ratios from various causes, overall, were

Infection:	
Cancer:	0.3
Leukemia/lymphoma:	8.0
Circulatory:	1.0
Cerebrovascular:	1.1
Respiratory:	0.9
Pneumonia:	5.3
Digestive:	1.5
Renal:	0.9
Rheumatoid arthritis:	12.9

The largest contribution to the SMR, 2.26, came from causes other than rheumatoid arthritis. Cardiovascular disease accounted for 361 and cerebrovascular disease 37 deaths; these two were the greatest causes of excess mortality. Interestingly, rheumatoid arthritis was mentioned on the death certificate in only 41 per cent of deaths. Also, although a primary cause of death in only 5.6 per cent of cases, gastrointestinal problems contributed to an additional 5.7 per cent of deaths.

32. Pincus, T., and Griffin, M.: Gastrointestinal disease associated with nonsteroidal anti-inflammatory drugs: new insights from observational studies and functional status questionnaires. Am. J. Med. 91:209, 1991.

This editorial includes a table of attributed causes of death in 2,262 patients with rheumatoid arthritis in 13 series. The cumulative totals, as percentages of deaths attributed to listed causes in all patients, are listed in Table 25–2 (see text).

33. Pincus, T., Brooks, R. H., and Callahan, L. F.: Prediction of long-term mortality in patients with rheumatoid arthritis

according to simple questionnaire and joint count measures. Ann. Intern. Med. 120:26, 1994.

This cohort study of 75 patients with rheumatoid arthritis from a university hospital outpatient clinic described mortality over 15 years. The following quantitative baseline measures were used:

Demographic (age, sex,* formal education*)

Clinical variables
   Duration of disease
   Morning stiffness
   Treatments
   Co-morbid cardiovascular disease*

Articular variables
   Joint count* (done with variable counts/patient)

Questionnaires about functional status*

Functional measurements
   Grip strength*
   Modified walking time*
   Button test*

The significant predictors of mortality are designated by asterisks. The mortality ratio at 15 years was 1.62, similar to findings in other studies. Causes of death were

Cardiovascular disease:	44%
Cancer:	21%
Gastrointestinal disease:	6%
Pulmonary disease:	12%
Infection:	15%
Rheumatoid arthritis:	3%

SECTION IX

GENERAL AND SPECIFIC TREATMENT OF RHEUMATOID ARTHRITIS

Therapy of rheumatoid arthritis begins with non-specific anti-inflammatory drugs and depending on the sophistication of the attending physicians, may become more complex. The trade-off to using potent agents is unfortunately, side effects. Each patient deserves to be a part of the therapeutic decision process, in a way that relates his or her degree of aversion to risk to potential benefit.

Joining standard medicinal pharmacology for treatment of rheumatoid arthritis are both monoclonal antibodies and products of recombinant DNA technology. It is crucial that the community of patients and their physicians deploy the available populations of patients for therapeutic trials that have the best apparent (probable) benefit:toxicity.

26

General Principles
of Therapy

Several important truths have emerged from outcome studies of rheumatoid patients observed over many years and exposed to diverse regimens of therapy:

1. No single therapeutic regimen has led to a marked or sustained improvement in clinical manifestations, or to a halt in the progression of loss of joint structure and function.[1]

2. Irreversible loss of articular cartilage begins, in many cases, within months of the onset of disease, and in most cases within a year of onset of continuously active synovitis. Analysis of radiographic data from several studies suggests that 50 per cent of the maximum damage to joints happens within the first 5 years of arthritis.[2,3] Use of MRI has enabled clinicians to pick up erosions early in the course of disease and long before they are visible on plain films.[4]

3. Side effects or complications of therapy lead all too often to increased morbidity or even death.

4. The only parameter that accurately identifies patients destined to develop severe erosive or extra-articular disease is the shared epitope, the QKRAA amino acid sequence in the third hypervariable region of the MHC class II *HLA-DRB1* chain.

5. Clinically available and effective predictors of prognosis (see Chapter 25) include the HAQ and its modifications, functional tests, acute-phase reactants, and the presence of and titer of rheumatoid factor.

6. Patients treated early in their disease course by rheumatologists tend to have a better long-term outcome than those treated by physicians who are not specialists in rheumatology, perhaps because rheumatologists are more likely to treat patients early and more aggressively. One study has confirmed the reluctance of primary care physicians to prescribe disease-modifying drugs. Although 73 per cent had heard of these drugs and were aware of their value, only 14 per cent used them in clinical practice.[5]

7. Not surprisingly, homeopathy is no more effective than placebo in treatment of rheumatoid arthritis,[6] although rheumatologists have long recognized the extraordinary power of placebo in clinical trials.

There are two parameters available to every clinician that can help determine the character of disease in individual patients:

• The degree of sustained synovitis
• The intensity of synovitis

Accurate assessment of these parameters gives physicians a crude index of the degree of urgency for instituting more aggressive therapy. Thus, the patient with intermittent flares of synovitis who is relatively symptom-free during partial remissions is not likely to go on to rapid loss of joint function or severe extra-articular disease. In contrast, the patient with continuous, active synovitis has a less good prognosis. Similarly, the intensity of disease activity, measured by clinical examination and laboratory tests as well as the patient's own assessment, is a useful predictor of risk for death or disability.

The challenge for treating rheumatoid arthritis is to begin early enough with therapy likely to down-regulate the disease process without causing morbidity or death from side effects of treatment. The goal is to alter, by treatment, the slope of the curve toward joint destruction.

There are a few solid reasons for optimism that an earlier, more aggressive therapeutic approach may be beneficial. One is that we know much more about the risk of long-term side effects of drugs than previously, and therefore we should be able to use them more carefully and effectively. For example, it is clear now that even a single daily dose of 5 mg prednisone has cumulative side effects, principally on bone density, and that higher doses are associated with increased mortality as well as morbidity. Nevertheless, proper use of prednisone may produce benefits that outweigh risk. Another reason for earlier therapy is that we are at a thresh-

TABLE 26–1. Rheumatoid Arthritis: Staging and Standard Therapy*

STAGE OF DISEASE	TIME AFTER ONSET OF SYNOVITIS	CLINICAL CHARACTERISTICS	LABORATORY FINDINGS	PATHOLOGIC PROCESS	BIOPATHOLOGY	MANAGEMENT
1	Days to several weeks	Onset may be relatively acute or gradual, over several weeks. Morning stiffness and fatigue are often first symptoms. Pain and swelling are variable. Wrists, MCP, PIP, and MTP joints are usually affected first. Anxiety at a high level. Joints are tender, grip strength slightly less than normal. Skin temperature over joints may be normal or warm. Fluid may be detectable in MCP-or PIP joints or knees. Hips are rarely involved now. Venous pattern may be prominent on skin over joints. Nodules rarely are present.	ESR/CRP usually a function of the severity, but rarely highly abnormal. RF helpful if positive. Platelet count, eosinophils may be increased. Radiographs are normal. Fever, occasionally.	In synovium, new capillaries begin to form near mononuclear cells; tissue is edematous and cells are scattered without a pattern. Synovial lining 2–4 cell layers deep. Electron micrographs could show APCs in contact with lymphocytes near capillaries. Macrophages begin to proliferate.	Antigen presented by class II MHC-bearing cells to CD4+ cells that have migrated to joints. Adhesion molecules in tall endothelium stop and fix rolling lymphocytes. PMN leukocytes begin to accumulate within increased amounts of synovial fluid produced by transudation from capillaries with added protein and hyaluronan from synovial cells. In response to angiogenic factors such as FGF, new capillaries sprout from existing ones.	Too early for a definite diagnosis. NSAIDs or, in selected cases, salicylates. Education about self-management. Physical therapy to keep muscle tone and full range of motion. Instruction in joint protection. **TESTS:** CBC RF ANA ESR and/or CRP *DRB1* sequence at third hypervariable region, if available, in a research setting Arthrocentesis if fluid is palpable
2	Approximately 6 weeks to 6 months	Although the symptoms may wax and wane, the overall course is one of continued joint swelling, morning stiffness, pain on motion, and fatigue. New joints, knees and elbows	70% will have positive test for RF by 3 months. ESR/CRP elevated. WBC and platelets increased. Radiographs may show early juxta-articular	Synovial lining cells proliferate. Lymphocytes accumulate in foci around proliferating capillaries. Plasma cells appear. Monocyte/macrophages begin to phagocytose debris. At insertion of synovium into subchondral bone,	Lymphokines from activated CD4+ cells and cytokines from macrophages generate synovial cell proliferation and activation. B cells are activated and begin synthesis of RF. Synovium may have 20- to 100-fold	**CRUCIAL STAGE OF THERAPY**† With a definite diagnosis made, a carefully designed, aggressive therapeutic regimen is indicated to halt the progressive synovial inflammation.

especially, may become symptomatic. Nodules may appear in active, aggressive disease with positive RF. Definite diagnosis possible at this time. demineralization. Arthrocentesis will give additional useful information about the level of inflammation in the joint.	proliferating synovium begins to invade bone and to encroach on peripheral surface of cartilage. Synovial effusions are often large, and contain from 5,000 to 100,000 WBC/mm^3.	the weight and volume of normal synovium. Early chondrocyte activation results in protease release and local degradation of proteoglycans. TNFα is the driving cytokine for IL-1β production.	NSAIDs or salicylates should be continued at maximal dose. In selected patients, prednisone, 5 mg/day, may be added. Hydroxychoroquine or—in particularly aggressive disease—addition of methotrexate is appropriate.‡ Appropriate exercise and protocols for joint protection, and continued education about the disease, are important. In patients who clearly have aggressive disease, the indications for combination therapy increase. The importance in measuring benefit-cost ratios and including the risks of additive toxicity become paramount. For example, it is not unwise to think of adding minocycline, 100 mg b.i.d., at this time, including sulfasalazine as a triple therapy, and injecting with glucocorticoids all joints that have tenderness and effusions.

Table continued on following page

TABLE 26–1. *Continued*

STAGE OF DISEASE	TIME AFTER ONSET OF SYNOVITIS	CLINICAL CHARACTERISTICS	LABORATORY FINDINGS	PATHOLOGIC PROCESS	BIOPATHOLOGY	MANAGEMENT
3	6–9 months to 2 years	If the synovitis has not subsided in response to therapy by this time, it has undergone substantial polarization and proliferation. Although it would be early for deformity to develop, loss of range of motion from soft tissue contracture is common, especially in knees and elbows. Muscle mass is diminished from disuse from pain. Functional tests reveal loss of dexterity and an increased time to accomplish simple tasks. Particular joints may cause special problems (e.g., loss of shoulder abduction or extension, very tender MTP joints). As a function of the degree of inflammation, generalized weakness and debilitation can be prominent. Extra-articular disease, such as vasculitis, Sjögren's syndrome, or Felty's syndrome, may develop.	Lab tests are more often needed to monitor therapy rather than to assess the disease process. Tests to monitor the activity of disease should be those found empirically that vary with clinical symptoms. RF is not likely to be an indicated test. Routine hemoglobins are needed to assess possible GI blood loss from NSAIDs.	The polarized synovitis has achieved a mass sufficient to invade subchondral bone, the periphery of cartilage, and the surface. Loss of proteoglycans from cartilage leaves the tissue susceptible to damage from weight bearing.	The proliferating synovial cells release stromelysin, gelatinase, and collagenase in large quantities, particularly at the cartilage-pannus junction. IgG deposits with antigen and complement components in the superficial layers of cartilage may serve as chemoattractants for this polarized, invasive pannus. Natural inhibitors in synovial fluid (e.g., $\alpha_2 M_1$) may be saturated, and TIMP levels may be inadequate to retard joint destruction. Depending on the degree to which the process expands beyond joints, lymphocytic infiltration may be found in the spleen (Felty's syndrome) or salivary and lacrimal glands (Sjögren's syndrome). IgG complexes in small arterioles can generate a vasculitis and be symptomatic in nerves, heart, lung, or GI tract.	When the disease has progressed this far, it is apparent that response to even aggressive therapy has been minimally effective. Before joint deformity develops, it is appropriate to use joint infections with a glucocorticoid such as triamcinolone hexacetonide. Gold or penicillamine should have been tried, and continued if efficacious. Methotrexate, and combinations of methotrexate with other drugs, should be used. **These patients are candidate for trials of biologic agents.** Orthopedic consultation should be retained earlier rather than later to prevent, as much as possible, loss of function.

4	Two to >25 years with active disease	These patients have developed deformity and have substantial loss of function. It is likely that side effects of medications have limited options for therapy or have produced anemia, kidney disease, leukopenia, or other problems. Risk for fracture and tendon rupture is high.	Complications of therapy often dominate any panels of abnormal laboratory tests. Radiographs show loss of cartilage, subluxed joints, erosions of bone, fractures, and osteopenia. Tolerance to therapy is known, and there are few surprises in laboratory tests. Anemia, hypoalbuminemia, hyperglobulinemia, and hypocemia can be caused by the disease itself. Proteinuria and bone marrow aplasias may reflect toxicity of therapy.	The changes here are extensions of those in stage 3. As all cartilage is lost from a particular joint, the synovitis may become less proliferative and luxuriant, and synovial effusions decrease. Granulomas invade bone that has become osteopenic. Fibrosis often increases over cellularity in the synovium. Tendon rupture may occur. Changes of osteoarthritis increase as the cellular synovitis diminishes.	The findings are an extension of those in stage 3. The downstream effects of TNFα dominate, producing cachexia as well as helping to accelerate destruction of cartilage, ligaments, and bone. "Reparative" cytokines (e.g., TGFβ) have only a mild effect.

Special problems such as cervical spine subluxation, fractures, flexion contractures, dysfunctional grasp, and severe pain from foot and ankle involvement may dominate the clinical picture.

Specific medications for arthritis should not be used unless a particular one is demonstrated to be effective; this is not likely considering that the disease has progressed so far. New compounds should be used with caution. Major emphasis should be on functional restoration through careful arthroplasty, osteotomy, tendon repairs, etc.

Modified from Harris, E. D. Jr.: Treatment of rheumatoid arthritis. *In* Kelley, W. N., Harris, E. D. Jr., Ruddy, S., and Sledge, C.B. (eds.): Textbook of Rheumatology, 5th ed. Vol. 1. Philadelphia, W. B. Saunders, 1996 (in press).

* Abbreviations: α_2M, α_2-macroglobulin; CBC, complete blood count; GI, gastrointestinal.

† Response of patients at this stage of disease is crucial if joint destruction is to be avoided. Although the process has a different rate of progression in each patient, the pathologic process in the synovium is well on its way to becoming cyclic and self-sustaining. Using the best predictors possible, the physician must weigh the possible side effects of medications against the risk of cartilage and bone loss. A complete remission is not a realistic goal, but a significant decrease in joint swelling, tenderness, and pain are appropriate objectives.

‡ The hydroxychloroquine or methotrexate can be given a full 2-month trial. If the therapy has not been efficacious, it will be appropriate to try additional cytotoxic drugs or, alternatively, to enlist the patient to join in a trial of biologic agents.

old of potential availability of biologic therapies that have targeted specificity within the pathophysiologic mechanisms that generate and sustain rheumatoid arthritis. Another factor is that combination therapies have been proved useful.

A reason for discouragement, or in the worst case therapeutic nihilism, is that the drugs we use are toxic, and it is rare for second-line drugs to be continued—either because of lack of efficacy or because of unacceptable side effects—for more than 2 or 3 years in any one patient.[2,7–10] Another discouraging reality is that no long-term analysis of radiographic progression of joint disease shows significant breaks in the curve toward inexorable joint destruction, regardless of therapy.

The most optimistic interpretation that can be taken from these data is the belief, mentioned earlier, that the only path available to effective delay or cessation of joint destruction in rheumatoid arthritis is to begin therapy early enough to prevent the amplified cycle of destructive elements from becoming self-sustaining.

STAGES OF RHEUMATOID ARTHRITIS AND IMPLICATIONS FOR THERAPY

Patients with rheumatoid arthritis are like fingerprints; although each may be similar to others, no two are identical. Of course, in every clinical trial, an effort must be made to fit patients into cohorts separable by some measurable parameter such as functional class or a radiographic index. In management of individuals, it is the subtleties of their particular disease pace and process, matched with elements of their personalities, that make each therapeutic challenge unique.

Many different schemes have been developed over the years in an attempt to put logic into therapeutic strategies for rheumatoid arthritis. The most used of these was the "therapeutic pyramid," in which the base was formed of education, physical therapy, occupational therapy, and salicylates. As one rose toward the peak of the pyramid, more potent drugs were added, and the capstone was usually cytotoxic drugs. This conceptualization may have done significant harm. It implied that, as the disease got worse, there were fewer and fewer modalities of therapy available, encouraging clinicians to hold back on aggressive therapy as long as possible. It resulted in physicians trying to catch up to rheumatoid arthritis rather than getting ahead of it. "Inversion" of the therapeutic pyramid was a concept that encouraged clinicians to use second-line drugs

early, and sometimes in combination.[3] This is closer to the "use what it takes" philosophy that has as its primary objective early suppression of disease activity.[11] The "sawtooth" strategy suggests sequential deployment of disease-modifying drugs, switching to the next drug on the list at the first hint of lack of or diminishing efficacy of the currently administered drug.[12] **Combination therapy** rests on the hypothesis that there is a greater additive (or synergistic) benefit from combining second-line drugs than additive or compounded risk from side effects of those drugs.

In order to provide a framework within which to focus on special qualities of each person's illness, a rheumatoid arthritis staging system has been devised using concepts partially developed previously[13,14] (Table 26–1). The pace of the process, the extent to which the synovitis is continuous, and the functional class can be matched with the pathology at the time that treatment options are presented. For each therapeutic modality or drug discussed in Table 26–1, there is a corresponding chapter in this section in which details of that management are stressed.

In future years, combination therapy is likely to be used early in the disease process. Patient preferences will play a larger role, and clinical trials will have relevant change for the better or toxicity as major end-points.

SURGERY IN RHEUMATOID ARTHRITIS

It should be noted that this book does not include discussions of surgery for rheumatoid arthritis. The absence of such discussions implies nothing other than a reluctance on the author's part to attempt to link medical and surgical approaches in one small text. No doubt exists: Surgery is an extremely important adjunct to the medical therapies discussed here. It is crucial to consult an orthopedic surgeon who is an expert on rheumatic diseases *early* in the course of deformity or joint destruction, not necessarily with expectations that surgery will be done then, but to give the consultant adequate time to join in evaluation.

The principles of surgery for rheumatoid arthritis have been outlined in a recent publication[15] and a textbook[16] based on years of experience at a hospital devoted exclusively to the medical, surgical, and rehabilitative care of joint disease. The following are important generalizations about operative care of patients with rheumatoid arthritis:

- Surgery is almost always elective, and planned over a long period of observation of the patient by a rheumatologist and orthopedic surgeon. Exceptions to this include operative stabilization of the cervical spine when C1–C2 subluxation occurs, and repair of extensor tendon rupture in the wrist.
- Surgery should be considered prophylactic as well as therapeutic. Focused tenosynovectomy, for example, may prevent tendon rupture.
- Surgery on a particular joint must be individualized in the context of other joint involvement and the patient's needs for activity.
- Evidence has accumulated about the effectiveness of similar procedures on different joints and should be taken seriously. For example, although total hip and knee arthroplasties generally produce high satisfaction in patients, total ankle and elbow replacements have a much higher failure rate.

THE COMPREHENSIVE THERAPEUTIC PLAN

The plan for an individual patient must be based on use of multiple disciplines (e.g., rheumatology, surgery, rehabilitation) and also on that particular patient's graph of time plotted against disease progression. Patients with rapid progression of continually active disease will warrant earlier intervention with second-line drugs and timely surgery. There is another important component in therapeutic decision making: patient preference. Although it takes much time by physicians and nurses, each patient must be given thorough explanations of the current status and probable prognosis of his or her arthritis, and the therapies proved useful in clinical trials that are appropriate at this stage. Along with potential benefit, the risks of each therapy must be laid out, and the patient can be helped in assessing how much risk is acceptable for the probability of achieving a beneficial effect.

REFERENCES

1. Ferraccioli, G., Salaffi, F., Nervetti, A., et al.: Slow acting drugs—outcome is no different than 15 years ago. J. Rheumatol. 117:1249, 1990.
2. Pincus, T., and Callahan, L. F.: The "side effects" of rheumatoid arthritis: joint destruction, disability and early mortality. Br. J. Rheumatol. 32(suppl. 1):28, 1993.
3. Fuchs, H. A., and Pincus, T.: Radiographic damage in rheumatoid arthritis: description by nonlinear models. J. Rheumatol. 19:1655, 1992.
4. Gilkeson, G., Polisson, R., Sinclair, H., et al.: Early detection of carpal erosions in patients with rheumatoid arthritis: a pilot study of magnetic resonance imaging. J. Rheumatol. 15:1361, 1988.
5. Stross, J. K.: Relationships between knowledge and experience in the use of disease-modifying antirheumatic agents: a study of primary care practitioners. JAMA 262: 2721, 1989.
6. Andrade, L. E. C., Ferraz, M. B., Atra, E., et al.: A randomized controlled trial to evaluate the effectiveness of homeopathy in rheumatoid arthritis. Scand. J. Rheumatol. 20: 204, 1991.
7. Pincus, T., Marcum, S. B., Callahan, L. F., et al.: Longterm drug therapy for rheumatoid arthritis in seven rheumatology private practices: I. Nonsteroidal antiinflammatory drugs. J. Rheumatol. 19:1874, 1992.

    Probabilities of continuation of a NSAID, including aspirin in various forms by 532 patients in seven rheumatologic practices were estimated. At 12 months, 48 per cent of patients who had started on a particular NSAID still were taking it, and at 24 months, 36 per cent continued. Interestingly, acetylated salicylates other than aspirin were continued longer than other types of NSAID.

8. Pincus, T., Marcum, S. B., and Callahan, L. F.: Longterm drug therapy for rheumatoid arthritis in seven rheumatology private practices: II. Second line drugs and prednisone. J. Rheumatol. 19:1885, 1992.

    The probability of continuing 1,077 courses of a second-line drug taken by 532 patients in seven rheumatology practices was examined. The number of months at which 50 per cent of patients would be still taking each drug was

Oral gold:	10
Hydroxychloroquine:	20
Penicillamine:	21
Parenteral gold:	25
Azathioprine:	27
Methotrexate:	60

    This study supports a meta-analysis that suggests that methotrexate may differ meaningfully in efficacy from other available second-line drugs in treatment of rheumatoid arthritis.

9. Pincus, T.: The case for early intervention in rheumatoid arthritis. J. Autoimmun. 5(suppl. A):209, 1992.
10. Wolfe, F., Hawley, D. J., and Cathey, M. A.: Termination of slow acting antirheumatic therapy in rheumatoid arthritis: a 14-year prospective evaluation of 1017 consecutive starts. J. Rheumatol. 17:994, 1990.
11. McCarty, D. J.: Suppress rheumatoid inflammation early and leave the pyramid to the Egyptians. J. Rheumatol. 17:1115, 1990.
12. Fries, J. F.: Reevaluating the therapeutic approach to rheumatoid arthritis: the "sawtooth" strategy. J. Rheumatol. 17(suppl. 22):12, 1990.
13. Harris, E. D. Jr.: Rheumatoid arthritis: pathophysiology and implications for therapy. N. Engl. J. Med. 322:1277, 1990.
14. Willkens, R. F.: Prognostic staging for therapy of rheumatoid arthritis. Semin. Arthritis Rheum. 21(2, suppl. 1):40, 1991.
15. Anderson, R. J.: The orthopedic management of rheumatoid arthritis. Arthritis Care Res. 9:223, 1996.
16. Sledge, C. B., Kelley, W. N., Harris, E. D. Jr., and Ruddy, S.: Arthritis Surgery. Philadelphia, W. B. Saunders, 1994.

27

Use of Patient Education and Physical Modalities in Early Treatment

The earliest therapy for rheumatoid arthritis is often the most important for outcome. It is then, even before a definite diagnosis can be made, that the patient begins adaptation to being sick and having pain, and becomes accustomed to a change of lifestyle with modulations in occupation, hobbies, diet, activity, and relationships. This is the time that an effective relationship with a physician interested in the details of management over months and years must be established.

This chapter deals with the therapies other than pharmacologic ones that can be initiated in the early weeks of symptoms, during Stage 1 of illness (see Table 26–1, Chapter 26). The patient has a polyarthritis; diagnosis is not yet possible. Much can be done at this time that will be useful for all patients, even those who will get better in weeks or months and never have a firm diagnosis. The areas for emphasis are the physician-patient contract, education about chronic arthritis, diet (see Chapter 28), and physical activity.

THE PHYSICIAN-PATIENT CONTRACT

The physician-patient "contract" is usually not a written one, and its nature is entirely dependent on the willingness of the patient to be thoroughly and responsibly involved in management of his or her disease, and yet have trust in the experience, judgment, and therapeutic plan of the physician. A valuable ally for successful development of this relationship is a nurse-practitioner or physician assistant, trained specifically to manage patients with chronic diseases and to work in close tandem with the physician. The nurse adds, among other assets, a crucial element of accessibility. Most of the new patient's questions and concerns are ones that can be readily and appropriately answered by the nonphysician professional partner.

LEARNED HELPLESSNESS: AN IMPEDIMENT TO EFFECTIVE MANAGEMENT OF RHEUMATOID ARTHRITIS

This model of a patient's reaction to chronic disease states that the patient believes that pain, disability, and other consequences of rheumatoid arthritis cannot be controlled by the physician or the patient because the cause of the disease is unknown, its course is unpredictable, and there is no cure.[1,2] The helpless state is marked by three types of deficits:

Emotional deficits: The patient readily develops anxiety, depression, fear of altered appearance, and loss of self-esteem.

Motivational deficits: The patient withdraws from attempts to engage in modified activities of daily living.

Cognitive deficits: The patient is unable to develop, even with guidance, new coping behaviors.

The end result of the confluence of these deficits is the noncompliant patient, one who readily tries unproven remedies, excessively relies on the health care system but rails against its perceived inadequacies, and takes few positive steps toward adaptation to illness. There is some evidence that helplessness is related to disability in a manner independent of disease severity, and more significantly than other psychosocial variables such as education and financial status.[3] Some data exist to support the belief that helplessness and depression are significantly related to joint counts.[4]

The only effective way to combat learned helplessness is to recognize the potential for it to develop in each patient, and to help prevent its development by education, reassurance, counseling, and—most important—early demonstration that prescribed therapy can alleviate symptoms.

Learned helplessness and depression are not components of the psyche of all rheumatoid patients. This is supported by a 10-year longitudinal study of 6,143 patients that showed no more depressive symptoms in rheumatoid patients than in other clinic patients.[5] Indeed, much depression in rheumatoid patients can be traced directly to deterioration of clinical status.[6] In an intriguing contrast with these data from the United States, however, a study of 42 Italian patients indicated that those with the highest depression scores showed more subsequent pain and disability.[7]

It should also be noted that, despite various degrees of depression that occur inevitably in the hurting rheumatoid patient, self-reports of functional status, such as the HAQ are reported to be a true measure of disability and not just a global, subjective, and emotionally colored index reflecting depression or the lack of it.[8,9]

Based on the accepted evidence that depression is more prevalent among women than among men, a study has examined the symptoms of emotional distress related to arthritis in men and women who do paid (not volunteer) work. The hypothesis was that higher levels of distress among women with rheumatoid arthritis would exist because women were exposed to more distressing work characteristics.[10] The results showed that women were more distressed because they reported more functional disability than men, not more exposure to stressful work characteristics. It can be inferred from these data that counseling and guidance about paid work in the context of each patient's disease activity should be part of any therapeutic plan for a rheumatoid patient. Indeed, the general management of "stress" can be helpful for rheumatoid patients. In one study,[11] a stress management approach emphasizing generalizability and maintenance of long-term benefits that utilized a computer-assisted method of program delivery and a 15-month follow-up was applied to 81 men and 60 women divided between a "standard care" group and those receiving only education about their disease. Findings were that (1) patients found stress management programs credible and educationally appealing, (2) the stress management program had an immediate effect on the psychological state of the participants, and (3) at the 15-month follow-up, the helplessness, pain, and health status scores were still lower in those who had received stress management than in those given standard care with or without educational programs.

STRESS AND THE IMMUNE RESPONSE

Is it possible that unhappiness, despair, stress, and pain can negatively influence immune functions? This study of "psychoneuroimmunology" has received significant scientific support from studies linking neuropeptides such as *substance P* as inducers of inflammation, proteases, and cytokines in rheumatoid arthritis.[12] In addition, several studies have actually demonstrated a correlation between stress and diminished immune responses.[12,13] One demonstrated that patients' perceptions of their abilities to manage the pain of arthritis correlated positively with the measured number of T-suppressor cells and negatively with helper-suppressor cell ratios.[13]

In one of the first studies to correlate a biologic marker of immune activity with psychological status, 14 patients with rheumatoid arthritis were assayed for mood disturbance, clinical indicators of disease, and serum soluble IL-2R. The data showed that changes in mood disturbance were unrelated to changes in joint inflammation, but that periods of worsening moods were linked with decreased soluble IL-2R levels and increases in reported joint pain.[14] If it is accepted that the soluble IL-2R assay is a quantitative measure of cell-mediated immune activation, it could be inferred that depressed mood correlates with depressed immune function in these patients (see Chapter 23).

EDUCATION ABOUT ARTHRITIS: A MAINSTAY OF THERAPY

One of the most interesting findings that relates various subsets of rheumatoid patients to poor outcome is the inverse correlation with formal education status and mortality.[15] Those patients with fewer years of schooling are more likely to die earlier than a well-educated patient, all other variables being relatively equal. Thus it is notable that an alternative to formal education—education in the clinic about what rheumatoid arthritis is, how it affects a person, and how it should be treated—has a positive effect on outcome of the disease. The Arthritis Self-Management Program (ASMP)—developed, tested, and implemented by Lorig and her colleagues at Stanford University—teaches patients and, equally important, enables them to be involved in therapy and therapeutic decisions from the beginning[16,17] of physician-supervised treatment. It is of importance that the beneficial outcomes of the Stanford self-management course are not adequately explained by behavioral change alone; some other factor must be working here, and as yet it is unknown.[18]

It is useful to compare the nature of rheumatoid arthritis with other diseases, and the opportunities for self-help among patients with those diseases. Rheumatoid arthritis, by its nature, gives the patient more opportunities to help himself or herself than do most other chronic processes. The afflicted individual must overcome the trials of a protracted course, discomfort, disability, and cost. In addition, medications constantly reveal the other edge of their sword: toxicity.

A patient's perceived self-efficacy to cope with the consequences of chronic arthritis correlates very well with the outcomes of the ASMP. Most encouraging has been the prolonged effect of the ASMP. Of 219 patients who completed phase I of the ASMP, 177 were studied 4 years later. During that interval, none had received any more formal help in self-management. Pain had declined a mean of 20 per cent and visits to physicians 40 per cent even though disability had increased 9 per cent. For each rheumatoid patient the estimated 4-year savings were $648.[19] Most people live with someone else. It has been demonstrated that participation of spouses in educational group sessions for patients with rheumatoid arthritis leads to additional beneficial effects.[20]

Physicians have the tendency to assume that their patients know more about the disease than they actually do know. In one study of 70 randomly selected patients with rheumatoid arthritis, 62 per cent knew that the cause of rheumatoid arthritis is, as yet, unknown but 27 per cent thought it could be caused by injury and 11 per cent by cold, damp weather. Fifty-two per cent had no idea why blood tests were necessary. In the realm of the rationale for, use of, and side effects of disease-modifying drugs, knowledge was abysmally inadequate.[21]

SEXUAL ACTIVITY OF RHEUMATOID PATIENTS

Although the changes in quantity and quality of sexual activity among patients with stable relationships is a sensitive measure of well-being or the lack of it, few physicians take a sexual history or record changes in sexuality as a routine part of follow-up visits. In a study of 102 men and 118 women with rheumatoid arthritis who were living with a spouse, it was found that physical disability, pain, and, to a lesser extent, depression were found to intrude on sexuality in 30 per cent of men and 36 per cent of women with this disease.[22] In a compre-hensive plan of therapy for each patient, there should be a component for sexual counseling and education. It should include teaching about how the disease and medications used to treat it alter mood and sexual responsiveness, how mutual masturbation and caressing can give pleasure without pain, and which positions for intercourse are least painful for each patient.

REST AND EXERCISE

As recently as the 1980s, patients with rheumatoid arthritis who had flares of disease activity were often admitted to general medical units or arthritis centers in hospitals, primarily for rest and supervised exercise. Although the long-term outcome may not have been changed by these interludes in a hospital, the short-term benefits were positive.[23,24] Close work with physical and occupational therapists and a "vacation" from home or the workplace was a tonic of encouragement for patients. It also was an ideal time for physicians to reassess drug therapy regimens and to check laboratory values to assay for disease activity and for early toxicity of medications. Patients who had comorbid disease, higher disability as measured by the HAQ, and lower hemoglobin on admission were more likely to have a prolonged admission.[25] These hospitalizations were often prolonged and, of course, very expensive.

Data appear to indicate that short-term benefit could accrue from stays in a hospital for as short as 2 weeks.[26] In a randomized study, 35 inpatients and 36 outpatients were measured and assessed at 19 weeks for all relevant costs and for outcome of clinical measures; inpatient therapy produced a sustained threefold increase in efficacy at a 2.5-fold increase in cost to society.[27]

Despite this study and other evidence that inpatient therapy of rheumatoid arthritis can be cost-effective, insurance companies and managed care health plans in the United States currently deny coverage for many if not most admissions for rest and therapy for rheumatoid patients unless there is a comorbid, acute process in evolution. Unfortunately, rest and exercise are modalities of therapy that must be managed and directed outside the hospital.

Titrating the proper amount of rest that a rheumatoid arthritis patient should take is a substantial challenge. Patients enter the disease process with different baselines of activity. Some are vigorous athletes or manual laborers, whereas others have had a lifestyle that never generates perspiration. An additional variable is individual sensitivity to pain.

Effects of Rest and Exercise

Disuse from sustained **rest**—induced by either pain, prescription, or volition—can cause loss of strength estimated at 8 per cent per week.[29] Full sustained rest is immobilization, and this leads to loss of strength plus joint contracture secondary to shortening of muscle and collagen in muscle tendons. Type II muscle fibers (those that have a fast contraction time) are particularly susceptible to atrophy from disuse, and are decreased in number and diameter in rheumatoid arthritis.[30] Sustained rest also generates a negative nitrogen balance (especially in patients on glucocorticoids), calciuria, and osteoporosis.[31]

There seems to be little argument that the proper amount of **exercise** is good for just about everyone. It increases or maintains range of motion, improves strength and endurance, preserves bone mineralization, cushions impact load, and distributes the forces of muscle contraction more evenly over joint surfaces. Globally, exercise increases the capacity of skeletal and cardiac muscle to do work; this can be measured as an increase in maximal oxygen consumption.

Some patients are made almost catatonic by their disease, whereas others either do not sense or ignore the pain of inflammatory synovitis and may go on to destroy joints while having few expressed symptoms (e.g., those with *arthritis robustus*). The challenge is to down-regulate activity of the athletes and vigorous workers, and up-regulate activity of the slothful patients.

In one series of patients with rheumatoid arthritis who had been referred for exercise training in Scandinavia, 38 per cent of the patients never or seldom exercised, whereas 72 per cent wished to increase their activity but were prevented by pain.[28] Lack of mobility can generate loss of self-confidence, and this can spiral down into a pseudo-catatonic depression for the hurting patient with polyarticular synovitis.

Techniques of Muscle Strengthening

Isometric Exercise

In isometric exercise, muscle is contracted in a fixed position against immobile resistance. It is particularly efficient when contraction occurs at the resting length of the muscle.[29] Maximum contrac-

tions, held for 6 seconds, repeated 5 to 10 times are generally recommended. Even brief isometric contraction (one contraction held for 6 seconds once a day) increases strength of a muscle.[32]

Dynamic Exercise

Increasing amounts of resistance applied during movement through the functional arc of a muscle is the standard approach for maximal increases in muscle strength and hypertrophy. In the **isokinetic** form of dynamic exercise, a dynamometer controls the velocity of contraction so that, with increasing velocity of contraction, the torque decreases. In **variable-resistance** exercise using isotonic contractions, the individual builds up to a maximal load on muscle throughout its full range of motion, and the rate of motion through the arc of movement is controlled by the user.

Exercise for the Patient with Inflammatory Synovitis

Long before the diagnosis is definitive for a patient with polyarthritis, much can be accomplished toward instructing him or her about exercise. For assessing the needs of patients, it has been shown that the standardized HAQ results correlate significantly with formal tests of muscle function.[33] Compliance is likely only if the exercise produces minimal discomfort during the workout and virtually none following it; pain control is the primary consideration in any rehabilitative program[34] (Table 27–1). For this reason, variable-resistance isotonic exercise is rarely appropriate for a patient with acutely inflamed joints. Isometric exercise has been shown to cause the least possible joint inflammation, increase in intra-articular pressure, and periarticular bone destruction.[35] The only negative aspect of isometric exercise is that the technique does produce an increase in blood pressure and demand on cardiac output; it must be used with caution in patients with cardiovascular disease.

For the patient with acutely and severely inflamed joints, either at the onset or during the course of rheumatoid arthritis, actual splinting to produce immobilization except for twice-daily full and slow passive movement through the range of motion to prevent soft tissue contracture may be all that is tolerated. For the more common patient with moderate synovitis, a prescribed isometric program is indicated for the involved joints that leads to well-supervised variable-resistance programs when the synovitis subsides.[36,37]

Under close supervision, isokinetic strength training can be appropriate for certain patients. In

TABLE 27–1. Principles and Aphorisms for Rehabilitative Therapies in Rheumatoid Arthritis

1. PAIN CONTROL is the first consideration in any rehabilitative regimen.
2. THE TREATMENT REGIMEN should be as brief and as simple as possible consistent with its goal (e.g., if 3 stretches of the shoulder one time daily will maintain the range of motion prescribed, 3 one-time daily and not 3 three-times daily, nor 30, etc., should be prescribed.
3. ADHERENCE (compliance) to a treatment regimen at the very least requires sufficient patient instruction to achieve an understanding of its specifics and to motivate its ongoing implementation. The motivation also requires understanding the patient and his or her style, fears, beliefs, and goals.
4. REST and restriction of skeletal motion can reduce inflammation but can also promote weakness and contractures. Rest must be balanced with appropriate movement whenever feasible.
5. JOINT PROTECTION PRINCIPLES:
   (a) Joints protected by splints, rest, or during activities should be positioned to avoid deformities.
   (b) Transferring skills (e.g., ability to arise from a chair or get into a car) must be taught to provide optimal independence, joint protection, safety, and energy conservation.
   (c) The strongest joints should be used insofar as possible during activities (e.g., shoulder strap versus a handle on a purse).
   (d) Planning and pacing activities to minimize prolonged or excessive joint use or to conserve energy.
6. EXERCISE therapy has many objectives, and typically only one objective is achieved optimally by any specific exercise.
   (a) Preserve motion
   (b) Restore lost motion
   (c) Increase strength and static endurance
   (d) Increase dynamic (kinetic) endurance
   (e) Enhance a feeling of well-being
   (f) Provide cardiovascular conditioning
   (g) Provide active recreation
7. SPLINTS should relieve pain or improve function, unless they are being used for specific postoperative positioning or on a temporary basis to reverse contractures.
8. THE HIERARCHY OF THERAPIES typically is
   (a) Pain control
   (b) Restoration of motion
   (c) Restoration of strength
   (d) Preservation of function

From Swezey, R. L.: Rheumatoid arthritis: the role of the kinder and gentler therapies. J. Rheumatol. 17:8, 1990. Used by permission.

one study, nine women with rheumatoid arthritis, all in functional stage II or III, underwent a low-intensity strengthening protocol using an isokinetic dynamometer with 48 repetitions at 50 per cent of maximal voluntary contraction, three times per week for 3 weeks. None had an increase in synovitis or joint pain, and the mean gain in strength was 21 per cent.[38]

The most persuasive evidence that well-monitored "aggressive" exercise programs have merit for rheumatoid patients comes from a controlled study of the feasibility of high-intensity progressive resistance training in elderly patients with rheumatoid arthritis, a group of healthy elderly subjects, and a group of healthy young subjects. The program was 12 weeks in duration; the control group of healthy elderly subjects performed only warm-up exercises. Progressive resistance was developed on pneumatic resistance equipment set at 80 per cent of maximal resistance overcome on one contraction for each muscle group for each individual on each day. The data showed a 54 to 75 per cent increase in maximal strength of all major exercised muscle groups without exacerbation of clinical disease activity,[39] and these patients reported reductions in perceived pain and fatigue and improved functional status. No changes in energy balance or body composition were noted.

If these data are accepted, the obstacles in providing monitored progressive-resistance training for patients are principally economic ones. The training requires supervision and expensive equipment. It will be a challenge to convince the providers of health insurance that, in the end, the costs expended on the therapy will save costs later.

So long as the exercise program is sustained and without significant postworkout pain, most data suggest that the outcome of appropriate exercise is improvement in one's ability to perform daily routines, less fatigue and weakness, improvement in global assessments and mood, and an increase in pain tolerance.[40,41] This appears to apply even to a dance-based aerobics program[42] and the ancient Chinese martial art and exercise, tai-chi chuan,[43] modalities that are particularly effective for groups of rheumatoid patients with disease at a similar stage.

Fortunate is the patient who has no foot, ankle, or knee involvement early in the disease process; these individuals can maintain active walking that permits general muscle tone and emotional well-being!

INSTRUCTION IN PERFORMING THE ACTIVITIES OF DAILY LIVING

The early phases of synovitis are an important moment to define for the patient how to use joints so as not to contribute in the years ahead to joint destruction. The basic principle underlying instruction in activities of daily living (ADL) supervised by occupational therapists should be to avoid as much as possible excessive force applied across the joint in both weight-bearing and non–weight-bearing joints. The concept is simple in the weight-bearing joints: avoiding jarring impact (e.g., running on hard surfaces) or forceful and repetitive quadriceps contracture during weight bearing (e.g., mountain climbing, heavy lifting, or skiing moguls).

For the non–weight-bearing joints, the key is avoiding powerful muscle contractions. Because more force is required to grasp a smaller than a larger handle, for example, pots, pans, and utensils with larger circumference handles are better for the patient with active synovitis, and it is better to lift with two hands rather than one hand. Another basic guideline is to avoid, as much as possible, repetitive motion that accentuates the force of gravity that normally works on joints. Lifting a pail of water, for example, drives the wrist and fingers into ulnar deviation, the common position of long-standing rheumatoid deformity.

The best instruction in ADL is given by occupational therapists. Home therapy by the Arthritis Society home service in Toronto was demonstrated in a prospective controlled trial to produce a statistically significant and clinically important improvement in function in patients with rheumatoid arthritis.[44] Interestingly, the same investigators were not able to demonstrate a difference in outcome in a similarly designed study of out-of-hospital physical therapy.[45]

TEMPERATURE MODALITIES

The rationale for using heat or cold is simple: they relieve pain.[34] Heat is the most commonly used modality, and there are many ways to apply it, including hot soaks, warm towels, heating pads, and more expensive methods such as diathermy or ultrasound. These latter techniques also may do more harm than good.[46]

There has been a debate regarding the use of heat therapy, focused by the evidence that collagen type II, the major cartilage of articular cartilage, is degraded significantly more rapidly by synovial collagenase at 37° to 39°C than at 33° to 36°C, the measured temperature of noninflamed joints.[47] Hot paraffin coating has been found to increase skin surface temperature by 8.9°C and the temperature within the underlying joint by 3.5°C[48] One study attempted to evaluate progression of erosions in 16 patients in a hand heated with electric mittens compared with the contralateral hand left out at room temperature. There were no differences in hand radiographs after the study,[49] so that, with our current state of knowledge, there is no confirmed contraindication to using daily or twice-daily heat therapy on rheumatoid joints.

The long-held belief that temperature within the knee actually goes down when heat is applied to the overlying skin appears to be false. Newer data show that, when ice is applied to the knee, the intra-articular temperature goes down, and when heat is applied, the temperature goes up.[50]

REFERENCES

1. Bradley, L. A.: Psychological aspects of arthritis. Bull. Rheum. Dis. 35:1, 1985.
2. Bradley, L. A., Young, L. D., Anderson, K. O., et al.: Psychological approaches to the management of arthritis pain. Soc. Sci. Med. 19:1353, 1984.
3. Lorish, C. D., Abraham, N., Austin, J., et al.: Disease and psychosocial factors related to physical functioning in rheumatoid arthritis. J. Rheumatol. 18:1150, 1991.
4. Parker, J., Smarr, K., Anderson, S., et al.: Relationship of changes in helplessness and depression to disease activity in rheumatoid arthritis. J. Rheumatol. 19:1901, 1992.
5. Hawley, D. J., and Wolfe, F.: Depression is not more common in rheumatoid arthritis: a 10-year longitudinal study of 6,153 patients with rheumatic disease. J. Rheumatol. 20:2025, 1993.
6. Wolfe, F., and Hawley, D. J.: The relationship between clinical activity and depression in rheumatoid arthritis. J. Rheumatol. 20:2032, 1993.
7. Cavalieri, F., Salaffi, F., and Ferraccioli, G. F.: Relationship between physical impairment, psychological variables and pain in rheumatoid disability: an analysis of their relative impact. Clin. Exp. Rheumatol. 9:47, 1991.
8. Peck, J. R., Smith, T. W., Ward, J. R., et al.: Disability and depression in rheumatoid arthritis: a multi-trait, multi-method investigation. Arthritis Rheum. 32:1100, 1989.
9. Pincus, T., Callahan, L. F., Bradley, L. A., et al.: Elevated MMPI scores for hypochondriasis, depression, and hysteria in patients with rheumatoid arthritis reflect disease rather than psychological status. Arthritis Rheum. 29:1456, 1986.

   This study used the scales for Hypochondriasis, Depression, and Hysteria of the Minnesota Multiphasic Personality Inventory (MMPI) in 70 randomly-selected patients with rheumatoid arthritis. The rheumatoid patients had higher scores on these scales, but these could be explained by five ''rheumatoid arthritis–related'' criteria in the MMPI statements. These statements correlated with results of measures of disease activity, such as painful function. The findings suggest that new criteria are needed for validation of the MMPI as a clinical tool for patients with rheumatoid arthritis.

10. Fifield, J., Reisine, S., Sheehan, T. J., and McQuillan, J.: Gender, paid work, and symptoms of emotional distress in rheumatoid arthritis patients. Arthritis Rheum. 39:427, 1996.
11. Parker, J. C., Smarr, K. L., Buckelew, S. P., et al.: Effects of stress management on clinical outcomes in rheumatoid arthritis. Arthritis Rheum. 38:1807, 1995.
12. Lotz, M., Vaughan, J. H., and Carson, D. A.: Effects of neuropeptides on production of inflammatory cytokines by human monocytes. Science 241:1218, 1988.

13. Zautra, A. J., Okun, M. A., Robinson, S. E., et al.: Life stress and lymphocyte alterations among patients with rheumatoid arthritis. Health Psychol. 8:1, 1989.

14. Harrington, L., Affleck, G., Urrows, S., et al.: Temporal covariation of soluble IL-2 receptor levels, daily stress, and disease activity in rheumatoid arthritis. Arthritis Rheum. 36:199, 1993.

15. Pincus, T., and Callahan, L. F.: Formal education as a marker for increased mortality and morbidity in rheumatoid arthritis. J. Chron. Dis. 38:973, 1985.

16. Lorig, K. R., Lubeck, D., Kraines, R. G., et al.: Outcomes of self-help education for patients with arthritis. Arthritis Rheum. 28:680, 1985.

17. Lorig, K.: Development and dissemination of an arthritis patient education course. Fam. Commun. Health 9:23, 1986.

18. Lorig, K., Seleznick, M., Lubeck, D., et al.: The beneficial outcomes of the arthritis self-management course are not adequately explained by behavioral change. Arthritis Rheum. 32:91, 1989.

19. Lorig, K. R., Mazonson, P. D., and Holman, H. R.: Evidence suggesting that health education for self-management in patients with chronic arthritis has sustained health benefits while reducing health care costs. Arthritis Rheum. 36:439, 1993.

20. Taal, E., Rasker, J. J., and Wiegman, O.: Patient education and self-management in the rheumatic diseases: a self-efficacy approach. Arthritis Care Res. 9:229, 1996.

21. Hill, J., Bird, H. A., Lawton, R. H., et al.: The development and use of a patient knowledge questionnaire in rheumatoid arthritis. Br. J. Rheumatol. 30:45, 1991.

22. Kraaimaat, F. W., Bakker, A. H., Janssen, E., and Bijlsma, J. W.: Intrusiveness of rheumatoid arthritis on sexuality in male and female patients living with a spouse. Arthritis Care Res. 9:120, 1996.

23. Mills, J. A., Pinals, R. S., Ropes, M. W., et al.: Value of bed rest in patients with rheumatoid arthritis. N. Engl. J. Med. 284:453, 1971.

24. Lee, P., Kennedy, A. C., Anderson, J., et al.: Benefits of hospitalization in rheumatoid arthritis. Q. J. Med. 43:205, 1974.

25. Sibley, J. T., Blocka, K. L. N., Haga, M., et al.: Clinical course and predictors of length of stay in hospitalized patients with rheumatoid arthritis. J. Rheumatol. 17:1623, 1990.

26. Spiegel, J. S., Spiegel, T. M., Ward, N. B., et al.: Rehabilitation for rheumatoid arthritis patients: a controlled trial. Arthritis Rheum. 29:628, 1986.

27. Helewa, A., Bombardier, C., Goldsmith, C. H., et al.: Cost-effectiveness of inpatient and intensive outpatient treatment of rheumatoid arthritis: a randomized, controlled trial. Arthritis Rheum. 32:1505, 1989.

28. Stenström, C. H., Lindell, B., Swanberg, E., et al.: Functional and psychosocial consequences of disease and experience of pain and exertion in a group of rheumatic patients considered for active training: result of a survey in Bollnäs Medical District. Scand. J. Rheumatol. 19:374, 1990.

29. Gerber, L. H.: Exercise and arthritis. Bull. Rheum. Dis. 39:1, 1990.

30. Wilson, C. H., and Maier, W. P.: Exercise mobilization techniques. In Leek, J. C., Gershwin, M. E., and Fowler, W. M., (eds.): Principles of Physical Medicine and Rehabilitation in the Musculoskeletal Diseases. New York, Grune & Stratton, 1986, pp. 11–23.

31. Galloway, M. T., and Jokl, P.: The role of exercise in the treatment of inflammatory arthritis. Bull. Rheum. Dis. 42:1, 1993.

32. Lieberson, W. T.: Brief isometric exercises in therapeutic exercise. In Basmajian, J. (ed.): Therapeutic Exercise. Baltimore, Williams & Wilkins, 1984, pp. 320–332.

33. Ekdahl, C., and Broman, G.: Muscle strength, endurance, and aerobic capacity in rheumatoid arthritis: a comparative study with healthy subjects. Ann. Rheum. Dis. 51:35, 1992.

34. Swezey, R. L.: Rheumatoid arthritis: the role of the kinder and gentler therapies. J. Rheumatol. 17:8, 1990.

   Basic principles for rehabilitative programs in rheumatoid arthritis should include each of the ingredients outlined in Table 26–1 (see text).

35. Jason, M., IV, and Dixon A. S. J.: Intra-articular pressure in rheumatoid arthritis of the knee. III. Pressure changes during joint use. Ann. Rheum. Dis. 29:401, 1970.

36. Nordemar, R., Edstrom, L., and Ekblom, B.: Changes in muscle fibre size and physical performance in patients with rheumatoid arthritis after short term physical training. Scand. J. Rheumatol. 5:70, 1976.

   Ten patients with rheumatoid arthritis were put into an intense training program of training in activities of daily living, workout on a stationary bicycle, quadriceps strengthening exercises, and stair climbing for 2 hours daily. By all parameters measured, physical performance increased and as shown by muscle biopsies, there was an increase in the size of types I and II muscle fibers. Most important, there was no observable deterioration in joint status by physical examination.

37. Nordemar, R., Berg, U., Ekblom, B., et al.: Changes in muscle fibre size and physical performance in patients with rheumatoid arthritis after 7 months physical training. Scand. J. Rheumatol. 5:233, 1976.

38. Lyngverg, K. K., Ramsing, B. U., Nawrocki, A., et al.: Safe and effective isokinetic knee extension training in rheumatoid arthritis. Arthritis Rheum. 37:623, 1994.

39. Rall, L. C., Meydani, S. N., Kehayias, J. J., et al.: The effect of progressive resistance training in rheumatoid arthritis: increased strength without changes in energy balance or body composition. Arthritis Rheum. 39:415, 1996.

40. Nordemar, R.: Physical training in rheumatoid arthritis: a controlled long term study II. Scand. J. Rheumatol. 10:25, 1981.

41. Harcom, T. M., Lampman, R. M., Banwell, B. F., et al.: Therapeutic value of graded aerobic exercise training in rheumatoid arthritis. Arthritis Rheum. 28:32, 1985.

42. Perlman, S. G., Connell, K. J., Clark, A., et al.: Dance-based aerobic exercise for rheumatoid arthritis. Arthritis Care Res. 3:29, 1990.

43. Kirsteins, A. E., Dietz, F., and Hwang, S.-M.: Evaluating the safety and potential use of a weight-bearing exercise, Tai-Chi Chuan, for rheumatoid arthritis patients. Am. J. Phys. Med. Rehabil. 70:136, 1991.

44. Helewa, A., Goldsmith, C. H., Lee, P., et al.: Effects of occupational therapy home service on patients with rheumatoid arthritis. Lancet 337:1453, 1991.

   Home service by occupational therapists was evaluated by randomizing 105 patients with rheumatoid arthritis on stable medical therapies. The groups received either a 6-week comprehensive program of occupational therapy or no such treatment, and at 6 weeks the control group received the occupational therapy home service as well. At 6 weeks, the functional score for the experimental group was significantly higher than for the control group, and the control patients at 12 weeks showed improvement similar to the experimental group.

45. Helewa, A., Smythe, H. A., and Goldsmith, C. H.: Can specially trained physiotherapists improve the care of pa-

tients with rheumatoid arthritis? A randomized health care trial. J. Rheumatol. 21:70, 1994.

46. Goddard, D. H., Revell P. A., Cason, J., et al.: Ultrasound has no anti-inflammatory effect. Ann. Rheum. Dis. 42:582, 1983.

47. Harris, E. D. Jr., and McCroskery, P. A. The influence of temperature and fibril stability on degradation of cartilage collagen by rheumatoid synovial collagenase. N. Engl. J. Med. 290:1, 1974.

48. Oosterveld, F. G. J., Rasker, J. J., Jacobs, J. W. G., et al.: The effect of local heat and cold therapy on the intraarticular and skin surface temperature of the knee. Arthritis Rheum. 35:146, 1992.

49. Mainardi, C. L., Walter, J. M., Spiegel, P. K., et al.: Rheumatoid arthritis: failure of daily heat therapy to affect its progression. Arch. Phys. Med. Rehabil. 60:390, 1968.

50. Oosterveld, F. G. J., and Rasker, J. J.: Effects of local heat and cold treatment on surface and articular temperature of arthritic knees. Arthritis Rheum. 37:1578, 1994.

28

Diet and Rheumatoid Arthritis

Few modalities of treatment for rheumatoid arthritis have more different options than food. The lists of ''arthritis diets'' and ''arthritis cookbooks'' are staggeringly long, and have been for many years. Are there any firm data to support the hypothesis that diet can beneficially affect rheumatoid arthritis?

The most obvious and most important principle of diet for this disease is regulating the *quantity* of food eaten and the weight of the patient eating it. Obesity is very harmful for arthritis in weight-bearing joints. Already depleted of proteoglycans by proteolytic enzymes from neutrophils in synovial fluid, synovium, and activated chondrocytes, articular cartilage is very much at risk of degenerative change. Added weight magnifies the degradative potential of weight bearing in patients with active synovitis.

As for the *quality* of food eaten, the data are much more controversial. It is probably more important for rheumatoid patients to have adequate vitamin supplements than the healthy population, but clear data to support this are lacking. The effect of malnourishment is also controversial. In one study, 26 per cent of patients with rheumatoid arthritis were malnourished,[1] and the malnourished were worse off clinically. In contrast, starvation has been demonstrated to have a suppressive effect on lymphocyte function; theoretically, a patient who is actively losing weight by caloric restriction might notice a decrease in inflammatory symptoms.

In considering all of the data about weight and arthritis, however, the best advice for physicians is to urge their patients to settle at a weight near the accepted mean for their sex and age. Although excess weight is more likely to damage cartilage by increasing impact load on weight-bearing joints, this is balanced by the knowledge that active synovitis is associated with cytokine production and release that often leads to a catabolic state in patients. Underweight rheumatoid patients often have a decreased axial bone mass.[2]

There is a scientific rationale for eliminating precursors of arachidonic acid from the diet: this leads to reductions in the inflammatory prostaglandins and leukotrienes. A number of studies using fish oil supplementation have given encouraging results,[3,4] and additional ones are discussed later. These fish oils exert measurable suppression of several inflammatory mediators produced by rheumatoid patients.[5] In a different approach with the same mechanism in mind, patients were put on a vegetarian diet in a controlled study. The vegetarians lost weight and improved in clinical and functional parameters.[6] (Studies similar to these are discussed later in the section on fatty acids.) Dietary manipulation is difficult to comply with, and, except for those patients who easily accept vegetarian regimens or fish oil supplements, a balance in diet, daily multivitamin supplements, and weight near to ''ideal'' weight would appear to be a good approach for all patients.

FOOD ALLERGIES AND RHEUMATOID ARTHRITIS

There are a number of forms of arthritis that are apparently induced in humans and other animals by specific foods or food additives (see ref. 7). That there may be a role of absorbed allergens in the activity of rheumatoid arthritis is supported by the fact that short-term fasting has been shown to have some benefit for rheumatoid patients.[8] However, the benefit of and measurable effects on inflammatory mediators (e.g., decreased activity of PMN leukocytes)[9] are not necessarily a direct result of the absence of a specific food, but rather could be related to changes brought about by the generic absence of calories.

A large number of anecdotal reports of food allergy and rheumatoid arthritis have been followed by a prospective, blind, controlled trial in a clinical research center to determine whether joint symptoms in patients already diagnosed as having rheumatoid arthritis could by exacerbated by certain foods.[10,11] Patients were challenged with potential food allergens. One patient exhibited marked, consistent objective and subjective improvement during fasting, but deteriorated rapidly and reproducibly when challenged with milk products but no other food families. In another group of 19 patients who claimed to have "allergic" arthritis, only 3 became asymptomatic while taking only elemental nutrition. Interestingly, all three had "seronegative rheumatoid arthritis" with nonerosive disease and intermittent (palindromic) symptom complexes.

In summary, there may be a very small subset of patients who have demonstrable flares of rheumatoid arthritis when ingesting certain foods, but it is both laborious and costly to weed them out from others also convinced that their arthritis is allergic in origin. In one study of 704 patients, 28 per cent of those surveyed reported on questionnaires some association between a specific food and clinical status.[12]

TRACE ELEMENTS AND AMINO ACIDS

Among the various low-molecular-weight supplements to diet advocated for rheumatoid arthritis are copper, selenium, zinc, iron, and histidine. Of these, none has been proven in controlled studies of diet supplementation to give significant benefit, although the scientific rationale for involvement of copper is the most interesting[7] (as discussed in chapter 31 in the section on D-penicillamine). It is not clear, however, whether copper depletion or supplementation would better help a rheumatoid patient; arguments can be made for both sides.

It is unlikely that well-controlled trials of any of these elements can be done effectively in rheumatoid populations in the United States. In the absence of better data, it is appropriate to recommend that vitamin supplements, in doses not much exceeding the minimum daily requirement, are not likely to hurt patients and may benefit certain aspects of physiology that could be helpful to global well-being. This recommendation may be particularly relevant in light of evidence that most rheumatoid patients in the Netherlands have calculated deficits against energy expenditure of carbohydrate, fat, and vitamin intake.[13]

FATTY ACIDS

There are two groups of essential fatty acids, those derived from linoleic acid and those derived

from α-linolenic acid. The pathways of their metabolism are shown in Figure 28–1.[14] Interventions in both the ω-3 and ω-6 pathways have been tried in patients with rheumatoid arthritis, and the rationales for their use are supported by animal and cell culture studies.

Omega-3 Pathway Manipulation

Addition to the diet of eicosapentaenoic acid (EPA), a polyunsaturated fatty acid that is abundant in fish oils, leads to a decrease in formation of arachidonic acid metabolites through the COX and lipoxygenase pathways. Instead of PGE_2 and LTB_4 being produced, PGE_3 and LTB_5, which are much less inflammatory, are generated. Diets enriched in fish oil also reduce generation of cytokines (e.g., PDGF, IL-1, and TNFα) by monocytes and suppress the chemotactic response of neutrophils to LTB_4[15–17] by more obscure mechanisms.

After several open studies gave encouraging results, 55 patients with rheumatoid arthritis were entered into a prospective, double-blind, randomized 30-week trial in which they received for 24 weeks either a high dose (54 mg/kg/day) of EPA plus a similar unsaturated fatty acid, docohexaenoic acid (DHA; 36 mg/kg/day), or a dose of both that was half that.[4] Then both groups received a placebo for 6 additional weeks. Both sets of EPA + DHA patients showed significant improvement in joint counts compared with placebo-treated patients. Similar results were observed in a smaller Dutch study.[18] In a study from Belgium, 2.6 g of ω-3 fatty acids helped patients improve in a 12-month study compared against supplemental olive oil.[19]

Those interested in advances in pathophysiology of rheumatoid arthritis must follow new findings in other chronic diseases as well. Accordingly, a publication that studied effects of an enteric-coated fish oil preparation on relapses in Crohn's disease has relevance to arthritis.[20] Seventy-eight patients who had a high risk of relapse were given either placebo or nine enteric-coated fish oil capsules containing a total of 2.7 g of ω-3 fatty acids (1.8 g of EPA and 0.9 g of DHA). The enteric coating made a controlled study possible and the fish oils acceptable; placebos contained caprylic acid and capric acid. Twenty-eight per cent of the fish oil group had relapses, whereas 69 per cent of the placebo group had relapses. Diarrhea was the only side effect (five cases in both groups). After a year of treatment, 59 per cent of the fish oil group were still in remission, compared with 26 per cent of the placebo group. Given that these oils are effective in rheumatoid arthritis but that the fish oil taste has

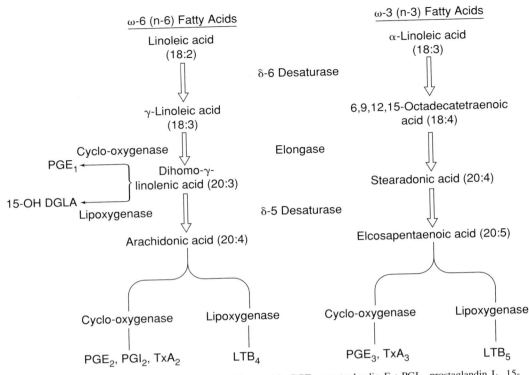

FIGURE 28–1. Metabolic pathways of essential fatty acids. PGE_2, prostaglandin E_2; PGI_1, prostaglandin I_1, 15-OH DGLA, 15-hydroxy-dihomo-γ-lineolenic acid; TxA_2, thromboxane A_2; LTB_4, leukotriene B_4. (From Zurier, B.: Essential fatty acids and inflammation. Ann. Rheum. Dis. 50:745, 1991. Used by permission. Copyright 1991 by BMJ Publishing Group.)

made them unpalatable, this enteric-coated preparation would be useful in rheumatoid patients.

Omega-6 Pathway Manipulation

As shown in Figure 28–1, dihomo-γ-linolenic acid (DGLA) is converted to PGE_1 and a 15-hydroxy-DGLA. This conversion is rapid, whereas the other desaturase pathway to arachidonic acid is sluggish.[14] Thus, the competition of DGLA with arachidonic acid is an effective one; if supplemental linolenic acid is given in the diet, PGE_1 levels rise appreciably and PGE_2 and LTB_4 levels do not change. In vitro, DGLA suppresses human synovial cell proliferation[21] by a PGE_1-dependent process, and IL-2–dependent human T-cell growth by a PGE-independent mechanism.[22] Both actions have relevance for intervention in rheumatoid arthritis, and for that reason, human studies with supplemental γ-linolenic acid (GLA) have been undertaken, first in an open study[23] and then in a more rigorous trial.

Thirty-seven patients with rheumatoid arthritis and active synovitis were enrolled in a randomized, double-blind, placebo-controlled study of 24 weeks' duration.[24] The treatment arm was 1.4 g/day GLA. The overall response assessment showed that seven treated but only one placebo patient had a meaningful improvement, whereas four placebo and none of the treated group deteriorated. Joint tenderness scores are shown in Figure 28–2. The benefit was not compromised by the fact that patients continued their NSAID and low-dose glucocorticoid treatment, suggesting either that production of PGE_1 was not completely inhibited, or that the therapeutic effect of NSAIDs was derived from prostaglandin-independent mechanisms (see ref. 22 and 23).

SUMMARY

This interesting work could be extended by trials of patients unable to take NSAIDs for one reason or another; also, these fatty acids could be added as supplements to other regimens in therapeutic trials. Indeed, it has been demonstrated that ω-3 fatty acid dietary supplementation permits patients to dimin-

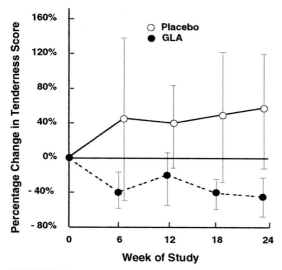

FIGURE 28–2. Joint tenderness scores in patients completing the study. Mean percentage change from baseline at each evaluation for placebo (○; $n = 13$) and γ-linolenic acid (GLA) treatment (●; $n = 14$) groups. Error bars are ± 1 standard error of the mean. (Modified from Leventhal, L. J., Boyce, E. G., and Zurier, R. B.: Treatment of rheumatoid arthritis with gammalinolenic acid. Ann. Intern. Med. 119:867, 1993. Used by permission.)

ish or discontinue NSAIDs without experiencing a flare in their disease.[25] There is no evidence that either EPA/DHA or GLA does harm to patients, something that cannot be said for our usual therapies in this disease.

REFERENCES

1. Helliwell, M., Coombes, E. J., Moody, B. J., et al.: Nutritional status in patients with rheumatoid arthritis. Ann. Rheum. Dis. 43:386, 1987.
2. Kroger, H., Honkanen, R., Saarikoski, S., et al.: Decreased axial bone mineral density in perimenopausal women with rheumatoid arthritis—a population based study. Ann. Rheum. Dis. 53:18, 1994.
3. Kremer, J. M., Michalek, A. V., Lininges, L., et al.: Effects of manipulation of dietary fatty acids on clinical manifestations of rheumatoid arthritis. Lancet 1:184, 1985.
4. Kremer, J. M., Jubiz, W., Michalek, A., et al.: Fish-oil fatty acid supplementation in active rheumatoid arthritis: a double-blinded, controlled, crossover study. Ann. Int. Med. 106:497, 1987.
5. Harris, E. D. Jr.: Treatment of rheumatoid arthritis. *In* Kelley, W. N., Harris, E. D. Jr., Ruddy, S., and Sledge, C. B. (eds.): Textbook of Rheumatology, 4th ed., Vol. 1. Philadelphia, W. B. Saunders, 1993, pp. 912–923.
6. Kjeldsen-Kragh, J., Borchgrevink, C. F., Laerum, E., et al.: Controlled trial of fasting and one-year vegetarian diet in rheumatoid arthritis. Lancet 338:899, 1991.
7. Buchanan, H. M., Preston, S. J., Brooks, P. M., et al.: Is diet important in rheumatoid arthritis? Br. J. Rheumatol. 30:125, 1991.
8. Palmblad, J., Hafstrom, I., and Ringertz, B.: Antirheumatic effects of fasting. Rheum. Dis. Clin. North Am. 17:351, 1991.
9. Hafstrom, I., Ringertz, B., Gyllenhammar, H., et al.: Effects of fasting on disease activity, neutrophil function, fatty acid composition, and leukotriene biosynthesis in patients with rheumatoid arthritis. Arthritis Rheum. 31:585, 1988.
10. Panush, R. S., Stroud, R. M., and Webster, E.: Food-induced (allergic) arthritis: inflammatory arthritis exacerbated by milk. Arthritis Rheum. 29:220, 1986.
11. Panush, R. S.: Food induced (''allergic'') arthritis: clinical and serological studies. J. Rheumatol. 17:291, 1990.
12. Tanner, S. B., Callahan, L. F., Panush, R., et al.: Dietary and allergic associations with rheumatoid arthritis: self-report of 704 patients. Arthritis Care Res. 3:189, 1990.
13. van de Laar, M. A. F. J., Nieuwenhuis, J. M., Former-Boon, M., et al.: Nutritional habits of patients suffering from seropositive rheumatoid arthritis: a screening of 93 Dutch patients. Clin. Rheumatol. 9:483, 1990.
14. Zurier, B.: Essential fatty acids and inflammation. Ann. Rheum. Dis. 50:745, 1991.
15. Sperling, R. I., Weinblatt, M., Robin, J. L., et al.: Effects of dietary supplementation with marine fish oil on leukocyte lipid mediator generation and function in rheumatoid arthritis. Arthritis Rheum. 30:988, 1987.
16. Endres, S., Ghorbani, R., Kelley, V. E., et al.: The effect of dietary supplementation with n-3 polyunsaturated fatty acids on the synthesis of interleukin-1 and tumor necrosis factor by mononuclear cells. N. Engl. J. Med. 320:265, 1989.
17. Fox, P. L., and DiCorleto, P. E.: Fish oils inhibit endothelial cell production of platelet-derived growth factor-like protein. Science 241:453, 1988.
18. van der Tempel, H., Tulleken, J. E., Limburg, P. C., et al.: Effects of fish oil supplementation in rheumatoid arthritis. Ann. Rheum. Dis. 49:76, 1990.

    Sixteen patients with rheumatoid arthritis were entered into a randomized, double-blind, placebo-controlled crossover design with 12-week treatment periods. Joint swelling and morning stiffness improved in the fish oil (containing a 2:1.3 ratio of EPA to DHA) group, but other studies did not reach statistical significance. Relative amounts of EPA and DHA that were incorporated into plasma cholesterol esters and neutrophil membrane phospholipid fractions increased at the expense of the ω-6 fatty acids.

19. Geusens, P., Wouters, C., Nijs, J., et al.: Long-term effect of omega-3 fatty acid supplementation in active rheumatoid arthritis. Arthritis Rheum. 37:824, 1994.

    Twenty patients were enrolled in each of three arms of this study that lasted 12 months and was double blind and randomized. One group received daily supplements of 2.6 g of ω-3 fatty acids, a second received 1.3 g of ω-3 fatty acids and 3 g olive oil, and the third received 6 g olive oil each day. Only the group taking 2.6 g ω-3 fatty acids improved, and they improved globally over the entire 12 months, reaching a final improvement of 27 per cent over baseline. Improvement in combined criteria (Ritchie Index, grip strength, and ESR) also was noted. The higher dose ω-3 group was able to decrease NSAID use during this period. It will be interesting to discover how long after ending the study the beneficial effects persist.

20. Belluzzi, A., Brignola, C., Campieri, M., et al.: Effect of an enteric-coated fish-oil preparation on relapses in Crohn's disease. N. Engl. J. Med. 334:1557, 1996.
21. Baker, D. G., Krakauer, K. A., Tate, G., et al.: Suppression of human synovial cell proliferation by dihomo-γ-linole-

nic acid. Arthritis Rheum. 32:1273, 1989.

DGLA inhibited synovial cell proliferation induced by recombinant IL-1. Indomethacin reduced this inhibitory effect. PGE_1 increased 14-fold, while there was a 70 per cent decrease in PGE_2. Exogenous PGE_1 inhibited cell growth, and the data suggested that DGLA exerted its suppressive effects by its capacity to increase PGE_1 production and subsequent cellular cAMP production.

22. Santoli, D., Phillips, P. D., Colt, T. L., et al.: Suppression of interleukin 2-dependent human T cell growth *in vitro* by prostaglandin E (PGE) and their precursor fatty acids: evidence for a PGE-independent mechanism of inhibition by the fatty acids. J. Clin. Invest. 85:424, 1990.
23. Pullman-Mooar, S., Laposata, M., Lem, D., et al.: Alteration of the cellular fatty acid profile and the production of eicosanoids in human monocytes by gamma linolenic acid. Arthritis Rheum. 33:1526, 1990.

Given to both normal controls and rheumatoid patients, GLA (1.1 g/day) increased its first metabolite, DGLA, in circulating mononuclear cells and caused significant reductions in PGE_2, LTB_4, and LTC.

24. Leventhal, L. J., Boyce, E. G., and Zurier, R. B.: Treatment of rheumatoid arthritis with gammalinolenic acid. Ann. Int. Med. 119:867, 1993.
25. Kremer, J. M., Lawrence, D. A., Petrillo, G. F., et al.: Effects of high-dose fish oil on rheumatoid arthritis after stopping nonsteroidal antiinflammatory drugs: clinical and immune correlates. Arthritis Rheum. 38:1107, 1995.

29

Nonsteroidal Anti-Inflammatory Drugs, Including Aspirin

It is estimated that 30 million people worldwide take NSAIDs.[1] These certainly are among the most frequently prescribed medicines in the United States. If, as calculated in one study, 100 million prescriptions are written each year[2] and the average 30-day supply costs $60, the total price tag for these drugs is between $3 and $4 billion per year.

It is appropriate and accepted practice to have all patients with rheumatoid arthritis on an NSAID throughout the course of their therapy. (Salicylates should be considered to be a NSAID.) Although it has never been rigorously tested, it is probable that the anti-inflammatory effects of NSAIDs are additive with most of the second-line drugs used in rheumatoid arthritis treatment.

As mentioned in Chapter 25, an NSAID ought to be made a staple of therapy at the first visit of the patient with arthritis, even before a diagnosis is possible. Prescribing an NSAID for the first time should be a teaching exercise for the physician, and an opportunity for the patient to learn some basic concepts about what joint inflammation is and how the NSAID may work to alleviate it. Equally important, however, is an honest accounting of the possible side effects. In a rather rigorous study of that crucial encounter between patient and physician when an NSAID was first prescribed, it was found that a mean of 1.7 side effects were mentioned by the physician. Epigastric discomfort was mentioned in 72 per cent of these encounters, but the others, including hepatic, renal, hematologic, and central nervous system toxicities, were brought up in less than 15 per cent of these initial prescribing sessions.[3]

Adequate knowledge of possible side effects, but not so much as to bewilder or frighten the patient, is the balanced objective. At a minimum, the patient should be warned about gastrointestinal distress, interaction with antihypertensive medications and other cardiac drugs, and central nervous system changes (e.g., depression, disorientation, headaches). Each patient should be encouraged to contact the physician or nurse when an abnormal sensation of any kind appears that did not predate starting the NSAID. A complete blood count, creatinine level, and basic liver function tests are the only ones essential to obtain before starting NSAID therapy.[4]

The goal of NSAID therapy in rheumatoid arthritis should be symptomatic relief of pain and swelling, and no more. NSAIDs have little effect on the proliferative lesion and, if synovitis persists, second-line drugs will be necessary. The cost of NSAIDs varies substantially, even among different salicylate preparations, and there is proven logic in the ''stepped formulary'' approach in which less expensive NSAIDs are prescribed before more expensive ones. Cost savings using this method can be up to 30 per cent of NSAIDs expense with no measurable detrimental effect upon patient care or patient satisfaction.[5]

SALICYLATES: STILL A REASONABLE FIRST CHOICE FOR ANTI-INFLAMMATORY ACTION

Although used by increasing numbers of citizens in small doses to ward off cardiac or peripheral thrombotic events, aspirin has lost favor among many physicians for chronic inflammatory arthritis. Why? Because of the convincing data that there is more gastrointestinal irritation than from other nonsteroidal compounds, the well-publicized hepatic and hepatorenal syndromes (e.g., Reye's syndrome) experienced by children taking aspirin, and the acetylation of proteins that makes many enzymes [e.g., cyclo-oxygenase (COX)] dysfunctional for many weeks. Nevertheless, there are several reasons to make salicylates the first NSAID given to patients:

1. Plasma salicylate levels are relatively inexpensive and are useful for gauging compliance with prescription orders.

2. Aspirin is inexpensive (although some of the enteric-coated and nonacetylated forms are not).

3. Salicylate levels correlate reasonably well with both therapeutic and toxic effects.

4. Toxicity of aspirin in its various forms is directly related to dose; 3 g/day has toxicity no greater than most nonsalicylate NSAIDs. These doses present an attractive alternative to other NSAIDs when used as adjunctive therapy to a second-line drug.[6]

5. Nonacetylated salicylates (e.g., salicylate, choline salicylate) do not interfere directly with cox activity but nevertheless have significant anti-inflammatory activity.

Bioavailability of salicylates, reflected by serum levels, differs from patient to patient and is affected by a number of variables. Factors that enhance the rate of dissolution will enhance the rate of absorption; these include

- Micronized aspirin
- Addition of antacids to the preparation
- Water-soluble salicylate salts, particularly those given in liquid form
- Drugs such as metoclopramide (because the bulk of absorption occurs in the upper small bowel)

In contrast, concurrent administration of glucocorticoids can lead to lower steady-state serum salicylate levels, probably as a result of an enhanced metabolic clearance.[7]

As serum levels of salicylates increase over 3 to 5 days during initiation of high-dose therapy for rheumatoid arthritis, the major metabolic pathways to salicylurate and salicylphenolic glucuronide become saturated. This means that, once therapeutic blood levels are reached, a single dose produces a larger increase in serum levels than would be expected (for a review of salicylate pharmacokinetics, see ref. 8). At higher blood levels, lengthening the interval between doses to 8 or 12 hours still will enable acceptable trough serum salicylate levels (between 150 and 300 μg/ml) to be sustained.

Enteric-coated aspirin or nonacetylated salicylates often are a logical first NSAID to prescribe. It has been established that absorption from the small bowel of one enteric-coated brand (Ecotrin) is efficient,[9] although the time of measuring salicylate levels after a dose should be 3, not 2 hours. Enteric-coated aspirin has no direct irritative effect on gastric mucosa; its side effects are related to the acetylation of proteins and glycoproteins and the diminished levels of prostaglandins secondary to this acetylation.

Nonacetylated salicylates are effective anti-inflammatory drugs when given in adequate doses[10] yet they have only a weak and reversible effect upon cox. This has led to studies demonstrating that, at concentrations below those needed to inhibit cox, salicylates interrupt signal transduction across cell membranes in such a way that activation of inflammatory pathways in cells such as the neutrophil is inhibited.[11] It will be essential to repeat the cox inhibition studies using assays to identify the inducible form of the enzyme, COX-2.

Another mechanism of action of sodium salicylate and aspirin is inhibition of the activation of the transcription factor nuclear factor-κB (NF-κB), which is critical for the inducible expression of multiple cellular genes involved in inflammation.[12] NF-κB is activated in response to IL-1, and TNFα, resulting in translocation of NF-κB from the cytoplasm to the nucleus, where it binds to DNA and regulates transcription of numerous other genes, including those coding for IL-6, IL-8, IL-1, TNFα, and cell adhesion molecules such as ELAM-1, ICAM-1, and VCAM-1.

Various preparations of aspirin and nonacetylated salicylates are listed in ref. 13. The dose of salicylates for rheumatoid arthritis should be sufficient to give blood levels of 20 to 30 mg/dl/day, or the dose just below that which produces tinnitus. Older patients often develop tinnitus at levels below the therapeutic level, and in such individuals salicylates cannot be used.

Treating Pain—a Challenge Different from Treating Inflammation

As has been emphasized in Chapter 16, the cycle of pain in rheumatoid arthritis often spreads, from activation of spinal pathways, to areas around joints much removed from sites of inflammation. The inference from this is that anti-inflammatory drugs should not be the only weapon against pain. Acetaminophen, for example, is an effective analgesic. It has little anti-inflammatory activity, but it produces no gastric or renal toxicity because it does not inhibit cox. It can be used in doses similar to salicylates and concurrent with salicylates and other NSAIDs.

It must be accepted, however, that NSAIDs and acetaminophen are often insufficient to control pain adequately in rheumatoid arthritis. A physician must be versed in the sophisticated techniques of using opiates in dosage patterns to avoid addiction, and should recognize that many psychological factors, including depression, amplify pain. Just as patients with *arthritis robustus* (see Chapter 19) experience little pain from erosive synovitis, there are other subsets who have pain out of proportion to inflammation. Severe pain may be an appropriate indication, in the absence of others, for surgical intervention on one or several joints, or for earlier use of second-line drugs such as methotrexate. In the future, centrally acting agents such as NMDA receptor antagonists (see Chapter 16) and alternative therapies including acupuncture may be appropriate analgesics in rheumatoid arthritis.[14]

Adverse Effects of Salicylates

Rather than generate an exhaustive list of side effects of these drugs, an attempt is made here to emphasize the more common adverse effects and give little attention to the less common or minor and idiosyncratic reactions. Most of these apply to the other NSAIDs as well.

Gastrointestinal Side Effects

Gastrointestinal side effects are the most common, and related to the aspirin-induced back-diffusion of hydrogen ions across the mucosa, producing inflammation and bleeding. Loss of effective concentrations of PGE_2 and prostacyclin top the list of damaging effects. Misoprostol can help prevent this gastritis or alleviate it once started, as can Histamine-2 (H_2) blockade (see later section on Prophylaxis and Treatment of NSAID-Induced Gastrointestinal Toxicity). Again, use of enteric-coated preparations or nonacetylated salicylates, particularly those formulated as a liquid, can minimize gastric damage.

Hematologic Side Effects

Bleeding from the irreversible incapacitation of platelets caused by acetylation of COX by aspirin is of particular concern for patients scheduled for a surgical procedure. The most appropriate strategy is to stop aspirin 10 to 14 days before surgery, replacing it with salicylsalicylic acid or another nonacetylated salicylate that does not affect platelets. For the same reasons, aspirin should be avoided during pregnancy of the rheumatoid patient. The bleeding time, often referred to as the gold standard for assessment of platelet function, is actually a difficult one to assay or reproduce and should be used only with these limitations in mind.

Renal Side Effects

Reduction of the glomerular filtration rate by 10 per cent or less is the rule for therapeutic doses of salicylates. This is rarely of consequence in patients with normal cardiovascular and renal function. However, those with abnormal renal function and those taking diuretics or other medications for the treatment of heart failure or hypertension are dependent upon renal prostaglandin production to counter the vasoconstrictive effects of the renin-angiotensin system and adrenergic activation.

It is helpful to be aware of the nature of the important contributions of prostaglandins to normal renal function.[15] The major effect is on the excretion of sodium. Prostaglandins increase renal blood flow by dilation of blood vessels, and this decreases reabsorption of sodium in the proximal tubules. In addition, prostaglandins directly inhibit sodium reabsorption at the thick ascending loop of Henle. The renal toxicity of NSAIDs, however, is more complex than the straightforward induction of resistance to diuretics by these drugs. NSAIDs produce three principal syndromes of renal impairment: (1) acute ischemic renal insufficiency, (2) acute interstitial nephritis, and (3) analgesic-associated nephropathy. Alone or in combination, these can lead to acute renal failure, the nephrotic syndrome, chronic renal failure, salt retention, hyponatremia, or hyperkalemia.

The **ischemic syndrome** occurs when NSAIDs are administered to patients in whom diseases or drugs have reduced the effective circulating blood volume and there is a compensatory increase in angiotensin II and catecholamine secretion. In these states, prostaglandins are needed to maintain adequate renal perfusion.[16] Administration of NSAIDs diminishes both renal blood flow and glomerular filtration rate.

Acute interstitial nephritis is rare (occuring in 1: 5,000 to 1: 10,000 patients on NSAIDs). Patients present with high serum creatinine levels (usually >6 mg/dl), edema, and proteinuria. This complication usually occurs in the elderly. Men older than 65 are particularly at risk, especially if they are heavy consumers of alcohol, have had a previous myocardial infarction, or have congestive heart failure.[17] Fenoprofen has been implicated in more than a third of cases. Subclinical damage sufficient to increase urinary pH and impair renal concentration capacity can be correlated with the cumulative intake of NSAIDs[18] (Table 29–1; Fig. 29–1).

Analgesic nephropathy is the most common form of drug-induced chronic renal failure.[19] Although most cases have been related to phenacetin abuse in middle-aged females with a characteristic psychological profile, there are numerous reports of its association with NSAIDs administered either alone or in combination with aspirin. Rarely, renal

TABLE 29–1. Laboratory Findings after 12-hr Fast in 104 Patients Receiving Long-term Treatment with NSAIDs and 123 Healthy Control Nonusers of NSAIDs*

PARAMETER†	PATIENTS	CONTROLS	p
Urinary pH	5.9 ± 0.7	5.2 ± 0.6	<0.05
Urinary density	1019 ± 5	1026 ± 5	<0.05
Urinary osmolality (mOsm/l)	502.1 ± 150.7	661.6 ± 157.6	<0.001
U_{Na}/U_{Cr}	14.6 ± 7.7	13.6 ± 6.7	NS
% FE_{Na}	0.78 ± 0.37	0.69 ± 0.26	NS
C_{Osm} (ml/m)	1.26 ± 0.25	1.83 ± 0.4	<0.001
Tc_{H_2O} (ml/m)	-0.21 ± 0.4	-0.98 ± 0.41	<0.001
Serum creatinine (mg/dl)	0.86 ± 0.16	0.79 ± 0.14	NS
C_{Cr} (ml/m)	94.4 ± 25.8	103.7 ± 21.2	NS

From Calvo-Alén, J. de Cos, M. A., Rodríguez-Valverde, V., et al.: Subclinical renal toxicity in rheumatic patients receiving long-term treatment with nonsteroidal antiinflammatory drugs. J. Rheumatol. 21:1742, 1994. Used by permission.

* Values are expressed as mean $\pm$ 1 SD. The results were analyzed by the 2-tailed Student's *t* test; $p < 0.05$ was considered statistically significant.

† Abbreviations: U_{Na}/U_{Cr}, urinary excretion of sodium/mmol of urinary creatinine; % FE_{Na}, fractional excretion of Na; C_{Osm}, osmolar clearance; Tc_{H_2O}, negative free water clearance; C_{Cr}, creatinine clearance.

papillary necrosis may be generated by analgesics or NSAIDs, probably as a result of renal blood flow away from the renal medulla. Chronic renal toxicity is probably more common than is generally appreciated. In a study in which patients treated with NSAIDs for rheumatoid arthritis and osteoarthritis were compared to a matched control arthritis population, the NSAID-treated patients had a rise in serum creatinine level from 1.28 to 2.58 mg/dl over a 4-year period; the control group creatinine concentrations did not change.[20] The initial values of creatinine imply that many of these patients had some renal insufficiency before going on the drugs, and this emphasizes the importance of using them sparingly in elderly patients. The elderly have diminished glomerular filtration rates and renal blood

flow, increased renal vascular resistance, decreased total body water, and a diminished hepatic capacity to metabolized drugs . . . each of which renders them susceptible to NSAID toxicity.

Analgesics that have no capacity to inhibit COX can also induce chronic nephropathy; one study showed that individuals taking more than one pill per day of acetaminophen (more than 1,000 pills lifetime) have twice the risk of developing end-stage renal disease.[21] If a physician must prescribe an NSAID to a patient with renal insufficiency, the best choices would be nonacetylated salicylates or sulindac. The unique metabolism of this drug[19] appears to spare renal prostaglandin syntheses; the trade-off is that sulindac is not a good drug to use in patients with compromised liver function.

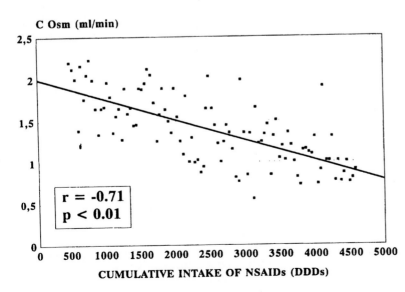

FIGURE 29–1. Relationship between the cumulative intake of NSAIDs and the osmolar clearance (C_{Osm}). The C_{Osm} was lower in those patients with a higher cumulative intake of NSAIDs ($r = -71, p < .01$). DDD = defined daily doses taken per month. (From Calvo-Alén, J., de Cos, M. A., Rodríguez-Valverde, V., et al.: Subclinical renal toxicity in rheumatic patients receiving long-term treatment with nonsteroidal antiinflammatory drugs. J. Rheumatol. 21: 1742, 1994. Used by permission.)

TABLE 29–2. Interaction of Salicylates with Other Drugs

DRUG	EFFECT
Furosemide Thiazide diuretics Spironolactone Triamterene β blockers Angiotensin-converting enzyme inhibitors	Hypertension, edema, hyperkalemia, congestive heart failure, especially in those with renal insufficiency
Lithium Digoxin Aminoglycosides	Particularly in those with diminished renal function, salicylate-induced reduction in glomerular filtration can lead to increased blood levels and direct toxicity
Methotrexate	Salicylates inhibit renal clearance of methotrexates, and both compete for binding sites on serum proteins
Cyclosporine	Aspirin or an NSAID plus cyclospo- rine can produce a marked decrease in glomerular filtration rates and ef- fective renal blood flow[23]
Chlorpropamide	Salicylates may potentiate the actions of this oral hypoglycemic drug[24]

TABLE 29–3. Chemical Classification of NSAIDs

Carboxylic acids	
Acetylated	Aspirin
Nonacetylated	Choline salicylate, diflunisal, magnesium salicylate, salicylamide, salicylate with magnesium salicylate, salsalate, and sodium salicylate
Acetic acids	Diclofenac,* indomethacin,* tolmetin,* sulindac,* and etodolac
Propionic acids	Flufenamic acid, mefenamic acid,* meclofenamic acid,* and niflumic acid
Enolic acids	Oxyphenbutazone, phenylbutazone,* piroxicam,* sudoxicam, tenoxicam, and isoxicam
Nonacidic compounds	Nabumetone, proquazone, and bufexamac

Data from Brooks and Day (1991).[2]
* Available in the United States.

Other Side Effects

Aspirin intolerance, asthma, and nasal polyposis is a syndrome related to compounds that inhibit prostaglandins. Serious reactions from nonacetylated salicylates in patients with aspirin-induced asthma have been reported as well.[22] It is wise to avoid these drugs in asthmatic patients and to accept the adverse effects of chronic low-dose glucocorticoids for the anti-inflammatory activity needed.

Interactions between salicylates and other drugs are often the cause of unexpected side effects of multiple medications in the rheumatoid patient. Some major interactions are listed in Table 29–2.

Tinnitus and reversible hearing loss may be a part of a more diffuse set of symptoms including malaise, sweating, restlessness, and anxiety. The hearing loss may be unrecognized by elderly patients and their relatives, and thus the symptom complex or components of it may elude diagnostic links to salicylates.

NONSALICYLATE NSAIDs

With so many NSAIDs available to choose from (Table 29–3), it is important for the physician confronted with a patient with polyarticular synovitis and a probable diagnosis of rheumatoid arthritis to choose among them wisely. All of these compounds inhibit COX, although, because they are derived from different chemical classes,[2] there are important differences in both actions and side effects. For example, several suppress lipoxygenase activity and potentially diminish leukotriene production.[2] Whereas piroxicam inhibits hydrogen peroxide production by activated neutrophils, ibuprofen does not.[25] Diclofenac significantly inhibits neutrophil migration (chemotaxis), but naproxen exerts a weaker effect in that system.[26] At this time, however, there is no useful way to extrapolate from these assays to the clinical realm by using these in vitro test results to choose an NSAID for use in individual patients. Cost is a very easy factor to assay, however, and can play a major role in patient compliance in taking one NSAID as opposed to another.[4]

Dosage Frequency: A Function of Plasma Half-Life

One of the principal barriers to compliance with some NSAIDs has been the necessity for four-times-per-day dosing. In one study, compliance was 78 per cent for once-a-day regimen but was only 60 per cent for four-times-daily dose schedules.[27] Therefore, emergence of drugs such as piroxicam, which has a serum half-life longer than 50 hours

TABLE 29–4. Mean (±SD) Plasma Half-Lives of Different NSAIDs*

DRUG	HALF-LIFE (hr)
Short half-life	
Aspirin	0.25 ± 0.03
Diclofenac	1.1 ± 0.2
Etodolac	3.0; 6.5 ± 0.3†
Fenoprofen	2.5 ± 0.5
Flufenamic acid	1.4; 9.0†
Flurbiprofen	3.8 ± 1.2
Ibuprofen	2.1 ± 0.3
Indomethacin	4.6 ± 0.7
Ketoprofen	1.8 ± 0.4
Pirprofen	3.8; 6.8†
Tiaprofenic acid	3.0 ± 0.2
Tolmetin	1.0 ± 0.3; 6.8 ± 1.5†
Long half-life	
Apazone	15 ± 4
Diflunisal	13 ± 2
Fenbufen	11.0
Nabumetone	26 ± 5
Naproxen	14 ± 2
Oxaprozin	58 ± 10
Phenylbutazone	68 ± 25
Piroxicam	57 ± 22
Salicylate	2–15‡
Sulindac (sulfide)	14 ± 8
Tenoxicam	60 ± 11

Adapted from Brooks, P. M., and Day, R. O.: Nonsteroidal antiinflammatory drugs—differences and similarities. N. Engl. J. Med. 324:1716, 1991. Copyright 1991, Massachusetts Medical Society. All rights reserved.

* Adapted from Day et al. (note 19) with the permission of the publisher.

† Elimination of this drug occurs in two phases (indicated by semicolon), of which the first is generally the most important.

‡ Elimination of this drug is dose dependent.

(see Table 29–4), has made single daily dosing possible. The problem with long-acting drugs, however, is that it takes longer to reverse toxicity, and a potential risk of gastrointestinal tract erosion exists if a pill sits long on a segment of mucosa. In addition, it takes longer (up to a week or more) for the longest acting drugs to achieve therapeutic plasma drug levels, and synovial concentrations of NSAIDs may be substantially different from those in plasma.[28] The active form of the drug may appear after metabolism of the compound given by mouth (e.g., sulindac), and the extent of protein binding may alter the true bioavailability of the drug given.

Which NSAID Should Be Used?

When a second-line drug (e.g., gold, methotrexate) is discontinued in rheumatoid patients, the reason is usually because there was unsatisfactory effi-

cacy or toxic side effects appeared. With NSAIDs there often is another reason: There are many NSAIDs, and there is a tendency among physicians (often urged by patients) to switch from one to another, even if symptoms are improved and no side effects have appeared. In a study in seven private rheumatologic practices of 1,775 courses of NSAIDs taken by 532 patients,[29] only 48 per cent were continued at 12 months and 36 per cent at 24 months. Interestingly, only acetylated salicylates other than plain aspirin were continued significantly longer than any other NSAID.

The best strategy for the physician prescribing a NSAID for a new patient with rheumatoid arthritis appears to be as follows:

- Assure the patient that the similarities among NSAIDs—in spite of what is presented in advertising—are greater than the differences.
- Plan to use one NSAID, beginning with one of the less expensive, using gradually increasing doses for at least 6 weeks or until an unacceptable side effect appears. If that NSAID fails, try another and then a third before giving up. Starting with an enteric-coated aspirin preparation, followed—if necessary—by a longer acting drug with a different dosage schedule, is a good alternative.
- Aim to supplement the NSAID relatively soon with a second-line drug such as hydroxychloroquine, but continue to stress to the patient who has responded satisfactorily to NSAID therapy that he or she should have one of these medications as a base of therapy for many years to come (see the box on opposite page.)

NSAID Toxicity: A Persistent Problem

As can be predicted from the mechanisms of action of these drugs, their side effects are similar. Many side effects have been reviewed in the section on salicylates earlier, but there appear to be some adverse reactions that are more common after non-aspirin NSAIDs are used than with salicylates:

- Ibuprofen may have a propensity to cause an aseptic meningitis.
- In a meta-analysis of gastrointestinal complications of NSAID therapy, piroxicam had a relative risk of 11.1, whereas that of ibuprofen was 2.3 and indomethacin 4.7.[33]
- Sulindac and nonacetylated salicylates probably have a lower incidence of prostaglandin-mediated renal side effects than do other NSAIDs (see earlier).
- Sulindac and diclofenac appear to cause more

Can NSAIDs Modify Rheumatoid Arthritis?

NSAIDs have been used for years in rheumatoid arthritis without evidence that they can actually modify the course of disease. It has been assumed that these drugs are useful for decreasing symptoms, but that they are incapable of suppressing the immunopathogenic mechanisms that drive rheumatoid synovitis.

Now there are data to indicate that, in a cohort of patients given a NSAID, some will have a clinical response. In those patients (but not the nonresponders), NSAID therapy is associated with a significant reduction in levels of IgM rheumatoid factor, a decrease in CRP level, an increase in the circulating numbers of lymphocytes, and a decrease in granulocytes[30] (Fig. 29–2). A second study of 18 patients given a washout period of NSAID and then restarted on the drugs revealed that 7 were responders and 11 nonresponders.[31] The responders showed an increase of CD3+, CD4+, and CD8+ cells along with reductions in ESR, CRP levels, and IgM rheumatoid factor titer and spontaneous synthesis of rheumatoid factor by lymphocytes in vitro.

These studies substantiate earlier data[32] finding that clinical improvement correlates with assays of immune function after NSAID use. Whether these changes in laboratory parameters are secondary to control of the disease activity, and not a primary effect upon immune cell function, must be determined. The conclusion must be, however, that NSAIDs can beneficially modulate the course of rheumatoid arthritis in a subset of patients.

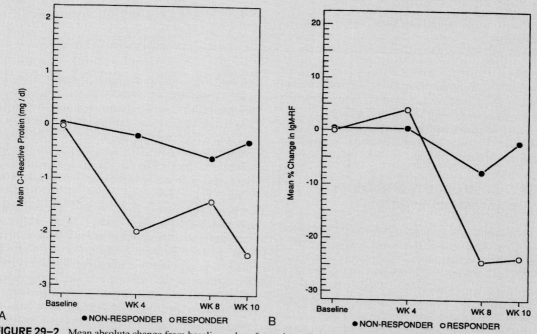

FIGURE 29–2. Mean absolute change from baseline values for various clinical parameters among responder and nonresponder rheumatoid arthritis populations during treatment with NSAIDs. *A*, CRP levels; values were significant for only the responders, at weeks 4 to 10 ($p < .05$). *B*, Serum IgM rheumatoid factor (IgM-RF) levels; values were significant for only the responders, at weeks 8 and 10 ($p < .05$). *C*, Granulocyte counts; values were significant for only the responders, at weeks 4 to 10 ($p < .05$). *D*, Lymphocyte counts; values were significant for only the responders, at weeks 8 and 10 ($p < .05$). (From Cush, J. J., Lipsky, P. E., Postlethwaite, A. E., et al.: Correlation of serologic indicators of inflammation with effectiveness of nonsteroidal antiinflammatory drug therapy in rheumatoid arthritis. Arthritis Rheum. 33:19, 1990. Used by permission.)

Illustration continued on following page

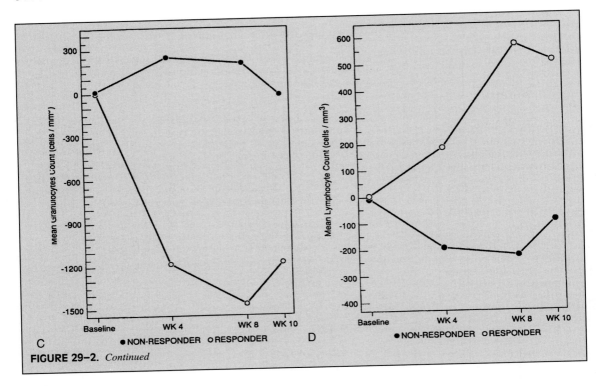

FIGURE 29–2. *Continued*

hepatitis than other NSAIDs,[34] whereas ibuprofen, indomethacin, ketoprofen, and naproxen were associated with the lowest incidence.

- Phenylbutazone and indomethacin are the only NSAIDs associated with agranulocytosis or aplastic anemia.[35]

NSAID Gastropathy and Other Gastrointestinal Events

Fortunately, the toxicities that could cause acute illness and drug-related death are, for the most part, very unusual occurrences. The exception to this is NSAID-related gastrointestinal events. The risk of gastrointestinal event–related death in patients taking NSAIDs for rheumatoid arthritis is estimated to be 0.19 per cent.[36] In elderly patients, the risk of death from gastrointestinal bleeding is high, and the rate of peptic ulcer disease is significantly increased. In a review of 1,415 patients hospitalized for confirmed peptic ulcer disease from 1984 through 1986 in Tennessee, the relative risk of ulcer disease in NSAID users compared with a case-control population of more than 7,000 patients was 4 to 8, depending on the dose of NSAID used.[37] In a nested case-control study of Medicaid enrollees age 60 or greater, 34 per cent of patients who died in a hospital from a peptic ulcer or gastrointestinal hemorrhage had filled a prescription for an NSAID within 30 days before the onset of illness, compared with 11 per cent of controls of the same age in a hospital who had no gastrointestinal event. This was extrapolated to an adjusted odds ratio of 4.7.[37]

From a large number of patients with rheumatoid arthritis in the ARAMIS data base, a gastrointestinal event score table for rheumatoid arthritis patients has been constructed that gives a rough estimate for any individual patient of the likelihood of hospitalization or death from a gastrointestinal event–related problem[36] (Fig. 29–3). Major risk factors for serious upper gastrointestinal complications include increasing age, history of a previous NSAID gastrointestinal side effect, disability index, the fraction of the maximum NSAID dose, cardiovascular disease, and current prednisone use.

There are two types of NSAID-associated mucosal lesions[38] (Table 29–5). Prognostically, the feature that most determines prognosis for an individual is the depth of the lesion. There is a dissociation of pain and endoscopic lesions in patients who use NSAIDs, much more than with non–NSAID-related ulcer disease, and a similar dissociation of symptoms and ulcer complications. In one study, 58 per cent of hemorrhages or perforations in NSAID users were silent, compared with 25 per cent of ulcers occurring in the absence of NSAID use.[39] It is important that not too much stress be placed on endoscopic evidence for asymptomatic ulcers, be-

GI EVENT SCORE TABLE FOR RA

AGE (years)	x 2 =
HISTORY OF PREVIOUS NSAID GI SIDE EFFECT	50 =
DISABILITY INDEX (0-3) OR (ARA CLASS-1)	x 10 =
NSAID DOSE (fraction of maximum recommended)	x 15 =
CURRENT PREDNISONE USE	40 =
TOTAL SCORE	————

GI EVENT RISK PER YEAR ON NSAIDS IN RA

RISK = (SCORE - 100) /40

FIGURE 29–3. Gastrointestinal (GI) event score table for rheumatoid arthritis (RA). Derived from logistic regression results, a simplified scheme is presented here: the sum of (1) patient age $\times$ 2; (2) 50 points if there is a prior history of NSAID dyspepsia; (3) 0 points for American Rheumatism Association (ARA) functional class 1 (normal), 10 for class 2 (adequate), 20 for class 3 (limited), or 30 for class 4 (unable); (4) 15 times the fraction, patient NSAID dose $\div$ manufacturer's highest recommended dose; and (5) 40 points for current prednisone use. When 100 is subtracted from this sum and the result divided by 40, the per cent risk of hospitalization or death from gastrointestinal events over the next 12 months is obtained. (From Fries, J. F., Williams, C. A., Bloch, D. A., et al.: Nonsteroidal anti-inflammatory drug-associated gastropathy: incidence and risk factor models. Am. J. Med. 91:213, 1991. Used by permission.)

cause of the evidence that many of these "come and go," (heal, then return). Clinical events (e.g., bleeding or perforation) are most important to follow (J.F. Fries, personal communication).

The mechanisms causing the NSAID gastropathy are multifactorial,[16,30,41] but most can be related to the inhibition of prostaglandin synthesis by these drugs that leads to the following:

- An increase in gastric acid synthesis
- Decreased production of the mucus barrier that coats gastric mucosa
- A decrease in glutathione synthesis resulting in less oxygen free radical scavenging
- Decreased bicarbonate biosynthesis
- Variable gastric mucosal blood flow

TABLE 29–5. Two Types of NSAID-Associated Mucosal Lesions

FEATURE	SUPERFICIAL LESIONS	ULCERS
Onset	Acute (persist for minutes)	Chronic (persist for days to years)
Site	Fundus > antrum	Antrum > fundus
Depth	Involves mucosa only	Penetrates submucosa
Mode	Topical contact, pH partition	Systemic, decreases PGs
Size	Smaller	Larger
Enteric coating	Decreases injury	May not decrease incidence
Clinical importance	Usually trivial	Sometimes critical (cause complications)
Healing	Rapid	Slow
Adaptation	Probably	Probably not

From Soll, A. H., Weinstein, W. M., Kurata, J., et al.: Nonsteroidal anti-inflammatory drugs and peptic ulcer disease. Ann. Intern. Med. 114:307, 1991. Used by permission.

Does *Helicobacter pylori* Infection Increase the Risk for NSAID Gastropathy?

Nonerosive (chronic active) gastritis is generally due to *H. pylori*, which is present in the gastric antrum of virtually all patients with duodenal ulcers and roughly 75 per cent of patients with gastric ulcer disease. If those taking NSAIDs are separated out of the gastric ulcer group, almost all patients with non–NSAID-related gastric ulcer have *H. pylori*. The inference is that NSAIDs are an independent risk factor for gastric ulcer.

In one of the most detailed studies on the subject, 61 patients with rheumatoid arthritis and 110 with osteoarthritis *not* taking NSAIDs were compared with 67 healthy volunteers and 50 rheumatoid patients on therapeutic doses of NSAIDs. Serology for *H. pylori* was obtained on all patients and almost all underwent esophagogastroduodenoscopy. Although *H. pylori* infection was clearly associated with both chronic and active gastritis, the rate of infection determined serologically was not different in the healthy control population or in rheumatoid patients taking NSAIDs.[40] In addition, it was demonstrated that, in the rheumatoid patients on NSAIDs, dyspeptic or other abdominal symptoms did not correlate with endoscopic evidence of significant mucosal damage.

NSAIDs and *H. pylori* are, it appears, independent and significant risk factors for gastroduodenal mucosal erosive disease.

In addition, NSAIDs may cause direct erosive injury by becoming trapped and concentrated within mucosal cells. Certain NSAIDs given as a prodrug (e.g., sulindac) that undergo enterohepatic recirculation may damage the gastric mucosa if and when biliary reflux occurs. Age and disability from longstanding rheumatoid arthritis appears to magnify and intensify all of the harmful effects of these drugs in the gastrointestinal tract. An alternative for future screening of patients both before and after starting NSAIDs to identify those at risk for gastropathy may be use of "permeability probes." One of these is sucrose. This complex sugar traverses gastroduodenal mucosa intact only when the mucosa is damaged, and after an oral dose its rate of excretion in the urine over the next hours can be quantitated and compared with normal rates. Those patients with high excretion probably should be considered for prophylactic therapy with misoprostol.[42]

Ulcerative disease of the colon, essentially indistinguishable from ulcerative colitis, is an unusual complication of NSAID therapy. Patients developing this toxicity are usually older, and the median latency period between drug exposure and onset of symptoms has been reported to be 3 months.[16,43]

PROPHYLAXIS AND TREATMENT OF NSAID-INDUCED UPPER GASTROINTESTINAL TOXICITY

It is a difficult concept for most physicians to give a drug only to prevent or blunt the side effects of another drug, but use of misoprostol to ward off NSAID gastroduodenopathy may be indicated in certain cases. Misoprostol is a prostaglandin E analogue. Early studies indicated that its use could prevent NSAID-induced gastric ulcer,[44] but it has been difficult to assess whether it diminished the clinically important outcomes of hemorrhage, perforation, and death. Initial data indicated that misoprostol was superior to H_2 antagonists in prevention of gastric damage but was of similar benefit in the duodenum (for review, see ref. 45). An annoying side effect is that misoprostol produces some degree of loose stool or actual diarrhea in many individuals.

A number of studies of the cost and benefit of misoprostol have been carried out.[46,47] In studies that formulated a decision analysis model based on patient preferences, charge data, and literature-derived probability estimates, it was concluded that prophylaxis was cost-saving if the ulcer complication rate was greater than 1.2 per cent[46] or 1.5 per cent[47] or if the 3-month price of misoprostol was less than $95. A formula exists for determination of the risk rate for serious gastrointestinal events or death (see Fig. 29–3).[36] From estimates within the Canadian health care system, prophylaxis costs an additional $650 for every additional gastrointestinal event prevented.[47]

If, as reported in an ARAMIS study of 2,747 patients, the excess risk of a serious gastrointestinal event is 15 to 16 per 1,000 patient-years,[36] the data[47] suggest that it would be necessary to prophylactically treat only 84 NSAID users to prevent one serious adverse gastrointestinal event.

To support this are data from 664 clinical practices in North America that enrolled 8,843 patients receiving continuous NSAID therapy.[48] Patients were randomly assigned to placebo or 200 μg misoprostol four times daily. Serious upper gastrointestinal complications were reduced by 40 per cent (odds ratio 0.598) among the misoprostol-treated patients during the 6-month trial.

Making decisions about a single patient is a different process from using decision analysis trees, and for that reason it is appropriate to consider misoprostol prophylaxis in patients older than 60 years who are NSAID responders, particularly if they have had dyspeptic symptoms, are taking concomitant low-dose prednisone, or have a positive sucrose permeability test. If diarrhea becomes annoying, misoprostol may have to be stopped and an H_2 blocker or omeprazole introduced. It is always wise to begin misoprostol with a lower dose of 100 μg given three or four times daily. In most patients receiving long-term NSAID therapy, 200 μg three times daily offers substantial protection against gastric and duodenal ulcers; this dose is better tolerated than 200 μg four times daily,[49] and, of course, costs less.

It has been common lore that misoprostol was the only pharmacologic deterrent against NSAID gastroduodenopathy, and that control of acid in the stomach would not prevent lesions if prostaglandins were not present. More recently it has been shown that an H_2 blocker, famotidine, in high doses (40 mg twice daily) significantly lowered the cumulative incidence of gastric ulcers and duodenal ulcers in patients receiving NSAID therapy over a 24-week period. Similar to other studies using endoscopic findings as end points, no data were available about clinically important events.[50] Unpublished reports from Scandinavia suggest that omeprozole provides a similar protective effect.

TENIDAP: SOMEWHERE BETWEEN NSAIDs AND SECOND-LINE DRUGS?

Tenidap, a compound that has a structure dissimilar to the available NSAIDs, is reported to inhibit COX, inhibit LTB_4 synthesis, and suppress release in vitro from macrophage cultures of IL-1, IL-6, and TNFα. In a double-blind, randomized, multicenter study, patients with active rheumatoid arthritis were treated with tenidap (120 mg/day) versus a combination of hydroxychloroquine and piroxicam, or piroxicam alone.[51] Tenidap proved to be better than piroxicam alone and equal in efficacy to the piroxicam-hydroxychloroquine mixture.

Tenidap and the combination regimen produced a decrease in serum CRP and plasma IL-6 levels. Six per cent of tenidap-treated patients developed a side effect not usually seen with NSAIDs: mild, reversible proteinuria. As expected of a drug that blocks COX, tenidap has gastrointestinal toxicity of about the magnitude of the standard NSAIDs.

Tenidap has not, as of the summer of 1996, been approved for marketing in the United States. The Food and Drug Administration (FDA) will decide whether it is presented as a second line drug or as yet another nonsteroidal anti-inflammatory compound. Good arguments have been made for declaring tenidap a drug with significant second-line activity. One reason is that the studies with tenidap have attributed sturdy decreases in acute-phase reactants such as CRP,[52] and it follows that a decrease in cytokine production must precede this.

CONCLUSION

Despite their toxicity, NSAIDs are useful for rheumatoid patients. They (this includes aspirin, as well) have side effects, but most are known and generally appreciated. They should be used early, and when and if other medications are added to suppress the arthritis, NSAIDs can usually be continued.

REFERENCES

1. Gibson, T.: Nonsteroidal anti-inflammatory drugs: another look. Br. J. Rheumatol. 27:87, 1988.
2. Brooks, P. M., and Day, R. O.: Nonsteroidal antiinflammatory drugs—differences and similarities. N. Engl. J. Med. 324:1716, 1991.

    This useful review catalogues actions, pharmacokinetics, and side effects of the NSAIDs. Sixteen are now available in the United States, and several are available as over-the-counter preparations. The chemical classifications are listed in Table 29–3 (see text). The plasma half-lives are used by industry and the FDA to establish dosage schedules for NSAIDs. Those with long (>6 hours) and shorter half-lives are listed in Table 29–4 (see text).

3. Katz, J. N., Daltroy, L. H., Brennan, T. A., et al.: Informed consent and the prescription of nonsteroidal antiinflammatory drugs. Arthritis Rheum. 35:1257, 1992.
4. Clements, P. J., and Paulnott, R.: Nonstreroidal antirheumatic drugs. In Kelly, W. N., Harris, E. D., Jr., Ruddy, S., and Sledge, C. B. (eds.): Textbook of Rheumatology, 5th ed., Vol. 1. Philadelphia, W. B. Saunders, 1996, pp. 707–740.
5. Jones, D. L., Kroenke, K., Landry, F. J., et al.: Cost savings using a stepped-care prescribing protocol for nonsteroidal anti-inflammatory drugs. JAMA 275:926, 1996.
6. Fries, J. F., Ramey, D. R., Singh, G., et al.: A reevaluation of aspirin therapy in rheumatoid arthritis. Arch. Intern. Med. 153:2465, 1993.

7. Day, R. O., Harris, G., Brown, M., et al.: Interaction of salicylate and corticosteroids in man. Br. J. Clin. Pharmacol. 26:334, 1988.

8. Day, R. O.: Aspirin and salicylates. *In* Kelley, W. N., Harris, E. D. Jr., Ruddy, S., and Sledge, C. B. (eds.): Textbook of Rheumatology, 4th ed., Vol. 1. Philadelphia, W. B. Saunders, 1993, pp. 681–691.

9. Paull, P., Day, R., Graham, G., et al.: Single dose evaluation of a new enteric-coated aspirin preparation. Med. J. Aust. 1:617, 1976.

10. Preston, S. J., Arnold, M. H., Beller, E. M., et al.: Comparative analgesic and anti-inflammatory properties of sodium salicylate and acetylsalicylic acid (aspirin) in rheumatoid arthritis. Br. J. Clin. Pharmacol. 27:607, 1989.

11. Abramson, S., and Weissmann, G.: The mechanisms of action of nonsteroidal anti-inflammatory drugs. Arthritis Rheum. 32:1, 1989.

12. Kopp, E., and Ghosh, S.: Inhibition of NF-κB by sodium salicylate and aspirin. Science 265:956, 1994.

13. American Medical Association: Drug Evaluations. Chicago, American Medical Association, 1994.

14. Bellamy, N., and Bradley, L. A.: Workshop on chronic pain, pain control, and patient outcomes in rheumatoid arthritis and osteoarthritis. Arthritis Rheum. 39:357, 1996.

15. Murray, M. D., and Brater, D. C.: Renal toxicity of the nonsteroidal anti-inflammatory drugs. Ann. Rev. Pharmacol. Toxicol. 32:435, 1993.

16. Simon, L. S.: Nonsteroidal anti-inflammatory drug toxicity. Curr. Opin. Rheumatol. 5:265, 1993.

17. Sandler, D. P., Burr, F. R., and Weinberg, C. R.: Nonsteroidal anti-inflammatory drugs and the risk for chronic renal disease. Ann. Intern. Med. 115:165, 1991.

18. Calvo-Alén, J., de Cos, M. A., Rodríguez-Valverde, V., et al.: Subclinical renal toxicity in rheumatic patients receiving long-term treatment with nonsteroidal antiinflammatory drugs. J. Rheumatol. 21:1742, 1994.

In this study, 104 patients treated for more than 2 years with NSAIDs and 123 controls were followed with urinalyses and assay of creatinine clearance, osmolar clearance, negative free water clearance, and urinary excretion of sodium. Although the serum creatinine and creatinine clearance values did not change, other values did in a way that was consistent with early dysfunction of the loops of Henle and distal nephron, involved in urinary acidification, concentration, and sodium conservation. These functional abnormalities support the concept that chronic treatment with NSAIDs produces renal damage consistent with subclinical interstitial nephropathy. Of particular relevance was the observation that the cumulative intake of NSAIDs was directly related to the dysfunction.

19. Palmer, B. F.: Renal complications associated with use of nonsteroidal anti-inflammatory agents. J. Invest. Med. 43: 516, 1995.

20. Rice, D., Turner, R., Felts, J., et al.: Renal failure in patients with rheumatoid arthritis and osteoarthritis on nonsteroidal antiinflammatory drugs. Fed. Proc. 43:1100, 1984.

21. Perneger, T. V., Whelton, P. K., and Klag, M. I.: Risk of kidney failure associated with the use of acetaminophen, aspirin, and nonsteroidal antiinflammatory drugs. N. Engl. J. Med. 331:1675, 1994.

22. Szczeklik, A., Nizankowska, E., and Dworski, R.: Choline magnesium trisalicylate in patients with aspirin-induced asthma. Eur. Respir. J. 3:535, 1990.

23. Altman, R. D., Perez, G. O., and Sfakianakis, G. N.: Interaction of cyclosporine A and nonsteroidal anti-inflammatory drugs on renal function in patients with rheumatoid arthritis. Am. J. Med. 93:396, 1992.

24. Richardson, T., Foster, J., and Mauer, G.: Enhancement by sodium salicylate of the blood glucose-lowering effect of chlorpropamide—drug interaction or summation of similar effects? Br. J. Clin. Pharmacol. 22:43, 1986.

25. Abramson, S., Korchak, H. M., Ludewig, R., et al.: Modes of action of aspirin-like drugs. Proc. Natl. Acad. Sci. U.S.A. 82:7227, 1985.

26. Scheja, A., Forsgren, A., Marsal, L., et al.: Inhibition of *in vivo* leukocyte migration by NSAIDs. Clin. Exp. Rheumatol. 3:53, 1985.

27. Jacobs, J., Goldstein, A. G., Kelly, M. E., et al.: NSAID dosing schedule and compliance. Drug Intelligence Clin. Pharm. 22:727, 1988.

28. Day, R. O., Graham, G. G., and Williams, K. M.: Pharmacokinetics of non-steroidal anti-inflammatory drugs. Baillières Clin. Rheumatol. 2:363, 1988.

29. Pincus, T., Marcum, S. B., Callahan, L. F., et al.: Longterm drug therapy for rheumatoid arthritis in seven rheumatology private practices: I. Nonsteroidal antiinflammatory drugs. J. Rheumatol. 19:1874, 1992.

30. Cush, J. J., Lipsky, P. E., Postlethwaite, A. E., et al.: Correlation of serologic indicators of inflammation with effectiveness of nonsteroidal antiinflammatory drug therapy in rheumatoid arthritis. Arthritis Rheum. 33:19, 1990.

In this study, 47 rheumatoid patients were given a NSAID for a 10-week trial. Of the 30 who completed at least 8 weeks of therapy, 12 were "responders" and 18 "nonresponders" by clinical parameters. Laboratory responses of CRP, IgM rheumatoid factor, and circulating lymphocytes and granulocytes are shown in Figure 29–2 (see text).

31. Cush, J. J., Jasin, H. E., Johnson, R., et al.: Relationship between clinical efficacy and laboratory correlates of inflammatory and immunologic activity in rheumatoid arthritis patients treated with nonsteroidal antiinflammatory drugs. Arthritis Rheum. 33:623, 1990.

32. Goodwin, J. S., Ceuppens, J. L., and Rodriguez, M. A.: Administration of nonsteroidal anti-inflammatory agents in patients with rheumatoid arthritis: effects on indexes of cellular immune status and serum rheumatoid factor levels. JAMA 250:2485, 1983.

33. Gabriel, S. E., Jakimainen, L., and Bombardier, C.: Risk for serious gastrointestinal complications related to use of NSAID: a meta-analysis. Ann. Intern. Med. 115:787, 1991.

34. Katz, L. M., and Love, P. Y.: NSAIDs and the liver. *In* Famaey, J. P., and Paulus, H. E., (eds.): Therapeutic Applications of NSAIDs: Subpopulations and New Formulations. New York, Marcel Dekker, 1992, pp. 862–894.

35. International Agranulocytosis and Aplastic Anemia Study Group: Risks of agranulocytosis and aplastic anemia. JAMA 256:1749, 1986.

36. Fries, J. F., Williams, C. A., Bloch, D. A., et al.: Nonsteroidal anti-inflammatory drug-associated gastropathy: incidence and risk factor models. Am. J. Med. 91:213, 1991.

The hazard ratio of patients taking NSAIDs to those not taking NSAIDs was 5.2 in this survey of 2,747 patients with rheumatoid arthritis and 1,091 patients with osteoarthritis. A rule is presented in Figure 29–3 (see text) that should help physicians in their decision analysis about whether or not to use NSAIDs in an individual patient. For example, a 70-year-old patient with previous dyspepsia from NSAIDs who is moderately disabled and is taking a maximum dose of NSAID in addition to a small prednisone dose has a 5.75 per cent risk of hospitalization or death from gastrointestinal complications in the next 12 months.

37. Griffin, M. R., Piper, J. M., Daugherty, J. R., et al.: Nonsteroidal anti-inflammatory drug use and increased risk for peptic ulcer disease in elderly persons. Ann. Intern. Med. 114:257, 1991.

38. Soll, A. H., Weinstein, W. M., Kurata, J., et al.: Nonsteroidal anti-inflammatory drugs and peptic ulcer disease. Ann. Intern. Med. 114:307, 1991.

39. Armstrong, C. P., and Blower, A. L.: Non-steroidal anti-inflammatory drugs and life threatening complications of peptic ulceration. Gut 28:527, 1987.

40. Loeb, D. S., Talley, N. J., Ahlquist, D. A., et al.: Long-term nonsteroidal anti-inflammatory drug use and gastroduodenal injury: the role of *Helicobacter pylori*. Gastroenterology 102:1899, 1992.

41. Loeb, D. S., Ahlquist, D. A., and Talley, N. J.: Management of gastroduodenopathy associated with the use of nonsteroidal anti-inflammatory drugs. Mayo Clin. Proc. 67:354, 1992.

42. Meddings, J. B., Sutherland, L. R., Byles, N. I., et al.: Sucrose, a novel permeability marker for gastroduodenal disease. Gastroenterology 104:1619, 1993.

43. Gibson, G. R., Whitacre, E. B., and Ricotti, C. A.: Colitis induced by nonsteroidal anti-inflammatory drugs. Arch. Intern. Med. 152:625, 1992.

44. Graham, D. Y., Agrawal, N. M., and Roth, S. H.: Prevention of NSAID-induced gastric ulcer with misoprostol: multicenter, double-blind, placebo-controlled trial. Lancet 2:1277, 1988.

45. Ballinger, A. B., Kumar, P. J., and Scott, D. L.: Misoprostol in the prevention of gastroduodenal damage in rheumatology. Ann. Rheum. Dis. 51:1089, 1992.

46. Gabriel, S. E., Campion, M. E., and O'Fallon, W. M.: A cost-utility analysis of misoprostol prophylaxis for rheumatoid arthritis patients receiving nonsteroidal antiinflammatory drugs. Arthritis Rheum. 37:333, 1994.

47. Gabriel, S. E., Jakimainen, R. L., and Bombardier, C.: The cost-effectiveness of misoprostol for nonsteroidal antiinflammatory drug-associated adverse gastrointestinal events. Arthritis Rheum. 36:447, 1993.

48. Silverstein, F. E., Graham, D. Y., Senior, J. R., et al.: Misoprostol reduces serious gastrointestinal complications in patients with rheumatoid arthritis receiving nonsteroidal anti-inflammatory drugs: a randomized, double-blind, placebo-controlled trial. Ann. Intern. Med. 123:241, 1995.

49. Raskin, J. B., White, R. H., Jackson, J. E., et al.: Misoprostol dosage in the prevention of NSAID-induced gastric and duodenal ulcers: a comparison of three regimens. Ann. Intern. Med. 123:344, 1995.

50. Taha, A. S., Hudson, N., Hawkey, C. J., et al.: Famotidine for the prevention of gastric and duodenal ulcers caused by nonsteroidal antiinflammatory drugs. N. Engl. J. Med. 334:1435, 1996.

51. Mlackburn, W. D. Jr., Prupas, H. M., Silverfield, J. C., et al.: Tenidap in rheumatoid arthritis. Arthritis Rheum. 38:1447, 1995.

52. Canvin, J. M. G., and Madhok, R.: Tenidap: not just another NSAID? Ann. Rheum. Dis. 55:79, 1996.

30

The Role of Glucocorticoids

In 1949, Hench and colleagues published observations on the beneficial effects of glucocorticoids on rheumatoid arthritis.[1] The first patient, a 29-year-old woman, was given three injections of 100 mg hydrocortisone, became asymptomatic, and rose from a bed in which she had been immobilized for 4 years. This paper triggered widespread use of natural and synthetic adrenocortical hormones for a wide variety of inflammatory diseases. Over the years, however, efficacy has been matched by a broad spectrum of toxic effects. Enthusiasm for glucocorticoids in large or moderate doses in treatment of rheumatoid arthritis waned appropriately as hypertension, osteoporosis, diabetes mellitus, and susceptibility to infection increased as a function of cumulative dose in patients.

A comparison of commonly used glucocorticoids is provided in Table 30–1.[2]

In the 1990s, there are the following indications for glucocorticoid therapy (almost always using prednisone) in rheumatoid arthritis:

- For **vasculitis** presenting as skin ulcers, mononeuritis multiplex, rapidly progressive pulmonary interstitial fibrosis, coronary arteritis, or severe systemic toxicity with fever and intense pain. Doses used (prednisone equivalents) are in the range of 40 to 120 mg daily, but initially the dose used should be whatever is needed to suppress the process.

- As a **bridge therapy** when NSAID therapy is insufficient to control the process, and second-line drugs have not yet had an effect. Doses used should be less than 7.5 mg given each day in the morning.

- To blunt the manifestations of **drug toxicity**, such as skin rash in D-penicillamine therapy.

- As short courses in doses greater than 60 mg/day for **severe flares of arthritis** or systemic complications of the disease.

- As **intra-articular injections** using a long-acting compound such as triamcinolone hexacetonide. This is particularly useful when a few joints are involved in a flare of disease.

ADRENAL FUNCTION IN RHEUMATOID PATIENTS: HORMONES AND THEIR RECEPTORS

Studies of daily secretion of cortisol by rheumatoid patients have yielded variable data through the years. When disease activity is integrated into the equations, not only is there a flattening of the usual circadian rhythm of cortisol secretion, but there is also a significant correlation between increased cortisol levels and the inflammatory activity of the rheumatoid arthritis[3] (Fig. 30–1). These data would not have been expected if humans with rheumatoid arthritis had the same blunting of corticotropin release in response to IL-1 that is manifested in rats susceptible to experimentally induced arthritis[4,5] (see Chapter 16).

A major factor in consideration of hormone action is the number and responsiveness of receptors for the particular hormone. Because circadian levels of circulating human lymphocytes are inversely related to cortisol plasma levels, this cell is a logical one to use in studying glucocorticoid receptors. One such study assayed glucocorticoid receptor density and affinity on lymphocytes from 90 patients with active rheumatoid arthritis and 100 controls; the patients had not taken glucocorticoids for at least 6 months.[6] Although single cortisol levels drawn between 8 and 9 A.M. were no different in rheumatoid patients and controls, density of receptors in patients (2,000/cell) was significantly less than in controls. Receptor affinity was not different, and there was no correlation of receptor density with the ESR. A subsequent study from the same group showed that, despite the lower density of glucocorticoid receptors in rheumatoid patients, the peripheral blood lymphocytes from these patients were at least as glucocorticoid sensitive as those from normal subjects. These data were consistent with the clinical observation that rheumatoid patients respond to these drugs.[7]

Another possible abnormality in rheumatoid patients is highlighted by the studies of CRH stimulation tests in patients treated chronically with low-

TABLE 30–1. Comparison of Commonly Used Glucocorticoids

DURATION OF ACTION	GLUCOCORTICOID	EQUIVALENT ORAL OR INTRAVENOUS DOSES (mg)	RELATIVE SODIUM-RETAINING ACTION
Short			
$t_{1/2}$ 8–12 h	Cortisone	25	0.8
	Cortisol	20	1
Intermediate			
$t_{1/2}$ 12–36 h	Prednisone	5	0.8
	Prednisolone	5	0.8
	Methylprednisolone	4	0.5
	Triamcinolone	4	0
Long			
$t_{1/2}$ 36–72 h	Paramethasone	2	0
	Dexamethasone	0.75	0
	Betamethasone	0.60	0

Modified from George, E., and Kirwan, J. R.: Corticosteroid therapy in rheumatoid arthritis. Baillière's Clin. Rheumatol. 4:621, 1990. Used by permission.

dose prednisone, compared with control patients.[8] Although substantial increases in adrenocorticotropic hormone (ACTH) and cortisol were induced with the CRH, the dose response in patients linking total ACTH and total cortisol was shifted to the right, suggesting that the patient group had a mildly deficient adrenocortical responsiveness; the defect appeared to be compensated for by elevated basal evening ACTH concentrations. This probably indicates mild suppression of the hypothalamic-pituitary-adrenal axis in these patients.

In addition, it appears that there are significant differences in individual responsiveness of rheumatoid patients to glucocorticoids. An assay that measures methylprednisolone suppression of concanavalin A–stimulated peripheral mononuclear cell proliferation correlates well with clinical responses to the same glucocorticoid.[9]

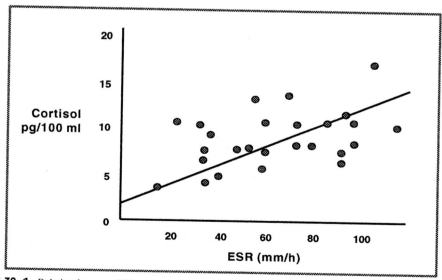

FIGURE 30–1. Relation between ESR as an indicator of inflammatory activity and the arithmetic mean value of cortisol as an indicator of adrenal secretory activity of 26 patients with rheumatoid arthritis. Cortisol levels were measured throughout a 24-hour cycle in 2-hour intervals (13 values for each patient). Linear regression analysis with a coefficient of regression $r = .63$ ($n = 26$) is significant ($p < .01$) (From Neeck, G., Federlin, K., Graef, V., et al.: Adrenal secretion of cortisol in patients with rheumatoid arthritis. J. Rheumatol. 17:24, 1990. Used by permission.)

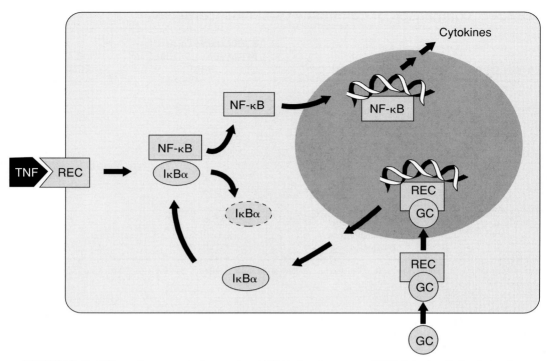

FIGURE 30–2. When an immune stimulator such as TNF binds to its receptor (REC), it leads to $I\kappa B\alpha$ destruction. NF-κB then moves into the nucleus, where it activates cytokines and other genes. By stimulating $I\kappa B\alpha$ production, the glucocorticoids (GC) may prevent this. (From Scheinman, R. I., Cogswell, P. C., Lofquist, A. K., et al.: Role of transcriptional activation of $I\kappa B\alpha$ in mediation of immunosuppression by glucocorticoids. Science 270:283, 1995; and Auphan, N., Di Donato, J. A., and Rosette, C.: Immunosuppression by glucocorticoids: inhibition of NF-κB activity through induction of $I\kappa B$ synthesis. Science 270:286, 1995. Used by permission. Copyright 1995 American Association for the Advancement of Science.)

MECHANISMS OF GLUCOCORTICOID ACTION IN SUPPRESSING INFLAMMATION AND IMMUNITY

Glucocorticoids enter the cell and bind to a receptor in the cytoplasm.[10] This receptor-glucocorticoid complex moves into the nucleus and acts as a transcription factor, binding to genes and either activating or suppressing them. In addition, glucocorticoids can prevent other transcription factors (e.g., AP-1) from binding to genes (e.g., the collagenase gene), thereby suppressing expression of the genes.

A major activator of immune response and inflammatory process genes is NF-κB. This factor is itself activated by phosphorylation, enabling it to migrate to the nucleus and activate target genes. Glucocorticoids increase expression of $I\kappa B\alpha$, a protein that prevents access of NF-κB to the nucleus (Fig. 30–2). This down-regulates many immunoinflammatory responses.[11,12]

There are significant gaps in knowledge of how the binding to DNA is translated into diminished cellular activity, but the following functions of glucocorticoids are definitely anti-inflammatory[10]:

- PMN leukocytes are inhibited from accumulation at sites of inflammation by inhibition of the leukocytes to endothelial cells.
- In macrophages

NF-κB and Immunoregulation

NF-κB is a heterodimer formed of p50 and p65 subunits. In response to inflammatory stimuli, repressor molecules such as the $I\kappa B$ family are rapidly degraded, allowing access of NF-κB to the cell nucleus. NF-κB induces many genes, including those coding for IL-1, IL-2, IL-3, IL-6, IL-8, TNFα, IFNγ, GM-CSF, MHC class I and II molecules, ELAM-1, and ICAM-1. Because the beneficial effects of glucocorticoids are dulled by their toxicity, it is an excellent strategy to search for compounds that specifically inhibit NF-κB.

- myelopoiesis is depressed
- class II MHC antigen expression is diminished
- cytokine release (e.g., IL-1, IL-6, TNFα) is blocked
- synthesis of prostaglandins and leukotrienes is blocked
- Eosinophils, basophils, and mast cells are inhibited from circulating and from accumulating in tissues.
- In endothelial cells
  - vascular permeability is diminished
  - activation is inhibited
  - expression of class II MHC antigens is inhibited
  - endothelial adhesion molecule expression is suppressed[13]
  - complement pathway component secretion is inhibited
- In fibroblasts
  - collagen and collagenase production is inhibited
  - fibronectin, IL-1, and TNFα synthesis is suppressed
  - in fibroblast arachidonic acid metabolism, PLA_2 is suppressed and COX-2 expression is inhibited
  - biosynthesis of plasminogen activator is inhibited
- In lymphocytes
  - T-cell activation is inhibited by depression of IL-2 production, and by inhibition of production of supplemental cytokines
  - B cell immunoglobulin catabolism is increased and its production decreased

EXPERIENCE WITH GLUCOCORTICOIDS IN RHEUMATOID ARTHRITIS

The "closet" use of glucocorticoids by rheumatologists is not unusual; physicians who publicly denounce their use because of toxicity sometimes start patients on prednisone, almost forgetting that they have! The reason is that, more than any drug used in arthritis, glucocorticoids are a two-edged sword. The immediate effect of their use is gratifying, yet the long-term toxicity can be very discouraging. For these reasons, it is not surprising that health care analysts have found great variation among rheumatologists in the patterns of their use of these drugs in rheumatoid arthritis.[14]

In the many clinical trials reported since 1954, very little clear-cut long-term benefit has been as-

cribed to use of prednisone or equivalent compounds. As pointed out in one study, the "lack of demonstrable long-term benefit with prednisone use in this and other studies is disconcerting."[15] In the 122 patients in this group compared retrospectively with a similar number of case controls, no benefit could be measured, and cataracts and fractures were much more common in the prednisone-treated group.

In a report of 18 trials of prednisone that had reasonable methodology, only 11 were longer than 6 weeks.[2] Using doses that are relatively safe, it will take longer than 6 weeks for the effects on other than acute inflammation to become manifest.

Any dose of glucocorticoids that provides symptomatic relief of active rheumatoid synovitis within 24 to 36 hours will, within a month, be associated with chronic and deleterious toxicity. In contrast, there rarely is immediate change in rheumatoid symptoms after institution of 5.0 mg prednisone given each day, but this dose may be sufficient to have some additive suppressive effects upon both inflammation and synovial proliferation after many weeks have gone by. This was exemplified in a 24-week double-blind, controlled study of 5 mg prednisone given daily to patients already taking NSAIDs but not second-line drugs.[16] There was some, but not significant, improvement in the prednisone group during the study but, in the 6-week period following abrupt cessation of prednisone in the treated patients, there was a significant deterioration of well-being and worsening of synovitis. It is unlikely that the deterioration could be ascribed simply to relative adrenal insufficiency, because there are good data to show that rheumatoid arthritis patients given 7.5 mg or less of prednisone per day for up to 40 months have no significant change in mean basal or peak levels of plasma cortisol or in mean peak levels of growth hormone in response to insulin challenge.[17] In addition, the flare of disease was not short lived, nor did it become manifest immediately on stopping the 5.0 mg prednisone each day. These observations are consistent with the marked recrudescence of pain, stiffness, and dysfunction that rheumatoid patients can experience when maintenance prednisone is cut only 1 mg/day, with a daily dose less than that of physiologic secretion (e.g., from 4 to 3 mg/day).

A much-needed study using low-dose oral prednisolone (7.5 mg daily for 2 years) in patients relatively *early* in the course of rheumatoid arthritis has been published[18] from the United Kingdom. This randomized, double-blind trial allowed use of other therapy. The primary outcome variables were the appearance of new hand joint erosions and the progression of pre-existing ones. Results can be summarized as follows:

1. Pre-existing erosions changed little in the prednisolone-treated group (0.72 units) but progressed much in the placebo group (5.37 units) (p = .004).
2. Twenty-two per cent of the prednisolone group and 46 per cent of the control group (p = .007) acquired new erosions during the 2 years.
3. As assayed by joint scores and disability indices, the prednisolone-treated group fared better.

Parenthetically, when the issue of whether or not a given patient on glucocorticoid therapy has adrenal suppression becomes important in management, it is appropriate to use either the pituitary-adrenal response to exogenous human CRH or an insulin hypoglycemia test, because pituitary-adrenal response cannot be reliably estimated from the dose of glucocorticoid, the duration of therapy, or the basal plasma cortisol concentration.[17]

The use of prednisone in elderly patients with rheumatoid arthritis has always presented a quandary to physicians. On the one hand, the drug may enable older patients to walk and handle activities of daily living more easily; on the other hand, toxicity can be amplified in this subset of patients. One study has compared use of either prednisone or chloroquine as the first second-line drug given to elderly patients.[19] Twenty-eight patients were in each group and all were older than 60 years; all were given an NSAID, 500 mg oral calcium, and cholecalciferol. The prednisone group was started on 15 mg/day, and this was decreased as low as possible after 1 month. Chloroquine was replaced in nonresponders after 3 months by intramuscular gold, and nonresponders in the prednisone group after 3 months were given chloroquine and, if needed, gold or sulfasalazine in addition to prednisone. Although complicated and nonblinded, this protocol produced interesting data:

1. Twelve of 28 in the prednisone group and 8 of 28 in the chloroquine group needed additional second-line therapy.
2. Functional capacity and disease activity improved in both groups, but earlier in the prednisone-treated group.
3. The excess bone loss in the prednisone group after 2 years (1.8 per cent in the spine and 1.5 per cent in the hip) was not significant.

In the aggregate, the data suggest that it is a valid strategy to use prednisone early in aged patients with rheumatoid arthritis if one accepts the probability that additional second-line therapy will be needed and it will be necessary to reduce the prednisone to minimal (~ 3 mg day or less) levels.

Glucocorticoid Treatment for Vasculitis of Rheumatoid Disease

There is little justification for use of glucocorticoid doses greater than 7 mg/day as long-term treatment of synovitis. The side effects are cumulative and often are amplified in the fragile sick.[2] However, in the vasculitic syndromes that can emerge in active rheumatoid patients (usually those with high concentrations of rheumatoid factor in blood), glucocorticoids must often be used in high doses (usually every 6 hours, frequently parenterally) or as pulse therapy. In vasculitic syndromes, the physician must deal with a different pathophysiology than with synovitis, and the beneficial effects of glucocorticoids are manifest in their effects on many cell types.

''Pulse'' therapy is considered as a large dose of methylprednisolone given intravenously over a period of 10 minutes or so, and was developed into a treatment for vasculitis of all etiologies by those who introduced it as acute therapy for organ transplant rejection. Although the standard dose has been 1.0 g given intravenously daily for 3 days, there is little evidence in the rheumatologic literature that 1.0 g has greater efficacy than 100 to 200 mg each day.[20] It is an unproved hypothesis that glucocorticoid pulsing can augment efficacy or decrease toxicity of gold salt or D-penicillamine therapy.[21]

Intrasynovial Glucocorticoid Therapy

Intrasynovial glucocorticoid therapy is used more by rheumatologists than by general internists or family physicians, not because of differing opinions about efficacy or toxicity but because the rheumatologists have more confidence in techniques of joint injection. There are several indications for intrasynovial glucocorticoid therapy[22]:

- Correction of soft tissue contractures secondary to synovitis
- Control of arthritis limited to several joints
- Control of prominent flares in one or several joints in patients with polyarticular disease
- Control of tendon sheath inflammation

TABLE 30–2. Contraindications to Intra-articular Corticosteroid Injections

Septic joint
Periarticular sepsis
Unstable joint
Intra-articular fracture
Marked juxta-articular osteorosis
Bacteremia
Blood-clotting disorders

From McCarthy, G. M., and McCarty, D. J.: Intrasynovial corticosteroid therapy. Bull. Rheum. Dis. 43:2, 1994. Used by permission. Copyright 1994 by the Arthritis Foundation.

TABLE 30–3. Amount of Triamcinolone Hexacetonide Used in Intrasynovial Injection Therapy

SIZE OF JOINT	EXAMPLES	DOSAGE (mg)
Large	Knee	40
	Ankle	30
	Shoulder	30
	Elbow	30
Medium	Subtalar	30
	Wrist	20
Small	Interphalangeal	5–10
	Metacarpophalangeal	
	Metatarsophalangeal	

From McCarthy, G. M., and McCarty, D. J.: Intrasynovial corticosteroid therapy. Bull. Rheum. Dis. 43:2, 1994. Used by permission. Copyright 1994 by the Arthritis Foundation.

Contraindications are listed in Table 30–2, and recommended amounts of triamcinolone are given in Table 30–3.[22]

In addition to suppressing inflammation, intra-articular glucocorticoids have the capability of "debulking" synovitis by inhibiting development of the proliferative aspects of rheumatoid arthritis; in relatively low concentrations, for example, these compounds inhibit growth factor synthesis and metalloprotease biosynthesis by synovial cells. Intra-articular injections may obviate the need for surgical synovectomy[23] in selected patients.

In one series of 956 injections given to 140 patients,[23] more than 75 per cent of injected joints or tendon sheaths remained in remission during a 7-year follow-up period. The rate of injection was about 2 per patient in the first year and 0.6 per patient-year for an additional 15 years. No clinical evidence of damage to cartilage (e.g., chondrolysis) was reported in this study, and other studies[24] indi-

cate the rarity of this complication so long as there is a suitable interval (3 or 4 months) between injections into the same joint. It has been shown that high initial levels of synovial fluid C4 and the percentage of neutrophils in the joint fluid correlated best with a decrease in circumference of injected knees.[25]

TOXICITY OF GLUCOCORTICOIDS

The full litany of glucocorticoid toxic side effects is not elaborated upon here; it is familiar to all physicians[2] (Table 30–5). Nevertheless, it is important to remember, in comparison, the toxicity of NSAIDs (Table 30–4). In addition, in low doses

TABLE 30–4. Relative Toxicity of NSAIDs: Data from Five ARAMIS Data Bank Centers (Standardized Toxicity Index Scores)

DRUG	NO. OF COURSES	MEAN	STANDARD ERROR	RANK
Salsalate	121	1.28	0.34	1
Ibuprofen	503	1.94	0.43	2
Naproxen	939	2.17	0.23	3
Sulindac	511	2.24	0.39	4
Piroxicam	790	2.52	0.23	5
Fenoprofen	161	2.95	0.77	6
Ketoprofen	190	3.45	1.07	7
Meclofenamate	157	3.86	0.66	8
Tolmetin	215	3.96	0.74	9
Indomethacin	386	3.99	0.58	10

From Fries, J. F., Williams, C. A., Ramey, D. R., et al.: The relative toxicity of alternative therapies for rheumatoid arthritis: implications for the therapeutic progression. Semin. Arthritis Rheum. 23(2, Suppl. 1): 68, 1993. Used by permission.

TABLE 30–5. Complications of Corticosteroid Therapy

Musculoskeletal
  Myopathy
  Osteoporosis—vertebral compression, fractures
  Aseptic necrosis of bone
Gastrointestinal
  Peptic ulceration (often gastric)
  Gastric hemorrhage
  Intestinal perforation
  Pancreatitis
Central nervous system
  Psychiatric disorders
  Pseudocerebral tumor
Ophthalmological
  Glaucoma
  Posterior subcapsular cataracts
Cardiovascular and renal
  Hypertension
  Sodium and water retention—edema
Metabolic
  Precipitation of clinical manifestations, including ketoacidosis of diabetes mellitus
  Hyperosmolar non-ketotic coma
  Hyperlipidemia
  Induction of centripetal obesity
Endocrine
  Growth failure
  Secondary amenorrhea
  Suppression of hypothalamic-pituitary-adrenal system
Inhibition of fibroplasia
  Impaired wound healing
  Subcutaneous tissue atrophy
Suppression of the immune response
  Superimposition of a variety of bacterial, fungal, viral, and parasitic infections in steroid-treated patients

From George, E., and Kirwan, J. R.: Corticosteroid therapy in rheumatoid arthritis. Baillière's Clin. Rheumatol. 4:621, 1990.

used by mouth for bridge therapy in rheumatoid arthritis, blatant toxic side effects such as hypertension and striae are rarely apparent. Development of cataracts is a problem for some patients and is poorly related to cumulative dose. Diabetes mellitus can be provoked in patients who are unaware that they are on the borderline of glucose intolerance.

One alleged side effect, development of peptic ulcer disease, appears not to be a true one. In a major meta-analysis of 93 double-blind, randomized, controlled trials of glucocorticoid therapy, clinically important peptic ulcer disease was found unlikely to be associated with steroid therapy alone[26] nor was there an increase in the risk of upper gastrointestinal bleeding in patients without a past history of such bleeding.[27] In contrast, persons receiving both corticosteroids and NSAIDs concur-

rently have a risk for peptic ulcer disease that is 15 times greater than that of nonusers of either class of drugs.[28]

Osteopenia and fractures, however, are serious and real toxic side effects, complications that are superimposed upon the inherent loss of bone mineral density associated with rheumatoid arthritis itself. These issues are discussed next in detail.

Osteopenia and Fractures: Major Toxic Side Effects of Long-Term Glucocorticoid Treatment

There are numerous mechanisms involved in osteoporosis caused by glucocorticoid therapy: osteoblast function is depressed, intestinal calcium absorption is decreased, and bone resorption is accelerated. These are superimposed upon the negative balance of bone remodeling associated intrinsically with rheumatoid arthritis. The result can be osteoporosis and fractures (Table 30–6). It is a major task of the physician to exploit the benefit of glucocorticoids without having the patient suffer pain or disability from toxicity. Rarely, glucocorticoid therapy can lead to avascular necrosis (see box).

By using doses of 7 mg/day or less of prednisone in rheumatoid arthritis, many of the side effects of the drug can be avoided. However, there is a direct relationship between the daily and cumulative dose

TABLE 30–6. Fractures Sites and Incidence

SITE	NUMBER
Ribs, collar bone	24
Arm (long bones)	13
Shoulder	8
Elbow	7
Wrist	12
Hand	12
Spine	46
Pelvis	15
Leg (long bones)	22
Hip	26
Knee	6
Foot, ankle	33
Other	2
Total	226

From Michel, B. A., Bloch, D. A., Wolfe, F., et al.: Fractures in rheumatoid arthritis: an evaluation of associated risk factors. J. Rheumatol. 20:1666, 1993. Used by permission.

Glucocorticoids and Avasacular Necrosis

Glucocorticoids have been implicated as a cause of avascular necrosis, but questions remain: how often does this complication occur? Which dose and preparations are likely to precipitate it? It does seem evident from reviewing case reports in the medical literature that dexamethasone is the preparation most often linked to the appearance of avascular necrosis. It can occur after prolonged treatment, including occasional pulse therapy, in renal transplant patients, but also has been seen after relatively short courses of therapy in cases of head trauma in which sustained doses of dexamethasone were used for periods less than 30 days.[29] The pathophysiology still is not known, but favored hypotheses are those that implicate fat buildup in a closed space (the bone) producing intraosseous pressures that exceed arteriolar blood pressure. In rheumatoid patients there is little risk from low-dose daily injections, but a real but not yet quantified risk from high-dose pulse therapy and too frequent injections of inflamed joints. In patients in whom the diagnosis is suspected, MRI is now the diagnostic modality of choice.

and the severe adverse events of fracture, serious infections, or a gastrointestinal bleed or ulcer. In a study of 112 rheumatoid patients receiving low-dose prednisone for greater than 1 year and matched against a control group, the risk factors for one of these serious adverse events were as follows[30]:

PREDNISONE DOSE	ODDS RATIO
10–15 mg/day	32.3
5–10 mg/day	4.5
0 to <5 mg/day	1.9

These and other data would appear to confirm the toxicity of chronic use of prednisone in doses greater than 5 mg/day, but still being argued is the impact of severe rheumatoid arthritis itself, and whether low-dose prednisone therapy that alleviates disease has a negative, positive, or neutral effect upon the odds ratio of developing fractures.

It is generally accepted that rheumatoid arthritis per se is associated with accelerated bone loss, with or without treatment with prednisone. As a corollary of this, it has been proposed that, if small doses of glucocorticoids can enable a patient to bear weight longer and be more active each day, the

osteopenic effects of the drug may be successfully counteracted by the bone-forming stimuli of exercise. For whatever reasons, the data have not been consistent enough to prove or disprove this. As noted (and referenced) by Laan et al.:

A negative association between duration of rheumatoid arthritis and bone mineral density was found in some . . . studies, but has not been confirmed by others. The degree of functional impairment has been suggested as an important risk factor for fracture by some workers, but not by all . . . Disease activity has also been suggested as a possible risk factor for osteopenia in patients with rheumatoid arthritis. Other workers found no such association.[31]

Effects of Rheumatoid Arthritis Per Se on Bone Mineral Density

The availability of dual-photon absorptiometry that can give measurement of BMD in the spine as well as in long bones has enabled relatively easy study of bones in a great variety of patients. In 147 patients with recent-onset rheumatoid arthritis who were followed for at least 3 months, no association was seen between BMD and joint counts, swollen joints, or degree of general health; however, a negative association was found between measurements of ESR and BMD.[31] This is consistent with the knowledge that cytokines and prostaglandins released by proliferating synovial cells in rheumatoid inflammation can be destructive to bone. It is probable that rheumatoid arthritis–dependent mechanisms such as this cause a gradual decrease in bone mass within the first 5 years of the disease. This study also revealed that the degree of functional impairment is related to BMD in the hip.[31] Bone histomorphometry indicates that bone formation is decreased in non–steroid-treated rheumatoid patients compared with controls.[32]

In a population-based study of BMD in rheumatoid and control patients in Finland, it was found that physical impairment and body weight were the major determinants of both spinal and femoral bone mass deficiency in rheumatoid patients, and, if the clinical activity of arthritis was factored into the equations, the effect of low-dose corticosteroid therapy on bone loss in rheumatoid patients was minimal.[33] The therapeutic lesson appears clear: Try to keep rheumatoid patients upright, mobile, and at average weight.

It has been suggested that the rapid periarticular bone loss in patients with rheumatoid arthritis involves interaction of normal amounts of parathyroid hormone with prostaglandins and cytokines produced in the adjacent joints.[34] Subchondral venous drainage could deliver these mediators to the periarticular bone, accelerating the loss of bone seen around inflamed joints relatively early in the disease. It is important to emphasize, however, that bone loss in rheumatoid arthritis can be generalized, affecting the entire skeleton, as well as occurring in a periarticular distribution.[35]

Supporting this are data from common laboratory tests. Rheumatoid patients who have never had glucocorticoid treatment differ from nonrheumatoid patients in having higher serum phosphorus, alkaline phosphatase, and osteocalcin, with normal measured concentrations of parathyroid hormone and calcitonin. Urinary excretion of hydroxyproline (an index of collagen breakdown) and proteoglycans is increased.[36] Taken together, these data indicate a generalized increased bone turnover in rheumatoid arthritis.

Studies of twins are the best for control of genetic factors in comparison of one variable to another. Accordingly, attention must be paid to studies of BMD, measured by dual-energy x-ray absorptiometry, in a monozygotic co-twin control study. None of the individuals studied was being treated with glucocorticoids. BMD was reduced at most skeletal sites in the twin with rheumatoid arthritis compared with the co-twin, and there were associated differences in lean soft tissue (i.e., muscle) at multiple sites.[37] These are important data, and support the thesis that reduced bone mass in rheumatoid arthritis may be secondary to loss of mobility or muscle mass associated with the disease, as well as to prostaglandins and inflammatory cytokines.

Prednisone, Bone Mineral Density, and Fractures

There is no doubt that factors other than prednisone use in rheumatoid patients put them at risk for fracture.[36,38] These include

- Postmenopausal state
- Previous diagnosis of osteoporosis
- Disability
- Age
- Lack of physical activity
- Female sex
- Family history of osteoporosis
- Disease duration
- Impaired grip strength
- Low body mass
- Fair complexion
- Cigarette smoking

Nevertheless, glucocorticoids do produce osteopenia in rheumatoid patients, and they damage trabecular bone more than cortical bone.

Several mechanisms appear to be operating. They include

1. Depressed osteoblast function
2. Decreased calcium absorption
3. Accelerated bone resorption, possibly secondary to a small amount of hyperparathyroidism.

Using serum osteocalcin as an index of bone formation and urinary collagen type I cross-links as a measure of bone resorption, it has been shown that in chronic rheumatoid arthritis bone formation and resorption become uncoupled; bone formation is reduced. In patients given prednisone, resorption increases as well, widening the gap between formation and resorption.[39]

In patients with rheumatoid arthritis, a previous diagnosis of osteoporosis and disability are more significantly associated than are other parameters with fracture. Patients with a higher disability index are more likely to be on prednisone, and this fact tends to confound data linking prednisone therapy to fractures.

One of the most puzzling pieces of data on fractures and rheumatoid arthritis is the study that showed increased fractures in patients treated with glucocorticoids, but no decrease in the bone mineral content of bone compared with nontreated rheumatoid arthritis patients, suggesting that corticosteroids might alter the quality and structure, rather than composition of bone in rheumatoid arthritis.[40,41] The percentage of patients who sustained vertebral or femoral neck fractures from minimal trauma was 16 per cent in the glucocorticoid group (mean prednisone dose, 8.9 mg/day for almost 5 years) and only 3.6 per cent in the untreated rheumatoid arthritis group. Similar results were recorded in an Australian study[42] of patients treated for up to 2 years with a mean dose of 6.6 mg/ prednisone per day. No increased loss of bone mineral density was found compared with untreated rheumatoid patients.

An interesting and important variation on these studies was one performed to determine the effects of a short course of glucocorticoids on bone mass.[43] BMD decreased abruptly in the treated patients but, more unusual, returned to almost normal levels in the 20 weeks following prednisone therapy (Fig. 30–3). If confirmed in independent studies, two main interpretations of these data are apparent:

- Loss of bone related to glucocorticoid therapy in postmenopausal women over the age of 50 begins

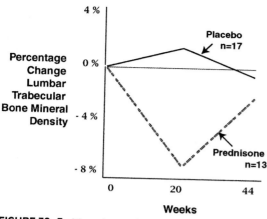

FIGURE 30–3. Mean changes in lumbar trabecular BMD during and after low-dose prednisone treatment in a subset of patients who did not use prednisone between weeks 20 and 44. The change (mean ± SE) in BMD was measured using dual-energy, quantitative CT. The prednisone dose was 10 mg/day from week 0 to week 12 and was tapered between weeks 12 and 20. (Modified from Laan, R. F. J. M., van Riel, P. L. C. M., van de Putte, L. B. A., et al.: Low-dose prednisone induces rapid reversible axial bone loss in patients with rheumatoid arthritis: a randomized, controlled study. Ann. Intern. Med. 119: 963, 1993. Used by permission.)

very soon after small doses are started. If a preventive strategy (e.g., vitamin D or calcitriol, calcium, biphosphonates) is going to be used, it should be initiated along with the prednisone.

- Contrary to general impressions, glucocorticoid-associated decreases in BMD can be partially reversed if the drug is stopped in relatively short time frame.

Observation of men with rheumatoid arthritis who have been treated with glucocorticoids removes the confounding variable of estrogens or the lack of them. One study has used dual-energy x-ray absorptiometry, believed to be more precise than dual-photon absorptiometry, in study of 20 men with rheumatoid arthritis who were receiving low-dose oral prednisolone (<10 mg/day), compared with 20 men with rheumatoid arthritis not treated with steroids and 20 healthy control men. Although prednisolone was genuinely associated with axial osteopenia (in anterior-posterior scans but not lateral scans) in rheumatoid men receiving glucocorticoids, rheumatoid men, on steroids or not, are were at risk for bone loss in the femoral heads.[44]

High-dose glucocorticoid pulse therapy in patients with rheumatoid arthritis has transient effects on bone metabolism. In a study of 17 patients treated with three doses of dexamethasone (200 mg, intravenously) over 8 days, bone formation (esti-

mated by tests on blood and urine, see Chapter 23), decreased slightly for a few days, whereas markers of bone resorption were unchanged.[45] A similar study, using serum osteocalcin as a measure of bone formation rate and urinary pyridinoline as a measure of bone resorption in patients given intra-articular administration of triamcinolone hexacetonide, also showed no net effect on bone resorption and only a transient effect on bone formation.[46]

Preservation of Bone in Glucocorticoid-Treated Patients

What are the options for preserving bone in patients being treated with glucocorticoids? In the postmenopausal woman, **estrogens** should be used whenever possible. (The mechanisms underlying osteopenia in estrogen deficiency are discussed in the Chapter 8 under IL-6.) Transdermal hormone replacement therapy has been well tolerated in rheumatoid patients, with increased well-being and increased lumbar spine bone density over a 1-year period in postmenopausal women with rheumatoid arthritis, matching findings in women without the disease.[47] It reduces the rate of bone resorption in postmenopausal rheumatoid women, whether or not they are taking steroids.[39] Hormone replacement therapy in postmenopausal women with rheumatoid arthritis who are taking low doses (mean daily dose, 6.9 mg prednisolone) of corticosteroids, preserved bone mass as well as in those not taking glucocorticoids.[48]

When estrogen is inappropriate, the antiresorptive **diphosphonates** can produce modest increases in bone mass that level off after a few years, and are appropriate adjuncts in patients in whom the risk and danger of developing more osteopenia is high. These compounds are inhibitors of bone resorption. Intermittent **etidronate** therapy given for 6 months to postmenopausal women receiving prednisone for temporal arteritis prevented vertebral bone loss.[49]

The aminobisphosphonate **alendronate** is a 100- to 500-fold more potent inhibitor of bone resorption than is etidronate and appears not to have detrimental effects upon mineralization. The presence of a nitrogen molecule in the secondary structure increases the antiresorptive potency. In a study of doses of 5 and 10 mg given daily for 2 years to postmenopausal osteoporotic women, alendronate reduced markers of bone remodeling and significantly increased BMD in the spine, hip, and total body.[50] Mild upper gastrointestinal intolerance led to cessation of therapy in 7 of 94 treated patients. No new vertebral fractures in either the treated or

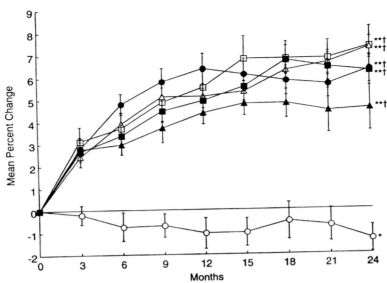

FIGURE 30–4. Mean (± SE) changes in BMD of the spine in postmenopausal women, as measured by dual-energy x-ray absorptiometry, in placebo (○), 5-mg (□), 10-mg (△), 20-mg/placebo (●), 40-mg/placebo (■), and 40-mg/2.5-mg (▲) alendronate treatment groups. *p <.05, **p < .01, both compared to baseline; †p < .001, alendronate-treated groups versus placebo. (From Chesnut, C. H. III, McClung, M. R., Ensrud, K. E., et al.: Alendronate treatment of the postmenopausal osteoporotic woman: effects of multiple dosages on bone mass and remodeling. Am. J. Med. 99: 144, 1995. Used by permission. Copyright 1995 by Excerpta Medica Inc.)

placebo group were noted (Fig. 30–4). A 3-year controlled study has confirmed the benefit of aledronate and has added the information that 10 mg/day is the optimal dose for cost and benefit.[51]

A similar molecule, **pamidronate**, has been used in 3-year randomized, double-blind trial of 300 mg/day compared with placebo in 105 patients with rheumatoid arthritis.[52] No patients taking glucocorticoids were included. The findings support the conclusion that pamidronate effectively prevents bone loss in the appendicular skeleton and increases bone mass in the axial skeleton. The mechanism for this beneficial effect, measured by urinary hydroxyproline, appeared to be a decrease in the rate of bone resorption, as expected. Yet another study is indicated to address the question: Can nitrogen-containing bisphosphonates halt loss of axial and appendicular bone in patients with rheumatoid arthritis on low-dose prednisone?

In a study of 103 patients starting long-term glucocorticoid therapy, it was found that **calcitriol** (1,25-dihydroxycalciferol, 0.6 μg/day) and 1,000 mg/day of **calcium**, with or without **calcitonin** (400 I.U./day) prevented more bone loss from the lumbar spine than did calcium alone.[53] To counter the benefit, however, a small but significant hypercalcemia developed in 25 per cent of the patients receiving calcitriol.

The complications of administering **sodium flu-**

oride in treatment or prevention of osteoporosis have been frequent and sometimes serious, including gastric bleeding and microfractures. A fluoride ion replaces a hydroxyl ion in the calcium hydroxyapatite crystal, and although this produces a substantial increase in bone mass, earlier studies reported no significant decrease in fracture rate in patients.[54] However, by use of a slow-release preparation of sodium fluoride given in 12-months cycles (2 months off) with continuous calcium citrate supplementation, compared with calcium citrate alone, new fractures were inhibited over a 2.5-year period, the mean spinal bone mass increased without loss of cortical bone, and there were no significant side effects.[55]

Although administering **human growth hormone** concomitant with prednisone prevents its protein catabolic effects,[56] it will not be cost-effective or practical to use this combination in the great majority of rheumatoid patients.

An alternative to prednisone in treatment of rheumatoid arthritis may be **deflazacort**, an oxazoline derivative of prednisone that has less suppression of intestinal absorption of calcium than does prednisone and induces less hypercalciuria.[57] It has been used with efficacy in treatment of polymyalgia rheumatica,[58] although one study indicated no calcium-sparing properties compared with prednisolone.[59] One study from Argentina has data to support use of deflazacort as a valid alternative to prednisone in rheumatoid arthritis.[60] Another series from Italy[61] had similar results: Postmenopausal patients with rheumatoid arthritis treated with low-dose prednisone (<10 mg/day) developed reduced levels of sex hormones and osteocalcin and reduced vertebral bone mass. Comparable doses of deflazacort showed only a mild inhibitory effect on sex hormones and osteocalcin, and did not show any detectable change in BMD.

Prevention of Bone Loss: The Appropriate Goal in Patients With Rheumatoid Arthritis Treated with Prednisone

Once the decision is made to use prednisone, even in small daily doses, a concomitant effort must be made to prevent osteoporosis and fractures. The reason is clear: Bone loss from glucocorticoids is greater in the first month or year of therapy than in subsequent periods. The following may be useful guidelines:

- Because prednisone-induced bone loss can be reversible if the drug is stopped within a 20-week period, a therapeutic plan should be in place that programs replacement of prednisone with onset of action of a second-line drug or more targeted and specific therapy.
- Menopausal or postmenopausal women all should be on estrogen replacement therapy, with or without progestins, unless there is a strong contraindication.
- The most cost-effective preventive therapy is a form of vitamin D and supplemental calcium. This should be given to women in addition to estrogen replacement, and to all men. Cost and availability will determine the best vitamin D formulation: 0.5 to 1.0 μg calcitriol/day plus 1.0 g of elemental calcium as the citrate, lactate, gluconate, or carbonate salt may be better than vitamin D_3 (50,000 I.U./week) and calcium, but is more expensive. Serum calcium levels greater than 11.0 mg/dl should be avoided.
- In patients with existing osteoporosis and compression fractures in whom prednisone is deemed unavoidable, it may be cost-effective to use one of the following adjuncts according to protocols described in the papers referenced in the text:
  - salmon calcitonin, intranasally
  - cyclic etidronate or daily alendronate
  - slow-release sodium fluoride

SUMMARY

There are good data to indicate that, for a short period (up to 2 years), supplemental low-dose prednisone can work additively with other antirheumatic drugs and help retard destruction of joints. This benefit is balanced by the long-term effect of bone loss. Patients given even low-dose prednisone ($\leq$ 7.5 mg/day) should be given bone-building therapy. The Task Force on Osteoporosis Guidelines of the American College of Rheumatology have published recommendations for prevention and treatment of glucocorticoid-induced osteoporosis.[62]

REFERENCES

1. Hench, P. S., Kendall, E. C., Slocomb, C. H., et al.: Effect of a hormone of the adrenal cortex (17 hydroxy-11 dehydrocorticosterone, compound E) and of pituitary adrenocortico-tropic hormone on rheumatoid arthritis: preliminary report. Proc. Staff Meet. Mayo Clinic 24:181, 1949.
2. George, E., and Kirwan, J. R.: Corticosteroid therapy in rheumatoid arthritis. Baillières Clin. Rheumatol. 4:621, 1990.
3. Neeck, G., Federlin, K., Graef, V., et al.: Adrenal secretion of cortisol in patients with rheumatoid arthritis. J. Rheumatol. 17:24, 1990.
4. Sternberg, E. M., Hill, J. M., Chrousos, G. P. et al.: Inflammatory mediator-induced hypothalamic-pituitary-adrenal axis activation is defective in streptococcal cell wall arthritis-susceptible Lewis rats. Proc. Natl. Acad. Sci. U.S.A. 86:2374, 1989.
5. Sternberg, E. M., Young, W. S., III, Bernardini, R., et al.: A central nervous system defect in biosynthesis of corticotropin-releasing hormone is associated with susceptibility to streptococcal cell wall-induced arthritis in Lewis rats. Proc. Natl. Acad. Sci. U.S.A. 86:4771, 1989.
6. Schlaghecke, R., Kornely, E., Wollenhaupt, J., et al.: Glucocorticoid receptors in rheumatoid arthritis. Arthritis Rheum. 35:740, 1992.
7. Schaghecke, R., Beuscher, D., Kornely, E., et al.: Effects of glucocorticoids in rheumatoid arthritis. Arthritis Rheum. 37:1127, 1994.
8. Cash, J. M., Crofford, L. J., Gallucci, W. T., et al.: Pituitary-adrenal axis responsiveness to ovine corticotropin releasing hormone in patients with rheumatoid arthritis treated with low dose prednisone. J. Rheumatol. 19:1692, 1992.
9. Kirkham, B. W., Corkill, M. M., Davidson, S. C., et al.: Response to glucocorticoid treatment in rheumatoid arthritis: In vitro cell mediated immune assay predicts in vivo responses. J. Rheumatol. 18:821, 1991.
10. Boumpas, D. T., Chrousos, G. P., Wilder, R. L., et al.: Glucocorticoid therapy for immune-mediated diseases: basic and clinical correlates. Ann. Intern. Med. 119:1198, 1993.
11. Scheinman, R. I., Cogswell, P. C., Lofquist, A. K., et al.: Role of transcriptional activation of $I\kappa B\alpha$ in mediation of immunosuppression by glucocorticoids. Science 270: 283, 1995.
12. Auphan, N., Di Donato, J. A., and Rosette, C.: Immunosuppression by glucocorticoids: inhibition of NF-κB activity through induction of $I\kappa$B synthesis. Science 270:286, 1995.
13. Cronstein, B. N., Kimmel, S. C., Levin, R. I., et al.: A

mechanism for the antiinflammatory effects of corticosteroids: the glucocorticoid receptor regulates leukocyte adhesion to endothelial cells and expression of endothelial-leukocyte adhesion molecule 1 and intercellular adhesion molecule 1. Proc. Natl. Acad. Sci. U.S.A. 89:9991, 1992.

14. Criswell, L. A., and Redfearn, W. J.: Variation among rheumatologists in the use of prednisone and second-line agents for the treatment of rheumatoid arthritis. Arthritis Rheum. 37:476, 1994.

15. McDougall, R., Sibley, J., Haga, M., et al.: Outcome in patients with rheumatoid arthritis receiving prednisone compared to matched controls. J. Rheumatol. 21:1207, 1994.

16. Harris, E. D. Jr., Emkey, R. D., and Nichols J. E.: Low dose prednisone therapy in rheumatoid arthritis: a double blind study. J. Rheumatol. 10:713, 1983.

17. Myles, A. B., Schiller, L. F. G., Glass, D., et al.: Single daily dose corticosteroid treatment. Ann. Rheum. Dis. 35:73, 1976.

18. Kirwan, J. R.: The effect of glucocorticoids on joint destruction in rheumatoid arthritis: the Arthritis and Rheumatism Council Low-Dose Glucocorticoid Study Group. N. Engl. J. Med. 333:142, 1995.

19. van Schaardenburg, D., Valkema, R., Dijkmans, B. A. C., et al.: Prednisone treatment of elderly-onset rheumatoid arthritis. Arthritis Rheum. 38:334, 1995.

20. Iglehart, I. W. III, Sutton, J. D., Bender, J. C., et al.: Intravenous pulsed steroids in rheumatoid arthritis: a comparative dose study. J. Rheumatol. 17:159, 1990.

21. Wong, C. S., Champion G., Smith, M. D., et al.: Does steroid pulsing influence the efficacy and toxicity of chrysotherapy? A double blind, placebo controlled study. Ann. Rheum. Dis. 49:370, 1990.

22. McCarthy, G. M., and McCarty, D. J.: Intrasynovial corticosteroid therapy. Bull. Rheum. Dis. 43:2, 1994.

This paper focuses on the use of triamcinolone hexacetonide as the least soluble crystal preparation that exhibits the longest duration of action and least systemic absorption. Good technique is essential, because injection outside the synovium or tendon sheath does no good and injection into tendons can cause atrophy and rupture. It is recommended to combine injection with prolonged (3 to 6 weeks) rest with once-daily full range of motion exercises.

23. McCarty, D. J., Harman, J. G., Grassanovich, J. L., et al.: Treatment of rheumatoid joint inflammation with triamcinolone hexacetonide. J. Rheumatol. 22:1631, 1995.

24. Malch, H. W., Gibson, J. M. C., and El-Ghobaref, A. F.: Repeated corticosteroid injections into knee joints. Rheumatol. Rehabil. 16:137, 1977.

25. Luukkainen, R., Hakala, M., Sajanti, E., et al.: Predictive value of synovial fluid analysis in estimating the efficacy of intra-articular corticosteroid injections in patients with rheumatoid arthritis. Ann. Rheum. Dis. 51:874, 1992.

26. Conn, H. O., and Poynard, T.: Corticosteroids and peptic ulcer: meta-analysis of adverse events during steroid therapy. J. Intern. Med. 236:619, 1994.

27. Carson, J. L., Strom, B. L., Schinnar, R., et al.: The low risk of upper gastrointestinal bleeding in patients dispensed corticosteroids. Am. J. Med. 91:223, 1991.

28. Piper, J. M., Ray, W. A., Daugherty, J. R., et al.: Corticosteroid use and peptic ulcer disease: role of nonsteroidal antiinflammatory drugs. Ann. Intern. Med. 114:735, 1991.

29. Wamuo, I. A., and Pitt, P. I.: The diagnostic challenge of acute polyarthritis. Ann. Rheum. Dis. 55:284, 1996.

30. Saag, K. G., Koehnke, R., Caldwell, J. R., et al.: Low dose long-term corticosteroid therapy in rheumatoid arthritis: an analysis of serious adverse events. Am. J. Med. 96:115, 1994.

31. Laan, R. F. J. M., Buijs, W. C. A. M., Verbeek, A. L. M., et al.: Bone mineral density in patients with recent onset rheumatoid arthritis: influence of disease activity and functional capacity. Ann. Rheum. Dis. 52:21, 1993.

32. Compston, J. E., Vedi, S., Croucher, P. I., et al.: Bone turnover in non-steroid treated rheumatoid arthritis. Ann. Rheum. Dis. 53:163, 1994.

33. Kroger, H., Honkanen, R., Saarikoski, S., et al.: Decreased axial bone mineral density in perimenopausal women with rheumatoid arthritis—a population based study. Ann. Rheum. Dis. 53:18, 1994.

34. Sambrook, P. N., Shawe, D., Hesp, R., et al.: Rapid periarticular bone loss in rheumatoid arthritis: possible promotion by normal circulating concentrations of parathyroid hormone or calcitriol (1,25-dihydroxyvitamin D_3). Arthritis Rheum. 33:615, 1990.

In this study of wrist joints in rheumatoid arthritis of disease duration ranging from 2 to 31 months, there were 17 rheumatoid patients and 14 age-matched controls (all were women; 12 in each group were postmenopausal). In the 2 to 3 years of observation, there was a 6.1 per cent rate of trabecular bone loss in the rheumatoid patients compared with 0.9 per cent in the control patients, but none in the radial midshaft or in the L2–L4 vertebrae. Joint scores, ESR, and radiographic joint analyses did not correlate with the radial head bone loss, but the plasma concentrations of calcitriol and immunoreactive parathyroid hormone did.

35. Kennedy, A. C., and Lindsay, R.: Bone involvement in rheumatoid arthritis. Clin. Rheum. Dis. 3:403, 1977.

36. Dequeker, J., and Geusens, P.: Osteoporosis and arthritis. Ann. Rheum. Dis. 49:276, 1990.

37. Sambrook, P. N., Spector, T. D., Seeman, E., et al.: Osteoporosis in rheumatoid arthritis: a monozygotic co-twin control study. Arthritis Rheum. 38:806, 1995.

38. Michel, B. A., Bloch, D. A., Wolfe, F., et al.: Fractures in rheumatoid arthritis: an evaluation of associated risk factors. J. Rheumatol. 20:1666, 1993.

In addition to a review of risk factors in rheumatoid arthritis for fracture, this paper, studying 879 women and 231 men with rheumatoid arthritis, lists the fracture sites and incidence in these patients, as shown in Table 30–5 (see text). It is interesting that foot and ankle fractures were second to spinal compression fractures; this addresses the importance of suitable footwear in these patients.

39. Hall, G. M., Spector, T. D., and Delmas, P. D.: Markers of bone metabolism in postmenopausal women with rheumatoid arthritis: effects of corticosteroids and hormone replacement therapy. Arthritis Rheum. 38:902, 1995.

40. Verstraeten, A., and Dequeker, J.: Vertebral and peripheral bone mineral content and fracture incidence in postmenopausal patients with rheumatoid arthritis: effect of low dose corticosteroids. Ann. Rheum. Dis. 45:852, 1986.

41. Peel, N. F. A., Moore, D. J., Barrington, N. A., et al.: Risk of vertebral fracture and relationship to bone mineral density in steroid treated rheumatoid arthritis. Ann. Rheum. Dis. 54:801, 1995.

42. Sambrook, P. N., Cohen, M. L., Eisman, J. A., et al.: Effects of low dose corticosteroids on bone mass in rheumatoid arthritis: a longitudinal study. Ann. Rheum. Dis. 48:535, 1989.

43. Laan, R. F. J. M., van Riel, P. L. C. M., van de Putte, L. B. A., et al.: Low-dose prednisone induces rapid reversible axial bone loss in patients with rheumatoid arthritis:

a randomized, controlled study. Ann. Intern. Med. 119: 963, 1993.

In this study, 40 patients with active rheumatoid arthritis being put on intramuscular gold therapy were randomly assigned to receive, in addition, either placebo or prednisone (10 mg/day tapered to zero after 20 weeks, giving a mean dose of 7.5 mg/day). The mean age of the patients was 54 years, and there were 28 women and 12 men. BMD was measured in the lumbar spine by dual-energy, quantitative CT during the 20-week period and up to 44 weeks. The bone density data are graphed in Figure 30–3 (see text). This 8 per cent decrease in BMD after 20 weeks was remarkable, and equally remarkable was the restoration of skeleton after the therapy was stopped. During the 20-week period the cumulative disease activity improved significantly in the prednisone group, but no mention is made of whether recrudescence occurred after the prednisone was stopped.

44. Garton, M. J., and Reid, D. M.: Bone mineral density of the hip and of the anteroposterior and lateral dimensions of the spine in men with rheumatoid arthritis: effects of low-dose corticosteroids. Arthritis Rheum. 36:222, 1993.
45. Lems, W. F., Gerrits, M. I., Jacobs, J. W. G., et al.: Changes in (markers of) bone metabolism during high dose corticosteroid pulse treatment in patients with rheumatoid arthritis. Ann. Rheum. Dis. 55:288, 1996.
46. Emkey, R. D., Lindsay, R., Lyssy, J., et al.: The systemic effect of intraarticular administration of corticosteroid on markers of bone formation and bone resorption in patients with rheumatoid arthritis. Arthritis Rheum. 39:277, 1996.
47. MacDonald, A. G., Murphy, E. A., Capell, H. A., et al.: Effects of hormone replacement therapy in rheumatoid arthritis: a double blind placebo-controlled study. Ann. Rheum. Dis. 53:54, 1994.
48. Hall, G. M., Daniels, M., Doyl, D. V., et al.: Effect of hormone replacement therapy on bone mass in rheumatoid arthritis patients treated with and without steroids. Arthritis Rheum. 37:1499, 1994.
49. Mulder, H., and Shelder, H. A. A.: Effect of cyclical etidronate regimen on prophylaxis of bone loss of glucocorticoid therapy in postmenopausal women. Bone Mineral Res. 17(Suppl 1):168, 1992.
50. Chesnut, C. H. III, McClung, M. R., Ensrud, K. E., et al.: Alendronate treatment of the postmenopausal osteoporotic woman: effect of multiple dosages on bone mass and remodeling. Am. J. Med. 99:144, 1995.
51. Liberman, U. A., Weiss, S. R., Bröll, J., et al.: Effect of oral alendronate on bone mineral density and the incidence of fractures in postmenopausal osteoporosis. N. Engl. J. Med. 333:1437, 1995.
52. Eggelmeijer, F., Papapoulos, S. E., van Paassen, H. C., et al.: Increased bone mass with pamidronate treatment in rheumatoid arthritis: results of a three-year randomized, double-blind trial. Arthritis Rheum. 39:396, 1996.
53. Sambrook, P., Birmingham, J., Kelly, P., et al.: Prevention of corticosteroid osteoporosis: a comparison of calcium, calcitriol, and calcitonin. N. Engl. J. Med. 328:1747, 1993.
54. Riggs, B. L., Hodgson, S. F., O'Fallon, M. W., et al.: Effect of fluoride treatment on the fracture rate in postmenopausal women with osteoporosis. N. Engl. J. Med. 322:802, 1990.
55. Pak, C. Y. C., Sakhaee, K., Piziak, V., et al.: Slow-release sodium fluoride in the management of postmenopausal osteoporosis: a randomized controlled trial. Ann. Intern. Med. 120:625, 1994.
56. Horber, F. F., and Haymond, M. W.: Human growth hormone prevents the protein catabolic side effects of prednisone in humans. J. Clin. Invest. 86:265, 1990.
57. Gennari, C., Imbimbo, B., and Montagniani, M.: Effect of prednisone and deflazacort on mineral metabolism and parathyroid hormone activity in humans. Calcif. Tissue Int. 36:245, 1984.
58. Cimmino, M. A., Moggiana, G., Montecucco, C., et al.: Long term treatment of polymyalgia rheumatica with deflazacort. Ann. Rheum. Dis. 53:331, 1994.
59. Krogsgaard, M. R., Thamsborg, G., and Lund, B.: Changes in bone mass during low dose corticosteroid treatment in patients with polymyalgia rheumatica: a double blind, prospective comparison between prednisolone and deflazacort. Ann. Rheum. Dis. 55:143, 1996.
60. Messina, O. D., Barreira, J. C., Zanchetta, J. R., et al.: Effect of low doses of deflazacort vs. prednisone on bone mineral content in premenopausal rheumatoid arthritis. J. Rheumatol. 19:1520, 1992.
61. Montecucco, C., Caporali, R., Caprotti, P., et al.: Sex hormones and bone metabolism in postmenopausal rheumatoid arthritis treated with two different glucocorticoids. J. Rheumatol. 19:1895, 1992.
62. American College of Rheumatology Task Force on Osteoporosis Guidelines. Recommendations for the prevention and treatment of glucocorticoid-induced osteoporosis. Arthritis Rheum. 39:1791, 1996.

These useful guidelines outline a comprehensive evaluation of a patient taking glucocorticoids who has a nontraumatic fracture. These guidelines include strong reliance on dual-energy x-ray absorptiometry to stratify the mineralization status of patients' bones. Since bone is lost most rapidly during the first 6 months of steroid use, a program for each patient who is beginning glucocorticoids for the first time is included.

31

Second-Line Treatment

The drugs used after it has become apparent that a rheumatoid patient's arthritis has become established and is not responding adequately to NSAIDs are most reasonably named "second-line drugs." Other names for this class of-drugs presume too much, particularly the phrase, "disease-modifying drugs." Most are relatively "slow-acting" (another term used extensively), but this characteristic may have little to do with mechanisms of action, rather reflecting the relatively low intensity or power of their actions on synovitis. Each has another characteristic: Their use in rheumatoid arthritis was not initiated by a prospective design based on a logical coalescence of the drug's actions and the pathophysiology of rheumatoid arthritis, but rather is founded on empirical, historical, and often serendipitous evidence that the compounds were effective. **Most important is that each of the standard and accepted second-line drugs can be effective, and any new therapies accepted for rheumatoid arthritis should clearly be demonstrated to be equally efficacious and less toxic than either intramuscular gold, D-penicillamine, hydroxychloroquine, or sulfasalazine.**[1] (Methotrexate, the drug currently used more than others as an initial second-line therapy, is considered in Chapter 32).

Just as both physician and patient must weigh carefully the potential risks of second-line drug therapy in rheumatoid arthritis, the expectations of the therapy must be to produce a significant improvement in signs and symptoms. (Table 31–1).[2] It is especially at this time that utility measures for patients to assess risk for their own particular approaches to life and lifestyles must be made a crucial part of the decision-making process.

Long-term studies have shown that, in a subset of patients, the second-line drugs are effective. In a group of 190 patients who had been on one of three second-line drugs (gold, D-penicillamine, or sulfasalazine) for 5 years, function improved; after this period they were still taking one of the drugs, and were still better off than before treatment was started.[3] The problem is that this subset only represented 30 per cent of those who began these clinical trials; inefficacy or toxicity led to stopping therapy in 70 per cent.

Using data on 2,888 patients followed in the AR-AMIS data bank from eight centers for up to 20 years, the question of whether a change in progression toward disability was obtained by using second-line drugs was addressed.[4] The data showed that increased second-line drug use was strongly associated with a better long-term disability index, and this association was strengthened when restricted to patients with more active disease at onset. Conservatively, there was at least a 30 per cent reduction in long-term disability with consistent second-line drug use. It is interesting that the use of prednisone had no correlation with outcome.

When planning a therapeutic regimen for a patient with rheumatoid arthritis, the physician—consciously or unconsciously—constructs a benefit-cost ratio for each scenario. The "cost" component of the ratio is composed of the potential toxicity, the dollar costs of the medication, and the dollar costs of monitoring for potential toxicity. In a careful audit of prices and practices, the dollar amounts for these three components for second-line drugs given for 6 months were determined[5] (Table 31–2). It will be appropriate for models such as these to be used in the development of practice guidelines to help define the most cost-effective way of providing care.

Perhaps the greatest differences among the second-line drugs are the patterns of toxicity. In a study of 2,479 patients from five centers in the ARAMIS system, the toxicity profile for each was different from the others[6] (Table 31–3). Of particular interest are the following findings[6]:

- Oral gold (auranofin) produced substantially more gastrointestinal toxicity (i.e., 399 diarrhea "events"/1,000 patient years).

- Methotrexate generated hepatotoxicity and mucosal ulcers (see Chapter 32), but it had the lowest discontinuation rate in the first 6 months.

- D-Penicillamine altered taste.

- Skin rash was seen with gold and D-penicillamine.

TABLE 31–1. Use of Disease-Modifying Antirheumatic Drugs for Rheumatoid Arthritis

Goal
  Remission or optimal control of inflammatory joint disease
Limitations
  May not prevent damage in spite of apparent clinical control
  May not have lasting efficacy
  May not be tolerated due to toxicity
Factors for selecting drugs
  Convenience and cost of medication and monitoring for toxicity
  Risk of adverse reactions, including frequency and seriousness
  Physician estimate of efficacy and disease prognosis
Monitoring efficacy
  Is disease in remission or optimally controlled?
Monitoring toxicity

From American College of Rheumatology Ad Hoc Committee on Clinical Guidelines: Guidelines for the management of rheumatoid arthritis. Arthritis Rheum. 39:713, 1996. Used by permission.

TABLE 31–2. Costs of Second-Line Drug Treatment

MEDICATION	COST/PATIENT/6 MONTHS*
Hydroxychloroquine	$939
Oral gold	$927
Azathioprine	$1,351
D-Penicillamine	$1,101
Methotrexate	$1,152
Injectable gold	$1,768

Data from Prashker and Meenan (1995).[5]
* In 1995 dollars.

Despite the recognized toxicities of these second-line drugs, it should be emphasized that NSAIDs are toxic as well. In one review[7] that applied a toxicity index to both classes of drugs (Table 31–4), a clear overlap among toxicities was found, indicating that there is a sound rationale for early use of second-line drugs in this disease.

These drugs can be used individually (Table 31–5) or in combination (the ''combination therapy'' approach is discussed in depth in Chapter 34). It is a sound approach to use the least toxic drug first, moving to more potent but complicated compounds if the more easily tolerated one or two fail, or else adding another second-line drug. Following this logic, hydroxychloroquine can be initiated first and relatively early in the course of disease, followed by methotrexate. Some rheumatologists will use gold salts rather than methotrexate, especially in patients with any form of liver disease or dependence upon alcohol. Enthusiasm for D-penicillamine is waning because of the complex toxicity of this drug, although it still has a role in special circumstances in rheumatoid arthritis. The place for sulfasalazine is still being defined. Some use it early, others find it toxic in rheumatoid patients, and it remains not yet approved for specific use in patients with rheumatoid arthritis by the FDA.

The question about whether second-line drugs should be started earlier or later in rheumatoid arthritis seems to be increasingly answered ''earlier.'' In an open but randomized clinical trial of 238 consecutive patients with recently diagnosed rheuma-

TABLE 31–3. Side Effect Ranks (Events/1,000 Patient Years)*

RANK	OH-CHLORO	IM GOLD	ORAL GOLD	D-PEN	AZA	MTX	CYCLO-
1	Rash (22)	Rash (115)	Diarrhea (391)	Rash (61)	Nausea (96)	Nausea (93)	Alopecia (180)
2	Nausea (21)	Mucosal ulcers (55)	Loose bowel movement (148)	Altered taste (40)	Vomiting (55)	Mucosal Ulcers (87)	Nausea (116)
3	Upper Abd pain (18)	Pruritus (51)	Nausea (117)	Mucosal ulcers (38)	Diarrhea (40)	Liver Abn (41)	Menstrual Abn (69)
4	Diarrhea (17)	Purpura (10)	Rash (100)	Nausea (35)	Mucosal ulcers (35)	Alopecia (37)	Diarrhea (59)
5	Blurred vision (17)	Diarrhea (10)	Upper Abd pain (98)	Pruritus (26)	Rash (30)	Rash (28)	Urticaria (58)
6	Photosensitivity (11)	Alopecia (9)	Lower Abd pain (76)	Low platelets (18)	Headache (20)	Upper Abd pain (27)	Dysuria (58)
7	Headache (10)	Nausea (7)	Mucosal ulcers (76)	Anorexia (18)	Low WBC (20)	Lower Abd pain (19)	Low WBC (30)
8	Alopecia (9)	Urticaria (7)	Flatulence (45)	Upper Abd pain (17)	Alopecia (15)	Increased infections (17)	Increased infections (20)
9	Pruritus (8)	Low Platelets (6)	Anorexia (40)	Alopecia (12)	Anorexia (15)	Diarrhea (16)	Dry Mouth (8)
10	Mucosal ulcers (8)	Low WBC (5)	Pruritus (31)	Pancytopenia (10)	Upper Abd pain (15)	Vertigo (16)	

From Singh, G., Fries, J. F., Williams, C. A., et al.: Toxicity profiles of disease modifying antirheumatic drugs in rheumatoid arthritis. J. Rheumatol. 18:188, 1991. Used by permission.
* Abbreviations: OH-CHLORO, hydroxychloroquine; IM Gold, intramuscular gold; D-PEN, D-penicillamine; AZA, azathioprine; MTX, methotrexate; CYCLO, cyclo-oxygenase; Abd, abdominal; Abn, abnormalities; WBC, white blood cell count.

TABLE 31–4. Relative Toxicity of DMARDs*: Data From Five ARAMIS Data Bank Centers (Standardized Toxicity Index Scores)

DRUG	NO. OF COURSES	MEAN	STANDARD ERROR	RANK
Hydroxychloroquine	639	1.38	0.15	1
Intramuscular gold	659	2.27	0.17	2
D-Penicillamine	496	3.38	0.36	3
Methotrexate	660	3.82	0.35	4
Azathioprine	190	3.92	0.39	5
Auranofin	409	5.25	0.32	6

From Fries, J. F., Williams, C. A., Ramey, D. R., et al.: The relative toxicity of alternative therapies for rheumatoid arthritis: implications for the therapeutic progression. Semin. Arthritis Rheum. 23 (2, Suppl. 1):68, 1993. Used by permission.
* DMARDs, disease-modifying antirheumatic drug.

toid arthritis,[8] patients received NSAIDs plus one of three second-line drugs (hydroxychloroquine, 400 mg/day; intramuscular gold, 50 mg/week; or pulse methotrexate, 7.5 to 15 mg/week), whereas the control group started with NSAIDs alone. Assessment was done every 3 months for a minimum of 12 months. Statistically significant advantages for the group started earlier on slow-acting drugs were found for disability, pain, joint score, and ESR, but they experienced more side effects (although none serious). Unfortunately, radiographic damage increased similarly (although minimally) in both groups; it was hoped that, by starting the more aggressive treatment early, radiographic change could be slowed. A very high number (92 per cent) of patients were receiving their initial therapy after 1 year, an impressive "drug survival rate."

Before discussing the individual drugs, it is appropriate to emphasize that virtually none of these drugs is known to be safe for use in pregnancy or lactation. During pregnancy, glucocorticoids are least likely to do harm to the fetus or mother (Table 31–6).[9]

ANTIMALARIAL DRUGS

Antimalarial drugs have been used for decades in rheumatoid arthritis. In one enthusiastic early report in 1960, 80 per cent of 107 patients who completed 1 year of chloroquine treatment had a definite "general improvement."[10] However, studies that linked an irreversible retinopathy with chloroquine therapy precipitated a distinct decline in use of these drugs in rheumatoid arthritis.[11] Recent dosage schedules that do not exceed 400 mg of hydroxychloroquine each day, and the fact that less than 20 cases of true retinopathy causing visual loss have been reported[12] have reassured clinicians that hydroxychloroquine is more safe than most other drugs and, in a subset of patients, efficacious. In most double-blind, controlled studies, antimalarials have clinical efficacy equal to gold salts or D-peni-

TABLE 31–5. Dosages of Antirheumatic Drugs Used in Second-Line Treatment of Rheumatoid Arthritis

TYPE OF DRUG	COMMONLY RECOMMENDED DOSAGE
Gold compounds	
Gold sodium thiomalate or aurothioglucose	Intramuscular; single doses of 10 mg, followed by 25 mg 1 week later to test for sensitivity and an initial course of 1.0 g; maintenance therapy, 50 mg weekly
Auranofin	Oral: 3–6 mg daily
Antimalarial drugs	
Hydroxychloroquine	Oral: 400 mg daily for 4–6 weeks, then 200 mg daily
Penicillamine	Oral: 125–250 mg daily, then increasing doses to a maximum of 750 mg daily
Sulfasalazine*	Oral: 500 mg daily, then increasing doses to a maximum of 3,000 mg daily

* Not approved by the FDA for use in patients with rheumatoid arthritis.

TABLE 31–6. Antirheumatic Drug Therapy in Pregnancy and Lactation, and Effects on Fertility*

DRUG	FDA USE-IN-PREGNANCY RATING[†]	CROSSES PLACENTA	MAJOR MATERNAL TOXICITIES	FETAL TOXICITIES	LACTATION	FERTILITY
Aspirin	C; D in third trimester	Yes	Anemia, peripartum hemorrhage, prolonged labor	Premature closure of ductus, pulmonary hypertension, ICH	Use cautiously; excreted at low concentration; doses >1 tablet (325 mg) result in high concentrations in infant plasma	No data
NSAIDs	B; D in third trimester	Yes	As for aspirin	As for aspirin	Compatible according to AAP	No data
Corticosteroids						
Prednisone	B	Dexamethasone and beta-methasone	Exacerbation of diabetes and hypertension, PROM	IUGR	5–20% of maternal dose excreted in breast milk; compatible, but wait 4 hours if dose >20 mg	No data
Dexamethasone	C					
Hydroxychloroquine	C	Yes: fetal concentration 50% of maternal	Few	Few	Contraindicated (slow elimination rate, potential for accumulation)	No data
Gold	C	Yes	No data	1 report of cleft palate and severe CNS abnormalities	Excreted into breast milk (20% of maternal dose); rash, hepatitis, and hematologic abnormalities reported, but AAP considers it compatible	No data
D-Penicillamine	D	Yes	No data	Cutis laxa connective tissue abnormalities	No data	No data
Sulfasalazine	B; D if near term	Yes	No data	No increase in congenital malformations, kernicterus if administered near term	Excreted into breast milk (40–60% maternal dose); bloody diarrhea in 1 infant; AAP recommends caution	Females: no effect; males: significant oligospermia (2 months to return to normal)

Table continued on following page

TABLE 31–6. *Continued*

DRUG	FDA USE-IN-PREGNANCY RATING†	CROSSES PLACENTA	MAJOR MATERNAL TOXICITIES	FETAL TOXICITIES	LACTATION	FERTILITY
Azathioprine	D	Yes	No data	IUGR (rate up to 40%) and prematurity, transient immunosuppression in neonate, possible effect on germlines of offspring	No data; hypothetical risk of immunosuppression outweighs benefit	Not studied; can interfere with effectiveness of IUD
Chlorambucil	D	Teratogenic effects potentiated by caffeine	No data	Renal angiogenesis	Contraindicated	No data
Methotrexate	X	No data	Spontaneous abortion	Fetal abnormalities (including cleft palate and hydrocephalus)	Contraindicated; small amounts excreted with potential to accumulate in fetal tissues	Females: infrequent long-term effect; males: reversible oligospermia
Cyclophosphamide	D	Yes: 25% of maternal level	No data	Severe abnormalities; case report: male twin developed thyroid papillary cancer at 11 years and neuroblastoma at 14 years	Contraindicated; has caused bone marrow depression	Females: age >25 years, concurrent radiation, and prolonged exposure increase risk of infertility; males: dose-dependent oligospermia and azoospermia regardless of age or exposure
Cyclosporin A	C	Yes	No data	IUGR and prematurity; 1 case report: hypoplasia of right leg; not an animal teratogen and unlikely to be a human one	Contraindicated due to potential for immunosuppression	No data

From American College of Rheumatology Ad Hoc Committee on Clinical Guidelines: Guidelines for monitoring drug therapy in rheumatoid arthritis. Arthritis Rheum. 39:723, 1996. Used by permission.

* ICH = intracranial hemorrhage; AAP = American Academy of Pediatrics; PROM = premature rupture of membranes; IUGR = intrauterine growth retardation; CNS = central nervous system; IUD = intrauterine device.

† Food and Drug Administration (FDA) use-in-pregnancy ratings are as follows: A = Controlled studies show no risk. Adequate, well-controlled studies in pregnant women have failed to demonstrate risk to the fetus. B = No evidence of risk in humans. Either animal findings show risk but human findings do not, or, if no adequate human studies have been performed, animal findings are negative. C = Risk cannot be ruled out. Human studies are lacking and results of animal studies are either positive for fetal risk or lacking as well. However, potential benefits may justify the potential risk. D = Positive evidence of risk. Investigational or post-marketing data show risk to the fetus. Nevertheless, potential benefits may outweigh the potential risk. X = Contraindicated in pregnancy. Studies in animals or humans, or investigational or post-marketing reports, have shown fetal risk which clearly outweighs any possible benefit to the patient.

TABLE 31–7. Numbers of Treatment Groups and Patients in the Meta-analysis of the Efficacy of Second-Line Drugs Used to Treat Rheumatoid Arthritis, According to Drug Treatment Group

	NO. OF TREATMENT GROUPS	NO. OF PATIENTS COMPLETING THE TRIAL
Antimalarial drugs	11	314
Auranofin	23	1,274
Injectable gold	29	656
Methotrexate	7	150
D-Penicillamine	19	511
Sulfasalazine	6	161
Placebo	22	891

From Felson, D. T., Anderson, J. J., and Meenan, R. F.: The comparative efficacy and toxicity of second-line drugs in rheumatoid arthritis: results of two metaanalyses. Arthritis Rheum. 33:1449, 1990. Used by permission.

cillamine.[13] In contrast, in one 36-week randomized, double-blind, placebo-controlled trial, there were no important differences in the side effects between hydroxychloroquine and placebo, although the treated patients improved significantly.[14] A study of the effects of low-dose cyclosporine compared with chloroquine has been carried out in a randomized, double-blind fashion in 44 patients with rheumatoid arthritis. The antimalarial drug was as effective as cyclosporine, producing statistically significant improvement between 4 and 24 weeks of therapy, particularly in patients with less severe disease.[15]

Meta-analysis of 66 short-term trials of second-line drugs (Table 31–7) showed that intramuscular gold was the most toxic and antimalarials and methotrexate the least toxic.[16] The relative benignity of hydroxychloroquine was confirmed in analysis of a large cohort of ARAMIS patients over a longer time period[17] (Table 31–8). Although in one meta-analysis[16] chloroquine was more effective than the hydroxylated derivative, most rheumatologists in the United States use hydroxychloroquine. When chloroquine is available in pharmacies, it may be reasonable to substitute it for hydroxychloroquine, particularly when 6-monthly ophthalmologic examinations are carried out.

Toxicity of Antimalarials

Skin rash and stomach pain have been the most bothersome side effects of antimalarials. The dropout rate for antimalarials in these studies averages out to be less than 8 per cent[16] (Fig. 31–1), or about twice that for placebo therapy.

The ocular toxicities of concern are a "bull's-eye" retinal pigmentation around the macula and pigmentary stippling of the macula as the drugs are deposited there. The appearance of these is an

TABLE 31–8. Comparative Toxicity of 6 DMARDs and 10 NSAIDs*

RANK	DMARD	STANDARDIZED TOXICITY INDEX (MEAN ± SEM)	NSAID	STANDARIZED TOXICITY INDEX (MEAN ± SEM)
1			Salsalate	1.28 ± 0.34
2	Hydroxychloroquine	1.38 ± 0.15		
3			Ibuprofen	1.94 ± 0.43
4			Naproxen	2.17 ± 0.23
5			Sulindac	2.24 ± 0.39
6	Intramuscular gold	2.27 ± 0.17		
7			Piroxicam	2.52 ± 0.23
8			Fenoprofen	2.95 ± 0.77
9	Penicillamine	3.38 ± 0.36		
10			Ketoprofen	3.45 ± 0.74
11	Methotrexate	3.82 ± 0.35		
12			Meclofenamate	3.86 ± 0.66
13	Azathioprine	3.92 ± 0.39		
14			Tolmetin	3.96 ± 0.74
15			Indomethacin	3.99 ± 0.58
16	Auranofin	5.25 ± 0.32		

From Fries, J. F., Williams, C. A., Ramey, D., et al.: The relative toxicity of disease-modifying antirheumatic drugs. Arthritis Rheum. 36:297, 1993. Used by permission.

* DMARDs, disease-modifying antirheumatic drugs.

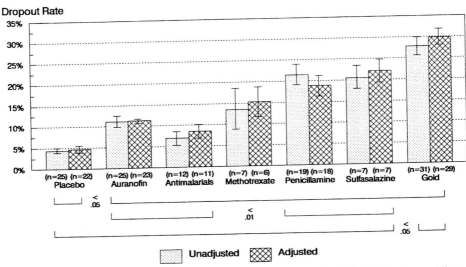

FIGURE 31–1. Rates of dropout because of drug toxicity from rheumatoid arthritis clinical trials of second-line agents, according to treatment group. Bars show the mean ± SEM (confidence intervals = 1.96 × SEM). (From Felson, D. T., Anderson, J. J., and Meenan, R. F.: The comparative efficacy and toxicity of second-line drugs in rheumatoid arthritis: results of two metaanalyses. Arthritis Rheum. 33:1449, 1990. Used by permission.)

indication to stop the drug. Although the risk of maculopathy is rare, patients with a visual field loss or decreased visual acuity should not be started on antimalarial drugs, and an ophthalmologic examination every 6 months after the drug is started is a reasonable course to follow[18] for all patients taking antimalarials.

SULFASALAZINE

In 1939, operating on the assumption that rheumatoid arthritis was caused by bacterial infection, Professor Nanna Svartz bound salicylic acid to sulfonamides. One of these, sulfasalazine, was effective in uncontrolled trials.[20] After decades of minimal use for rheumatoid arthritis, it has once again become a drug of interest for this disease. After oral administration, colonic bacteria reduce it to sulfapyridine and 5-aminosalicylic acid (mesalamine); these are absorbed (Fig. 31–2). Which of the two metabolites is the more active in arthritis is still being debated.[21]

As with the antimalarials, searches for the mechanisms of action of sulfasalazine followed demonstration of its efficacy. Do results from any assay have true relevance? There are no definitive answers, but the drug or its metabolites have been shown to scavenge oxygen radicals and inhibit production of arachidonic acid products,[21] and it is possible (see Chapter 32) that, similar to methotrexate, sulfasalazine facilitates accumulation of the anti-inflammatory molecule adenosine in cells. In addition, treatment for periods of 16 weeks or longer results in decreased serum concentrations of IgA and IgG that correlate with reduced concentrations of IL-6, but no change in immunoglobulin

---

Mechanisms of Action of Antimalarials

Studies of the actions of antimalarials followed the common use of the drugs in rheumatoid arthritis. As assays related to pathophysiology of the disease were developed, the antimalarials were added to them. It is not surprising, therefore, that many effects of the drug have been demonstrated, but that there are few leads to indicate which effect may be most important. Inhibition of phagocytosis and chemotaxis, stabilization of lysosomal membranes, and inhibition of lymphocyte function are a few documented activities of this class of drug.[13]

Recent work has shown that the antimalarials inhibit IL-2 production by a CD4+ T-cell line in response to a specific APC.[19] These drugs are weak bases that can diffuse into acidic vacuoles, become protonated, and raise the pH of vacuoles in which processed antigen peptides bind to the MHC. The higher pH could alter the molecular assembly of MHC-peptide complexes, leading to a decreased stimulation of autoimmune CD4+ T cells.

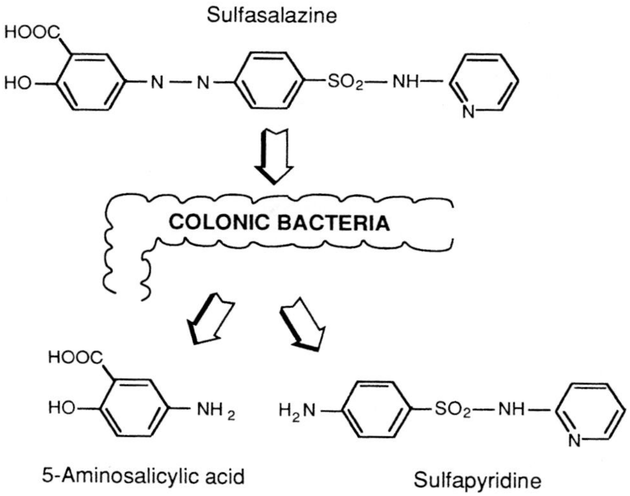

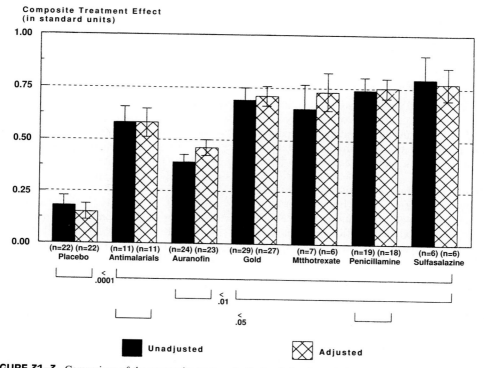

Sulfasalazine

COLONIC BACTERIA

5-Aminosalicylic acid   Sulfapyridine

FIGURE 31–2. Chemical structure of sulfasalazine. (From Day, R. D.: Sulfasalazine. In Kelley, W. N., Harris, E. D., Jr., Ruddy, S., and Sledge, C. B. [eds.]: Textbook of Rheumatology, 4th ed., Vol. 1. Philadelphia, W. B. Saunders, 1993, pp. 692–699. Used by permission.)

levels in saliva or jejunal fluid is noted. Circulating IgA and IgM rheumatoid factor levels diminish as well.[22]

Sulfasalazine appears to exert a beneficial effect earlier (within 4 weeks after starting the drug)[23]

than antimalarials, gold, or D-penicillamine, but not as soon as methotrexate. Although in some patients it may be as efficacious as gold or methotrexate[16] (Fig. 31–3), with significant improvement noted in joint swelling and tenderness, grip strength, morn-

Composite Treatment Effect (in standard units)

FIGURE 31–3. Comparison of the composite treatment effects of placebo and six second-line drugs used to treat rheumatoid arthritis. The composite treatment effect is the mean of "standardized change" in the tender joint count, ESR, and grip strength. Bars show the mean ± SEM improvement with treatment. (From Felson, D. T., Anderson, J. J., and Meenan, R. F.: The comparative efficacy and toxicity of second-line drugs in rheumatoid arthritis: results of two metaanalyses. Arthritis Rheum. 33:1449, 1990. Used by permission.)

ing stiffness, and pain scores, the withdrawals because of nausea or vomiting have generated a high dropout rate.[16,24] Recently developed enteric-coated preparations have improved tolerance.

In a study versus placebo, 80 patients with the diagnosis of rheumatoid arthritis for less than 1 year were randomized to placebo (plus NSAIDs and low-dose glucocorticoids) or sulfasalazine (500 mg increasing to 2,000 mg, when tolerated, in 4 weeks).[23] The sulfasalazine-treated group improved modestly more than the control group, and seronegative rheumatoid arthritis patients improved more than seropositive patients. There were fewer erosive changes in the sulfasalazine-treated group, but not significantly so. In contrast, several studies have suggested that sulfasalazine has the capability to slow progression of erosive disease, even in chronically active and destructive disease.[25,26] In a study comparing hydroxychloroquine (200 mg/day) and sulfasalazine (2,000 mg/day) assessed by using a Dutch modification of the HAQ, there was a significant difference in favor of the sulfasalazine group in the physical disability score after 48 weeks.[27]

One intriguing study that measured gastrointestinal blood loss and studied gastroduodenal endoscopic biopsies has suggested that sulfasalazine reduces both intestinal inflammation and blood loss inflicted by NSAIDs, whereas gold, D-penicillamine, and hydroxychloroquine do not.[28] This presents a rationale for use of sulfasalazine relatively early in rheumatoid arthritis in conjunction with baseline NSAIDs.

Despite differences in toxicity and putative mechanisms of action, a study of hydroxychloroquine and sulfasalazine alone and in combination showed no benefit of the combination over each given separately in a randomized double-blind trial.[29]

In summary, if the annoying nausea and vomiting generated by sulfasalazine will be bypassed or minimized by enteric-coated preparations for oral administration, the demonstrated efficacy of the drug could be exploited effectively, and it could be used early in the disease course, as is methotrexate.

GOLD SALTS

In the early 1960s, the drug therapy for rheumatoid arthritis was limited to salicylates, phenylbutazone, hydroxychloroquine, and gold salts. The latter appeared to be the most potent, and a study of gold salt therapy carried out by the Empire Rheumatism Council[30] supported use of injectable gold

salts as an effective therapy in rheumatoid arthritis. This double-blind study was one of the first well-controlled trials in rheumatology. A growing cadre of rheumatologists in Europe, Great Britain, and the United States began using aurothiomalate or aurothioglucose with enthusiasm. Although using gold salts meant having patients come into the physicians' offices or clinics once each week for checks of blood and urine and the weekly injection, this system was remarkably well tolerated by both patients and the health insurance companies.

Similar to the other second-line drugs that were introduced several decades ago, there had been no convincing demonstration of a mechanism of action for gold salts in rheumatoid arthritis; use was empirical. It became apparent that there was a delay of 2 to 4 months before beneficial effects were seen, but a therapeutic response rewarded up to 60 per cent of patients who tolerated the parenteral therapy.[31] Those patients who did benefit often maintained a good response when the interval between injections was widened to as long as 4 weeks.

The Mechanism of Action of Gold Salts

The monocyte/macrophage is the most likely target for action of gold salts, and the effects upon lymphocytes may be secondary to suppression of essential macrophage contribution to lymphocyte activation by blocking antigen presentation and other components of macrophage function.[32] Macrophages and synovial cells sequester gold salts; the concentration within these cells is 5- to 10-fold that found in serum of treated patients, and these levels are sufficient to inhibit monocyte/macrophage-derived angiogenic activity.[33]

Use of focused technology with monoclonal antibodies to identify macrophage cytokine expression demonstrated a decrease in IL-1, IL-6, and TNFα expression 12 weeks after starting intramuscular gold.[34] There was an associated reduction in macrophages in the synovial lining without change in numbers of T or B lymphocytes.

Both gold salts and D-penicillamine suppress the in vitro development of colonies of myeloid cells from progenitor cells in mouse and human bone marrow; this mechanism could explain some of the efficacy of both of these drugs as well as the rare episodes of marrow aplasia associated with therapy[35,36] (Fig. 31–4)

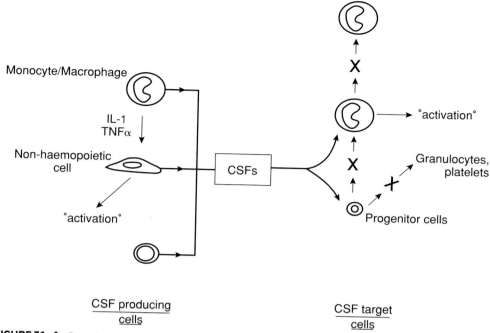

FIGURE 31–4. Opposing actions of hematopoietic growth factors and slow-acting antirheumatic drugs (X) in rheumatoid arthritis. (From Hamilton, J. A.: Rheumatoid arthritis: opposing actions of haemopoietic growth factors and slow-acting anti-rheumatic drugs. Lancet 342:536, 1993. Used by permission. © by The Lancet Ltd. 1993.)

The cumbersome need for injections of gold salts stimulated development of an oral preparation of gold. Auranofin—the first drug developed specifically for use in rheumatoid arthritis—was introduced in mid-1980s.[37] Although auranofin has significantly less of the serious toxicities that injectable preparations have, it has less efficacy as well. In a meta-analysis of 66 clinical trials and 117 treatment groups,[16] auranofin tended to have less efficacy than methotrexate, injectable gold, D-penicillamine, or sulfasalazine.

The side effects of auranofin are very different from those of injectable gold. Whereas the injectable preparations more often cause the more serious problems of thrombocytopenia and proteinuria, a reversible but annoying syndrome of loose stools related to a mild enterocolitis is common with auranofin. Indeed, although the toxicity index for auranofin was quite high in one large study,[17] the poor showing was almost entirely due to a high incidence of relatively minor symptoms (e.g., diarrhea, nausea, and skin rash).

The rationale for developing a toxicity index that can be applied to all NSAIDs and second-line drugs is a sound one, and the process for its construction is reviewed in ref. 17. Although it is not likely that there will be clinical utility of correlating HLA class II genes with toxicity, a component of

$DQ\alpha1*0501$—associated previously with idiopathic membranous nephropathy—appears to be an important gene for the development of gold-induced nephropathy.[38]

It is generally held that a less toxic drug can be used earlier in treatment sequences for rheumatoid arthritis, and in one study of 83 patients with active disease for less than 2 years, evidence emerged that early treatment with auranofin could enable patients to continue working and postpone early retirement or declaration of permanent disability.[39] Seventy-five of these patients were followed for another 3 years. At the second year, almost all had been switched to one or another second-line drug. The critical data are that continued improvement in the group started early on second-line drugs was seen and differences between the two groups were maintained with regard to clinical variables, outcome measures, and radiographic evaluation.[40] If this Scandinavian study could be confirmed in the United States, the benefit-cost ratio for early treatment with auranofin, antimalarials, or methotrexate would increase strikingly.

Despite the serious toxicities of parenteral gold, which occur uncommonly, it appears from a study in Finland of 573 patients with rheumatoid arthritis treated first during the period 1961 to 1966 that gold therapy was not associated with premature death in these patients. To the contrary, long-term gold therapy was associated with improved survival.[41] However, the difficulty patients have in tolerating gold therapy is significant. In a retrospective 10-year follow-up of parenteral gold therapy in 376 patients, 42 per cent, 55 per cent, 74 per cent, and 92 per cent had discontinued the drug after 1, 2, 5, and 10 years, respectively.[42] Mucocutaneous side effects were the main cause of discontinuing the drug during the first 3 years, and inefficacy dominated after 4 years. There were no deaths in this study, and serious toxicity was rare.

Does Gold Therapy Really Help?

The difficulties in evaluating therapy in a chronic disease such as rheumatoid arthritis were highlighted by a prospective observational study of patients over a 5-year period under the care of community rheumatologists in the San Francisco Bay Area.[43] A total of 822 patients with rheumatoid arthritis entered the study; outcomes were compared in those receiving gold therapy for no less than 2 years with those patients who did not receive parenteral gold at any time during the 5 years of the study. At the end of the study, 574 patients still participated, and there were no differences at enrollment between those who remained and those who dropped out.

The data showed that functional disability assessed by the HAQ and the number of painful joints in the 574 patients was, on average, unchanged over 5 years and was unaffected by use of gold therapy. Although the average duration of disease was more than 10 years, there were no differences in the function score and painful joints in those patients whose disease duration was less than 2 years, whether or not gold therapy was given.

These data are different from others reviewed here and in other chapters in two important respects: (1) gold was not efficacious, and (2) there was no deterioration of function in any group of patients. In contrast, most studies demonstrate a relentless deterioration of patients with rheumatoid arthritis over time. The data in the Bay Area study attest more to the effective treatment of *all* patients in this group, rather than to the failure of gold therapy.[44]

No parameter for assessing outcome of therapy is more convincing to rheumatologists than evidence that a treatment regimen decreases the progression of erosions. Therefore, a recent study compared 13 patients receiving a course of gold salts (gold sodium thiomalate) early in the course of disease (mean duration 8 ± 5 months), along with NSAIDs, to 10 patients in whom the gold therapy was delayed 6 months.[45] To assay progression of erosions, quantitative microfocal radiography of hand joints was used to produce high magnification and spatial resolution. The results were significant and encouraging: Earlier treatment produced delay in erosion progression by 6 months in the group treated early, but both groups benefited after 1 year of the study. In all, 16 patients showed either no progression of erosions or erosion repair, and those receiving gold early did slightly better than those receiving it on the delayed protocol. This study helps build the case for earlier rather than delayed therapy with second-line drugs. Quantitative microradiography of hand joints should be used in trials of other second-line drugs, including methotrexate.

Practical Use of Gold Salts

The following specific points about the use of gold salts are helpful for any physician considering these drugs:

- In patients with early but active synovitis who are either intolerant to methotrexate (with or without concomitant hydroxychloroquine therapy) or in whom methotrexate is contraindicated because of liver disease or alcoholism, parenteral gold is the best choice for a second-line drug.
- ''Bridge'' therapy with prednisone (<7 mg/day) during the weeks to months that are needed for gold to have demonstrable efficacy is appropriate. After benefit of gold salts has been achieved, the goal should be to taper prednisone to no more than 2 or 3 mg/day.
- Gold can be used in patients with neutropenia from Felty's syndrome, or eosinophilia associated with active disease.
- Because pre-existing proteinuria or dermatitis can mimic side effects of gold therapy, they are relative contraindications to initiation of gold therapy.
- If improvement achieved by a 6-month course of weekly injections of 50 mg is not maintained by monthly injections, re-establishment of benefit may be achieved by return to weekly therapy.[46]
- Four times as many patients withdraw from intramuscular gold as from oral gold because of intolerance.
- A ''nitritoid'' reaction (weakness, dizziness, nausea, sweating, and facial flushing) is not uncommonly seen with gold thiomalate but is rare with gold thioglucose.
- Although most patients who develop the nephrotic syndrome on parenteral gold generally recover completely, auranofin is a better choice in patients with proteinuria or chronic renal failure.

- Consistent with the impression that *HLA-DR3* is associated with an enhanced cellular immune or autoimmune response are studies of MHC class II alleles in patients developing toxicity to gold. *HLA-DR3* is found in 85 per cent of patients who develop thrombocytopenia on intramuscular gold, whereas it is found in only 30 per cent of the general population.[31] *HLA-DR3* was found in 59 per cent of 27 patients who developed gold-induced nephropathy, compared with only 14 per cent of those who received gold without developing nephropathy.[38] Balancing these data somewhat is the evidence that *HLA-DR3* may be associated with a better response to gold therapy.[47] Patients with rheumatoid arthritis who develop dermatitis following treatment with aurothiomalate have T cells that proliferate in an HLA-DR–restricted manner to oxidized gold salts, the form most likely found within phagolysosomes.[48]

- Consistent monitoring of WBC count, peripheral blood smear, and urinalysis during gold therapy does not prevent toxicity but allows early detection, enabling a better outcome.

- Rare but disturbing side effects of gold therapy include a pulmonary hypersensitivity presenting as acute respiratory distress, enterocolitis (particularly in older women), and neurologic complications resembling encephalopathy, Guillain-Barré syndrome, or cranial nerve palsies.[49]

D-PENICILLAMINE

Use of D-penicillamine in rheumatoid arthritis was fostered first by Dr. Israeli Jaffe of New York during the 1960s. Jaffe reasoned that this thiol-containing derivative of cysteine (Fig. 31–5) could break the disulfide bonds linking μ chains of IgM rheumatoid factor and thereby have a beneficial effect on the disease. His early therapeutic trials were positive, especially in patients with vasculitis.[50,51] The efficacy of the compound for rheumatoid ar-

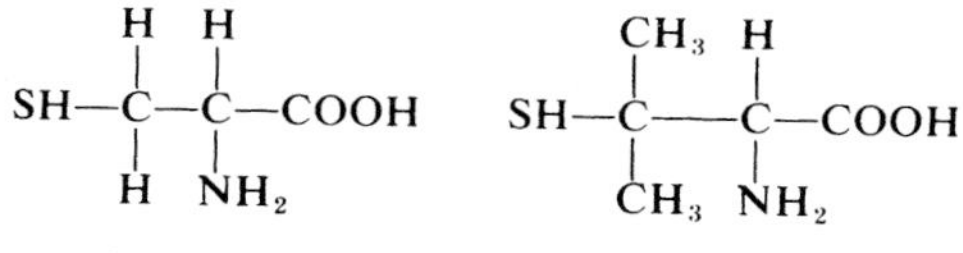

FIGURE 31–5. The chemical structure of penicillamine. The drug is an analogue of the naturally occurring amino acid cysteine, with CH_3 groups replacing H^+ at the β-carbon position. (From Jaffe, I.: Penicillamine. *In* Kelley, W. N., Harris, E. D. Jr., Ruddy, S., and Sledge, C. B. [eds.]: Textbook of Rheumatology, 4th ed., Vol. 1. Philadelphia, W. B. Saunders, 1993, pp. 760–766. Used by permission.)

thritis was established by the United Kingdom Multi Center trial in 1973,[52] and since then it has been approved by the FDA for use in rheumatoid arthritis.

The niche for D-penicillamine in treatment of rheumatoid arthritis is in patients who have failed or cannot tolerate hydroxychloroquine, methotrexate, or gold salts, or combinations of those, and in whom disease is still active. In patients with active vasculitis involving skin or internal organs, it often is used as primary therapy. The same applies to rheumatoid patients with manifestations that are fibrotic in nature (e.g., pulmonary interstitial fibrosis, soft tissue contractures). The rationale for this use is that D-penicillamine inhibits collagen cross-links and could slow down collagen deposition in fibrotic processes.[53,54]

There are many similarities of D-penicillamine to gold salts in terms of response patterns and toxicity. D-penicillamine must be taken each day for 2 to 4 months before a beneficial response is obtained. Because of the general feeling that rheumatoid pa-

---

Mechanisms of Action of D-Penicillamine

As with the other drugs introduced for therapy in rheumatoid arthritis without a prospective mechanism of action that has held up under scrutiny, D-penicillamine has ''worked'' in almost every assay system used. Which of these may have primary relevance in rheumatoid patients? Most evidence points to the activity of the reactive thiol group[57,58] as being responsible for both biologic actions and toxicity. Catalyzed by transition metals (e.g., copper), oxidation of the thiol moiety generates disulfide bonds with other proteins. In addition, D-penicillamine reacts with aldehydes or ketones to form a thiazolidine. By this mechanism it interferes with normal cross-link formation of collagen.[54]

D-Penicillamine is not anti-inflammatory, and it does not inhibit B or $CD8^+$ lymphocytes or macrophage function. In the presence of copper ions, D-penicillamine causes a selective decrease in $CD4^+$ T-helper/inducer cells.[57] In addition, D-penicillamine suppresses human fibroblast proliferation in vitro[59] and inhibits new blood vessel formation in vivo. Thus, the drug inhibits selectively a crucial phase of the immune response and can also suppress the proliferative reaction of fibrovascular tissue in the synovium. It is a pity that D-penicillamine is so toxic.

tients were more likely to develop untoward side effects from D-penicillamine, the recommended dose was dropped to 500 to 1,000 mg/day, and development of toxicity could often be obviated if therapy was started with only 125 mg/day and gradually increased to 750 to 1,000 mg/day over a period of 6 to 8 weeks. This is the ''go low, go slow'' principle.

Meta-analysis showed that, in a composite treatment effect analysis, D-penicillamine is as effective as intramuscular gold, methotrexate, and sulfasalazine; slightly more efficacious than hydroxychloroquine; and significantly more effective than oral gold.[16] Progression of joint space narrowing or bone erosions is not retarded,[55] but this could be related to the fact that, once synovitis has been active for 2 years or more, irreversible changes are set in motion that inexorably destroy connective tissue. In patients who respond clinically, acute-phase reactants decrease and hemoglobin increases, implying a definite suppression of disease activity.[56]

Special Toxicity of D-Penicillamine

The toxicity of D-penicillamine is at once disturbing and fascinating. One class of side effects are similar to those seen in gold therapy:

- Urticarial, macular or papular eruptions are the majority of skin side effects.
- Excretion of 0.5 g/day of protein in the urine occurs in approximately 9 per cent of patients, and uncommonly the nephrotic syndrome develops. Previous proteinuria during gold therapy and the presence of HLA-B8 increase the risk of this complication[52]; a membranous glomerulonephritis is usually present, and usually resolves after stopping the drug.
- Thrombocytopenia and neutropenia can occur at any time, perhaps as a result of a suppressive effect on stem cell maturation. Neutropenia is the most common fatal complication of D-penicillamine therapy.[60]

The other class of side effects are unusual ones that probably are related to the reactive thiol group in D-penicillamine. One, a taste disturbance characterized by a metallic taste and diminished ability to taste food, is related to chelation of zinc within enzymes essential for taste. Others, fortunately rare, are autoimmune in their presentation, and often serious:

- *Myasthenia gravis:* it may take over 1 year to resolve after stopping D-penicillamine.

- *Dermatomyositis/polymyositis:* this usually resolves rapidly after stopping the drug.
- *Systemic lupus erythematosus:* this form of SLE resembles more that occurring secondary to procainamide rather than the idiopathic form, although glomerulonephritis or neurologic involvement occasionally is seen. Use of D-penicillamine may be the cause of some cases of the ''Rufus'' syndrome, in which a patient with definite rheumatoid arthritis presents years later with a classical SLE syndrome.
- *Pemphigus:* this complication is associated with significant mortality secondary to infection of exposed dermis and fluid and electrolyte disturbances. In serious cases, plasmapheresis and systemic glucocorticoid therapy may be needed.

REFERENCES

1. Capell, H. A., Porter, D. R., Madhok, R., et al.: Second line (disease modifying) treatment in rheumatoid arthritis: which drug for which patient? Ann. Rheum. Dis. 52:423, 1993.
2. American College of Rheumatology Ad Hoc Committee on Clinical Guidelines: Guidelines for the management of rheumatoid arthritis. Arthritis Rheum. 39:713, 1996.
3. Porter, D. R., McInnes, I., Hunter, J., et al.: Outcome of second line therapy in rheumatoid arthritis. Ann. Rheum. Dis. 53:812, 1994.
4. Fries, J. F., Williams, C. A., Morfeld, D., et al.: Reduction in long-term disability in patients with rheumatoid arthritis by disease-modifying antirheumatic drug-based treatment strategies. Arthritis Rheum. 39:616, 1996.
5. Prashker, M. J., and Meenan, R. F.: The total costs of drug therapy for rheumatoid arthritis. Arthritis Rheum. 38:318, 1995.
6. Singh, G., Fries, J. F., Williams, C. A., et al.: Toxicity profiles of disease modifying antirheumatic drugs in rheumatoid arthritis. J. Rheumatol. 18:188, 1991.

   This study develops a profile of toxicity that can help physicians in their initial prescribing patterns. In Table 31–3 (see text) the side effects are numbered as events/1,000 patient years.

7. Fries, J. F., Williams, C. A., Ramey, D. R., et al.: The relative toxicity of alternative therapies for rheumatoid arthritis: implications for the therapeutic progression. Semin. Arthritis Rheum. 23(2, suppl. 1):68, 1993.

   The relative toxicities of NSAIDs and second-line drugs are tabulated in Table 31–4 (see text). The Toxicity Index developed by these authors include components of symptoms, laboratory tests, and hospitalizations. The side effects range from 0 to 10 and are multiplied by the severity factor: 0.5 for mild, 1.0 for moderate, and 1.5 for severe. The same is used for laboratory side effects. This is an arbitrary but well-reasoned approach.

8. van der Heide, A., Jacobs, J. W. G., Bijlsma, J. W. J., et al.: The effectiveness of early treatment with ''second-line'' antirheumatic drugs: a randomized, controlled trial. Ann. Intern. Med. 124:699, 1996.
9. American College of Rheumatology Ad Hoc Committee on Clinical Guidelines: Guidelines for monitoring drug

therapy in rheumatoid arthritis. Arthritis Rheum. 39:723, 1996.

10. Freedman, A., and Steinberg, V. L.: Chloroquine in rheumatoid arthritis: a double-blindfold trial of treatment for one year. Ann. Intern. Med. 19:243, 1960.
11. Hobbes, H. E., Sorsby, A., and Freedman, A.: Retinopathy following chloroquine therapy. Lancet 2:478, 1959.
12. Bernstein, H. N.: Ocular safety of hydroxychloroquine. Ann. Ophthalmol. 23:292, 1991.
13. Rynes, R. I.: Antimalarial drugs. In Kelley, W. N., Harris, E. D. Jr., Ruddy, S., and Sledge, C. B. (eds.): Textbook of Rheumatology, 4th ed., Vol. 1. Philadelphia, W. B. Saunders, 1993, pp. 731–742.
14. HERA Study Group: A randomized trial of hydroxychloroquine in early rheumatoid arthritis: the HERA study. Am. J. Med. 98:156, 1995.
15. Landewe, R. B. M., The, H. S. G., van Rijthoven, A. W. A. M., et al.: A randomized, double-blind, 24-week controlled study of low-dose cyclosporine versus chloroquine for early rheumatoid arthritis. Arthritis Rheum. 37:637, 1994.
16. Felson, D. T., Anderson, J. J., and Meenan, R. F.: The comparative efficacy and toxicity of second-line drugs in rheumatoid arthritis: results of two metaanalyses. Arthritis Rheum. 33:1449, 1990.

Clinical trials were collected from January 1966 through August 1989. The studies used were on adults with rheumatoid arthritis, and randomized assignment to treatment regimens was generally essential. Numerical values for joint count, ESR, and grip strength were required, and these were found to be most sensitive to change (see Fig. 31–3 text). In toxicity analysis, the proportion of subjects who dropped out was defined as the proportion of all those who entered a study arm and who dropped out by the end of the trial. The numbers of treatment groups and patients are shown in Table 31–8 (see text). The dropout rate according to treatment group is shown in Figure 31–1 (see text). The difference between efficacy of chloroquine and hydroxychloroquine was unexpected; the former was significantly more effective, even at a dosage ratio of 1:2.

17. Fries, J. F., Williams, C. A., Ramey, D., et al.: The relative toxicity of disease-modifying antirheumatic drugs. Arthritis Rheum. 36:297, 1993.

Toxicity Index scores computed from symptoms, laboratory abnormalities, and hospitalizations attributed to second-line drugs were assessed in 2,747 patients with rheumatoid arthritis receiving 3,053 courses of six drugs and 1,309 courses of prednisone over 7,278 patient-years. The Toxicity Indices, going from lowest (least toxic) to highest (most toxic), were

Hydroxychloroquine:	1.33
Intramuscular gold:	2.36
D-Penicillamine:	3.49
Methotrexate:	3.95
Azathioprine:	3.86
Auranofin:	5.91
Prednisone:	5.35

Comparative toxicities of six second-line drugs and 10 NSAIDs are shown in Table 31–9 (see text).

18. Mazzuca, S. A., Yung, R., Brandt, K. D., et al.: Current practices for monitoring ocular toxicity related to hydroxychloroquine (Plaquenil) therapy. J. Rheumatol. 21:59, 1994.
19. Fox, R. I., and Kang, H.-I.: Mechanism of action of antima-larial drugs: inhibition of antigen processing and presentation. Lupus 2(suppl. 1):S9, 1993.
20. Svartz, N.: Salazopyrin, a new sulfanilamide preparation. Acta Med. Scand. 110:577, 1942.
21. Day, R. O.: Sulfasalazine. In Kelley, W. N., Harris, E. D. Jr., Ruddy, S., and Sledge, C. B. (eds.): Textbook of Rheumatology, 4th ed., Vol. 1. Philadelphia, W. B. Saunders, 1993, pp. 692–699.
22. Kanerud, L., Engstrom, G. N., and Tarkowski, A.: Evidence for differential effects of sulphasalazine on systemic and mucosal immunity in rheumatoid arthritis. Ann. Rheum. Dis. 54:256, 1995.
23. Hannonen, P., Mottonen, T., Hakola, M., et al.: Sulfasalazine in early rheumatoid arthritis: a 48-week double-blind, prospective, placebo-controlled study. Arthritis Rheum. 36:1501, 1993.
24. Pinals, R., Kaplan, S., Lawson, J., et al.: Sulphasalazine in rheumatoid arthritis: a double-blind placebo controlled trial. Arthritis Rheum. 29:1427, 1986.
25. van der Heijde, D., van Riel, P., Nuver-Zwart, E., et al.: Sulphasalazine versus hydroxychloroquine in rheumatoid arthritis: 3-year follow-up. Lancet 335:539, 1990.
26. Pullar, T., Hunter, J., and Capell, H.: Effect of sulphasalazine on the radiological progression of rheumatoid arthritis. Ann. Rheum. Dis. 46:398, 1987.
27. van der Heijde, D. M. F. M., van Riel, P. L. C. M., and van de Putte, L. B. A.: Sensitivity of a Dutch health assessment questionnaire in a trial comparing hydroxychloroquine vs. sulphasalazine. Scand. J. Rheumatol. 19:407, 1990.
28. Haylar, T., Smith, T., MacPherson, A., et al.: Nonsteroidal antiinflammatory drug-induced small intestinal inflammation and blood loss. Arthritis Rheum. 37:1146, 1994.
29. Faarvang, K. L., Egsmose, C., Kryger, P., et al.: Hydroxychloroquine and sulphasalazine alone and in combination in rheumatoid arthritis: a randomised double blind trial. Ann. Rheum. Dis. 52:711, 1993.
30. Research Sub-committee of the Empire Rheumatism Council: Gold therapy in rheumatoid arthritis: report of a multi-centre controlled trial. Ann. Rheum. Dis. 19:95, 1960.
31. Gordon, D. A.: Gold compounds in the rheumatic diseases. In Kelley, W. N., Harris, E. D. Jr., Ruddy, S., and Sledge, C. B. (eds.): Textbook of Rheumatology, 4th ed., Vol. 1. Philadelphia, W. B. Saunders, 1993, pp. 743–759.
32. Lipsky, P. E., and Ziff, M.: Inhibition of antigen- and mitogen-induced human lymphocyte proliferation by gold compounds. J. Clin. Invest. 59:455, 1977.
33. Koch, A. E., Burrows, J. C., Polverini, P. J., et al.: Thiol-containing compounds inhibit the production of monocyte/macrophage-derived angiogenic activity. Agents Actions 34:350, 1991.
34. Yanni, G., Nabil, M., Garahat, M. R., et al.: Intramuscular gold decreases cytokine expression and macrophage numbers in the rheumatoid synovial membrane. Ann. Rheum. Dis. 53:315, 1994.
35. Hamilton, J. A., and Williams, N.: In vitro inhibition of myelopoiesis by gold salts and D-penicillamine. J. Rheumatol. 12:892, 1985.
36. Hamilton, J. A.: Rheumatoid arthritis: opposing actions of haemopoietic growth factors and slow-acting anti-rheumatic drugs. Lancet 342:536, 1993.

The hypothesis is advanced here that the colony-stimulating factors have an important role in rheumatoid arthritis as regulators of myelopoiesis and as activators of inflammatory leukocytes, and that gold salts, D-penicillamine, and perhaps the antimalarial drugs act principally by opposing the actions of these hematopoietic factors. The logic of this is presented in Figure 31–4 (see text).

37. Abruzzo, J. L.: Auranofin: a new drug for rheumatoid arthritis. Ann. Intern. Med. 105:274, 1986.

38. Sakkas, L. I., Chikanza, I. C., Vaughan, R. W., et al.: Gold induced nephropathy in rheumatoid arthritis and HLA class II genes. Ann. Rheum. Dis. 52:300, 1993.

39. Borg, G., Allander, E., Berg, E., et al.: Auranofin treatment in early rheumatoid arthritis may postpone early retirement: results from a 2-year double blind trial. J. Rheumatol. 18:1015, 1991.

40. Egsmose, C., Lund, B., Borg, G., et al.: Patients with rheumatoid arthritis benefit from early 2nd line therapy: 5 year followup of a prospective double blind placebo controlled study. J. Rheumatol. 22:2208, 1995.

41. Lehtinen, K., and Isomäki, H.: Intramuscular gold therapy is associated with long survival in patients with rheumatoid arthritis. J. Rheumatol. 18:524, 1991.

42. Bendix, G., and Bjelle, A.: A 10 year follow up of parenteral gold therapy in patients with rheumatoid arthritis. Ann. Rheum. Dis. 55:169, 1996.

43. Epstein, W. V., Henke, C. J., Yelin, E. H., et al.: Effect of parenterally administered gold therapy on the course of adult rheumatoid arthritis. Ann. Intern. Med. 114:437, 1991.

44. Pincus, T., and Wolfe, F.: Treatment of rheumatoid arthritis: challenges to traditional paradigms. Ann. Intern. Med. 115:825, 1991.

45. Buckland-Wright, J. C., Clarke, G. S., Chikanza, I. C., et al.: Quantitative microfocal radiography detects changes in erosion area in patients with early rheumatoid arthritis treated with myocrisine. J. Rheumatol. 20:243, 1993.

46. Sagransky, D. M., and Greenwald, R. A.: Efficacy and toxicity of retreatment with gold salts: a retrospective view of 25 cases. J. Rheumatol. 7:474, 1980.

47. Speerstra, F., van Riel, P. L. C. M., Reekers, P., et al.: The influence of HLA phenotypes on the response to parenteral gold in rheumatoid arthritis. Tissue Antigens 28:1, 1987.

48. Verwilghen, J., Kingsley, G. H., Gambling, L., et al.: Activation of gold-reactive T lymphocytes in rheumatoid arthritis patients treated with gold. Arthritis Rheum. 35:1413, 1992.

49. Fam, A. G., Gordon, D. A., Sarkozi, J., et al.: Neurologic complications associated with gold therapy for rheumatoid arthritis. J. Rheumatol. 11:700, 1984.

50. Jaffe, I. A.: Comparison of the effect of plasmapheresis and penicillamine on the level of circulating rheumatoid factor. Ann. Rheum. Dis. 22:71, 1963.

51. Jaffe, I. A.: Rheumatoid vasculitis: report of a second case treated with penicillamine. Arthritis Rheum. 11:585, 1968.

52. Multi-Center Trial Group: Controlled trial of D-penicillamine in severe rheumatoid arthritis. Lancet 1:275, 1973.

53. Nimni, M. E., and Bavetta, L. A.: Collagen defect induced by penicillamine. Science 150:905, 1965.

54. Harris, E. D. Jr.: Effect of penicillamine on human collagen and its possible application to treatment of scleroderma. Lancet 2:996, 1966.

55. Scott, D. L., Greenwood, A., Bryans, R., et al.: Progressive joint damage during penicillamine therapy for rheumatoid arthritis. Rheumatol. Int. 8:135, 1988.

56. Dixon, A. S. T. J., Pickup, M. E., Lowe, J. R., et al.: Discriminatory indices of response in patients with rheumatoid arthritis treated with D-penicillamine. Ann. Rheum. Dis. 34:416, 1980.

57. Joyce, D. A.: D-Penicillamine pharmacokinetics and action. Agents Actions 23S:197, 1988.

58. Bird, H. A., Le Gallez, P., Dixon, J. S., et al.: A clinical and biochemical assessment of a nonthiol ACE inhibitor (pentopril; CGS-13945) in active rheumatoid arthritis. J. Rheumatol. 17:603, 1990.

59. Matsubara, T., and Hirohata, K.: Suppression of human fibroblast proliferation by D-penicillamine and copper sulfate in vitro. Arthritis Rheum. 31:964, 1988.

60. Kay, A.: Myelotoxicity of D-penicillamine. Ann. Rheum. Dis. 38:232, 1979.

32

Methotrexate

The use of oral methotrexate in a low dose given once weekly has become the mainstay of therapy for active and sustained rheumatoid arthritis. There are a number of reasons for this:

- Patients are more likely to be taking methotrexate from 2 to 5 years after it is first prescribed than any second-line or cytotoxic/immunosuppressive drug.
- It acts relatively quickly after being initiated, often within several weeks.
- Methotrexate is inexpensive, and monitoring for routine toxicity is less expensive than for gold, D-penicillamine, or other cytotoxic drugs.
- Most important, it appears to have genuine efficacy.

CLINICAL USE

Physicians first used the folic acid antagonist aminopterin for treatment of rheumatoid arthritis in 1951, having noted amelioration of joint symptoms when the drug was used for severe psoriasis. The more stable and better tolerated *N*-10-methylaminopterin, or methotrexate, was introduced in low-dose treatment regimens for rheumatoid arthritis. By ''low dose'' is meant weekly doses of 7.5 to 20 mg by mouth. Doses greater than 20 mg/week are administered parenterally to gain better bioavailability.

In the late 1970s, reports of efficacy of methotrexate with an acceptable safety profile in rheumatoid patients began to appear. Four randomized, short-term, placebo-controlled studies were published.[1-4] Analysis of these four trials showed the following[5]:

- Joint pain and swelling improved in 25 per cent of treated patients
- Morning stiffness improved 46 per cent on average in treated patients
- The ESR fell by 15 per cent on average in treated patients

Additional trials have shown improvement and a satisfactory tolerance of the drug by most patients over more than 4 years. Willkens and Watson studied 67 patients for up to 10 years.[6] Although 16 patients did not respond to therapy, 49 had demonstrable benefit. In a prospective study designed to study the effects of methotrexate on liver function and histology,[7] clinical improvement was noted in the joint count, morning stiffness, grip strength, and walking time in assessments of both physicians and patients. Improvement often began within a month after beginning therapy and was sustained over more than 2 years. In an extension of the study,[8] after a mean of 53 months of therapy, 25 of 29 patients remained on therapy. The overall efficacy was good and side effects were minimal.

Weinblatt and colleagues studied 26 patients in an open study[9,10] (Weinblatt et al., Abstract 675) first evaluated at 36 weeks. The oral dose was no more than 15 mg/week. Patients had withdrawn from the study for the following reasons: (1) one died after open heart surgery, (2) eight failed to, or did not want to, adhere to protocol, and (3) one had no efficacy from methotrexate. As in other studies, the maximal effect was noted after 6 months. Sixty per cent of patients had improvement in joint counts. In 14 patients taking prednisone at baseline, reduction from a mean of 7.1 to 2.9 mg/day was possible. Radiographic analyses showed worsening in six, no change in three, and a decrease in size of erosions but continued loss in joint space in five. Adverse side effects were noted in 62 per cent, but toxicity was not the reason for withdrawal from the study for any patient. An increase in the size of rheumatoid nodules was seen in three patients. Liver biopsies of 17 patients at 24 months showed no evidence of fibrosis or cirrhosis in any sample. After 45 months of therapy in this same cohort (16 remained in the study), sustained improvement continued[11] after a mean cumulative dose of 2.1 g. One patient biopsied had mild fibrosis in the liver. This study, the longest prospective study of any disease-modifying antirheumatic drug, has been completed after 11 years of treatment (Weinblatt et al., Abstract 675). Of the 26 patients enrolled in 1983, 10 still remained on methotrexate (mean dose, 10 mg/week) and a significant improvement in function still was present.

TABLE 32–1. Toxicities Requiring Cessation of Treatment in a Long-Term Study of Methotrexate

SIDE EFFECT	NO. OF PATIENTS
Gastrointestinal system	32
Oral ulceration	10
Intractable nausea	22
Pneumonitis	3*
Hematologic toxicity	12†
Pancytopenia	9
Anemia	1
Thrombocytopenia	1
Anemia and thrombocytopenia	1
Elevated transaminase	7
Miscellaneous (not serious)	5

Data from Buchbinder et al.[14]

* One patient also had pancytopenia and died from a *Pneumocystis carinii* infection.

† Eleven of the 12 had complete resolution of hematologic indices when methotrexate was removed and folinic acid added.

A total of 123 patients who had never had gold therapy were enrolled in a 5-year prospective study of methotrexate.[12] An impressive and sustained improvement compared with baseline was noted in all clinical disease variables, functional status, and ESR. Thirty-six per cent withdrew during the study, 7 per cent for lack of efficacy and 7 per cent as a result of adverse experiences. At 5 years, 64 per cent of patients were still taking methotrexate. In another study,[13] 30 per cent continued to take methotrexate after 10 years.

Results in community practices with methotrexate are not quite as encouraging as those from university clinics but are still positive. In a life table analysis of 587 patients in eight rheumatologic practices in Australia, 75 per cent of patients assessed 70 months from commencement of therapy were still taking methotrexate.[14] Older patients were three times more likely to terminate the drug because of toxicity than younger ones. The specific toxicities requiring cessation of therapy are listed in Table 32–1. Most toxicity occurred within the first 2 to 3 years of therapy.

Other studies have, in general, confirmed these observations. Particularly encouraging is the high percentage of patients remaining in ongoing methotrexate studies (Fig. 32–1).[10] This tolerance and efficacy of methotrexate is in marked contrast to experience with most of the other antirheumatic drugs used.

There is histologic evidence, as well, to support the efficacy of methotrexate. Compared with biopsies from 12 patients taking naproxen, synovial samples from 11 patients on methotrexate had fewer $CD3^+$, $CD4^+$, and $HLA-DR^+$ cells, a finding that correlated with improvements in clinical criteria.[15]

It is not clear why some patients given methotrexate have no beneficial response at all. One reason might be a diminished bioavailability of the drug; a high interindividual variability of the half-life of the drug in plasma has been noted.[16]

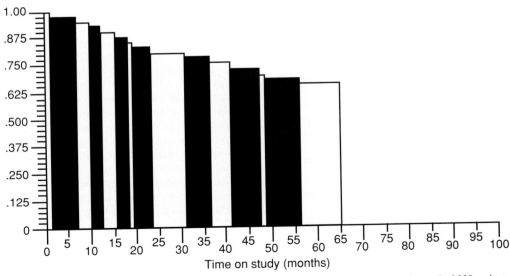

FIGURE 32–1. Proportion of patients projected to remain in ongoing methotrexate studies. A total of 230 patients enrolled in the study. Life table analysis was performed. (From Weinblatt, M. E. and Maier, A. L.: Longterm experience with low dose weekly methotrexate in rheumatoid arthritis. J. Rheumatol. 17[suppl. 22]:33, 1990. Used by permission.)

The relative success of methotrexate in diminishing evidence for inflammation in patients with rheumatoid arthritis has renewed interest of investigators in examining whether radiographic stability or improvement could be associated with methotrexate therapy. There is little agreement among different studies, but the data may be confounded by the differences in time after onset of rheumatoid arthritis that the methotrexate was started. It has been emphasized throughout this book that irreversible destruction of articular cartilage (and, probably, bone) begins within 1 year of the onset of synovitis, and therefore studies that enroll patients much after a year or two of disease onset have little hope of reversing or stabilizing loss of cartilage. For example, one study treated 41 patients with severe and longstanding rheumatoid arthritis (mean duration: 12.9 years). After 24 months, 84 per cent had deterioration of radiographic indices (the Larsen score).[17] In another study, radiologic progression was less in patients treated with methotrexate than in those treated with gold.[18] In this group of 31 patients, the mean duration of disease at baseline was 8.1 years, with a range of 1 to 26 years. Methotrexate was started because the patients had failed to respond to gold. Methotrexate also appears to be superior to azathioprine in its capability to retard appearance of new erosions, and this has correlated with improvement in joint scores.[19] Radiologic "stabilization" after 48 weeks of therapy was recorded in 10 per cent of the azathioprine group and 29 per cent of those taking methotrexate. A trend toward a slowing of radiographic progression in patients treated with methotrexate was noted in the Cooperating Clinics study comparing methotrexate and auranofin.[20]

In a meta-analysis of 11 studies including a total of 558 patients, each of whom had quantitation of bone erosions at joint margins, methotrexate-treated patients had slower rates of disease progression than those treated with azathioprine, but not slower than those treated with gold salts.[21] The problem in this analysis, consistent with the hypothesis that early treatment is the key to cartilage protection, is that some methotrexate- and gold-treated patients had been ill at baseline for less than 2 years, whereas no azathioprine-treated patient had rheumatoid arthritis for less than 8.7 years at the start of therapy. The challenge is to have a cohort of methotrexate-treated and "other" patients enrolled in a radiographic progression study after less than 1 year of active disease.

Refinements of our understanding of the use of methotrexate include the following:

- The clinical response is somewhat dose dependent.

- Folic acid, 1 mg each day, may diminish mucocutaneous side effects of methotrexate without diminishing efficacy of the therapy.

- There is mild but definite renal toxicity of methotrexate, particularly when given with NSAIDs.

- Some patients can continue to benefit from methotrexate by taking the medication on an every-other-week basis.

- In patients treated with high-dose regimens of methotrexate for malignant disease, there appears to be a definite osteopenia induced by the therapy. The mechanism for this, explored in mouse bone cells, appears to be an inability of osteoblasts exposed to low-dose methotrexate to synthesize and calcify matrix, perhaps through a defective production of osteocalcin.[22] The limited data on patients receiving low-dose regimens are contradictory. One report suggests that methotrexate can induce low BMD,[23] whereas another found no evidence for methotrexate-induced osteopenia (West et al., Abstract 955).

SIDE EFFECTS AND TOXICITY

Despite perceptions that low-dose therapy with methotrexate has relatively few complications, toxicity was the most frequent reason for discontinuing the drug in a 10-year study of 152 patients.[13] Nevertheless, methotrexate-treated patients had no higher mortality than other cohorts of rheumatoid patients. Infection was the major complication and cause of excess death, while cirrhosis of the liver and cancer occurred no more than expected in the general rheumatoid population not treated with immunosuppression.

Fibrosis in the Liver

One of the benefits of methotrexate to both physician and patient is that the most common side effects, gastrointestinal distress and mouth soreness, rarely are incapacitating or lead to the need for extensive laboratory testing or hospitalization. This is in contrast to gold and D-penicillamine use, which requires frequent monitoring of peripheral blood counts and urinalyses. It seems conclusive that, if patients are willing to forego alcohol, the risk of significant or progressive fibrosis in the liver is small, and that of actual cirrhosis rare. It has been calculated that the risk of serious liver disease among rheumatoid patients is less than 1:1,000 cases after 5 years of treatment.[24] The increased risk of progressive histologic change is 2.5 to 5 times greater in patients with "heavy" use of alcohol who also take methotrexate,[21] but data on heavy alcohol users who are not taking methotrexate are not available. A meta-analysis of 15 studies[21] suggests that 1 in 5 patients who take a cumulative dose of at least 3 g of methotrexate will experience progression of at least one grade on liver biopsy, and about 1 in 35 will experience advanced changes.

Using a decision-analytic model to assess the cost and benefit associated with using liver biopsy to detect methotrexate-induced liver disease in rheumatoid arthritis patients, it has been demonstrated that liver biopsy after 5 years of methotrexate treatment results in a minimal increase in life expectancy, and that the cost for all patients eligible to receive the drug—$1,891,830—is extremely high.[25]

The most extensive data on liver histopathology in methotrexate-treated patients have been gathered on 27 patients on methotrexate who were subjected to a mean of 6.3 liver biopsies per patient over a mean follow-up period of 8.2 years.[26] The following observations were made on these patients and biopsies:

- No progression toward cirrhosis was found in patients whose methotrexate dose each week was altered as a function of serum albumin and aspartate aminotransferase (if aspartate aminotransferase levels become abnormal, the methotrexate dose should be lowered by 2.5 mg/week).
- Collagen deposition in the perisinusoidal space of Disse does not progress.
- Other changes of liver pathology were never significant.

It is appropriate to agree with the authors that methotrexate ''is the most effective drug in current use for rheumatoid arthritis'' when prescribed with appropriate monitoring and pacts of agreement about the importance of alcohol avoidance.[26]

Recommendations for monitoring patients with psoriasis who are receiving methotrexate include a liver biopsy after a cumulative dose of 1.5 g and thereafter at 1.0 to 1.5-g intervals. For obscure reasons, liver disease in psoriatic patients exposed to methotrexate is more common than it is in patients with rheumatoid arthritis. Therefore, the ACR recommendations do not make biopsy routine.[27] These recommendations are summarized in Table 32–2.[28] A dermatologist and rheumatologist treating a patient with psoriatic arthritis must reach a common view about the monitoring of therapy! (See the box on page 383.)

Pulmonary Complications

Pneumonitis can be expected to occur in 2 to 5 per cent of patients taking low doses of methotrex-

TABLE 32–2. Recommendations for Monitoring Hepatic Toxicity in Patients with Rheumatoid Arthritis (RA) Receiving Methotrexate

A. Baseline
  1. Tests for all patients
    a. Liver blood tests (aspartate aminotransferase [AST], alananine aminotransferase [ALT], alkaline phosphatase, albumin, bilirubin), hepatitis B and C serological studies
    b. Other standard tests, including complete cell count and serum creatinine
  2. Pretreatment liver biopsy (Menghini suction-type needle) only for patients with:
    a. Prior excessive alcohol consumption
    b. Persistently abnormal baseline AST values
    c. Chronic hepatitis B or C infection
B. Monitor AST, ATL, albumin at 4–8 week intervals
C. Perform liver biopsy if:
  1. Five of nine determinations of AST within a given 12 month interval (six of 12 if tests are performed monthly) are abnormal (defined as an increase above the upper limit of normal)
  2. There is a decrease in serum albumin below the normal range (in the setting of well controlled RA)
D. If results of liver biopsy are:
  3. Roenigk grade I, II, or IIA, resume methotrexate and monitor as in B, C1, and C2 above
  4. Roenigk grade IIIB or IV, discontinue methotrexate
E. Discontinue methotrexate in patients with persistent liver test abnormalities, as defined in C1 and C2 above, or who refuse liver biopsy

From Hassan, W.: Methotrexate and liver toxicity: role of surveillance liver biopsy. Conflict between guidelines for rheumatologists and dermatologists. Ann. Rheum. Dis. 55:273, 1996. Used by permission.

ate for rheumatoid arthritis.[31] Diagnosis of definite methotrexate pneumonitis requiers the presence of at least six of the nine criteria listed in Table 32–3.[32]

The pathology suggests that methotrexate pneumonitis is a hypersensitivity reaction, although arguments have been put forth that it is idiosyncratic (perhaps involving a specific cellular immune response in some individuals).[33] Interstitial pneumonitis and bronchiolitis are found in tissue samples. In fluid recovered from bronchoalveolar lavage, lymphocytes and eosinophils are present. The lung pathology is not prevented by folinic acid treatment, and it may occur after a single first dose of methotrexate. In peripheral blood, moderate leukocytosis and eosinophilia may be present.

These patients present with cough and sometimes fever. The symptoms are usually nonspecific, resembling at first a viral upper respiratory infection. The most important entity to rule out is

Preventing Methotrexate-Associated Fibrosis in the Liver

Physicians also should realize that not only does the combination of salicylates and methotrexate greatly increase the frequency of abnormal liver enzyme values, but the addition of hydroxychloroquine to a regimen of either methotrexate or salicylates can possibly eliminate serum transaminase abnormalities.[29] This effect may be related to the high concentrations of the antimalarial compounds in the liver or, alternatively, to a decrease or change in bioavailability.[30] Before advocating addition of hydroxychloroquine to methotrexate if transaminases rise beyond mild elevations in early days following the weekly methotrexate dose, a prospective evaluation of methotrexate along with hydroxychloroquine in the context of liver function must be performed.

In contrast, another second-line drug used in treatment of rheumatoid arthritis, sulfasalazine, is also an inhibitor of folate-dependent enzymes that methotrexate inhibits. Therefore, it is possible that combination therapy with methotrexate and sulfasalazine (see Chapter 34) may produce additive or synergistic toxicity.

TABLE 32–3. Criteria for Diagnosis of Methotrexate Pneumonitis

1	Acute onset of shortness of breath
2	Fever $> 38.0°C$
3	Tachypnea ≥ 28/min and a nonproductive cough
4	Radiological evidence of pulmonary interstitial or alveolar infiltrates
5	White cell count $\leq 15.0 \times 10^9$/l
6	Negative blood and sputum cultures (obligatory)
7	Pulmonary function tests demonstrating restrictive pulmonary function with decreased diffusion capacities
8	$pO_2 < 55$ mm Hg on room air at time of admission
9	Histopathology consistent with bronchitis or interstitial pneumonitis
Definite	6 or more criteria present
Probable	5 of 9 present
Possible	4 of 9 present

From Searles, G., and McKendry, R. J. R.: Methotrexate pneumonitis in rheumatoid arthritis: potential risk factors. Four case reports and a review of the literature. J. Rheumatol. 14:1164, 1987. Used by permission.

infection with *Pneumocystis carinii* because this organism is increasingly found among immunocompromised patients with rheumatic disease, and the clinical characteristics, dominated by an acute onset of dyspnea and fever in the setting of bilateral interstitial infiltrates on radiographs, are the same for both. If there is doubt about ruling out *P. carinii* infection, bronchoscopy and transbronchial biopsy should be done immediately. Many clinicians recommend that all patients being started on methotrexate also be given standard prophylaxis against *P. carinii*.

An interstitial pneumonia caused by cytomegalovirus in a patient treated with 10 to 15 mg/week (total dose, 230 mg) has been described that precisely mimicked the hypersensitivity reaction.[34]

Treatment of presumed methotrexate pneumonitis, even while waiting for special stains, cultures, or tissue sections from bronchoscopic biopsy, should be glucocorticoids, 1 to 1.5 mg/kg/day of prednisone equivalence, given intravenously or by mouth. No delay is necessary, because glucocorticoids are currently used routinely in *P. carinii* infections of the lung. Empirical antibiotic treatment can be used until infectious causes are ruled out.

Because methotrexate pneumonitis can progress rapidly to an obliterative bronchiolitis and respiratory distress syndromes, and because therapy with glucocorticoids is so effective in halting progression and allowing resolution of this process, the patient being started on methotrexate should have the prescribing physician's home phone or pager number, and be urged to call immediately if cough, fever, or "flu" symptoms appear.

There are increasing reports of *P. carinii* pneumonitis appearing in patients being treated with low-dose weekly methotrexate. The physician directing therapy must decide for each patient whether or not to recommend prophylaxis with trimethoprim/sulfamethoxazole (TMP/SMX) or pentamadine against this organism. More and more, this is accepted therapy. Weighing in against prophylaxis is the potential toxicity of the prophylactic drugs, including the specter of pancytopenia.

Malignant Transformation

When methotrexate was first used in patients with rheumatoid arthritis, there was optimism that there was little risk of inducing malignancies similar to those that evolve in patients treated with azathioprine or cyclophosphamide.[7,35] However, it appears that methotrexate will not escape culpability in generating malignant change. Clear-cut examples are development of lymphomas associated with EBV that occur during methotrexate therapy for rheumatoid arthritis, some of which are reversible when the drug is removed.[36] Indeed, patients with rheumatoid arthritis being treated with methotrexate who develop an EBV-associated lymphoproliferative disorder deserve a trial of discontinuation of immunosuppression before chemotherapy is considered.[37] However, lymphomas not associated with EBV have been described in methotrexate-treated patients as well (Davies et al., Abstract 312). A case of a large-cell lymphoma of the choroid in the eye in a patient on methotrexate for rheumatoid arthritis also has been reported.[38] It is possible that patients with rheumatoid arthritis who have an abnormally elevated frequency of EBV-infected lymphocytes and in whom there appears to be a defect in the ability of T cells to suppress proliferation of these cells[39] have a predisposition for such malignant transformation.

The largest review of this issue has been the retrospective analysis of 16,263 patients who registered at the Mayo Clinic with rheumatoid arthritis from 1976 through 1992 compared with patients registered during the same period with a hematologic malignancy. Thirty-nine patients who had been treated with a disease-modifying drug subsequently developed a hematologic malignancy; 12 had been given methotrexate. The characteristics of those who received methotrexate, including the type of malignancy, did not differ from those of patients who received other disease-modifying antirheumatic drugs.[40]

The risk of malignancy is real, but it is a very small risk, so small that, with our current state of knowledge, it will rarely influence decisions about whether and when to begin methotrexate therapy in rheumatoid arthritis.

Pancytopenia

Severe, and occasionally fatal, pancytopenia may occur in up to 7 in 100,000 patients each year of those receiving low-dose weekly methotrexate. In a MEDLINE literature search combined with personal experience, 70 such cases were found.[41] Twelve resulted in death; of these, 10 had renal impairment as a predisposing factor, although the lesion is probably multifactorial, including advanced age, displacement of methotrexate from plasma proteins, competition with NSAIDs for tubular excretion, concomitant antibiotic therapy (e.g., TMP/SMX), and hidden alcohol intake.

Dihydrofolate Reductase Inhibition

One major effect of methotrexate is to inhibit dihydrofolate reductase. Using 1 mg/day supple-

mentation with folic acid, the fully oxidized form of the vitamin, a 50 per cent decrease in mouth ulcers without a decrease in efficacy was observed.[42] Although there have been reports that use of folinic acid (leucovorin, the form of folate used for toxicity rescue in cancer patients treated with very large doses of the drug) blocked efficacy of methotrexate in rheumatoid arthritis,[43] it appears from a multicenter, randomized, double-blind, placebo-controlled trial that this does not happen.[44] In addition to giving physicians a wider window of dose range for methotrexate, these data indicate that the mechanism of action of methotrexate in rheumatoid arthritis may be other than, or in addition to, inhibition of dihydrofolate reductase.

Alternate Dosing to Reduce Toxicity

Experience with gold salts has indicated that, when a patient responds well to the drug, the injections can often be given biweekly or, in some cases, monthly, without losing efficacy. A similar rationale was used in a study of methotrexate given every other week in hopes of maintaining efficacy while reducing toxicity.[45] In this series, 12 of 23 patients receiving every-other-week therapy were able to complete 6 months of this treatment without experiencing a disease flare, while the other 11 withdrew early because of a flare of disease. It is not known whether prompt resumption of weekly treatment in such patients would restore efficacy.

MECHANISMS OF ACTION OF METHOTREXATE IN RHEUMATOID ARTHRITIS

Like gold and D-penicillamine, low-dose methotrexate was first used empirically, without a defined molecular rationale. This is much different from use of drugs such as captopril that were custom-designed to inhibit a specific enzyme. Therefore, investigators have placed methotrexate into multiple types of assays searching for positive effects of the drug. It is not surprising, perhaps, that many have been found, including

- Slight reduction in IgM rheumatoid factor in serum.[46]
- A decreased capacity of ex vivo stimulated PMN leukocytes to produce LTB_4 from exogenous arachidonic acid[47,48] by an effect upon the 5-lipoxygenase enzyme. However, these data were not confirmed in another study.[49]

- Inhibition of neutrophil chemotaxis, possibly related to the suppression of LTB_4 and of endothelial cell proliferation.

- Inhibition of clonal growth of T and B cells in vitro, but not adherent synovial cells. The mechanism appears to be directly related to inhibition of de novo purine synthesis in the lymphocytes, whereas synovial cells may utilize the salvage pathway of purine synthesis for synthesis of nucleotides.[50]

- Inhibition of endothelial cell proliferation[51] and neovascularization.

- A decrease in the gene expression of mRNA levels for collagenase in biopsies of synovium from methotrexate-treated patients compared with pretreatment biopsies. Expression of mRNA for neither collagenase inhibitor (TIMP-1) nor the protease stromelysin was affected. Because collagenase expression by cultured fibroblasts in vitro exposed to methotrexate was not diminished, it was concluded that the effect of methotrexate was on the cytokines that regulate synovial collagenase biosynthesis.[52]

- A decrease in the number of leukocytes, the number and proportion of neutrophils, and concentrations of IL-1β in synovial fluid. This may reflect a decrease in the migration of leukocytes into the inflamed synovium.[53]

- Peripheral blood mononuclear cells from patients treated effectively with low-dose methotrexate[54] exhibit the following activities that are different from pretreatment assay: stimulation of IL-1ra and soluble TNFR, increase of IL-1ra–IL-1β ratio, and inhibition of IL-8 production.

Whether any or all of these effects have relevance to the benefit produced by low-dose methotrexate in rheumatoid patients is, of course, unknown. There are data on a basic mechanism of methotrexate within cells that may be relevant to each and all of the purported actions of the drug that have been described experimentally. The therapeutic benefit may be linked to the capacity of methotrexate to promote the release of adenosine from cells. The rationale and support for this hypothesis, are discussed in the next section.

Methotrexate and the Anti-inflammatory Effects of Adenosine

New understanding of the metabolism of methotrexate and of the biologic effects of its metabolites has generated good support for the hypothesis that methotrexate acts by increasing adenosine release from cells, and that subsequent binding of adenosine to A_2 receptors initiates multiple anti-inflammatory and antiproliferative effects in patients.

As shown in Figure 32–2, methotrexate, after rapid uptake by cells, is metabolized to a family of polyglutamated derivatives that persist intracellularly. These MTX_{GLU} compounds are probably the biologically active forms of the drug. MTX_{GLU} inhibits dihydrofolate reductase, but perhaps more important is its ability to inhibit metabolism of an important intermediate of de novo purine biosynthesis, AICARibotide, by inhibition of AICARibotide transformylase. Thus, AICARibotide accumulates in cells, and it has been shown that this enhances synthesis and release of adenosine by human fibroblasts into the extracellular space.[55,56]

Through binding to A_2 receptors on cells, adenosine initiates the following functions in several systems:

- Inhibition of neutrophil adhesion to connective tissue cells and down-regulation of several functions (e.g., the ability to generate free radicals of oxygen)

- In lymphocyte function, decrease in proliferative capacity and increased suppressor cell function

- In macrophage/monocyte function, decreased TNF secretion and decrease in superoxide generation.

- Protection of endothelial cells from damage by activated neutrophils

- Inhibition of neutrophil accumulation at inflamed sites[56]

- Selective down-regulation of collagen gene expression (Boyle, et al., Abstract 1142)

In addition to its relationship to effects of methotrexate, adenosine may mediate the anti-inflammatory effects of sulfasalazine as well. The proposed mechanism is similar: increasing intracellular AICAR (see Fig. 32–2), which enhances adenosine release at inflammatory sites (Gadangi, et al., Abstract 1308).

Pharmacologic use of adenosine is limited by its effects on the cardiovascular system as well as by its half-life in plasma of several seconds. Other strategies to enhance adenosine release at inflamed sites include clinical trials with AICAR and inhibitors of adenosine deaminase or adenosine kinase.

A specific inhibitor of adenosine kinase (GP-1-515) has been developed that does not inhibit adenosine deaminase, nor does it bind to adenosine receptors (A_1 or A_2). Because adenosine is rapidly taken up by cells and phosphorylated by adenosine kinase, inhibition of this enzyme increases intracellular adenosine concentrations (Fig. 32–3). In ex-

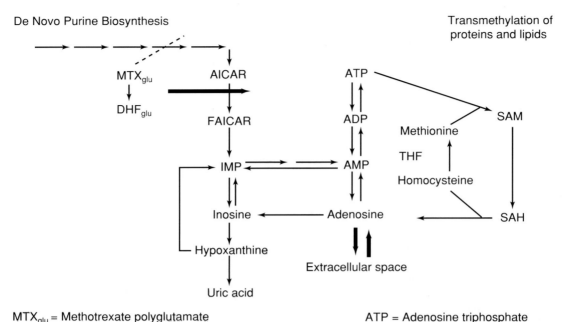

De Novo Purine Biosynthesis

Transmethylation of proteins and lipids

MTX$_{glu}$ = Methotrexate polyglutamate
DHF$_{glu}$ = Dihydrofolate polyglutamate
AICAR = Aminoimidazolecarboxamidoribonucleotide
FAICAR = Formylaminoimidazolecarboxamidoribonucleotide
IMP = Inosine monophosphate

ATP = Adenosine triphosphate
ADP = Adenosine diphosphate
AMP = Adenosine monophosphate
SAM = S-adenosylimethionine
SAH = S-adenosylhomocysteine
THF = Tetrahydrofolate (reduced folate)

FIGURE 32–2. Effects of methotrexate on purine biosynthesis. Polyglutamated derivatives of methotrexate promote release of adenosine from fibroblasts by inhibiting metabolism of a purine biosynthesis intermediate (AICARibotide). (From Cronstein, B. N., Eberle, M. A., Gruber, H. E., et al.: Methotrexate inhibits neutrophil function by stimulating adenosine release from connective tissue cells. Proc. Natl. Acad. Sci. U.S.A. 88:2441, 1991. Used by permission.)

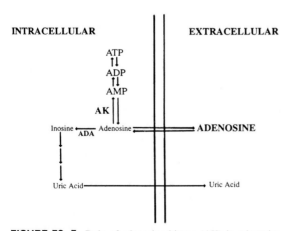

FIGURE 32–3. Role of adenosine kinase (AK) in adenosine metabolism. ADA, adenosine deaminase. (From Cronstein, B. N., Naime, D., and Firestein, G.: The anti-inflammatory effects of an adenosine kinase inhibitor are mediated by adenosine. Arthritis Rheum. 38:1040, 1995. Used by permission.)

perimental models of arthritis, anti-inflammatory activity has proved to be mediated by adenosine.[57]

Specific blockade of adenosine receptors is a goal, and a worthy one, for the future. Methotrexate may be one of the first agents that has as its major anti-inflammatory mechanism the enhancement of adenosine production. Mechanisms of action aside, methotrexate can be considered as a NSAID when given in low doses on a weekly basis to rheumatoid patients.[56]

LEFLUNOMIDE: A DRUG SIMILAR TO METHOTREXATE

Leflunomide is an ixoxazole drug with immunosuppressive and antiproliferative properties. It inhibits the pyrimidine rather than the purine synthesis pathway in rapidly dividing cells. It has the potential for liver toxicity similar to methotrexate, but patients receiving it have not developed signs or symptoms suggestive of interstitial pneumonitis.

In a randomized and placebo-controlled trial of leflunomide in 402 patients with rheumatoid arthritis,[58] the drug was effective at the $p < 0.05$ level versus placebo. As in many studies, there was a substantial placebo effect.

REFERENCES

1. Williams, H., Willkens, R. F., Samuelson, C. O. Jr., et al.: Comparison of low dose oral pulse methotrexate and placebo in the treatment of rheumatoid arthritis: a controlled clinical trial. Arthritis Rheum. 28:721, 1985.
2. Weinblatt, M. E., Coblyn, J. S., Fox, D. A., et al.: Efficacy of low dose methotrexate in rheumatoid arthritis. N. Engl. J. Med. 312:818, 1985.
3. Andersen, P. A., West, S. G., O'Dell, J. R., et al.: Weekly pulse methotrexate in rheumatoid arthritis: clinical and immunologic effects in a randomized double blind study. Ann. Intern. Med. 103:489, 1985.
4. Thompson, R. N., Watts, C., Edelman, J., et al.: A controlled two center trial of parenteral methotrexate therapy for refractory rheumatoid arthritis. J. Rheumatol. 11:760, 1984.
5. Tugwell, P., Bennett, K., and Gent, M.: Methotrexate in rheumatoid arthritis: indications, contraindications, efficacy and safety. Ann. Intern. Med. 197:358, 1987.
6. Willkens, R. F., and Watson, M. A.: Methotrexate: a perspective of its use in the treatment of rheumatic disease. J. Lab. Clin. Med. 100:314, 1982.
7. Kremer, J. M., and Lee, J. K.: The safety and efficacy of the use of methotrexate in long-term therapy for rheumatoid arthritis. Arthritis Rheum. 29:822, 1986.
8. Kremer, J. M., and Lee, J. K.: A long term prospective study of the use of methotrexate in rheumatoid arthritis, update after a mean of fifty-three months. Arthritis Rheum. 31:577, 1988.

After a mean of 53 months, 25 of 29 patients still were in the study. The average weekly dose of methotrexate was 14.6 mg. Nine of 21 patients were able to discontinue prednisone, and all had been able to decrease their daily dose. Other changes included

- Painful joints decreased from 15 to 7 on average per patient
- Swollen joints decreased from 17 to 12 on average per patient
- Morning stiffness decreased from 162 to 63 minutes
- Hemoglobin values increased and ESR decreased
- Eight of 22 patients had deterioration of radiographic status

Toxicity was predictable; gastrointestinal intolerance was most common, including soreness of the mouth. Leukopenia did not require discontinuation of therapy.

9. Weinblatt, M. E., Trentham, D. E., Fraser, P. A., et al.: Long term prospective trial of low dose methotrexate in rheumatoid arthritis. Arthritis Rheum. 31:167, 1988.
10. Weinblatt, M. E., and Maier, A. L.: Longterm experience with low dose weekly methotrexate in rheumatoid arthritis. J. Rheumatol. 17(suppl. 22):33, 1990.
11. Weinblatt, M. E., Fraser, P. A., Holdsworth, D. E., et al.: Long term prospective study of methotrexate in rheumatoid arthritis: 45 month update [Abstract]. Arthritis Rheum. 31:S115, 1988.
12. Weinblatt, M. E., Kaplan, H., and Germain, B. F.: Metho-

trexate in rheumatoid arthritis. Arthritis Rheum. 37:1492, 1994.
13. Alarcón, G. S., Tracy, I. C., Strand, G. M., et al.: Survival and drug discontinuation analyses in a large cohort of methotrexate treated rheumatoid arthritis patients. Ann. Rheum. Dis. 54:708, 1995.
14. Buchbinder, R., Hall, S., Sambrook, P. N., et al.: Methotrexate therapy in rheumatoid arthritis: a life table review of 587 patients treated in community practice. J. Rheumatol. 20:639, 1993.

Toxicity sufficient for withdrawal of methotrexate was as shown in Table 32–1 (see text)

15. Balsa, A., Gamallo, C., Martín-Mola, E., et al.: Histologic changes in rheumatoid synovitis induced by naproxen and methotrexate. J. Rheumatol. 20:9, 1993.
16. Lebbe, C., Beyeler, C., Gerber, N. J., et al.: Interindividual variability of the bioavailability of low dose methotrexate after oral administration in rheumatoid arthritis. Ann. Rheum. Dis. 53:475, 1994.
17. Sany, J., Kaliski, S., Couret, M., et al.: Radiologic progression during intramuscular methotrexate treatment of rheumatoid arthritis. J. Rheumatol. 17:1636, 1990.
18. Rau, R., Herborn, G., Karger, T., et al.: Retardation of radiologic progression in rheumatoid arthritis with methotrexate therapy: a controlled study. Arthritis Rheum. 34:1236, 1991.
19. Jeurissen, M. E. C., Boerbooms, A. M. T., van de Putte, L. B. A., et al.: Influence of methotrexate and azathioprine on radiologic progression in rheumatoid arthritis: a randomized, double-blind study. Ann. Intern. Med. 114:999, 1991.
20. López-Méndez, A., Daniel, W. W., and Reading, J. C.: Radiographic assessment of disease progression in rheumatoid arthritis patients enrolled in the Cooperative Systematic Studies of the Rheumatic Diseases program randomized clinical trial of methotrexate, auranofin, or a combination of the two. Arthritis Rheum. 36:1364, 1993.
21. Alarcón, G. S., López-Méndez, A., Walter, J., et al.: Radiographic evidence of disease progression in methotrexate treated and nonmethotrexate disease modifying antirheumatic drug treated rheumatoid arthritis patients: a meta-analysis. J. Rheumatol. 19:1868, 1992.
22. May, K. P., Mercill, D., McDermott, M. T., and West, S. G.: The effect of methotrexate on mouse bone cells in culture. Arthritis Rheum. 39:489, 1996.
23. Preston, S. J., Diamond, T., Scott, A., et al.: Methotrexate osteopathy in rheumatic disease. Ann. Rheum. Dis. 52:582, 1993.
24. Walker, A. M., Funch, D., Dreyer, N. A., et al.: Determinants of serious liver disease among patients receiving low-dose methotrexate for rheumatoid arthritis. Arthritis Rheum. 36:329, 1993.
25. Bergquist, S. R., Felson, D. T., Prashker, M. J., et al.: The cost-effectiveness of liver biopsy in rheumatoid patients treated with methotrexate. Arthritis Rheum. 38:326, 1995.
26. Kremer, J. M., Kaye, G. I., Kaye, N. W., et al.: Light and electron microscopic analysis of sequential liver biopsy samples from rheumatoid arthritis patients receiving long-term methotrexate therapy. Arthritis Rheum. 38:1194, 1995.
27. Kremer, J. M., Alacron, G. S., Lightfoot, R. W., et al.: Methotrexate for rheumatoid arthritis: suggested guidelines for monitoring liver toxicity. Arthritis Rheum. 37:316, 1994.
28. Hassan, W.: Methotrexate and liver toxicity: role of surveillance liver biopsy. Conflict between guidelines for

rheumatologists and dermatologists. Ann. Rheum. Dis. 55:273, 1996.

29. Fries, J. F., Singh, G., Lenert, L., et al.: Aspirin, hydroxychloroquine, and hepatic enzyme abnormalities with methotrexate in rheumatoid arthritis. Arthritis Rheum. 33:1611, 1990.

30. MacKenzie, A. H.: Pharmacologic actions of 4-aminoquinoline compounds. Am. J. Med. 75(suppl.):5, 1983.

31. Carroll, G. J., Thomas, R., Phatouros, C. C., et al.: Incidence, prevalence and possible risk factors for pneumonitis in patients with rheumatoid arthritis receiving methotrexate. J. Rheumatol. 21:51, 1994.

In a survey from Western Australia, 10 definite cases of methotrexate pneumonitis were found. It was concluded that pre-existing lung disease may confer increased risk, but no difference was observed between methotrexate pneumonitis and rheumatoid factor, duration of rheumatoid arthritis, use of tobacco, dose of methotrexate, serum creatinine, or treatment with aspirin, other NSAIDs, or prednisolone.

32. Searles, G., and McKendry, R. J. R.: Methotrexate pneumonitis in rheumatoid arthritis: potential risk factors. Four case reports and a review of the literature. J. Rheumatol. 14:1164, 1987.

33. Barrera, P., Laan, R. F. J. M., van Riel, P. L. C. M., et al.: Methotrexate-related pulmonary complications in rheumatoid arthritis. Ann. Rheum. Dis. 53:434, 1994.

34. Aglas, F., Rainer, F., Hermann, J., et al.: Interstitial pneumonia due to cytomegalovirus following low-dose methotrexate treatment for rheumatoid arthritis. Arthritis Rheum. 38:291, 1995.

35. Hazleman, B.: Incidence of neoplasms in patients with rheumatoid arthritis exposed to different treatment regimens. Am. J. Med. 78(suppl. 1A):39, 1985.

36. Kamel, O. W., van de Rijn, M., Weiss, L. M., et al.: Brief report: reversible lymphomas associated with Epstein-Barr virus occurring during methotrexate therapy for rheumatoid arthritis and dermatomyositis. N. Engl. J. Med. 328:1317, 1993.

In this paper from Stanford, one patient had large-cell lymphoma and the other presented with nodular sclerosing Hodgkin's disease. Both were associated with EBV. In both the tumor regressed after methotrexate was stopped. It is generally accepted that the lack of immune surveillance in these patients allows the proliferation of EBV-transformed B lymphocytes. The process initially is polyclonal. Then, after the most proliferative clone predominates, a monoclonal tumor can be identified.

37. Bachman, T. R., Sawitzke, A. D., Perkins, S. L., et al.: Methotrexate-associated lymphoma in patients with rheumatoid arthritis: report of two cases. Arthritis Rheum. 39: 325, 1996.

38. Zimmer-Galler, I., and Lie, J. T.: Choroidal infiltrates as the initial manifestation of lymphoma in rheumatoid arthritis after treatment with low-dose methotrexate. Mayo Clin. Proc. 69:258, 1994.

39. Depper, J. M., Bluestein, H. G., and Zvaifler, N. J. Impaired regulation of Epstein-Barr virus-induced lymphocyte proliferation in rheumatoid arthritis is due to a T celld efect. J. Immunol. 127:1899, 1981.

40. Moder, K. G., Tefferi, A., Cohen, M. D., et al.: Hematologic malignancies and the use of methotrexate in rheumatoid arthritis: a retrospective study. Am. J. Med. 99:276, 1995.

41. Gutierrez-Ureña, S., Molina, J. F., García, C. O., et al.: Pancytopenia secondary to methotrexate therapy in rheumatoid arthritis. Arthritis Rheum. 39:272, 1996.

42. Morgan, S. L., Baggott, J. E., Vaughn, W. H., et al.: The effect of folic acid supplementation on the toxicity of low-dose methotrexate in patients with rheumatoid arthritis. Arthritis Rheum. 33:9, 1990.

43. Tishler, M., Caspi, D., Fishel, B., et al.: The effects of leucovorin (folinic acid) on methotrexate therapy in rheumatoid arthritis patients. Arthritis Rheum. 31:906, 1988.

44. Shiroky, J. B., Neville, C., Esdaile, J. M., et al.: Low-dose methotrexate with leucovorin (folinic acid) in the management of rheumatoid arthritis: results of a multicenter randomized, double-blind, placebo-controlled trial. Arthritis Rheum. 36:795, 1993.

In this multicenter randomized, double-blind, placebo-controlled trial of leucovorin, 2.5 to 5.0 mg orally, given 24 hours after the single weekly oral dose of methotrexate, patients were evaluated for 52 weeks for disease activity and side effects. Forty-four patients were in the leucovorin arm, and 48 in the placebo group. Seventeen patients who had placebo withdrew because of side effects, whereas only 6 of the leucovorin patients withdrew because of side effects. Clinical variables improved equally in both groups. The adverse reactions necessitating withdrawal were gastrointestinal distress, oral ulcers, transaminase elevations, or combinations of all three. The mean dose of methotrexate was 13.6 mg in the placebo group and 12.0 mg in the leucovorin group.

45. Kremer, J. M., Davies, J. M. S., Rynes, R. I., et al.: Every-other-week methotrexate in patients with rheumatoid arthritis. Arthritis Rheum. 38:601, 1995.

46. Alarcón, G. S., Schrohenloher, R. E., Bartolucci, A. A., et al.: Suppression of rheumatoid factor production by methotrexate in patients with rheumatoid arthritis: evidence for differential influences of therapy and clinical status on IgM and IgA rheumatoid factor expression. Arthritis Rheum. 33:1156, 1990.

47. Leroux, J. L., Damon, M., Chavis, C., et al.: Effects of a single dose of methotrexate on 5- and 12-lipoxygenase products in patients with rheumatoid arthritis. J. Rheumatol. 19:863, 1992.

48. Sperling, R. I., Benincaso, A. I., Anderson, R. J., et al.: Acute and chronic suppression of leukotriene B_4 synthesis *ex vivo* in neutrophils from patients with rheumatoid arthritis beginning treatment with methotrexate. Arthritis Rheum. 35:376, 1992.

49. Hawkes, J. S., Cleland, L. G., Proudman, S. M., et al.: The effect of methotrexate on *ex vivo* lipoxygenase metabolism in neutrophils from patients with rheumatoid arthritis. J. Rheumatol. 21:55, 1994.

50. Nakajima, A., Hakoda, M., Yamanaka, H., et al.: Divergent effects of methotrexate on the clonal growth of T and B lymphocytes and synovial adherent cells from patients with rheumatoid arthritis. Ann. Rheum. Dis. 55:237, 1996.

51. Hirata, S., Matsubara, T., Saura, R., et al.: Inhibition of *in vitro* vascular endothelial cell proliferation and *in vivo* neovascularization by low-dose methotrexate. Arthritis Rheum. 32:1065, 1989.

These studies used human umbilical vein endothelial cells and found both basal and growth factor–stimulated incorporation of deoxyuridine into the cells at a concentration of 5×10^{-9} molar, equal to that found in serum of treated patients. Using a rabbit corneal model of neovascularization, methotrexate suppressed new blood vessel formation.

52. Firestein, G. S., Paine, M. M., and Boyle, D. L.: Mechanisms of methotrexate action in rheumatoid arthritis: selective disease in synovial collagenase gene expression. Arthritis Rheum. 37:193, 1994.

53. Thomas, R., and Carroll, G. J.: Reduction of leukocyte and interleukin-1B concentrations in the synovial fluid of rheumatoid arthritis patients treated with methotrexate. Arthritis Rheum. 36:1244, 1993.

54. Seitz, M., Loetscher, P., Dewald, B., et al.: Methotrexate action in rheumatoid arthritis: stimulation of cytokine inhibitor and inhibition of chemokine production by peripheral blood mononuclear cells. Br. J. Rheumatol. 34:602, 1995.

55. Cronstein, B. N., Eberle, M. A., Gruber, H. E., et al.: Methotrexate inhibits neutrophil function by stimulating adenosine release from connective tissue cells. Proc. Natl. Acad. Sci. U.S.A. 88:2441, 1991.

56. Cronstein, B. N., Naime, D., and Ostad, E.: The antiinflammatory mechanism of methotrexate: Increased adenosine release at inflamed sites diminishes leukocyte accumulation in an *in vivo* model of inflammation. J. Clin. Invest. 92:2675, 1993.

57. Cronstein, B. N., Naime, D., and Firestein, G.: The antiinflammatory effects of an adenosine kinase inhibitor are mediated by adenosine. Arthritis Rheum. 38:1040, 1995.

58. Mladenovic, V., Domljan, Z., Rozman, B., et al.: Safety and effectiveness of leflunomide in the treatment of patients with active rheumatoid arthritis: results of a randomized, placebo-controlled, Phase II study. Arthritis Rheum. 38:1595, 1995.

Cytotoxic, Immunosuppressive, and Biologic Therapy

Cytotoxic, immunosuppressive, and biologic agents are the broad class of compounds that are attracting the most interest in physicians, clinical investigators, and biotech/pharmaceutical corporations. The initial drugs used were cytotoxic, borrowed from medical oncology because they effectively destroyed many types of cells that were in a relatively rapid phase of division and multiplication. Among the cells killed were immunocytes. More recently the lymphocytes and their functions have been targeted more specifically, both by drugs with more focused action and by monoclonal antibodies (mAbs) and products of recombinant DNA technology. In addition, increasing understanding of the pathogenic pathways involved in amplification of the immune and proliferative responses in rheumatoid arthritis have brought into play biologic substances that act to blunt effects of cytokines that drive these pathways.

Although there are many similarities between rheumatoid arthritis and a localized malignancy, many data suggest that the disease is not simply the product of one or several aberrant clones of cells, so that, if they could be scourged from the system, the disease would regress. Somewhat cruel experiments of nature have helped define this. One woman with seropositive, erosive rheumatoid arthritis developed aplastic anemia. After bone marrow transplantation from an HLA-identical brother, only donor cells could be identified in her blood or marrow. During induction, marrow ablation, transplantation, and engraftment, the rheumatoid arthritis went into complete remission. After 2 years, however, the synovitis returned and her rheumatoid factor titers, which had dropped to zero, rose again.[1] This patient's marrow had been repopulated with identical APCs and stem cell precursors of T and B lymphocytes. The fact that she "reacquired" rheumatoid arthritis indicates that the combination of environmental and host factors were once again

in line to permit recurrence of the disease. Not yet attempted in any systematic study is *autologous* stem cell transplantation, a procedure that would result in repopulation of marrow with different immunogenetic markers. The great initial expense, the difficulty in selecting the optimal patients, and the need for assurance that ablation of marrow takes with it all memory T cells are major obstacles in the path of this work. **It appears not to be primary immunoproliferation, but rather an antigen-driven response in the context of MHC restriction, that governs the appearance and persistence of rheumatoid arthritis.**

A PROGRESSION TOWARD SPECIFIC IMMUNOTHERAPY

As noted in the earlier chapters in this section, prednisone and the second-line drugs have immunomodulating functions. It still is debated whether methotrexate is anti-inflammatory or immunosuppressive or both, and diets that have an inhibitory effect upon immune function can be used appropriately in rheumatoid arthritis. Pulsed steroids, which may work by redistributing lymphocytes to the marrow and lymph nodes and by suppressing lymphokine production, are immunosuppressive. Thoracic duct drainage, a technique of lymphocyte depletion that cannot be used because of technical and economic reasons as well as costs of complications, is, despite its unwieldiness, a focused and targeted form of immunotherapy.[2]

Total Lymphoid Irradiation

In 1981, two studies treated intractable and severe rheumatoid arthritis with total lymphoid irradiation, using fields and dosages that had been introduced for treatment of Hodgkin's disease.[3,4] The results from both centers were very good at 1 year, but then remissions and complications occurred. Rheumatoid patients, many of them frail, were susceptible to infections by bacteria and viruses, and bothered by xerostomia, pericarditis, cutaneous vasculitis, and other annoying problems. Evolution of amyloidosis may have been accelerated in some patients, and the specter of delayed lymphoid malignancy still exists as a feared possibility.

After radiotherapy, there was a marked decrease in the numbers and function of peripheral blood helper/inducer T lymphocytes and in the spontaneous secretion of IL-1 by synovial biopsy samples, whereas products of B lymphocytes (ANAs, IgM, IgA, and IgG rheumatoid factor) and C3 concentrations did not change.[5,6] The lymphopenia induced by total lymphoid irradiation can persist up to 3 years. CD4[+] T cells are primarily depleted, and the CD8[+]–CD4[+] cell ratio increases. Lymphocytes harvested from peripheral blood of these patients respond poorly to mitogens, and NK cell activity is depressed.[7,8]

Total lymphoid irradiation is no longer appropriate therapy in rheumatoid arthritis for any but the most desperate situations. Its legacy is one of an effective treatment too toxic for general use.

AZATHIOPRINE, CYCLOPHOSPHAMIDE, AND CHLORAMBUCIL

Of these three drugs, chlorambucil has been used much less than the other two. However, with the advent of increased and earlier use of methotrexate, the use of all three is decreasing. Specificity is lacking, and the short- and long-term toxicities are significant.

Azathioprine is a purine analogue that interferes with the synthesis of adenosine and guanine in the construction of nucleic acids. In doses of 1.5 to 2.5 mg/kg/day, it has been used singly and in combination in rheumatoid arthritis. It has an established benefit of enabling glucocorticoid doses to be tapered in patients who are becoming cushingoid.[9,10] It is not effective in doses of less than 1.0 mg/kg/day. Although it has no greater early toxicity than gold or D-penicillamine, it is not measurably more efficacious than these two. There are as yet no convincing data to implicate azathioprine given as treatment for rheumatoid arthritis in the pathogenesis of lymphoma.[11] Monitoring during therapy of the circulating WBC count is essential; marrow suppression with neutropenia is the most common complication. It has been determined that defi-

TABLE 33–1. Immunosuppressive Effects of Chronically Administered Cyclophosphamide Therapy in Humans

Absolute lymphocytopenia of both T and B lymphocytes, with early preferential depletion of B lymphocytes

Significant suppression of in vitro lymphocyte blastogenic responses to specific antigenic stimuli, with only mild suppression of responses to mitogenic stimuli

Suppression of antibody response and cutaneous delayed hypersensitivity to a new antigen, with relative sparing of established cutaneous delayed hypersensitivity

Reduction of elevated serum immunoglobulin levels as well as occurrence of hypogammaglobulinemia in patients treated for extended periods of time (years)

Selective suppression of in vitro B-lymphocyte function, with diminution of increased spontaneous immunoglobulin production of individual B lymphocytes as well as suppression of mitogen-induced immunoglobulin production

From Fauci, A. S., and Young, K. R. Jr.: Immuno-regulatory agents. *In* Kelley, W. N., Harris, E. D. Jr., Ruddy, S., and Sledge, C. B. (eds.); Textbook of Rheumatology, 4th ed., Vol. 1. Philadelphia, W. B. Saunders, 1993, pp. 797–821. Used by permission.

ciency of enzymes involved in purine metabolism, particularly thiopurine methyltransferase, may be responsible for severe azathioprine-related bone marrow toxicity in certain rheumatoid patients receiving 1.5 to 2.0 mg/kg/day.[12] In the general population, approximately 1:300 has a complete deficiency and 1:10 has intermediate activity, so that this becomes a significant factor for concern as therapeutic strategies for rheumatoid patients are planned.

Cyclophosphamide is an alkylating agent that cross-links DNA, affecting cells in all phases of their growth cycle. Its immunosuppressive effects are shown in Table 33–1.[13] The usual dose is 2 mg/kg orally. Intravenous pulse therapy with doses of 750 to 1,000 mg/m[2] are being used frequently in aggressive SLE, Wegener's granulomatosis, and systemic vasculitis; however, no benefit for severe synovitis in rheumatoid arthritis was found in one study.[14] In general, the toxicity of cyclophosphamide is greater than most patients with rheumatoid synovitis and their physicians are willing to accept. The major side effects are[13]

- Marrow suppression—predominantly neutropenia
- Gonadal suppression—oligospermia, ovarian dysfunction
- Alopecia
- Gastrointestinal intolerance

A link between cyclophosphamide therapy of rheumatoid patients and subsequent development

TABLE 33–2. Malignancies Seen in Cyclophosphamide (CPA)-Treated Patients

MALIGNANCIES*	CPA-TREATED PATIENTS		CONTROLS	
	11-YEAR FOLLOW-UP	20-YEAR FOLLOW-UP	11-YEAR FOLLOW-UP	20-YEAR FOLLOW-UP
Bladder	6	9	0	0
Leukemia	2	2	0	0
NHL	2	2	0	0
CLL	0	0	1	0
MM	1	1	0	0
Skin	10	19	0	6

Modified from Radis, C. D., Kahl, L. E., Baker, G. L., et al.: Effects of cyclophosphamide on the development of malignancy and on long-term survival of patients with rheumatoid arthritis: A 20-year follow-up study. Arthritis Rheum 38:1120, 1995. Used by permission.
* NHL, non-Hodgkin's lymphoma; CLL, chronic lymphocytic leukemia; MM, multiple myeloma.

of malignancy is fairly strong, particularly for hematologic, skin, and bladder tumors[15,16] (Table 33–2). Bladder toxicity caused by acrolein, a metabolite of cyclophosphamide, is counteracted by mesna, a sulfhydryl-containing compound, but data are not available to indicate whether the protective effect applies to daily oral dosing as well as intravenous administration.

Chlorambucil is a bifunctional alkylating agent, as is cyclophosphamide. Except for a period of popularity in France in the 1960s,[17] it has been used infrequently in rheumatoid arthritis. No intravenous preparation is available, ruling out the possibility of pulse therapy. Delay in onset of action was as long as 2 to 3 months in the French series. The fact that, in one retrospective series, 11 malignancies (8 cutaneous, 3 hematologic) occurred in a series of 39 patients receiving the drug for a mean of 25 months[18] makes it unlikely that chlorambucil will ever be recommended for use in rheumatoid arthritis before azathioprine or cyclophosphamide.

In summary, although intravenous cyclophosphamide may be indicated in an aggressive case of rheumatoid vasculitis, and although azathioprine is appropriately used as a "steroid-sparing agent" in selected cases, the short-term toxicity as well as the possibility of a malignancy developing with use of these cytotoxic drugs with broad action makes them poor choices for rheumatoid arthritis.

CYCLOSPORINE: A MORE SELECTIVE CYTOTOXIC AND IMMUNOSUPPRESSIVE DRUG

Cyclosporine A acts more specifically upon the immune system than do the other cytotoxic/ immu-

nosuppressive drugs discussed earlier. It is a fungal peptide and is used widely in organ transplantation to prevent graft rejection. It has the following known effects on lymphocytes:

- Blockade of IL-2 mRNA within CD4+ and CD8+ T lymphocytes
- Inhibition of production of IFNγ and IL-4
- Inhibition of CD40L gene expression (CD40L [p33] is a membrane glycoprotein expressed on activated T cells that is a ligand for a B-cell receptor CD40 and has a role in B-cell activation.[19]) CD40-associated signal transduction is essential for immunoglobulin isotype switching from IgM to IgG and IgA. The mechanism appears to be by inhibition of the Ca^{2+}/calmodulin-dependent protein phosphatase calcineurin after it complexes with cyclophilin.

Cyclosporin A was initially popularized for rheumatoid arthritis in Europe. In an early double-blind study[20] from Paris, treatment with 5 mg/kg/day was considered "good or very good" by 14 of 26 treated patients but by only 2 of 26 placebo-treated patients. In treated patients, improvements were seen on five of seven clinical assessment criteria. A similar study from the National Institutes of Health and Georgetown University used daily doses of 10 mg/kg versus 1 mg/kg; after 6 months, 10 of 15 high-dose and 4 of 16 low-dose patients had improved by subjective and objective criteria.[21] Although the numbers were small, anergic patients appeared to respond better than nonanergic patients to cyclosporin A.

The major problem with cyclosporin A is renal toxicity[21] (Table 33–3). Both glomerular filtration and decreased renal plasma flow occur concomitantly, probably driven by an increase in renal vas-

TABLE 33-3. Side Effects in Patients Receiving High-Dose and Low-Dose Cyclosporin A Therapy

	THERAPY GROUP	
	HIGH-DOSE* (*n* = 15)	LOW-DOSE† (*n* = 16)
Nephrotoxicity	15 (2)‡	12 (0)
Neurotoxicity	15 (0)	9 (2)
Hypertension	4 (1)	2 (0)
Hepatotoxicity	7 (0)	3 (0)
Infection	0 (0)	1 (1)
Endocrine§	5 (0)‖	1 (0)¶
Fatigue	10 (0)	7 (0)
Gastrointestinal	10 (0)	7 (0)
Hypertrichosis	8 (0)	4 (0)

Modified from Yocum, D. E., Klippel, J. H., Wilder, R. L., et al.: Cyclosporin A in severe, treatment-refractory rheumatoid arthritis. Ann. Intern. Med. 109:863, 1988. Used by permission.

* The dosage of cyclosporin A in this group was 10 mg/kg body weight per day.

† The dosage of cyclosporin A in this group was 1 mg/kg per day.

‡ Numbers in parentheses indicate the number of patients in whom therapy was discontinued due to toxicity.

§ All patients were premenopausal.

‖ The total number of patients was 13.

¶ The total number of patients was 14.

cular resistance.[21–23] Loss of renal function was greater in patients given both cyclosporin A and NSAIDs.[24] In a trial of 6 months using 5 mg/kg/day, there was an irreversible loss of about 15 per cent of renal function,[25] and results such as these led to trials using 2.5 mg/kg/day.[26]

When the use of cyclosporine is contemplated, it also must be remembered that increased effective concentrations of the drug are induced by various mechanisms if other drugs (e.g., erythromycin, ketoconazole, diltiazem, verapamil, even grapefruit juice) are administered concurrently. The "statin" forms of cholesterol-lowering compounds given along with cyclosporine may increase a risk for myositis.

By beginning therapy with a lower dose, it has been possible to use the drug earlier in the disease, to compare cyclosporin A against other second-line drugs, and to combine it with drugs that act at other sites. For example, a randomized, double-blind study compared cyclosporin A (2.5 mg/kg initially, then increasing to a median dose of 3.6 mg/kg/day) against chloroquine (300 mg/day initially, decreasing to 100 mg/day) in 44 patients with a mean disease duration of 6 months.[27] Both drugs were efficacious, neither more than the other, and, by lowering the cyclosporin A dose, the toxicity of both was similar (Table 33–4).

Hypertension occurs in approximately 25 per cent of patients receiving cyclosporine for rheumatoid arthritis, an effect usually controlled by either lowering the dosage or treating with antihypertensive drugs. Pre-existing hypertension should be a contraindication to using cyclosporine in rheumatoid arthritis as should significant renal or hepatic dysfunction. Hypertrichosis is a bothersome side effect, more to some patients than others.

In a study of patients only partially responsive to either gold or methotrexate, cyclosporin A was added at a dose of 2.5 mg/kg/day. All measures of

TABLE 33-4. Adverse Events, by Treatment Group

ADVERSE EVENTS	CYCLOSPORINE (*n* = 22)	CHLOROQUINE (*n* = 22)
Gastrointestinal complaints	11	11*
Paresthesia	11	4
Serum creatinine >130%	7†	3
Gingival symptoms	4	0
Hyperkalemia	4	0
Exanthema	0	4
Edema	3	0
Headache	3	2
Hypomagnesemia	2	0
Hypertrichosis	1	1
Tremor	1	0
Liver function abnormalities	1	1

From Landewé, R. B. M., Thè, H. S. G., van Rijthoven, A. W. A. M., et al.: A randomized, double-blind, 24-week controlled study of low-dose cyclosporine versus chloroquine for early rheumatoid arthritis. Arthritis Rheum. 37:637, 1994. Used by permission.

* Symptoms led to premature discontinuation in one patient.

† All values normalized after dosage reduction.

efficacy showed statistically and clinically significant improvements, and, after cyclosporin A was tapered off at 6 months, all patients had clinical flares of arthritis and a return of rheumatoid nodules that had diminished or disappeared while they were on the combination therapy[28] (see Chapter 34 for further discussion). In this vein, patients with necrotizing scleritis and corneal melting appear to respond to cyclosporin A when other drugs do not work.[29]

Radiographic examination has shown that cyclosporine was capable of retarding joint destruction in a double-blind and placebo-controlled study that included 122 patients followed for 46 weeks of treatment (5 mg/kg/day).[30] Clinical improvement in tender joints, swollen joints, morning stiffness, and functional capabilities were noted as well. Only two had to be withdrawn from the study because of rising creatinine levels, although five needed antihypertensive therapy. Although enthusiasm for these results must be tempered by the absence of formal proof that function and disability are directly related to joint damage, another study from Italy supports these observations. Blinded evaluation of hand and foot radiographs in 167 patients treated with 3 mg/kg/day cyclosporin A and 173 patients treated with conventional slow-acting drugs (excepting methotrexate) after 1 year showed highly significant decreases in progression of erosion and in appearance of new erosion in the cyclosporine group.[31]

In a meta-analysis of second-line drugs, 70 trials of cyclosporine and other drugs were found acceptable for comparison (Felson, et al., Abstract 778). The data put cyclosporine in the mid-range of drug efficacy, as shown in Table 33–5. The efficacy in group A in Table 33–5 was based on measures of tender and swollen joints, grip strength, and ESR. Toxicity is not a variable. The removal of the ESR from the data improves cyclosporine and azathioprine results considerably.

The use of cyclosporine should be reserved for patients with good renal function and severe progressive disease. As discussed further in Chapter 34, cyclosporine is more effective, and no more toxic, when given along with methotrexate in patients only partially responsive to methotrexate. It is wise to stop administration of NSAIDs (except low-dose prednisone) in such patients to prevent additive adverse effects upon renal blood flow. The monitoring of serum creatinine level and blood pressure every 2 weeks initially, then monthly, is essential. If the creatinine level creeps up to values 30 per cent or more above initial measurements, the cyclosporine dose can be decreased by 0.5 to 1.0 mg/kg/day or more to prevent further loss of renal function. Most patients will have a gradual return of renal function to normal after cyclosporine doses are decreased or when the drug is stopped.

The immunosuppressant FK 506 has a mode of action similar to that of cyclosporine. It may be as much as 100 times more potent than cyclosporin A in selective inhibition of IL-2, IL-3, and IL-4 production. It has been very successful in liver transplantation.[32] The degrees of its renal toxicity and other side effects, in comparison with cyclosporin A, have not yet been clarified in patients who are not recipients of organ transplants.

TARGETED IMMUNOTHERAPY

Preceding chapters have outlined many of the pathways that coalesce to produce the cyclic amplification of chronic inflammation that is rheumatoid arthritis. In design of therapy to intervene and block this process, the goal is to affect the earliest pathways in the immunoproliferative pathology without endangering natural defenses against infection or neoplasia. The challenge is formidable. Where are the avenues appropriate for attack?

The Ternary Complex (Fig. 33–1)

Intervention could include any of the following:

- Use of a low-molecular-weight inhibitor of the MHC that would lead to a decrease in HLA-DR–antigen complexes (to below an essential minimum of ~1,000/cell), producing a corre-

TABLE 33–5. Efficacy of Second-Line Antirheumatic Drugs

	REGRESSION (HIGHER IS BETTER)	
	A With ESR Effect	**B** Without ESR Effect
Methotrexate	0.59 (0.08)	0.57 (0.08)
Sulfasalazine	0.55 (0.09)	0.50 (0.09)
Penicillamine	0.50 (0.07)	0.42 (0.07)
Gold	0.48 (0.06)	0.42 (0.06)
Azathioprine	0.48 (0.10)	0.55 (0.10)
Antimalarials	0.46 (0.08)	0.48 (0.08)
Cyclosporine	0.41 (0.13)	0.50 (0.12)
Auranofin	0.32 (0.05)	0.29 (0.05)

Data from Felson et al. (Abstract 778).

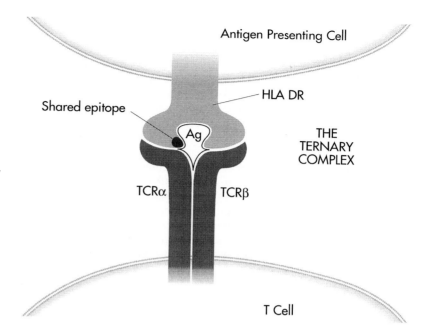

FIGURE 33–1. The ternary complex as a target for immunotherapy.

sponding reduction in activated T lymphocytes. A low-molecular-weight drug that could gain access to lysosomal/endosomal pathways is what is needed; the difficulty of a biologically derived peptide gaining such access is formidable. *The potential problem with this strategy is that it could be too broadly immunosuppressive.*

- Use of an autoantigen as an immunogen to produce antigen-specific tolerance. *Problems here are first, the need to identify the antigen or autoantigen, then the risk of exacerbating the disease. Determining the ideal route of delivery would be crucial.*

- Use of an exogenous antigen as a vaccine. *What is the antigen? None has emerged, despite intense investigation of multiple classes of infectious organisms.*

- Use of modified peptides as either TCR agonists or antagonists.

- Use of antibodies directed against the TCR on cells involved in T helper activity. *Many published efforts along this line have been accomplished. Few have given sustained improvement, and the risk of immune suppression sufficient to permit opportunistic infection is a real one.*

- Use of a vaccine formed of subpathogenic doses of disease-promoting T cells. *The lack of firm evidence for oligoclonal α/β T-cell clonal expansion makes this strategy a difficult one.*

The Cytokines

Cytokines produced by monocyte-macrophages, endothelial cells, synovial lining cells, and lymphocytes have a major role in modification as well as amplification of the immune and proliferative components of rheumatoid arthritis. For these reasons, therapy to block action of the following cytokines could prove useful: TNFα, IL-1, IL-6, GM-CSF, IL-2, and IFNγ.

Four major approaches to therapy against cytokines can be taken:

1. Inhibition of cytokine synthesis
2. Inhibition of cytokine release from cells
3. Inhibition of cytokine action
4. Inhibition of the intracellular signaling process activated by cytokines

The challenge here is determining which are the leaders in the pathologic process and which are less relevant followers, and which may have beneficial effects (e.g., TGFβ) that outweigh harmful effects.

Several characteristics common to most trials of biologic compounds in rheumatoid arthritis reflect the actions of these drugs and give guidelines for future strategies of therapy[33]:

- Beneficial effects are usually maximal within a few weeks of administration.

- Expected, measured biologic effects of the injections (e.g., a decrease in CD4$^+$ cells after administration of anti-CD4) do not necessarily correlate with clinical benefit.
- Systemic "flu-like" symptoms are frequent acute associations of the administration of biologics, and are attributed to activation of the cytokine network. For example, transient elevation of circulating IL-6 has been noted following treatment with some agents.[34]
- Even "humanized" mAb can evoke an immunogenic response in patients by provoking antibody development to the idiotype on the antibody.
- Dose-efficacy relationships may not be linear; a higher dose of a biologic compound may give less efficacy than a lower dose, reflecting poorly understood interactions with receptors or circulating molecules.

The following discussion moves from the theoretical to the summary of biologic interventions given trials in rheumatoid arthritis. These approaches have been outlined elsewhere by Strand and Keystone[35] and by Kingsley et al.[36]

Intervention against the Ternary Complex (Ag/MHC/TCR)

V$_\beta$17 TCR Peptide Vaccination

As reviewed in earlier chapters, there is only suggestive evidence for oligoclonality in rheumatoid T cells. Nevertheless, with the data that V$_\beta$17 may be overrepresented in rheumatoid arthritis, a pilot study examined V$_\beta$17 peptide intramuscular vaccination.[37] Mild improvement in joint count was noted at 1 year and there were no untoward side effects. In three of four patients given 300 μg of the peptide, there was a 20 per cent decrease in peripheral IL-2R–positive T cells reactive to the V$_\beta$17 peptide up to 6 weeks after vaccination.

Vaccination with CDR3 Peptides from V$_\beta$ Chains

CDR3 peptides could elicit anti-idiotypic immune responses that could inactivate T cells by inhibiting the TCR interaction with antigen-MHC complexes. These specific therapies, or CDR3-based antisense oligonucleotide therapy, might have to be customized for individual patients and are in early stages of development.

Anti-DR4

A murine mAb to the DR4 susceptibility gene product has been tried in nine patients with rheumatoid arthritis, five of whom benefited clinically.[38]

Oral Tolerance

Considering the enormous number of antigens presented to our gut mucosa each day, it is surprising, in view of this antigen overload, that we do not develop active and aggressive immunity against multiple peptides absorbed there. Despite the very large immune system in Peyer's patches and in gut epithelium, there is very little immunologic memory in the gut, and this is probably related to the activation by absorbed antigen of cells capable of suppressing a systemic immune response to that antigen. This, by definition, is oral tolerance. Although characterization in biology of the elusive "T-suppressor cell" has been difficult, it is in the induction of oral tolerance in the gut to multiple antigens that a role for such suppressor cells would have the firmest foundation.[39,40] Suppressor activity also could be initiated by inhibitory cytokines, including IL-4, IL-10, and TGFβ.

Although there are still multiple gaps in the data base for explaining oral tolerance, there is increasing interest in using type II collagen as an oral tolerAgen. In Lewis rats it was demonstrated that adjuvant arthritis could be suppressed by oral administration of type II collagen.[41] In humans, multiple sclerosis was one of the first diseases to be approached by attempting to induce clinical benefit by giving antigen by mouth. In a double-blind pilot trial of giving either bovine myelin or a placebo to patients with multiple sclerosis for 1 year, 12 of 15 placebo-fed patients had major multiple sclerosis attacks, whereas only 6 of the 15 given myelin had attacks.[39]

In rheumatoid arthritis, using doses of chicken type II collagen (100 μg/day for 1 month, increasing to 500 μg/day during months 2 and 3), there was significant improvement over placebo controls ($p < .05$) in joint counts and the patient assessment. A total of 28 patients were in the collagen group and 31 in the placebo cohort. Four patients in the collagen group had "complete remission" of their disease.[42] Because there are no data to indicate that type II collagen is the primary cause of rheumatoid arthritis, the beneficial effects are ascribed to "antigen-driven bystander suppression."

In a larger study from Berlin,[43] 90 patients with rheumatoid arthritis (disease duration less than 3 years) were enrolled in an oral collagen study for 12 weeks. The dose schedule was much higher than in the study mentioned previously.[42] Thirty patients received 1 mg/day, 30 received 10 mg/day, and 30 received a placebo in a double-blind and randomized study. There was no overall difference in the results, although 3 patients in the 10-mg type II collagen group had a "very good" response (including disappearance of anti-collagen antibodies), whereas none had a similar improvement in other groups.

Many unanswered questions exist about the future of tolerization with collagen. What is the optimal dose? Is it very small (<50 μg/day) or much higher (>10 mg/day)? Would inhalation of the antigen give a better result? Would recombinant human type II collagen be a more effective toleragen?

Another possibility for tolerization with collagen type II would be use of the apparent "immunodominant" region of human type II collagen. It is a peptide that spans residues 250 to 270 in the type II α-chain. It confers tolerance when given orally in mouse models of collagen-induced arthritis.[44]

Bacterial Peptides

An extract of *Escherichia coli* containing one of the hsp60 family of heat shock proteins that could act as a cross-reacting superantigen in a disease such as rheumatoid arthritis has been administered to rheumatoid patients in a double-blind study. It was reported that the disease was partially ameliorated.[45] As with collagen, there is no evidence that there must be absolute specificity of the antigen to produce symptomatic down-regulation of the immune response. As an accessory immune stimulus, heat shock proteins could induce suppressor cells sufficient to modulate down-regulation of multiple T-cell clones.

Antibodies against T-Cell Surface Antigens

Anti-CD5 Immunoconjugate

CD5 is a glycoprotein expressed on most human T cells and B cells as well. A mAb linked to ricin A (an effective ribosome inhibitor) against CD5 has been engineered. Work from in vitro studies led to enthusiasm for use of the mAb in patients. Anti-CD5 inhibited recombinant IL-2–induced synovial fluid T-cell proliferation, but in similar experiments actually stimulated peripheral blood T-cell growth[46] (Fig. 33–2).

Clinical benefit in 60 to 75 per cent of 76 patients was observed in 1 month but was prolonged to 3 to 6 months in less than 25 per cent.[47] Patients with relatively early disease responded better than did patients sick for more than 3 years. T-cell and CD5 B-cell depletion occurred but normalized in 1 to 2 months. Side effects included rash, nausea, fever,

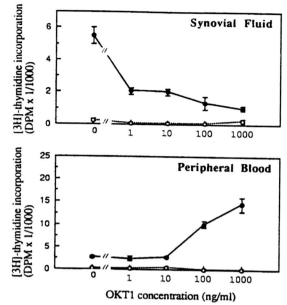

FIGURE 33–2. Dose dependence of the anti-CD5 monoclonal antibody (OKT1) inhibition of IL-2–induced proliferation in synovial fluid (SF) T cells and induction of IL-2 proliferative response in peripheral blood (PB) T cells. SF and PB T cells (0.25×10^6 ml) were incubated for 5 days with (solid circles) or without (open circles) rIL-2 (10 units/ml) on goat anti-mouse IgG-coated plates, with various concentrations of OKT1 (from 1 ng/ml to 1 μg/ml). Data shown are from a representative rheumatoid arthritis patient. Proliferation was measured as ^{3}H-thymidine incorporation. Values are the mean + SD of quadruplicate cultures. (From Verwilghen, J., Kingsley, G. H., Ceuppens, J. L., et al.: Inhibition of synovial fluid T cell proliferation by anti-CD5 monoclonal antibodies: A potential mechanism for their immunotherapeutic action *in vivo*. Arthritis Rheum. 35:1445, 1992. Used by permission.)

fatigue, myalgias, and hypoalbuminemia. No in vitro tests of T-cell function were disturbed.[48]

Anti-CD4 mAb

There is sound logic behind the strategy of devising therapy aimed at this membrane glycoprotein on T-helper/inducer cells, which stabilizes the T cell–MHC class II–antigen ternary complex, leading to T-cell activation. The first use of a murine anti-CD4 mAb was by Herzog and colleagues.[49] A series of uncontrolled, open-label trials indicated that clinical improvement in joint counts for up to 1 year after the therapy with a murine mAb occurred in a majority of patients[35] (Table 33–6), and those who did not respond to one course frequently obtained benefit from a second.[50]

In one series of 10 patients treated with murine anti-CD4, no significant depletion in total or CD4+ T cells in peripheral blood was seen.[51] In contrast,

TABLE 33–6. Anti-CD4 mAbs: Summary of Clinical Trials in Rheumatoid Arthritis*

| | MURINE ANTI-CD4 | | | | | CHIMERIC ANTI-CD4 | |
	TOTAL	MAX 16H5 IgG1	BF-5 IgG1	BL4 IgG2a	MT151/VIT4 IgG2a	OPEN TRIALS	RANDOMIZED CONTROL TRIALS
# Reports	14	6	3	1	4	8	1
# RCT	0	0	0	0	0	—	2
# Patients	75	9	25	7	17	88	124
Doses	.15–.75 mg/kg × 3–10 days	0.3 mg/kg × 7 days	.15, .2, .3, .4 .75 mg/kg × 10 days	.3–.6 mg/kg × 3–10 days	.15–.3 mg/kg × 7 days	10–100 mg 10–100 × 3–7 days	45, 90, 450 mg or P
TOTAL DOSE	45–525 mg	100–150 mg	75–525 mg	45–450 mg	50–150 mg	50–700 mg	45–450 mg
Population:							
Disease Duration	Variable	NR	8 yrs	NR	NR	11.5 yrs +	8.7 yrs
DMARDs Failed	Variable	NR	3	NR	NR	>4; >5	NR
Concomitant Rx	NSAIDs, Pred					MTX in 25	MTX in 64
Outcome Measure	Ritchie index	Ritchie	Ritchie	Ritchie	Ritchie	≥50% TJC, SJC	≥50% SJC, TJC
Clinical Response	60–75%	7/9	23/25	5/6	11/17	60–75%	12–19%
Response Duration	3–6 mos	1–6 mos	1–12 mos	>30 days	1–12 mos	3–6 mos	3 mos
ESR/CRP	Only p BF-5 & MAX 16H5	Decr ESR	Decr CRP 15/17	NE	NE	NE	NE
Biologic Effect	CD4 cytopenia	50% decr CD4 ≥2 mos; Decr prolif to PHA, Con A	75% decr CD4 normalize 24 hr; Nl prolif to Ag at 1 mo	50% decr CD4; DTH decr in 3	50–80% decr CD4; Decr prolif DTH neg 4/10	>50% decr CD4 ≥30 months w/MTX; 60% baseline CD4 12 mos w/o MTX	>50% decr CD4; Decr prolif to Ag, mitogens at 60 d
Tolerability	Constitutional	Constitutional incr TNF, IL-2	Chills, dyspnea nonsevere in 25	AEs in 1/7	Fever	Constitutional	Constitutional AEs 12–31% v. 13% P
Deaths	0	0	0	0	0	1	0
Antibody Resp	33–66%	6/9	6/25	4/6	9/15 (MT 151) 3/3 (VIT4)	40–50%	NR
ReRx	Yes	4/9	1	NR	Anaphylactic rxn—1 (MT 151)	Yes	Yes
Response	No RCT						Not superior to P

From Strand, V., and Keystone, E. C.: Biologic interventions in rheumatoid arthritis. J. Biotechnol. Health Care 1:283, 1994. Used by permission.

* RCT, randomized controlled trials; P, placebo; DMARDs, disease-modifying antirheumatic drugs; Pred, prednisolone; MTX, methotrexate; TJC, tender joint counts; SJC, swollen joint counts; PHA, phytohemagglutinin; Con A, concanavalin A; Ag, antigen; AEs, adverse effects; NR, not reported; NE, no effect.

observations on one patient indicated that anti-CD4 could diminish for a long period the capacity of the CD4$^+$ T-helper cell pool to regenerate; in this patient, CD4$^+$ T-cell numbers stayed as low as 200 to 500/μl for more than 2 years.[51] No infections occurred. No evidence for humoral or cellular immune reactivity against CD4$^+$ cells was found (an expected response if, indeed, the immune response to new antigens was effectively deadened by the anti-CD4$^+$). The anti-CD4 mAb provided no clinical benefit, but at the time that CD4$^+$ cell counts were very low, a small dose of chlorambucil (2 mg/day) was added for 5 months, and this resulted in significant improvement.

Host antibodies could be measured in many patients, leading to development of chimeric "humanized" mAb to enable retreatment and increase efficacy. Using a chimeric antibody, a randomized controlled trial was carried out in which 64 patients also receiving methotrexate were given 3 monthly courses of anti-CD4 mAb in total doses of 45 to 450 mg, or a placebo.[52] After 3 months, 13 to 18 per cent of the treated group had a significant response, as did 13 per cent of the placebo group. The principal side effect, as seen in most mAb studies, was a mild flu-like syndrome.

Similar to most of the murine mAbs, the chimeric forms of anti-CD4 mAb cause a depletion of CD4$^+$ cells in peripheral blood that begins, as recorded in one open-label study,[53] within 1 hour of mAb administration. In this same study there was no correlation of clinical benefit with CD4$^+$ cell numbers or with the dose of mAb; 50 mg given each day for 1 week appeared to have more benefit than did 10 or 100 mg given each day for 1 week. Although depletion of circulating CD4$^+$ T cells was transient in studies using murine anti-CD4 monoclonal antibodies, the chimeric monoclonal anti-CD4 produced a prolonged depletion; all 23 patients had continued low levels at 30 months after the infusions.[54] It may be that, within the CD4$^+$ subset, the activated/memory cells are relatively spared from depletion and account for most of the CD4$^+$ cell repopulation (van der Lubbe et al., Abstract 194). This could also explain the lack of clinical effect.

In a subsequent trial of the hybrid anti-CD4 (murine antigen-binding region plus human constant IgGIκ regions), 60 patients in a randomized, double-blind, placebo-controlled study over 9 months were given monthly mAb (highest dose, 50 mg/day for 5 days).[55] The circulating CD4$^+$ cells fell to about 200/μl in the treated patients, most of whom had recent-onset disease and had not been treated with disease modifiers. The gnawing concern about this study is that insufficient doses of the mAb were given.

The chimeric anti-CD4 monoclonal antibody cM-T412 was used in a group of patients concomitantly treated with methotrexate. In contrast to patients given cyclosporine along with methotrexate, no significant clinical efficacy (compared with the placebo group) was seen.[56] No opportunistic infectious complications occurred.

In a subsequent study of patients treated with cM-T412 who benefited clinically, a correlation could be made between the percentage of lymphocytes in synovial fluid coated with cM-T412 and the degree of clinical improvement noted.[57] No correlation with monoclonal antibody coating of peripheral blood lymphocytes and improvement could be made. Interestingly, it was only after 5 days of daily injections (the "induction" course) that antibody-coated T cells were found. The authors concluded that "in order to achieve significant disease improvement, the dose and the treatment regimen must deliver high concentrations of cM-T412 into the joints."

Perhaps the most optimistic work that supports the concept of targeted therapy using biologic substances or antibodies is the study in established collagen-induced arthritis that there is *synergy* between anti-CD4 and anti-TNF in the amelioration of this arthritis.[58] These data help confirm our biases that, by attacking different arms of the inflammatory and proliferative lesion in rheumatoid arthritis, successful intervention can be achieved. The initial promise that anti-CD4 alone would be a focused "silver bullet" for rheumatoid arthritis has not been realized.

CAMPATH-1H

CAMPATH-1H is a "humanized" form of a rat mAb against the CDw52 surface antigen expressed on human peripheral blood monocytes and lymphocytes. A randomized, blinded study compared CAMPATH-1H against standard therapies. Clinical responses that occurred in approximately half of the 41 patients were sustained up to 4 months in some patients.[59] This mAb definitely has more toxicity than those discussed previously; high fevers with chills, nausea, and hypotension were observed concurrent with administration, and a persistent lymphopenia was observed, with CD4$^+$ and CD8$^+$ counts being less than 10 per cent of baseline for up to 18 months.[60]

Results from another open-label study of 30 patients, expressed with refreshing brevity and clarity, were that "[p]atients receiving C1H developed profound lymphopenia, mild to moderate acute drug toxicity, and transient improvement in arthritis manifestations."[61] It is interesting that, despite fusing the rat antibodies to a human IgG1 backbone to minimize an immune response against the mAb being produced, serum antibodies to CAMPATH-1H developed in 54 per cent of patients.

Infection has been a common adverse effect, and at least two patients treated with CAMPATH-1H have died from infection secondary to immunocompromization. After depletion, the peripheral T-cell compartment was reconstituted, very slowly, by clonal proliferation of surviving antigen-primed memory T cells and not by de novo generation of T cells. Dominant clonotypes, restricted in number, emerged. Were these a selective expansion of disease-relevant clonotypes that could promote synovial inflammation in spite of peripheral lymphopenia? The synovial tissue in these patients was infiltrated by CD4[+] T cells to an extent similar to that seen in untreated patients.[62] It follows that such global T-cell depletion as was accomplished by CAMPATH-1H therapy could actually result, after repopulation of lymphocytes, in a dominance of harmful T cells.

Synovial biopsies in several patients treated with the mAb CAMPATH-1H contained significant T-lymphocytic infiltrates at a time when circulating T lymphocytes were markedly depleted.[63] Is this related to poor access of the antibody to tissues, or to a differential effect of the antibody on peripheral and tissue-localized T cells? The answer is not known. As noted by the authors in the intravenous dose-escalation study,[60] "[t]he entire role of depleting monoclonal antibody therapy in the treatment of this disease must now be re-examined in light of the sustained lymphopenia observed following infusion with both CAMPATH-1H and lytic Mab directed at CD4[+] cells."

Anti-CD7 mAb

The CD7 glycoprotein is found on 70 per cent of T lymphocytes and is increased on activated T cells. It is one of the co-stimulatory factors for T-cell proliferation. A chimeric IgG1 mAb was constructed with complement-fixing and antibody-dependent cellular cytotoxicity functions. A dose-ranging study showed clinical improvement with low doses, not higher ones,[64] and overall the benefit was not as much as that gained with anti-CD4. In 9 of the 10 treated patients, fever and chills occurred within an hour of beginning the infusion.

In summary, although some short-lived efficacy was demonstrated with this and the previously discussed mAbs against surface antigens of T cells, the toxicity from prolonged lymphopenia suggests that it is unwise to use such broadly active antibodies that can deplete multiple clones of activated and resting lymphocytes.

Soluble CTLA4

As discussed in Chapters 3 and 6, CTLA4 is an essential co-stimulator expressed with CD28 on T cells and interacting with the B7-1/B7-2 molecules on APCs. Signaling that results from this interaction prevents induction of anergy in T-cell clones, augments T-cell–mediated cytotoxicity, and leads to B-cell differentiation.[65] Murine lupus can be modified by blocking the B7–CD28-CTLA4 interaction with a soluble form of CTLA4. It is possible that similar blockade in rheumatoid patients would lead to clonal anergy of relevant T cells rather than to clonal proliferation.

Biologic Therapy Directed Against Antigens Involved in Activation of T Lymphocytes
(Table 33–7)

DAB486 IL-2

This interesting protein is a fusion of the active fragment of diphtheria toxin and recombinantly expressed sequences for human IL-2. Once the fusion protein binds to the IL-2R, it is internalized and the diphtheria toxin inhibits protein synthesis, causing cell death. By targeting cells that have open IL-2Rs, only the cells activated by antigen or superantigen should be affected, giving much more potential specificity to the therapy. Nineteen patients proven refractory to methotrexate were placed in an open-label trial using various doses of this IL-2 fusion toxin.[66] Doses were given for 5 or 7 consecutive days, and 13 patients were given additional courses. Nine of the 19 appeared to respond modestly with higher doses. The maximal clinical effect was noted by 14 days after therapy. Antibodies to diphtheria toxin developed or were enhanced in all patients. In 45 longstanding and refractory rheumatoid arthritis patients given either placebo or DAB486, clinical benefit was observed after 1 month in 4 of 22 treated patients and none of the placebo group.[67]

Adverse events occurred in about 50 per cent of patients and included transient fever and chills, nausea/vomiting, elevated levels of transaminases, and increased joint pain. Despite predictions, no differences from controls in the numbers of peripheral blood-activated lymphocytes were found.

Logically, DAB486 would be more effective in

TABLE 33–7. T-Cell–Targeted Agents: Summary of Clinical Trials in Rheumatoid Arthritis*

	MURINE ANTI-CD4 (TOTAL)	CHIMERIC ANTI-CD4 (RCTs)		CD5 RICIN CONJUGATE	CAMPATH 1H	DAB486 IL-2	DAB389 IL-2	
# Reports	14	1	5	—	6	1	1	1
# RCT	0	2	—	1	0	—	1	1
# Patients	75	124	92	120	106	19	45	55
Doses	.15–.75 mg/kg × 3–10 days	45, 90, 450 mg	.2–.33 mg/kg × 5 days	8 mg/m² × 4 days	0.3–10 mg × 10; 6–40 mg × 5–10	.04–.1 mg/kg × 5–7 days	.07 mg/kg × 5 days or P	75–300 ku/kg × 5 days
TOTAL DOSE	45–525 mg	45–450 mg or P	50–125 mg	45–60 mg or P	30–400 mg	14–50 mg	17.5–25 mg or P	18,750–105,000 ku or P
Population:								
Disease Duration	Variable	Early: 8.7 yrs	≤3.5; 10.8	<8 yrs	8; 13 yrs	10 yrs	9.6 yrs	11.8 yrs
DMARDs Failed	Variable	Variable	≥3	<2	≥4; ≥5	4.5	4.7	5.9
Concomitant Rx	NSAIDs, Pred	0; MTX in 64	MTX, AZA	0	NSAIDs, Pred	NSAIDs, Pred	NSAIDs, Pred	NSAIDs, Pred
Outcome Measure	Ritchie index	≥50% SJC, TJC	Paulus 20%	Paulus 20%	Paulus 20%	Seragen index	Seragen index	Seragen index
Clinical Response	60–75%	12–19%	60–75%	NR	60–75%	25% 1st	4/22 v 0/23	2/37 v 2/13
Response Duration	3–6 mos	3 mos	3–6 mos	NR	1–2 mos	33–40% ReRx	33% ReRx	16% ReRx
ESR/CRP	Only p BF-5 & MAX 16H5	NE	±	NR	NE	NE	NE	NE
Biologic Effect	CD4 cytopenia	>50% decr CD4, decr prolif to Ag, mitogens at 60 d	Transient CD3 depletion	NR	Sig CD4 cytopenia >18 months	NE	NE	NE
Tolerability	Constitutional	Constitutional AEs 12–31% v. 13% P	Constitutional myopathy	NR	Constitutional hypotension	Constitutional incr LFTs	Constitutional incr LFTs	Constitutional incr LFTs, rash
Deaths	0	0	0	0	3	0	0	0
Antibody Response	33–66%	NR	100%	NR	90%	100%	100%	100%
ReRx	Yes	Yes	Yes	NR	Yes	Yes	Yes	Yes
Response	No RCT	Not superior to P	—	NR	No RCT	—	>P for 1st course	=P for 1st course

From Strand, V., and Keystone, E. C.: Biologic interventions in rheumatoid arthritis. J. Biotechnol. Health Care 1:283, 1994. Used by permission.

* RCT, randomized controlled trials; P, placebo; DMARDs, disease-modifying antirheumatic drugs; Pred, prednisolone; MTX, methotrexate; AZA, azathioprine; SJC, swollen joint counts; TJC, tender joint count;

Ag, antigen; AEs, adverse effects; LFTs, liver function test values; NR, not reported; NE, no effect.

patients with early disease rather than those in whom a cyclic automaticity of disease is entrenched. The same applies to use of mAb against the IL-2R (also known as CD25 or TAC).[68] When there is evidence that these agents clearly do not cause dangerous immunosuppression, the way toward trials in early disease will be cleared.

Anti-IL-2R mAb

Rat IgG2b mAb (also known as CAMPATH 6) was one of the first mAbs used in trials of treatment in rheumatoid arthritis.[69] There is sound logic in this approach; high-affinity IL-2Rs (CD26) are expressed on activated T lymphocytes, not resting cells. Only three patients were treated (25 mg over 10 consecutive days); all three noted reductions in pain scores, morning stiffness, and joint swelling. Two patients had benefits lasting for 3 months, but the third relapsed after 4 weeks. From the justifiable concern about developing serious immunity to rat proteins, this approach was tabled, awaiting chimeric mAb.

Therapeutic Regulation of Autoimmunity by Altering Plasma Immunoglobulin

Intravenous immunoglobulin is being used for treatment of many different diseases, most of which have an apparent autoimmune component of pathogenesis. In addition to evidence that the IgG down-regulates autoantibody production or binding to antigen, T-cell–mediated disease has been alleviated as well; the number of exacerbations of multiple sclerosis was reported to decrease in patients given long-term infusions of IgG.[70] The same investigators published data showing that intravenous IgG inhibited the active induction of adjuvant arthritis.[70] It also was effective when given just at the onset of clinical disease. A diminished production of TNFα by spleen cells from treated animals was noted.

Most studies in rheumatoid patients have been uncontrolled ones, including one in which six of eight treatment-refractory patients who received high-dose intravenous immunoglobulin reported clinical improvement.[71] A pilot study, but a randomized, double-blind, and placebo-controlled one, was conducted to assess the use of low-dose intravenous immunoglobulin in 20 patients with refractory rheumatoid arthritis. The study patients received 5 mg/kg every 3 weeks for 15 weeks; placebo patients received the same dose of albumin.[72] In this dose, intravenous immunoglobulin had no beneficial clinical effect, nor did it effect a change in the ESR or CRP level.

Placenta-eluted gamma globulin (PEGG) has been used for therapy based on the hypothesis that alloantibodies to class II HLA antigens in the PEGG would down-regulate disease.[73] It is also possible that natural antibodies against cytokines (see Chapter 8) could be partially responsible for the beneficial effect. In a series of 10 patients with active rheumatoid arthritis and prior unsuccessful treatment with at least one slow-acting antirheumatic drug, 400 mg/kg of intravenous immunoglobulin was given for 3 days and then once monthly for 12 months. Clinical improvement occurred, but not for 6 months. The benefit was associated with a decrease in serum TNFα and a late but significant reduction in soluble IL-2R concentrations.[74] In a recent study, four patients who had failed to improve on conventional therapy, received intravenous immunoglobulin 1 mg/kg/day for 2 days each month for 3 months (Maksymowych et al., Abstract 779). None improved, and TNFα production in whole blood actually increased. The high cost of the therapy and lack of proven efficacy makes intravenous immunoglobulin a poor candidate for further trials.

Selective Extracorporeal Immunoabsorption

When bound to an inert silica matrix, purified staphylococcal protein A has the capacity to bind selectively IgG, IgM, and immune complexes from plasma. This modality has been used with some success in treatment of immune thrombocytopenia. The technique has also been used on rheumatoid patients. Eleven individuals with refractory rheumatoid arthritis were given weekly treatments over a 12-week period.[75] Most patients had a clinical improvement and experienced few side effects. No decrease in the ESR or CRP level or change in serum concentrations of immunoglobulins or rheumatoid factor were noted during the study. The beneficial effects, quite striking and significant initially, were beginning to wear off 9 weeks after completing the last immunoabsorption. It is unfortunate that ''sham'' procedures were not carried out on a control group, because the powerful placebo effect of hooking up a patient to such an apparatus has been demonstrated years ago with plasmapheresis alone. In addition, the high cost and relatively transient duration of this treatment relegates its potential use in rheumatoid patients to situations of life-threatening vasculitis.

Therapy Targeted against the Cytokine System (Table 33–8)

Interferon

The evidence that low levels of IFNγ are found in rheumatoid synovium,[34] along with data that this protein can down-regulate expression by synovial cells of prostaglandins and collagenase, led to trials of infusing recombinant preparations of IFNγ in rheumatoid patients. After open-label trials, modest benefit in placebo randomized controlled trials were reported in one study[76] and more positive results in another.[77]

It must be remembered, of course, that cyclosporine and FK506 inhibit biosynthesis of IFNγ as well as IL-2, IL-3, and IL-4 by mechanisms that inhibit the calmodulin-dependent protein kinase calcineurin and the subsequent activation of the nuclear lymphokine transcription factor.

Interleukin-1

Data supporting evidence that IL-1 is a major force in the amplification of rheumatoid synovitis are presented in Chapters 8 and 9. Inhibiting this cytokine is a logical strategy for treatment. The purification and characterization of IL-1ra led to clinical trials in a number of disease processes, even though its molar concentration must be at a 100-fold excess of IL-1β to exert significant inhibition (Fig. 33–3). Gene transfer technology has enabled investigators to insert the IL-ra gene into synovial lining, with its subsequent active expression being sufficient to block experimental arthritis.[78]

Clinical trials of IL-1ra, given by subcutaneous injection, have showed moderate efficacy. In a randomized, blinded study in 175 patients comparing varying dosage schedules, beneficial effects upon swollen and tender joints were observed in patients receiving the most intensive initial treatment courses.[79] Injection site reactions were common, but were the only significant side effect. An additional study, as yet not published, was carried out in Europe and had similar encouraging results, including the suggestion that progression of erosions in the treated group was retarded. Because injection site reactions are a small price of toxicity to pay for relief in this disease, it may be that many patients would be willing to accept giving themselves subcutaneous injections each day in return for an efficacious therapy.

Low-molecular-weight inhibitors of IL-1 include the prototype glucocorticoids,[80] including **tenidap**, one of a new class of drug not yet ready for marketing.

As noted in Chapter 5, the enzyme responsible for conversion of the inactive precursor of IL-1β to the active form, ICE, is an attractive target for inhibition, much as angiotensin-converting enzyme was, because of the specificity of action. Pentamidine isethiocyanate (the antiprotozoal drug), and a few other experimental compounds, appear to inhibit the release of IL-1 from cells.[81]

An alternative strategy to using IL-1ra is administering recombinant soluble human IL-1R (type I) (rHuIL-1RI) to rheumatoid patients. Twenty-three patients with active disease have been part of a randomized double-blind study using subcutaneous injections of either rHUIL-1RI or a placebo for 28 consecutive days.[82] No significant clinical improvement was seen, although treatment with the soluble receptor did result in a reduction of monocyte cell surface IL-1α. I1-1RI binds IL-1α and I1-1β less avidly than it does IL-1α, raising the possibility that, particularly at low doses, rHuIL-1RI might exacerbate the disease. The likelihood of this is increased, in theory, because of the weaker binding affinity of IL-1ra for cell-associated IL-1R, compared with the affinity of IL-1β for its receptor.

Tumor Necrosis Factor α

Strong support has been building for setting up TNFα as one of the principal initiators of the inflammatory and proliferative pathology in rheumatoid arthritis. In rheumatoid synovial cell cultures the production of IL-1[83] and GM-CSF[84] could be blocked by anti–TNFα. In a mouse transgenic for the human TNFα gene that reproducibly developed arthritis, anti–TNFα could prevent the arthritis.[85] In vitro, the sustained presence of anti-TNF actually enhances proliferative responses of T cells and increases lymphokine production. This was noted as well in ex vivo experiments in rheumatoid patients; those treated with anti-TNF had a return toward normal of proliferative responses of their peripheral blood mononuclear cells to mitogens and recall antigens.[86] One IgG chimeric anti-human TNF monoclonal antibody, cA2, binds with high affinity to transmembrane TNFα, an event that results in efficient killing by both antibody-dependent and complement-dependent cytotoxicity.[87]

A chimeric human-mouse monoclonal anti–TNFα antibody was created by linking the constant regions of human IgG1 to the Fc region of a high-affinity mouse anti-human TNFα antibody.[88] In an open-label trial, 20 patients with a disease duration of more than 3 years and a history of failed therapy with standard second-line drugs were given either two or four infusions of anti-TNF for a total dose of 20 mg/kg. The following observations from this study are particularly relevant:

TABLE 33–8. Other Biologic Agents: Summary of Clinical Trials in Rheumatoid Arthritis*

	IL-1ra	sIL-1R	ch ANTI-TNF	sTNFaR:Fc	mu ANTI–ICAM-1	Vb17 PEPTIDE	ORAL TOLERANCE
# Reports	2	1	1	1	1	1	1
# RCT	0	1	0	1	0	0	1
# Patients	195	16	20	16	31	15	60
Doses	0.5–6 mg/kg × 7 20–200 mg × 3–9	25–500 µg/knee	10 mg/wk × 2 5 mg/5 days × 4	4–32 mg/m² × 1 2–16 mg/m² × 8	10–70 mg/1–5 days	10–300 µg IM q 4 wks × 2	0.1 mg QD × 1 mo 0.5 mg QD × 2 mo
TOTAL DOSE	140–500 mg	25–500 µg	20 mg	20–160 mg/m²	140–560 mg	20–600 µg IM	33 mg
Population: Disease Duration	NR	NR; ACR I–III	10 yrs	8.5 yrs	15 yrs	9.6 yrs; ACR II–III	10 yrs; ACR II–III
DMARDs Failed	NR	NR	4.2	≥1	4.3	NR	NR
Concomitant Rx	NSAID, Pred	NR	NSAID, Pred	NSAID, Pred	NSAID, Pred	NSAID, Pred, Plaq	NSAID, Pred
Outcome Measure	# tender jts ≥ 50% SJC, TJC	Joint eval; walk time; lab	Ritchie Paulus 20%	≥40% SJC ≥ 3/7 parameters	Paulus 20%	TJC, SJC	TJC, SJC
Clinical Response	At 70 mg × 7 doses	Improved at 250 µg	100% at 6 weeks	5/9 active 2/3 placebo	13/24	Trend at 52 wks	4/31 active 4/28 P
Response Duration	3–7 weeks	48 hrs + 7 days	8–25 weeks	NR	3 months	52 wks	3 mos
ESR/CRP	CRP decr during weekly treatment	Decr ESR at 250 µg	Decr CRP in 17	Decr ESR (32%)	NE	NR	NE
Biologic Effect	None evident	NR	IL-6 decr 17/19 anti-DNA Abs—2	NR	Lymphocytosis incr CD4, CD 25 6 anergic during Rx	≥20% decr IL-2R+ Vβ-reactive T cells ≥3 × incr T cell prolif to Vβ 17 in 6/15	NR
Tolerability	Injection site rxn 58% serious infx 4%	Contact derm—1 incr effusion—1	Mild infection—2	Injection site rash—2	Fever, HA, N + V in 74%	No AEs	No AEs
Deaths	0	0	0	0	0	0	0
Antibody Response	NE	NR	Yes, NR	NR	Yes, NR	NR	NE
ReRx	Yes	No	Yes	2×/wk × 4	Yes	Yes	Daily dosing
Response	No RCT		No RCT	Response = P	No RCT	No RCT	Magnitude of resp > P

From Strand, V., and Keystone, E. C.: Biologic interventions in rheumatoid arthritis. J. Biotechnol. Health Care 1:283, 1994. Used by permission.

* RCT, randomized controlled trials; ACR I–III, American College of Rheumatology stages I–III; DMARDs, disease-modifying antirheumatic drugs; Pred, prednisolone; SJC, swollen joint count; TJC, tender joint counts; Abs, antibodies; N + V, nausea and vomiting; AEs, adverse effects; NR, not reported; NE, no effect.

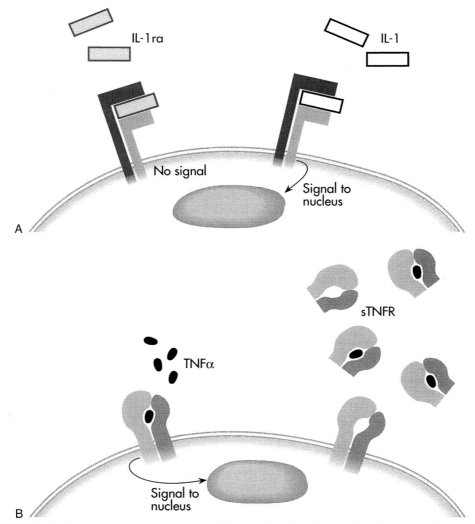

FIGURE 33–3. Two mechanisms for endogenous inhibitory action of cytokines. *A*, IL-1ra blocks signal transduction by binding as a nonactivating ligand to the IL-1R. *B*, In contrast, TNFα may be regulated in vivo by soluble portions of the TNFα receptor that binds TNFα before it can lock into its cell surface receptor.

- There were no acute manifestations of "flu-like" toxicity, and only one patient had a transient fall in the peripheral blood lymphocyte count.

- Joint counts and other major clinical assessments improved over a 6-week period after administration of anti–TNFα (Fig. 33–4). Improvement in some lasted as long as 25 weeks.

- Unlike other trials with biologics, the ESR and CRP level fell significantly, as did serum amyloid A (another acute-phase reactant) levels. After anti–TNFα therapy, plasma levels of IL-6 and stromelysin decreased, as did markers in the urine (e.g., pyridinoline, a marker of collagen cross-links; and collagen type I *N*-telopeptide) of colla-

gen metabolism in bone (Choy et al., Abstract 198).

- Biopsies of synovial membranes before and after anti-TNF therapy showed a decrease in the thickness of lining cells and in the mononuclear cell infiltration.

- Patients treated with repeated cycles of the chimeric monoclonal antibody to TNFα had a response (measured by the Paulus criteria)[89] following each of four treatment cycles, each lasting for approximately 3 months.[88]

- Repeated doses of anti–TNFα (10 mg/kg, 8 weeks apart) have proved as safe and effective as the original therapy (Rankin et al., Abstract 197).

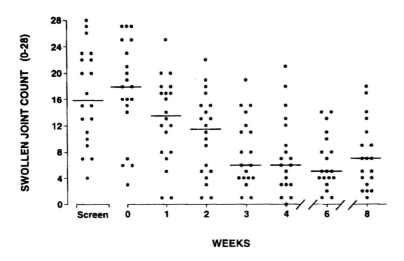

FIGURE 33–4. Swollen joint counts (maximum 28), as recorded by a single observer, in 20 patients with rheumatoid arthritis treated with the chimaeric anti-TNF antibody cA2. The screening time point was within 4 weeks of entry to the study (week 0); data from patient 15 were not included after week 2 (dropout). Significance of the changes, relative to week 0, were determined by Mann-Whitney test (adjusted): $p > .05$ at week 1, $p < .02$ at week 2, $p < .002$ at weeks 3 and 4, and $p < .001$ at weeks 6 and 8. Bars show median values. (From Elliot, M. J., Maini, R. N., Feldman, M., et al.: Treatment of rheumatoid arthritis with chimeric monoclonal antibodies to tumor necrosis factor α. Arthritis Rheum. 36:1681, 1993. Used by permission.)

These early data are important, and support a role for TNFα in early establishment of disease. Part of the effects of inhibiting TNFα may rest in mechanisms other than the "traditional" cytokine effects; because TNFα is a potent inducer of COX-2, inhibiting this cytokine may diminish by direct means the synovial inflammation.

The strategy of competing for TNF by overloading the system with soluble receptors that could be rapidly cleared after binding TNF was implemented by creation of a fusion protein (two type I TNFα receptors on an IgG1 Fc backbone) (Fig. 33–3). This was well tolerated and provided modest efficacy in a dose-escalation study.[90] An extension of this research has been a large placebo-controlled,

double-blind study of the use of subcutaneous TNFR:Fc. Injections of placebo or TNFR:Fc—0.25 mg/m^2 (low dose), 2 mg/m^2 (medium dose), and 16 mg/m^2 (high dose)—were given twice weekly for 12 weeks.[91] Most patients had had rheumatoid arthritis for over 5 years, had active disease, and had failed one to four disease-modifying antirheumatic drugs and were given only NSAIDs or prednisone (<10 mg/day) during the study. Some of the data from this study are presented in Table 33–9.

Local skin reactions at the injection site were the only side effect. No patient developed an antibody response against any component of the fusion protein. As could be predicted from other studies of recombinant agents or mAbs in rheumatoid arthri-

TABLE 33–9. Results of a Trial of Varying Doses of Subcutaneously Injected TNFR:Fc

	PLACEBO	DOSE		
		Low	Medium	High
Number of patients	44	46	46	44
Patients who completed study (%)	52	61	74	93
Disease exacerbation during study (%)	43	4	2	0
Change in painful joints (%)	−28	−24	−45	−63
Change in swollen joints (%)	−24	−16	−32	−58
Change in ESR (mm/hr)	+27	+10	−10	−31
Response by ACR criteria				
≥20% improvement (%)	14			75
≥50% improvement (%)	11			68

Data from Baumgartner et al.[91]

tis, after the study all patients began a slow but steady return to baseline levels.

This study supports two primary theses:

1. TNFα plays a central role in rheumatoid pathophysiology.

2. Even the most effective therapies, when discontinued, are followed by exacerbation of disease.

Further studies of longer duration and in patients with early disease are indicated while the search for agents that block TNFα but are given by mouth continues.

Anti–IL-6 mAb

IL-6 can be thought of as a major effector cytokine that is triggered for expression by IL-1 and then induces production of proteases, acute-phase reactants, and other proteins by multiple different organs. A murine IgG1 anti–IL-6 mAb has been developed and, in open-label Phase I trials, provided some transient relief of symptoms in five patients with rheumatoid arthritis.[92]

Blockade of Intercellular Adhesion Molecules with Anti–ICAM-1 mAb

The receptor-counterreceptor pair that plays a central role in adhesive interactions that mediate the transendothelial migration of T lymphocytes is LFA-1 (CD11a/CD18), which binds with ICAM-1 (CD54). ICAM-1 is highly expressed in rheumatoid synovium,[93] and its concentration in serum of active rheumatoid patients is increased, presumably from shedding of the receptor into the circulation[94] (reviewed in Chapter 7) (Fig. 33–5).

A murine IgG2a mAb against CD54, the ICAM receptor for LFA-1, has been created and used in patients with longstanding rheumatoid arthritis.[95,96] Thirty-two patients with active disease for at least 4 years who had failed at least two second-line drugs were studied and assessed by the Paulus criteria.[89] The principal adverse effect was a serum sickness–like reaction. A second course of this murine mAb to ICAM-1 was given to eight of these patients. Six had a serum sickness–like reaction, and the clinical response was less than the initial one (Kavanaugh et al., Abstract 765). A human mAb or mouse-human mAb will be needed for any future trials of anti–ICAM-1.

Thirteen of the 23 patients who received 5 days of intravenous therapy demonstrated clinical improvement through 4 weeks, and 9 of these had sustained improvement through 8 weeks. A transient inhibition (3 days) of delayed cutaneous hy-

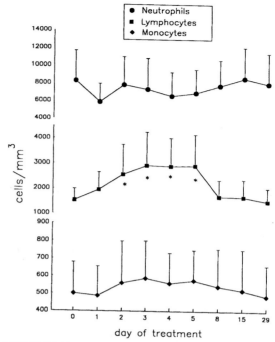

FIGURE 33–5. Alterations in blood leukocyte numbers as a result of therapy with anti–ICAM-1. Values are the mean and SD for 32 patients with rheumatoid arthritis. *, $p < .0005$ versus day 0 and day 1 (pretreatment). (From Kavanaugh, A. F., Davis, L. S., Nichols, L. A., et al.: Treatment of refractory rheumatoid arthritis with a monoclonal antibody to intercellular adhesion molecule 1. Arthritis Rheum. 37:992, 1994. Used by permission.)

persensitivity during therapy suggests that recirculation of T cells with enhanced migratory capacity was being inhibited. Because the clinical improvement in some patients persisted long after the therapy, additional studies on patients ex vivo were performed. A decrease in IL-2 production by circulating T cells in the treated patients was noted in some patients up to 5 months after treatment with anti–ICAM-1 mAb.[97]

As of November 1996, the initial data on targeted immunotherapy lead one to the following conclusions and strategy for the future:

- **Monoclonal antibodies against CD4, because of their equivocal results and difficulty of administration, are not likely to be useful in therapy unless a dose and preparation could evolve that would have a beneficial effect for at least one month after a single intravenous injection, and not predispose the recipient to opportunistic infection.**

- **The most promising biologies are recombinant products (e.g., IL-1ra and TNFR:Fc) because** they appear to be effective, and can be given subcutaneously, as is insulin.

- **Combinations of IL-1ra or TNFR:Fc with methotrexate, or with cyclosporine, or with a biologic product that inhibits CD4$^+$ (Th1) cell activation or leukocyte transmigration should be the next approaches for study in double blind clinical trials.**

REFERENCES

1. Jacobs, P., Martell, V., and Martell, R. W.: Prolonged remission of severe refractory rheumatoid arthritis followed allogenic bone marrow transplantation for drug-induced aplastic anemia. Bone Marrow Transplant. 1:237, 1986.
2. Vaughan, J. H., Fox, R. I., Abresch, R. J., et al.: Thoracic duct drainage in rheumatoid arthritis. Clin. Exp. Immunol. 58:645, 1984.
3. Kotzin, B. L., Strober, S., Engleman, E. G., et al.: Treatment of intractable rheumatoid arthritis with total lymphoid irradiation. N. Engl. J. Med. 305:969, 1981.
4. Trentham, D. E., Belli, J. A., Anderson, R. J., et al.: Clinical and immunologic effects of fractionated total lymphoid irradiation in refractory rheumatoid arthritis. N. Engl. J. Med. 305:976, 1981.
5. Gaston, J. S. H., Strober, S., Solovera, J. J., et al.: Dissection of the mechanisms of immune injury in rheumatoid arthritis using total lymphoid irradiation. Arthritis Rheum. 31: 21, 1988.
6. Tanay, A., Shiffma, N., and Strober, S.: Effect of total lymphoid irradiation on levels of serum autoantibodies in systemic lupus and in rheumatoid arthritis. Arthritis Rheum. 29:26, 1986.
7. Kotzin, B. L., Kansas, G. S., Engleman, E. G., et al.: Changes in T cell subsets in patients with rheumatoid arthritis treated with total lymphoid irradiation. Clin. Immunol. Immunopathol. 27:250, 1983.
8. Kotzin, B. C., Strober, S., Kansas, G. S., et al.: Suppression of pokeweed mitogen stimulated immunoglobulin production in patients with rheumatoid arthritis after treatment with total lymphoid irradiation. J. Immunol. 132: 1049, 1984.
9. Luqmani, R. A., Palmer, R. G., and Bacon, P. A.: Azathioprine, cyclophosphamide and chlorambucil. Baillières Clin. Rheumatol. 4:595, 1990.
10. Mason, M., Currey, H. L. F., Barnes, C. G., et al.: Azathioprine in rheumatoid arthritis. Br. Med. J. 1:420, 1969.
11. Cash, J. M., and Klippel, J. H.: Malignancy and rheumatoid arthritis (in press).
12. Kerstens, P. J. S. M., Stolk, J. N., De Abreu, R. A., et al.: Azathioprine-related bone marrow toxicity and low activities of purine enzymes in patients with rheumatoid arthritis. Arthritis Rheum. 38:142, 1995.
13. Fauci, A. S., and Young, K. R. Jr.: Immunoregulatory agents. In Kelley, W. N., Harris, E. D. Jr., Ruddy, S., and Sledge, C. B. (eds.): Textbook of Rheumatology, 4th ed., Vol. 1. Philadelphia, W. B. Saunders, 1993, pp. 797–821.
14. Walters, M. T., and Cawley, M. I. D.: Combined suppressive drug treatment in severe refractory rheumatoid disease: an analysis of the relative effects of parenteral methylprednisolone and cyclophosphamide. Ann. Rheum. Dis. 47:924, 1988.
15. Baker, G. L., Kahl, L. E., Zee, B. C., et al.: Malignancy following treatment of rheumatoid arthritis with cyclo-

phosphamide: long-term case-control follow-up study. Am. J. Med. 83:1, 1987.
16. Radis, C. D., Kahl, L. E., Baker, G. L., et al.: Effects of cyclophosphamide on the development of malignancy and on long-term survival of patients with rheumatoid arthritis: a 20-year followup study. Arthritis Rheum. 38: 1120, 1995.

This study is the 20-year follow-up of the patients described in ref. 15 at 11 years. A total of 119 cyclophosphamide-treated rheumatoid arthritis patients and 119 matched controls were followed. Most of both groups had been treated with gold and glucocorticoids. Cash and Klippel[11] have summarized the data from both papers (Table 33–2; see text). After 20 years there was a relative risk of cancer for those treated with cyclophosphamide of 1.5.

17. Kahn, M. F., Bedoisear, M., and de Seze, S.: Immunosuppressive drugs in the management of malignant and severe rheumatoid arthritis. Proc. R. Soc. Med. 60:130, 1967.
18. Patapanian, H., Graham, S., Sambrook, P. N., et al.: The oncogenicity of chlorambucil in rheumatoid arthritis. Br. J. Rheumatol. 27:44, 1988.
19. Fuleihad, R., Ramesh, N., Horner, A., et al.: Cyclosporin A inhibits CD40 ligand expression in T lymphocytes. J. Clin. Invest. 93:1315, 1994.
20. Dougados, M., Awada, H., and Amor, B.: Cyclosporin in rheumatoid arthritis: a double blind, placebo controlled study in 52 patients. Ann. Rheum. Dis. 47:127, 1988.
21. Yocum, D. E., Klippel, J. H., Wilder, R. L., et al.: Cyclosporin A in severe, treatment-refractory rheumatoid arthritis. Ann. Intern. Med. 109:863, 1988.

The side effects, not the efficacy, of cyclosporin A are the major issue with this drug. Those found in this study of high and low doses are listed in Table 33–3 (see text). Results of insulin clearance studies are shown in Figure 33–5. An unusual side effect, hypertrichosis, is bothersome to many patients.

22. Curtis, J. J., Luke, R. G., Dubovsky, E., et al.: Cyclosporin in therapeutic doses increases renal allograft vascular resistance. Lancet 2:477, 1986.
23. Dougados, M., Duchesne, L., Awada, H., et al.: Assessment of efficacy and acceptability of low dose cyclosporin in patients with rheumatoid arthritis. Ann. Rheum. Dis. 48: 550, 1989.
24. Altman, R. D., Perez, G. O., and Sfakianakis, G. N.: Interaction of cyclosporine A and nonsteroidal anti-inflammatory drugs on renal function in patients with rheumatoid arthritis. Am. J. Med. 93:396, 1992.
25. van Rijthoven, A. W. A. M., Dijkmans, B. A. C., Thè, H. S. G., et al.: Longterm cyclosporine therapy in rheumatoid arthritis. J. Rheumatol. 18:19, 1991.
26. Dijkmans, B. A. C., Landewé, R. B. M., van Rijthoven, A. W. A. M., et al.: Cyclosporine in rheumatoid arthritis (RA): State of the art, with emphasis on the treatment of early RA. Reumatismo 44:35, 1992.
27. Landewé, R. B. M., Thè, H. S. G., van Rijthoven, A. W. A. M., et al.: A randomized, double-blind, 24-week controlled study of low-dose cyclosporine versus chloroquine for early rheumatoid arthritis. Arthritis Rheum. 37:637, 1994.

In this study, both drugs caused gastrointestinal complaints more than others. In the cyclosporine-treated group, the increases in serum creatinine returned to normal after the study.

28. Bensen, W., Tugwell, P., Roberts, R. M., et al.: Combination

therapy of cyclosporine with methotrexate and gold in rheumatoid arthritis (2 pilot studies). J. Rheumatol. 31: 2034, 1994.

29. McCarthy, J. M., Dubord, P. J., Chalmers, A., et al.: Cyclosporine A for the treatment of necrotizing scleritis and corneal melting in patients with rheumatoid arthritis. J. Rheumatol. 19:1358, 1992.
30. Førre, Ø., and Norwegian Arthritis Study Group: Radiologic evidence of disease modification in rheumatoid arthritis patients treated with cyclosporine. Arthritis Rheum. 37: 1506, 1994.
31. Pasero, G., Priolo, F., Marubini, E., et al.: Slow progression of joint damage in early rheumatoid arthritis treated with cyclosporin A. Arthritis Rheum. 39:1006, 1996.
32. Macleod, A. M., and Thomson, A. W.: FK 506: an immunosuppressant for the 1990s? Lancet 337:25, 1991.
33. Strand, V.: Are there special considerations relevant to trials of biologic agents? J. Rheumatol. 21:41, 1994.
34. Moreland, L., Pratt, P., Sanders, M., et al.: Experience with a chimeric monoclonal anti-CD4 antibody in the treatment of refractory rheumatoid arthritis. Clin. Exp. Rheumatol. 11:S153, 1993.
35. Strand, V., and Keystone, E. C.: Biologic interventions in rheumatoid arthritis. J. Biotechnol. Health Care 1:283, 1994.
36. Kingsley, G., Panayi, G., and Lanchbury, J.: Immunotherapy of rheumatoid diseases—practice and prospects. Immunol. Today 12:177, 1991.
37. Moreland, L. W., Heck, L. W. Jr., Koopman, W. J., et al.: Vβ_{17} T-cell receptor peptide vaccine: results of a phase 1 dose-finding study in patients with rheumatoid arthritis. Arthritis Rheum. 37:R28, 1994.
38. Quaghata, F., Schenkelaars, E. J., and Ferrone, S.: Immunotherapeutic approach to rheumatoid arthritis with anti-idiotypic antibodies to HLA-DR4. Isr. J. Med. 39:154, 1993.
39. Weiner, H. L., Friedman, A., Miller, A., et al.: Oral tolerance: immunologic mechanisms and treatment of animal and human organ-specific autoimmune diseases by oral administration of autoantigens. Annu. Rev. Immunol. 12: 809, 1994.
40. Husby, S., Mestecky, J., Moldoveanu, Z., et al.: Oral tolerance in humans: T cell but not B cell tolerance after antigen feeding. J. Immunol. 152:4663, 1994.
41. Zhang, Z. J., Lee, C. S. Y., Lider, O., et al.: Suppression of adjuvant arthritis in Lewis rats by oral administration of type II collagen. J. Immunol. 145:2489, 1990.
42. Trentham, D. E., Dynesius-Trentham, R. A., Orav, E. J., et al.: Effects of oral administration of type II collagen on rheumatoid arthritis. Science 261:1727, 1993.
43. Sieper, J., Kary, S., Sörensen, H., et al.: Oral type II collagen treatment in early rheumatoid arthritis: a double-blind, placebo-controlled, randomized trial. Arthritis Rheum. 39:41, 1996.
44. Khare, S. D., Krco, C. J., Griffiths, M. M., et al.: Oral administration of an immunodominant human collagen peptide modulates collage-induced arthritis. J. Immunol. 155: 3653, 1995.
45. Vischer, T. L.: A double-blind multicenter trial of OM-8990 and auranofin in rheumatoid arthritis. Ann. Rheum. Dis. 47:582, 1988.
46. Verwilghen, J., Kingsley, G. H., Ceuppens, J. L., et al.: Inhibition of synovial fluid T cell proliferation by anti-CD5 monoclonal antibodies: a potential mechanism for their immunotherapeutic action *in vivo*. Arthritis Rheum. 35:1445, 1992.

The opposite effects of anti-CD5 on peripheral blood and synovial fluid T cells from rheumatoid patients are shown in Figure 33–2 (see text). A mAb directed against CD28 did not influence IL-2–dependent synovial fluid T-cell proliferation, even though CD5 and CD28 share similar properties in resting T cells. The most noticeable difference between peripheral blood and synovial fluid T cells is that the latter are generally at a higher level of activation than the former in rheumatoid patients. An additional factor, not assayed in these experiments, is that the subset ratios of T cells are likely to be different between peripheral blood and synovial fluid. The authors made the reasonable conclusion that ''the immunotherapeutic properties of mAb [may] depend not on T cell depletion, but on other, as-yet-uncharacterized, mechanisms which may involve preferential inhibition or killing of pre-activated synovial fluid T cells'' (p. 1450).

47. Strand, V., Lipsky, P. E., Cannon, G. W., et al.: Effects of administration of an anti-CD5 immunoconjugate in rheumatoid arthritis. Arthritis Rheum. 36:620, 1993.
48. Fishwild, D., and Strand, V.: Treatment with an anti-CD5 immunoconjugate: effect on peripheral T cells and *in vitro* assays of immune function in patients with rheumatoid arthritis. J. Rheumatol. 21:596, 1994.
49. Herzog, C., Walker, C., Pichler, W., et al.: Monoclonal anti-CD4 in arthritis. Lancet 2:1461, 1987.
50. Horneff, G., Burmester, G. R., Emmrich, F., et al.: Treatment of rheumatoid arthritis with an anti-CD4 monoclonal antibody. Arthritis Rheum. 34:129, 1991.
51. Horneff, G., Emmrich, F., Reiter, C., et al.: Persistent depletion of CD4$^+$ T cells and inversion of the CD4/CD8 T cell ratio induced by anti-CD4 therapy. J. Rheumatol. 19: 1845, 1992.

Although anti-CD4 mAb reduced CD4$^+$ counts in this patient, clinical benefit was not apparent until a small dose (2 mg/day) of chlorambucil was added.

52. Moreland, L. W., Pratt, P., Mayes, M., et al.: Minimal efficacy of a depleting chimeric anti-CD4 (CM-T412) in treatment of patients with refractory rheumatoid arthritis (RA) receiving concomitant methotrexate (MTX). Arthritis Rheum. 36:S39, 1993.
53. van der Lubbe, P. A., Reiter, C., Breedveld, F. C., et al.: Chimeric CD4 monoclonal antibody cM-T412 as a therapeutic approach to rheumatoid arthritis. Arthritis Rheum. 36:1375, 1993.
54. Moreland, L. W., Pratt, P. W., Bucy, R. P., et al.: Treatment of refractory rheumatoid arthritis with a chimeric anti-CD4 monoclonal antibody: long-term followup of CD4$^+$ T cell counts. Arthritis Rheum. 37:834, 1994.
55. van der Lubbe, P. A., Dijkmans, B. A. C., and Markusse, H. M.: A randomized double-blind, placebo-controlled study of CD4 monoclonal antibody therapy in early rheumatoid arthritis. Arthritis Rheum. 38:1097, 1995.
56. Moreland, L. W., Pratt, P. W., Mayes, M. D., et al.: Double-blind, placebo-controlled multicenter trial using chimeric monoclonal anti-CD4 antibody, cM-T412, in rheumatoid arthritis patients receiving concomitant methotrexate. Arthritis Rheum. 38:1581, 1995.
57. Choy, E. H. S., Pitzalis, C., Cauli, A., et al.: Percentage of anti-CD4 monoclonal antibody-coated lymphocytes in the rheumatoid joint is associated with clinical improvement. Implications for the development of immunotherapeutic dosing regimens. Arthritis Rheum. 39:52, 1996.
58. Williams, R. O., Mason, L. J., Feldman, M., et al.: Synergy between anti-CD4 and anti-TNF in the amelioration of established collagen-induced arthritis. Proc. Natl. Acad. Sci. U.S.A. 91:2762, 1994.
59. Isaacs, J. D., Manna, V. K., Hazleman, B. L., et al.: CAM-

PATH 1H in RA—a study of multiple IV dosing. Arthritis Rheum. 36:S40, 1993.

60. Weinblatt, M. E., Maddison, P. J., Bulpitt, K. J., et al.: CAMPATH-1H, a humanized monoclonal antibody, in refractory rheumatoid arthritis: an intravenous dose-escalation study. Arthritis Rheum. 38:1589, 1995.

61. Matteson, E. L., Yocum, D. E., and St. Clair, E. W.: Treatment of active refractory rheumatoid arthritis with humanized monoclonal antibody CAMPATH-1H administered by daily subcutaneous injection. Arthritis Rheum. 38:1187, 1995.

62. Jendro, M. C., Ganten, T., and Matteson, E. L.: Emergence of oligoclonal T cell populations following therapeutic T cell depletion in rheumatoid arthritis. Arthritis Rheum. 38:1242, 1995.

63. Ruderman, E. M., Weinblatt, M. E., and Thurmond, L. M.: Synovial tissue response to treatment with CAMPATH-1H. Arthritis Rheum. 38:254, 1995.

64. Kirkham, B. W., Thien, F., Pelton, B. K., et al.: Chimeric CD7 monoclonal antibody therapy in rheumatoid arthritis. J. Rheumatol. 19:1348, 1992.

65. Clark, E. A., and Ledbetter, J. A.: How B and T cells talk to each other. Nature 367:425, 1994.

66. Sewell, K. L., Parker, K. C., Woodworth, T. G., et al.: DAB 486 IL-2 fusion toxin in refractory rheumatoid arthritis. Arthritis Rheum. 36:1223, 1993.

67. Moreland, L. W., Sewell, K. L., and Trentham, D. E.: Interleukin-2 diphtheria fusion protein (DAB_{486} IL-2) in refractory rheumatoid arthritis. Arthritis Rheum. 38:1177, 1995.

68. Junghans, R. P., Waldmann, T. A., Landolfi, N. F., et al.: Anti-Tac-H, a humanized antibody to the interleukin 2 receptor with new features for immunotherapy in malignant and immune disorders. Cancer Res. 50:1495, 1990.

69. Kyle, V., Coughlan, R. J., Tighe, H., et al.: Beneficial effect of monoclonal antibody to interleukin 2 receptor on activated T cells in rheumatoid arthritis. Ann. Rheum. Dis. 48:428, 1989.

70. Achiron, A., Pras, E., Gilad, R., et al.: Open controlled therapeutic trial of intravenous immune globulin in relapsing-remitting multiple sclerosis. Arch. Neurol. 49:1233, 1992.

71. Muscat, C., Betotto, A., Ercolani, R., et al.: Long term treatment of rheumatoid arthritis with high doses of intravenous immunoglobulins: effects on disease activity and serum cytokines. Ann. Rheum. Dis. 54:382, 1995.

72. Kanik, K. S., Yarboro, C. H., Naparstek, Y., et al.: Failure of low-dose intravenous immunoglobulin therapy to suppress disease activity in patients with treatment-refractory rheumatoid arthritis. Arthritis Rheum. 39:1027, 1996.

73. Moynier, M., Cosso, B., Brochier, J., et al.: Identification of class II HLA alloantibodies in placenta-eluted gamma globulins used for treating rheumatoid arthritis. Arthritis Rheum. 30:375, 1987.

74. Muscat, C., Bertotto, A., Ercolani, R., et al.: Long term treatment of rheumatoid arthritis with high doses of intravenous immunoglobulins: effects on disease activity and serum cytokines. Ann. Rheum. Dis. 54:382, 1995.

75. Wiesenhutter, C. W., Irish, B. L., and Bertram, J. H.: Treatment of patients with refractory rheumatoid arthritis with extracorporeal protein A immunoadsorption columns: a pilot trial. J. Rheumatol. 21:804, 1994.

76. Cannon, G. W., Pincus, S. H., Emkey, R. D., et al.: Double blind trial of recombinant γ interferon versus placebo in the treatment of rheumatoid arthritis. Arthritis Rheum. 32:964, 1989.

77. Machold, K. P., Neumann, K., and Smolen, J. S.: Recombinant human interferon γ in the treatment of rheumatoid

arthritis: double blind placebo controlled study. Ann. Rheum. Dis. 51:1039, 1992.

Thirty-three patients with rheumatoid arthritis who could not tolerate or received no efficacy from "established disease modifying drugs" after at least 6 months of treatment were enrolled. All had been off such therapy for at least 4 weeks. The treated group received 0.1 mg IFNγ (2×10^6 I.U.) subcutaneously three times each week of the study. Eight of 16 treated patients and 2 of the 15 placebo group patients improved after the first 4 months of therapy. A second crossover component of the study was impossible to evaluate statistically because of technical problems. Febrile reactions were the only toxic effect.

78. Bandara, G., Mueller, G. M., Galea-Lauri, J., et al.: Intraarticular expression of biologically active interleukin-1 receptor antagonist protein by *ex vivo* gene transfer. Proc. Natl. Acad. Sci. U.S.A. 90:10704, 1993.

79. Lebsack, M. E., Paul, C. C., and Bloedow, F. X.: Subcutaneous IL-1 receptor antagonist in patients with rheumatoid arthritis. Arthritis Rheum. 34:S45, 1991.

80. Henderson, B.: Therapeutic modulation of cytokines. Ann. Rheum. Dis. 54:519, 1995.

81. Dougados, M., Combe, B., Beveridge, T., et al.: IX 207–887 in rheumatoid arthritis: a double-blind clinical trial. Arthritis Rheum. 35:999, 1992.

82. Drevlow, B. E., Lovis, R., Haag, M. A., et al.: Recombinant human interleukin-1 receptor type I in the treatment of patients with active rheumatoid arthritis. Arthritis Rheum. 39:257, 1996.

83. Brennan, F. M., Chantry, D., Jackson, A., et al.: Inhibitory effects of TNFα antibodies on synovial cell interleukin-1 production in rheumatoid arthritis. Lancet 2:244, 1989.

84. Haworth, C., Brennan, F. M., Chantry, D., et al.: Expression of granulocyte-macrophage colony-stimulating factor (GM-CSF) in rheumatoid arthritis: regulation by tumour necrosis factor-α. Eur. J. Immunol. 21:2575, 1991.

85. Keffer, J., Probert, L., Cazlaris, H., et al.: Transgenic mice expressing human tumour necrosis factor: a predictive genetic model of arthritis. EMBO J. 10:4025, 1991.

86. Cope, A. P., Londei, M., Chu, N. R., et al.: Chronic exposure to tumor necrosis factor (TNF) in vitro impairs the activation of T cells through the T cell receptor/CD3 complex: reversal in vivo by anti-TNF antibodies in patients with rheumatoid arthritis. J. Clin. Invest. 94:749, 1994.

87. Scallon, B. J., Moore, M. A., Trinh, H., et al.: Chimeric anti-TNF-alpha monoclonal antibody cA2 binds recombinant transmembrane TNF-alpha and activates immune effector functions. Cytokine 7:251, 1995.

88. Elliott, M. J., Maini, R. N., Feldmann, M., et al.: Treatment of rheumatoid arthritis with chimeric monoclonal antibodies to tumor necrosis factor α. Arthritis Rheum. 36:1681, 1993.

One of the most interesting results of this study was that, in addition to clinical improvement, acute-phase reactant levels fell and remained low for as long as 8 weeks. Similarly, IL-6 levels, elevated significantly in 17 of 20 patients at study entry, fell over the first 2 weeks after anti-TNF administration.

89. Paulus, H. E., Egger, M. J., Ward, J. R., et al.: Analysis of improvement in individual rheumatoid arthritis patients treated with disease-modifying antirheumatic drugs, based on the findings in patients treated with placebo. Arthritis Rheum. 33:477, 1990.

90. Moreland, L. W., Margolies, G. R., Heck, L. W., et al.: Soluble tumor necrosis factor receptor (STNFR): results of a phase I dose-escalation study in patients with rheumatoid arthritis. Arthritis Rheum. 37:R27, 1994.

91. Baumgartner, S., Moreland, L. W., Schiff, M. H., et al.: Double blind, placebo controlled trial of tumor necrosis factor receptor fusion protein in active rheumatoid arthritis. J. Invest. Med. 44:235A, 1996.
92. Wendling, D., Racadot, E., and Wijdenes, J.: Treatment of severe rheumatoid arthritis by anti-interleukin 6 monoclonal antibody. J. Rheumatol. 20:259, 1993.
93. Lindsley, H. B., Smith, D. D., Davis, L. S., et al.: Regulation of the expression of adhesion molecules by human synoviocytes. Semin. Arth. Rheum. 21:330, 1992.
94. Cush, J. J., Rothlein, R., Lindsley, H. B., et al.: Increased levels of circulating intercellular adhesion molecule 1 in the sera of patients with rheumatoid arthritis. Arthritis Rheum. 36:1098, 1993.
95. Kavanaugh, A. F., Davis, L. S., Nichols, L. A., et al.: Treatment of refractory rheumatoid arthritis with a monoclonal antibody to intercellular adhesion molecule 1. Arthritis Rheum. 37:992, 1994.

The doses chosen for administration of anti–ICAM-1 were based on data from renal allograft recipients. Most of the increase in T-cell numbers reflected an increase in $CD4^+$ cells, both memory ($CD45RA^-$) and naive ($CD45RA^+$). The lack of suitability of the therapy for repeat or long-term dosing was made obvious by the development of IgG human anti-mouse antibodies by day 15 of follow-up in all patients so tested. Transient cutaneous anergy was noted in six patients during therapy.

96. Davis, L. S., Kavanaugh, A. F., Nichols, L. A., et al.: Immunoregulatory changes induced by treatment of RA patients with a monoclonal antibody to intercellular adhesion molecule-1. Arthritis Rheum. 36:S129, 1993.
97. Davis, L. S., Kavanaugh, A. F., Nichols, L. A., and Lipsky, P. E.: Induction of persistent T cell hyporesponsiveness in vivo by monoclonal antibody to ICAM-1 in patients with rheumatoid arthritis. J. Immunol. 154:3525, 1995.

34

Combination Therapy

In the context of this book, ''combination therapy'' will be defined as use of two or more drugs at the same time in the hope of adding efficacy without compounding toxicity. In previous chapters, several examples of this have been mentioned:

- The possibility that use of antimalarials with methotrexate can minimize liver toxicity from the methotrexate.
- The use of sulfasalazine not only as a second-line drug in its own right but as one that reduces inflammation and bleeding in the gastrointestinal tract secondary to NSAIDs.
- Mini-pulse glucocorticoids given at initiation of gold salt therapy in an effort to decrease minor skin and systemic reactions to the gold and hasten a decrease in disease activity.

Not included in these discussions is the use of one drug (e.g., misoprostol) to counteract the potential for adverse effects of others (e.g., NSAIDs).

RATIONALE

One rationale for combining drugs has come from evidence that rheumatoid arthritis becomes destructive and entrenched more rapidly than previously appreciated. In an effort to reassess therapeutic approaches, the concept of ''inverting the pyramid'' by using more potent therapy early in the disease and combining more than one drug in an effort to induce a long-lasting remission has been embraced by a number of investigators. Additional support for the idea has been scientifically based: **If two drugs target different arms of the inflammatory/immune response that is rheumatoid arthritis, is there not logic in trying to cut off more than one arm at the same time?**

After a 10-year observation period, McCarty and Carrera reported in 1982 results of a personal series using cyclophosphamide, azathioprine, and hydroxychloroquine in combination.[1] Good results were blunted by the unacceptable toxicity of even the low dose of cyclophosphamide used (30 mg/day), leading to substitution of methotrexate for

cyclophosphamide. Results of treating 169 patients with three different regimens for at least 1 year (mean for the entire group, 7 years) have been published.[2] Improvement in 80 per cent of the variables measured, leading to remission in 69 per cent of the methotrexate-azathioprine-hydroxychloroquine cohort, was recorded, although the disease flared in patients when the therapies were tapered or stopped. Survival was no different from that in the general population. Herpes zoster flared in 17 patients. The mean prednisone dose could be lowered from 9.3 to 5.9 mg/day. As noted by the authors, the general principle of the multidrug regimen was to use ''whatever it takes'' to produce disease remission, including intrasynovial glucocorticoid injections, the use of D-penicillamine in patients taking methotrexate in whom multiple rheumatoid nodules appeared, and, when necessary, prescription of 2 to 3 g/day sulfasalazine or 500 mg/day hydroxyurea.

One of the most important lessons from this study is that patients respond to a physician as well as a drug. Caring optimism linked with judgment, skill, and experience can help greatly in care of a chronic disease such as rheumatoid arthritis. In addition, this study emphasizes the difficulties involved in duplicating encouraging results such as these in rigorously controlled double-blind studies in which the drugs used and doses prescribed are fixed. As pointed out by Pincus,[3] ''intrinsic limitations, including patient selection, insufficient patient numbers, and a short time frame, may render it difficult (or impossible) to document the efficacy of combination therapy in rheumatoid arthritis using standard randomized controlled clinical trials.''

This is reinforced by results of a meta-analysis of published trials that evaluated combinations of full-dose second-line drugs compared to single drugs at full dose.[4] Five trials were found that met inclusion criteria. In all, 749 entering patients and 516 completing patients were found. Differences in efficacy between combination and single-drug therapy were clinically marginal, and 9 per cent more combination therapy patients experienced side effect–related discontinuation of therapy than patients on single-drug therapy. From these reviews of combination therapy, one trend is clear: non-blinded, nonrandomized studies are likely to be enthusiastically positive about combination therapy, whereas the double-blind, randomized controlled studies seldom show either significant efficacy or comparative safety of combinations.

The rationale for combination therapy is clear. Because the pathophysiology of rheumatoid arthritis is very complicated, involving many different pathways of inflammation and destruction, it is sensible to attempt to intervene and down-regulate the multiple different pathways involved. Perhaps the best approach to controlled studies of combination therapy in rheumatoid arthritis is to set up trials that push a dose to either benefit or toxicity with one drug, and then add a second drug for those patients who have failed. The important number is how many patients have a marked improvement on one or another form of therapy pushed to maximal tolerance. That also is the approach used by rheumatologists in treating patients not enrolled in therapeutic studies.

CLINICAL RESULTS IN CONTROLLED TRIALS OF COMBINATION THERAPY

Are there any combinations for which there is some logic for study? The most likely to succeed would be combinations of less toxic drugs. One possibility would be antimalarials and enteric-coated sulfasalazine superimposed on full-dose NSAIDs.

Another lead worth exploring has been using misoprostol for its immunosuppressive effects rather than (or in addition to) its gastric cytoprotection; it has been reported that misoprostol improves renal function and safely reduces the incidence of acute rejection in renal transplant recipients treated concurrently with cyclosporine and prednisone.[5] Both interesting and important are the evidence that, given by itself, misoprostol does not exhibit immunosuppressive activity, but that it can safely amplify effects of concurrently administered immunosuppressive drugs. Unfortunately, in another randomized, double-blind study of misoprostol versus placebo in rheumatoid patients on low-dose cyclosporine (<5 mg/kg/day),[6] the serum creatinine became elevated to 27 per cent above baseline in the misoprostol group and 13 per cent above baseline in the placebo group after 12 weeks. This was not a positive study; 23 of the 50 patients in the five

participating centers withdrew, usually because of adverse effects of cyclosporine.

It is becoming apparent that one of the better strategies for testing therapies in rheumatic diseases is to use consortiums of rheumatologists from different medical centers, or groups of rheumatologists located around one central core center. In an example of the former strategy, 209 patients with active rheumatoid arthritis were collected from 17 practices (academic centers and community offices) to assess the relative efficacy of methotrexate, azathioprine, and their combination.[7] The drugs were assigned randomly, but this was not a double-blinded study. A total of 110 patients remained on the initially assigned regimen at 48 weeks. Responders were defined as those who had 30 per cent or more improvement in three of four variables. The group treated with methotrexate alone had 45 per cent responders, which was better than the combined group (38 per cent) or the azathioprine-treated group (26 per cent). The patients treated with methotrexate alone had a noticeable trend toward decreased radiologic progression. The combined use of methotrexate and azathioprine must be tempered by the data showing that, in 43 patients who had azathioprine added to a stable methotrexate regimen, 4 developed an acute febrile toxic reaction characterized by fever, leukocytosis, and cutaneous leukocytoclastic vasculitis.[8]

Two studies, both randomized and double-blind, are prototypes for studies of combination therapy. In one trial, cyclosporine (2.5 to 5 mg/kg) was added to methotrexate given at the maximal tolerated dose to patients who had only a partial response to methotrexate and NSAIDs.[9] A total of 148 patients were in the full study that lasted 6 months. As compared with the placebo group, the treated group had a net improvement of variables as follows:

- Tender joint count: 24 per cent
- Swollen joint count: 25 per cent
- Physician assessment: 19 per cent
- Patient assessment: 21 per cent
- Joint pain: 23 per cent
- Improvement in disability: 26 per cent

Thirty-six patients (48 per cent) of the cyclosporine group and 12 patients (16 per cent) of the placebo group met the 1993 criteria for improvement by ACR standards. A key to minimizing renal toxicity was in lowering cyclosporine doses if the creatinine level rose to more than 30 per cent of initial values.

In another study, centered at the University of Nebraska,[10] 102 patients with rheumatoid arthritis and poor responses to at least one second-line drug were randomized to a 2-year, double-blind, randomized study of methotrexate alone (7.5 to 17 mg/week), the combination of sulfasalazine (500 mg twice daily) plus hydroxychloroquine (200 mg twice daily), or all three drugs. Of the 50 patients (about half) who had at least a 50 per cent improvement for the 2-year period without evidence of major toxicity, 24 (of 31) had received all three drugs, 12 (of 36) were treated with methotrexate alone, and 14 (of 35) had received hydroxychloroquine and sulfasalazine. Of great importance was that there was no incremental toxicity from the combination therapies, although 13 patients dropped out because of drug toxicity. Not answered by this study is how to treat those patients who drop out because of lack of efficacy (37 patients overall). It is interesting that, in another study comparing cytokine measurements in patients receiving methotrexate alone or in combination with sulfasalazine, it was only the combined group that showed decreased production of IL-1β, IL-1ra, and soluble TNF receptors; both groups had diminished IL-6 and soluble IL-2R levels.[11]

There are several lessons to be learned from these trials:

- Combination therapy need not be associated with additive toxicity.

- Methotrexate as a base therapy, adding hydroxychloroquine/sulfasalazine or cyclosporine with the goal of achieving efficacy by increasing doses if need be unless toxicity supervenes, is a good approach.

- The combination of methotrexate and azathioprine appears to have additive toxicity, including the danger of acute febrile reactions with vasculitis.

Most critical about these studies are the standard they set for biologic therapy. If 50 per cent of patients with active disease can significantly improve according to ACR criteria by taking combination therapy, the data from more expensive and less familiar biologic molecules must be very compelling to merit their serious development and use as effective therapy in rheumatoid arthritis.

REFERENCES

1. McCarty, D. J., and Carrera, G. F.: Treatment of intractable rheumatoid arthritis with combined cyclophosphamide, azathioprine and hydroxychloroquine. JAMA 255:2215, 1982.
2. McCarty, D. J., Harman, J. G., Grassanovich, J. L., et al.: Combination drug therapy of seropositive rheumatoid arthritis. J. Rheumatol. 22:1636, 1995.
3. Pincus, T.: Rationale for combination therapy in rheumatoid arthritis: Limitations of randomized clinical trials to recognize possible advantages of combination therapies in rheumatic diseases. Semin. Arthritis Rheum. 23(2, suppl. 1):2, 1993.
4. Felson, D. T., Anderson, J. J., and Meenan, R. F.: The efficacy and toxicity of combination therapy in rheumatoid arthritis: A meta-analysis. Arthritis Rheum. 37:1487, 1994.
5. Moran, M., Mozes, M. F., Maddux, M. S., et al.: Prevention of acute graft rejection by the prostaglandin E1 analogue misoprostol in renal-transplant recipients treated with cyclosporine and prednisone. N. Engl. J. Med. 322:1183, 1990.

    In this study of renal transplant patients, 77 allograft recipients were enrolled in a randomized, double-blind, placebo-controlled trial. They received either misoprostol (200 μg four times daily) or placebo for the first 12 weeks after transplantation in addition to cyclosporine and prednisone. Serum creatinine and creatinine clearance values improved significantly, and acute rejection occurred in 10 of 38 treated patients and 20 of 39 of the placebo group.
6. Weinblatt, M. E., Germain, B. F., Kremer, J. M., et al: Lack of a renal-protective effect of misoprostol in rheumatoid arthritis patients receiving cyclosporin A. Results of a randomized, placebo-controlled trial. Arthritis Rheum. 37:1321–1325, 1994.
7. Willkens, R. F., Sharp, J. T., Stablein, D., et al.: Comparison of azathioprine, methotrexate, and the combination of the two in the treatment of rheumatoid arthritis: a forty-eight–week controlled clinical trial with radiologic outcome assessment. Arthritis Rheum. 38:1799, 1995.
8. Blanco, R., Martinez-Taboada, V. M., Gonzalez-Gay, M. A., et al.: Acute febrile toxic reaction in patients with refractory rheumatoid arthritis who are receiving combined therapy with methotrexate and azathioprine. Arthritis Rheum. 39:1016, 1996.
9. Tugwell, P., Pincus, T., Yocum, D., et al.: Combination therapy with cyclosporine and methotrexate in severe rheumatoid arthritis. N. Engl. J. Med. 333:137, 1995.
10. O'Dell, J. R., Haire, C. E., Erikson, N., et al.: Treatment of rheumatoid arthritis with methotrexate alone, sulfasalazine and hydroxychloroquine, or a combination of all three medications. N. Engl. J. Med. 334:1287, 1996.
11. Barrera, P., Haagsma, C. J., Boerbooms, A. M. T., et al.: Effect of methotrexate alone or in combination with sulphasalazine on the production and circulating concentrations of cytokines and their antagonists: longitudinal evaluation in patients with rheumatoid arthritis. Br. J. Rheumatol. 34:747, 1995.

35

Antibiotics and Other Novel Therapies

Tetracyclines, often in combination with other drugs, were advocated for treatment of rheumatoid arthritis by T. McPherson Brown for many years, based upon the hypothesis that mycoplasma were the cause, just as group A streptococci were linked to rheumatic fever. No data have directly linked mycoplasma to rheumatoid arthritis but, in recent years, data have accumulated that tetracyclines might benefit rheumatoid patients. Most relevant was their capacity to inhibit biosynthesis and activity of matrix metalloproteases by mechanisms unrelated to their antibiotic capabilities.[1] In addition to preventing cartilage matrix resorption by metalloprotease inhibition, doxycycline stimulates cartilage growth and disrupts the terminal differentiation of chondrocytes.[2] Bone resorption is similarly repressed in various models, and some evidence suggests that the inhibitory capability of these drugs is related to chelating capacity for divalent cations (e.g., calcium and zinc) essential for maintaining intact molecular conformation of the metalloproteases.[3] It has been shown in vitro that the presence of doxycycline during activation of human neutrophil procollagenase caused fragmentation of the enzyme and loss of its activity, presumably by altering molecular conformation of the proenzyme sufficiently to render it susceptible to proteolysis.[4]

Somewhat surprisingly, tetracyclines can suppress human neutrophil function and can inhibit phospholipase A_2 pathways, leading to decreased production by these cells of leukotrienes and prostaglandins.[5] Minocycline, the tetracycline preparation most often used over the last several years in rheumatoid arthritis trials, inhibits synovial T-cell proliferation and cytokine production. These tetracycline derivatives have many actions that could be beneficial in treatment of inflammatory processes that are unrelated to their antimicrobial activities. In addition, they have the advantage of some definite tropism for connective tissue.

Two double-blind, placebo-controlled trials of **minocycline** in rheumatoid arthritis have been reported.[6,7] From the Netherlands came a report of 80 patients with active rheumatoid arthritis randomized to placebo or minocycline, 100 mg twice daily.[6] Concurrent second-line drugs and prednisone (10 mg/day) were permitted. Sixty-five patients completed the study. Although no patients in either group had a decrease in progression of radiographic abnormalities, there were 15 responders in the minocycline group and 7 in the placebo group. (Responders were defined as those experiencing greater than 25 per cent improvement in two of these three parameters: Ritchie articular index, number of swollen joints, and CRP level. A failure constituted 25 per cent or more deterioration in two of the three efficacy parameters.) There were no failures in the minocycline group and nine failures in the placebo group. No improvement in either group was found in the following parameters: pain, fatigue, morning stiffness, or grip strength. The laboratory test changes—similar to the findings in the studies testing anti–TNFα—were most interesting: the ESR, CRP, hemoglobin, and IgM rheumatoid factor titers all improved significantly.

In a larger, multicenter trial of 219 patients[7] with a similar patient profile and concomitant therapeutic regimen including second-line drugs, similar results were obtained. Fifty-four per cent of the minocycline group noted a 50 per cent improvement in swollen joints or tender joints. The minocycline dose was 200 mg/day. A remarkable 39 and 41 per cent improvement in joint swelling and tenderness, respectively, was noted in the placebo group. There was no serious toxicity in this study although many of both minocycline-treated and placebo-treated patients complained of ''dizziness'' and liver toxicity is a threat. Recent reports of ''lupus-like'' illnesses in patients taking tetracyclines must be taken seriously.

The obvious question about minocycline treatment is: What would be the results from a blinded and controlled trial if patients early in disease being treated only with NSAIDs were the cohort randomized and tested? This has been answered in part by a study of 48 patients in a double-blind, randomized,

415

placebo-controlled trial of 100 mg minocycline given twice daily (O'Dell et al., Abstract 771). All patients had disease duration of less than 1 year. Of 40 patients completing the trial, 12 of 20 minocycline-treated and 3 of 20 placebo-treated patients met 50 per cent improvement criteria.

It is reasonable to consider minocycline concomitant with NSAID therapy early in disease.

CALCITONIN

Calcitonin, a hormone with primary effects upon bone cells, has been advanced as a valid therapy for rheumatoid arthritis. Using eel calcitonin, patients derived clinical benefit and had associated decreases in ESR, CRP level, and levels of IgM rheumatoid factor. Prior therapy with corticosteroids blunted beneficial effects,[8] and other data suggest that the efficacy is related to down-regulation of monocyte function.[9]

RIFAMPIN

Rifampin, the antituberculous drug, has been a logical choice for therapeutic trials in rheumatoid arthritis because of its fundamental action within pathways of synthesis of RNA. There have been anecdotal reports of improvement in subsets of patients treated with the drug,[10] and a double-blind, controlled trial of patients with early disease is indicated.

RETINOIDS

Retinoids are analogues of vitamin A, and have multiple effects on biologic systems. One of these is suppression in vitro of metalloprotease production by rheumatoid synovial cells.[11] Early trials suggested that etretinate, used frequently in psoriasis, also benefitted the arthritis associated with this disease. An open and uncontrolled trial of one of the synthetic retinoids, N-(4-hydroxyphenyl)retinamide, was recently given to 12 patients with severe and longstanding disease. None improved, and paired synovial biopsies done in two patients (before and after therapy) revealed no decrease in mRNA for procollagenase or prostromelysin.[12] It may be useful, however, to try other retinoid compounds as they are developed and proven to have little significant toxicity.

RADIATION SYNOVECTOMY WITH DYSPROSIUM 165–FERRIC HYDROXIDE MACROAGGREGATES

This mode of synovectomy has been tailor-made to provide β emissions with a short half-life and tissue penetration of less than 6 mm. After a single injection into the knees of 270 mCi, an 86 per cent improvement in patients with relatively early radiographic changes was noted after 1 year.[13] In a subsequent study, 13 patients who failed to respond to an initial injection had a repeat injection, and among these, 54 per cent of the knees were better 1 year later.[14] Limited to centers with an adjacent source of short-lived isotopes, this therapy is useful for patients with one or two severely active joints.

TRIPTERYGIUM WILFORDII HOOK F

A number of studies in China have confirmed that *T. wilfordii* Hook F (thunder god vine) is useful therapy for rheumatoid arthritis and other autoimmune diseases.[15] In vitro experiments in the United States[16] have shown that an ethanol extract of the vine inhibited T- and B-cell proliferation and IL-2 production without causing toxicity to the cells. Further trials should await chemical characterization of the active ingredient.

ERYTHROPOIETIN

Seventeen patients with rheumatoid arthritis with stable hematocrits of 34 per cent or less received various doses (50 to 150 U/kg) of recombinant human erythropoietin three times weekly.[17] Expected increases in hematocrits were found without significant toxicity, but no improvement in overall rheumatologic clinical status was found.

CONCLUSION

New ideas for therapy in rheumatoid arthritis will be generated with each passing year. Some may be simple compounds used for other illnesses (e.g., tetracyclines). Others may be designed specifically to inhibit or down-regulate one particular arm of the complex pathophysiology of this disease (e.g., IL-Ira). By whatever route these therapies appear, it is incumbent upon physicians and allied health professionals to be sure that good therapies are not

TABLE 35–1. Type and Frequency of Adverse Effects in 80 Rheumatoid Arthritis Patients, by Treatment Group*

ADVERSE EFFECT	MINOCYCLINE ($n = 40$)	PLACEBO ($n = 40$)
Gastrointestinal	23 (4/4)	6 (0/0)
Nausea	20 (4/4)	5 (0/0)
Vomiting	1 (0/1)	1 (0/0)
Increased appetite	10 (2/0)	0
Change of taste	7 (2/0)	0
Dizziness	16 (6/4)	6 (0/1)
Leading to major event	2 (1/0)†	0
Skin eruption	0	1 (1/0)
Allergic pneumonitis	1 (0/1)	0
Headache	1 (0/0)	0
Miscellaneous	0	3 (0/0)
Candida esophagitis	0	1 (0/0)
Herpes zoster	0	2 (0/0)

From Kloppenburg, M., Breedveld, F. C., Terwiel, J. P., et al.: Minocycline in active rheumatoid arthritis: A double-blind, placebo-controlled trial. Arthritis Rheum. 37:629, 1994. Used by permission.

* Values are the number of patients with adverse effects leading to (dose reduction/premature discontinuation). Several patients had more than one adverse effect.

† One patient had a fracture of the elbow, another a fracture of the humerus.

ignored because they are not put in effective trials, or that mediocre therapies are not given the status of good treatments for the same reasons. Our patients deserve no less.

REFERENCES

1. Greenwald, R. A., Golub, L. M., Lavietes, B., et al.: Tetracyclines inhibit synovial collagenase *in vivo* and *in vitro*. J. Rheumatol. 14:28, 1987.
2. Cole, A. A., Chubinskaya, S., Luchene, L. J., et al.: Doxycycline disrupts chondrocyte differentiation and inhibits cartilage matrix degradation. Arthritis Rheum. 37:1727, 1994.
3. Yu, L. P. Jr., Smith, G. N., Hasty, K. A., et al.: Doxycycline inhibits type XI collagenolytic activity of extracts from human osteoarthritic cartilage and of gelatinase. J. Rheumatol. 18:1450, 1991.
4. Smith, G. N. Jr., Brandt, K. D., and Hasty, K. A.: Activation of recombinant human neutrophil procollagenase in the presence of doxycycline results in fragmentation of the enzyme and loss of enzyme activity. Arthritis Rheum. 39:235, 1996.
5. Gabler, W. L., and Creamer, H. R.: Suppression of human neutrophil function by tetracyclines. J. Periodontol. Res. 26:52, 1991.
6. Kloppenburg, M., Breedveld, F. C., Terwiel, J. P., et al.: Minocycline in active rheumatoid arthritis: A double-blind, placebo-controlled trial. Arthritis Rheum. 37:629, 1994.
7. Tilley, B., Alarcon, G., Heyse, S., et al.: Minocycline in rheumatoid arthritis: A 48-week, double-blind, placebo-controlled trial. Ann. Intern. Med. 122:81, 1995.
8. Aida, S., and Shimoji, K.: Effects of calcitonin on rheumatoid arthritis and the relation with corticosteroids. Pain Res. 5:85, 1990.
9. Aida, S., Okawa-Takatsuji, S., Aotsuka, S., et al.: Calcitonin inhibits production of immunoglobulins, rheumatoid factor and interleukin-1 by mononuclear cells from patients with rheumatoid arthritis. Ann. Rheum. Dis. 53:247, 1994.
10. Gabriel, S. E., Conn, D. L., and Luthra, H.: Rifampicin therapy in rheumatoid arthritis. J. Rheumatol. 17:163, 1990.
11. Brinckerhoff, C. E., McMillan, R. M., Dayer, J.-M., et al.: Inhibition by retinoic acid of collagenase production in rheumatoid synovial cells. N. Engl. J. Med. 303:432, 1980.
12. Gravallese, E. M., Handel, M. L., Coblyn, J., et al.: N-(4-hydroxyphenyl) retinamide in rheumatoid arthritis. Arthritis Rheum. 39:1021, 1996.
13. Sledge, C. B., Zuckerman, J. D., Zalutsky, M. R., et al.: Treatment of rheumatoid synovitis of the knee with intra-articular injection of dysprosium 165-ferric hydroxide macroaggregates. Arthritis Rheum. 29:153, 1986.
14. Vella, M., Zuckerman, J. D., Shortkroff, S., et al.: Repeat radiation synovectomy with dysprosium 165-ferric hydroxide macroaggregates in rheumatoid knees unresponsive to initial injection. Arthritis Rheum. 31:789, 1988.
15. Tao, X. L., Shi, Y. P., Cheng, X. H., et al.: Mechanism of treatment of rheumatoid arthritis with *Tripterygium wilfordii* Hook F. I. Effect of T2 on secretion of total IgM and IgM-RF by PBMC. Acta Acad. Med. Sin. 10:361, 1988.
16. Tao, X., Davis, L. S., Lipsky, P. E.: Effect of an extract of the Chinese herbal remedy *Tripterygium wilfordii* Hook F on human immune responsiveness. Arthritis Rheum. 34:1274, 1991.
17. Pincus, T., Olsen, N. J., Russell, I. J., et al.: Multicenter study of recombinant human erythropoietin in correction of anemia in rheumatoid arthritis. Am. J. Med. 89:161, 1990.

The results in this study are especially noteworthy for the decrease in acute-phase reactants, which were more impressive for minocycline-treated patients than were improvement in clinical measures. Perhaps this was related to the longstanding disease in all patients (mean, 12 to 14 years) and the fact that all could continue a basic drug regimen during the study that included second-line drugs. The adverse effects are shown in Table 35–1. The discontinuation percentage was 12.5. Dizziness from vestibular effects, a problem with minocycline, was annoying and caused fractures from falls in two patients.

Appendix

Cited Abstracts of the 1995 ACR National Scientific Meeting

The following abstracts appear in *Arthritis and Rheumatism*, Volume 38, No. 9 (Supplement), September 1995. In the text, each is listed by the author's name and abstract number.

Amin, A. R., Vvas, P., Attur, M., et al.: A novel mechanism of action for nonsteroidal anti-inflammatory drugs: effects on inducible nitric oxide synthase. Abstract 1144.

Bjarnason, I., Macpherson, A., Schupp, J., and Hayllar, J.: A randomised, double blind, crossover comparative endoscopy study on the tolerability of flosulide, a selective cyclo-oxygenase-2 inhibitor, and naproxen. Abstract 761.

Boyle, D. L., Sajjada, F. G., and Firestein, G. S.: Selective down regulation of collagenase gene expression by adenosine. Abstract 1142.

Brezinschek, R. I., Lipsky, P. E., Wisby, H., et al.: Characterization of human T cell migration through rheumatoid synovial endothelium. Abstract 205.

Choy, E. H., S., Kassimos, D., Kingsley, G. H., et al.: The effect of an engineered human anti-tumour necrosis factor alpha (TNFα) antibody (Ab) on interleukin-6 (IL-6) and bone markers in rheumatoid arthritis (RA) patients. Abstract 198.

Davies, J. M. S., Kremer, J. M., and Furst, D. E.: Lymphomatous changes during methotrexate therapy. Abstract 312.

Devlin, J., Gough, A., Huissoon, A., et al.: The acute phase and function in early rheumatoid arthritis: CRP levels correlate with functional and radiological outcome. Abstract 617.

Dolhain, R. J. E. M., van der Heiden, A. N., ter Haar, N. T., et al.: Dominance of T helper (Th)-1 over Th-2 cytokine producing lymphocytes in synovial fluids of patients with rheumatoid arthritis (RA). Abstract 492.

El-Gabalawy, H., Oen, K., and Wilkins, J.: Coexpression of macrophage and fibroblast markers by RA synovial lining cells in culture and in situ. Abstract 24.

Felson, D. T., Anderson, J. J., Chernoff, M. C., and Meenan, R. F.: The comparative efficacy of cyclosporine (CS) and other second line drugs in rheumatoid arthritis (RA): update of a meta-analysis. Abstract 778.

Fujisawa, K., Aono, H., Hasunama, T., et al.: Fas ameliorates chronic inflammatory arthritis in HTLV-1 *tax* transgenic mice. Abstract 1328.

Gadangi, P., Longaker, M., Naime, D., et al.: The antiinflammatory action of sulfasalazine (SSA) is mediated by adenosine (ADO). Abstract 1308.

Gonzalez-Gay, M. A., Zanelli, E., Khare, S. D., et al.: DRB1*1502-DR2Dw12 transgene protects mice against arthritis: implications in the role of DRB1 molecules in rheumatoid arthritis. Abstract 937.

Handel, M. L., McMorrow, L. B., and Gravallese, E. M.: Transcription factor NF-κB in rheumatoid synovium. Abstract 238.

Ibberson, M., So, A., Péclat, V., et al.: Genetic susceptibility to rheumatoid arthritis is linked to the T-cell receptor alpha locus and interacts with HLA-DR4. Abstract 204.

Jonas, B. L., Gonzalez, E. B., Callahan, L., et al.: The shared epitope is not associated with disease severity in an African-American population with rheumatoid arthritis. Abstract 246.

Kavanaugh, A., Davis, L., Nichols, L., and Lipsky, P.: Retreatment of rheumatoid arthritis (RA) patients with an anti-ICAM-1 monoclonal antibody. Abstract 765.

Maksymowych, W. P., Avina-Zubieta, A., Luong, M., and Russell, A. S.: High dose intravenous immunoglobulin (IVIg) in severe refractory rheumatoid arthritis (RA): no evidence for efficacy. Abstract 779.

McInnes, I. B., Al-Mughales, I., Huang, F. P., et al.: A role for interleukin-15 in T cell migration and activation in rheumatoid arthritis (RA). Abstract 490.

Morita, Y., Yamamura, M., and Harada, S.: Anti-inflammatory properties of interleukin-13 in rheumatoid synovial inflammation. Abstract 1197.

Nabozny, G. H., Baisch, J. M., Cheng, S., et al.: Induction of collagen induced arthritis (CIA) in HLA-DQw8 transgenic mice: a unique model to dissect the role of HLA-DQ molecules in human rheumatoid arthritis (RA). Abstract 206.

O'Dell, J., Haire, C., Erikson, N., et al.: Efficacy of triple DMARD therapy in RA patients with suboptimal responses to MTX: results of an open-label study. Abstract 201.

O'Dell, J., Haire, C., Erikson, N., et al.: Successful treatment of early rheumatoid arthritis (RA) with minocycline: results of a double-blind trial. Abstract 771.

Pincus, T., Brooks, R. H., Callahan, L. F.: Measures of inflammatory activity in rheumatoid arthritis may indicate no change or improvement over 5 years while measures of damage indicate disease progression: implications for assessment of long-term outcomes. Abstract 630.

Rankin, E. C. C., Choy, E. H. S., Sopwith, M., et al.: Repeated doses of 10 mg/kg of an engineered human anti-TNFα antibody, CDP571, in RA patients are safe and effective. Abstract 197.

Schmidt, D., Goronzy, J. J., and Weyand, C. M.: A male and a female pattern in rheumatoid arthritis. Abstract 816.

Schulze-Koops, H., Lipsky, P. E., Kavanaugh, A. F., and Davis, L. S.: Elevated Th1-like cytokine mRNA in the peripheral circulation of patients with rheumatoid arthritis: modulation by treatment with a monoclonal antibody to ICAM-1. Abstract 825.

Sieper, J., Kary, S., Eggens, U., et al.: Treatment of rheumatoid arthritis with oral collagen type II: results of a double-blind placebo-controlled randomized trial. Abstract 957.

Sugiyama, E., Taki, H., Kuroda, A., et al.: Interleukin-4 inhibits prostaglandin E_2 production by freshly prepared rheumatoid synovial cells via inhibition of biosynthesis and gene expression of cyclooxygenase II but not those of cyclooxygenase I. Abstract 1193.

Thomas, R., Quinn, C., and Wong, R.: Dendritic cell differentiation in rheumatoid synovium: CD86 is a marker of functional dendritic cell activation. Abstract 378.

van der Lubbe, P. A., Miltenburg, A. M., Tak, P. P., et al.: Immunological effects of a chimeric CD4 monoclonal antibody (cM-T412) in patients with early rheumatoid arthritis. Abstract 194.

Vita, R., Brezinschek, R. I., Lipsky, P. E., and Oppenheimer-Marks, N.: Interleukin-15 increases the transendothelial migration of human T cells. Abstract 491.

Walmsley, M., Katsikis, P. D., Abney, E., et al.: IL-10 treatment inhibits disease progression in established collagen-induced arthritis. Abstract 767.

Weinblatt, M., Maier, A., Blotner, S., and Coblyn, J.: Long term prospective study of methotrexate (MTX) in rheumatoid arthritis (RA): update at 11 years. Abstract 675.

West, S. G., Hugler, R., Battafarano, D., et al.: Low-dose weekly methotrexate (MTX) does not cause osteoporosis in rheumatoid arthritis (RA) patients. Abstract 955.

Wolfe, F., and Sharp, J. T.: Long term radiographic outcome of patients seen early in the course of rheumatoid arthritis. Abstract 1056.

INDEX

Note: Page numbers in *italics* refer to illustrations; page numbers followed by t refer to tables.

ISBN 0-7216-5249-2